Handbuch der
experimentellen Pharmakologie

Handbook of
Experimental Pharmacology

Heffter-Heubner   New Series

Herausgegeben von/Editorial Board

O. Eichler   **A. Farah**   **H. Herken**   **A. D. Welch**
Heidelberg   Rensselaer, NY   Berlin   Princeton, NJ

Beirat/Advisory Board

E. J. Ariëns · Z. M. Bacq · P. Calabresi · S. Ebashi · E. G. Erdös
V. Erspamer · U. S. von Euler · W. S. Feldberg · G. B. Koelle
O. Krayer · T. A. Loomis · H. Rasková · M. Rocha e Silva · F. Sakai
J. R. Vane · P. G. Waser · W. Wilbrandt

Vol. XVI/11 B

Springer-Verlag Berlin · Heidelberg · New York 1973

Erzeugung von Krankheitszuständen durch das Experiment

Teil 11 B

Infektionen IV

Bearbeitet von

B. Babudieri · R.-E. Bader · U. Ullmann
H. Werner · H. Winkler

Herausgeber

Oskar Eichler

Mit 29 Abbildungen

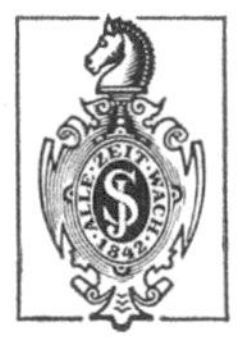

Springer-Verlag Berlin · Heidelberg · New York 1973

Herausgeber Professor Dr. OSKAR EICHLER, Pharmakologisches Institut
der Universität, 6900 Heidelberg, Hauptstraße 47—51

ISBN-13: 978-3-642-65606-4   e-ISBN-13: 978-3-642-65605-7
DOI: 10.1007/978-3-642-65605-7

Inhaltsverzeichnis

Experimental Infections by Spirochaetas
  B. Babudieri. With 8 Figures

Experimental Infections by Spirilla
B. BABUDIERI. With 1 Figure

A Study of the Chemotherapeutics Active on Syphilis
B. BABUDIERI

Experimentelle Infektionen durch Vibrionen
HILDEGARD WINKLER und UWE ULLMANN. Mit 6 Abbildungen

Experimentelle Infektionen durch Bakteroidazeen

Herbert Werner. Mit 10 Abbildungen

Verhütung von Laboratoriumsinfektionen

RICHARD-ERNST BADER. Mit 4 Abbildungen

Mitarbeiterverzeichnis

Professor Dr. BRENNO BABUDIERI†, Istituto Superiore di Sanita, Viale Regina Elena, 299, I-00161 Roma

Professor Dr. RICHARD-ERNST BADER, Direktor, Hygiene-Institut der Universität, 7400 Tübingen, Silcherstr. 7

Dr. med. UWE ULLMANN, Wiss. Assistent, Hygiene-Institut der Universität, 7400 Tübingen, Silcherstr. 7

Professor Dr. HERBERT WERNER, Institut für Medizinische Mikrobiologie und Immunologie der Universität, 5300 Bonn-Venusberg

Dr. med. HILDEGARD WINKLER, Akad. Oberrätin, Hygiene-Institut der Universität, 7400 Tübingen, Silcherstr. 7

Experimental Infections by Spirochaetas

B. Babudieri

With 8 Figures

Order Spirochaetales: Systematic

The order of *Spirochaetales* Buchanan (1918), comprises microorganisms which, according to Bergey's Manual of Determinative Bacteriology, have the following characteristics:

"Slender, flexuous bodies, 6 to 500 microns in length, in the form of spirals with at least one complete turn. Some forms may show an axial filament, a lateral crista, or ridge, or transverse striations; otherwise there is no significant protoplasmic pattern. Smaller forms may have a lower refractive index than that of true bacteria, and therefore they can be seen only with darkfield illumination. Some forms take aniline dyes with difficulty; Giemsa's stain is uniformly successful. Granules are formed in some species which are found in vector hosts. All forms are motile. In the true bacteria, motility is effected by flagella endowed with a lashing movement; however, no such structures exist among the spirochetes. Terminal projections, whether derived from the periplast or from the axial filament, may assist in the movements, and it is possible that the crista has a similar function, although neither of these structures can explain the violent motion of the spirochetes. This motility consists of a rapid whirling or spinning about the long axis, which activity drives the organism forward or backward, there being no anteroposterior polarity. In addition the spirochetes make violent, lashing movements, curling and uncurling their spirals. Multiplication is by transverse fission, no sexual cycle being known. Free-living, saprophytic and parasitic forms."

Also according to Bergey's Manual, the *Spirochaetales* are subdivided into two Families. The first one: that of *Spirochaetaceae*, is characterized represented by coarse, spiral organisms, 30 to 500 microns in length, with definite protoplasmatic structures. Found in stagnant, fresh or salt water and in the intestinal tracts of bivalve mollusks (*Lamellibranchiata*). The second one: that of *Treponemataceae* is made up of spirochetas with coarse or slender spirals, 4 to 16 microns in length; longer forms are due to incomplete or delayed division. The spirals may be regular or irregular, and flexible or comparatively rigid. The protoplasm possesses no obvious structural features. Some cells may show terminal filaments. Some cells are visible only under darkfield illumination. Many of these organisms can be cultured. With few exceptions, parasitic in vertebrates. Some are pathogenic.

The family *Spirochaetaceae* comprises three Genera:

I. *Spirochaeta*, with no obvious periplast membrane and no cross-striation,

II. *Saprospira*, with periplaste membrane present and cross-striations in stained specimens. Free-living in marine ooze,

III. *Cristispira*, with periplaste membrane present and cross-striation in stained specimens. Parasitic on lamellibranch mollusks. Cristae are prominent.

The family *Treponemataceae* comprises three Genera:

I. *Borrelia,* which stains easily with ordinary aniline dyes,

II. *Treponema,* which stains with difficulty except with Giemsa's stain or silver impregnation and is anaerobic,

III. *Leptospira,* which stains with difficulty except with Giemsa's stain or silver impregnation and is aerobic.

We should mention also the more recent classification proposed by Babudieri, 1954, according to which the Order *Spirochaetales* is divided into two Families: I. *Saprospiraceae,* supplied with cross-septa, and: II. *Spirochaetaceae,* with no cross-septa.

The first Family is subdivided into two Genera: *Cristispira,* characterized by a prominent undulating membrane, and *Saprospira,* without any undulating membrane.

The second Family is subidivided into six Genera, characterized by the following morphologic features:

Axistyle present	Flagellum present			1. *Spirella*
	Flagellum absent	Volutin present	2. *Spirochaeta*
		Volutin absent	3. *Leptospira*
Axistyle absent	Crista present	Flagellum present	4. *Treponema*
		Flagellum absent	5. *Cristispirella*
	Crista absent		6. *Trichospira*

The taxonomy of spirochaetas is presently the subject of debate and agreement in this field has not yet been reached.

There is a tendency to believe that the genus *Saprospira,* and perhaps also *Cristispira,* should not be classed as *Spirochaetales* and that the genera *Treponema* and *Borrelia* should be classed as a single genus: the *Treponema.*

Anyway, the genera *Cristispira, Saprospira, Spirella, Spirochaeta, Cristispirella* and *Trichospira* only include saprophytic or commensal spirochaetas and are as such of no interest for present purposes. Parasitic, pathogenic spirochaetas are contained in only two genera:

Treponema (+ *Borrelia*) and *Leptospira.*

I. Experimental Infections with Treponemata

A. Genus Treponema Schaudinn (1905)

Bergey's Manual defines this genus, as follows: "Cells, 3 to 18 microns in length, with acute, regular or irregular spirals; longer forms are due to incomplete division. Terminale filament may be present. Some species stain only with Giemsa's stain. Weakly refractive by dark-field illumination in living preparations. Cultivated under strictly anaerobic conditions. Some are pathogenic and parasitic for man and other animals. Generally produce local lesions in tissues."

The type species is *Treponema pallidum* (Schaudinn and Hoffmann, 1905), Schaudinn, 1905.

Research using the electron microscope has shown that the spirochaetas of the genus *Treponema* normally have a rounded end and a pointed one. They are surrounded by an enveloping membrane made up of three layers. A bundle of thin fibrils, varying in number according to the species starts from each end of the Spirochaeta. Each fibril arises from a disc-like end-knob. The two bundles, starting from opposite ends, overlap in the middle part of the Spirochaeta (Listgarten and Socransky, 1964; Swain and Anderson, 1972), and are covered with an expansion of the enveloping membrane, which thus forms the so-called "crista" (BABUDIERI and BOCCIARELLI, 1943, 1948).

The bundle of fibrils starting from the sharp end and enveloped by the membrane, extends beyond the rounded end of the spirochaeta, forming a sort of thick flagellum. These fibrillar formations are exceedingly delicate and subject to easy alterations in compounds not prepared with particular care.

The genus *Treponema* comprehends saprophytic species (*T. zuelzerae*, *T. elusum*, etc.) living in fresh or salt water, and others commensal and practically harmless, which are found in the oral cavity, in the intestine and on the mucous membranes of man and animals, including some insects [*T. microdentium*, *T. macrodentium*, *T. mucosum*, *T. calligyrum*, *T. genitalis*, *T. (Borrelia) buccalis*, *T. (Borrelia) vincentii*, *T. (Borrelia) refringens*, *T. termitidis*, *T. parrum*, etc.].

Some of these species have been supposed to exert, in particular conditions, a certain pathogenic action. This may be said especially of the species present in the oral cavity, particularly for *T. mucosum*, which is found with particular abundance in cases of pyorrhea or around decayed teeth. It is probable, however, that, more than being a cause of disease, these species of spirochaetas find inflammatory states of the mucous membranes, caused by other pathogenic agents especially favourable to their growth.

The same can probably also be said, of those treponemas described in septic lesions associated with pyogenic microorganisms (*T. refringens*, *T. phagedenis*, *T. gangrenosum nosocomiale*, etc.) (NOGUCHI, 1912a–c, e).

Other species of the genus *Treponema*, in contrast, are definitely pathogenic and are the cause of important diseases. They are:

T. pallidum, causative agent of syphilis,
T. pertenue, causative agent of yaws,
T. carateum, causative agent of pinta or carate,
T. cuniculi, causative agent of spirochaetosis in the rabbit.

Besides these, the list of pathogenic species of the genus *Treponema*, should include the spirochaetas which cause relapsing fevers in man and which some people think should be included in the genus *Borrelia*.

The spirochaetas of relapsing fevers (blood treponematoses) have been divided into numerous species but the validity of this classification is rather questionable. In fact, they cannot be distinguished from one another by any particular morphological characteristics or any well-defined and consistent antigenic patterns (see HINDLE, 1931).

These species have been essentially distinguished from one another according to the species of arthropod which is their carrier and customary spreader (xenodiagnosis). Of some species, isolated only once from single patients (*T. novyi*, *T. kochii*) or from animals (*T. harveyi*) it is not even known which arthropod transmits them, and therefore their individuality is very dubious.

The species *T. recurrentis* may be considered valid enough. It is transmitted by the louse and shows rather particular biological characteristics.

T. carteri, which is very similar and perhaps even identical to it must also be mentioned.

The numerous species borne by ticks or more frequently by ticks belonging to the genus *Ornithodorus* need scarcely be distinguished from one another (*T. berbera*, *T. hispanica*, *T. hermsii*, *T. duttoni*, *T. parkeri*, *T. venezuelensis*, *T. persica*, *T. turicatae*, *T. caucasica*, *T. brasiliensis*, etc.). In fact, some of them are borne by more than one species of tick, or else they may be adopted by ticks that usually do not lodge them. Their antigenic constitution is not very specific and may vary widely even between strains isolated in the same place and from the same species of ticks.

It seems advisable to consider all spirochaetas causing relapsing tickborne fevers in man as belonging to a single species.

In various animals blood spirochaetas have been observed, some only in single cases, which from a morphological point of view, are likely to belong to the genus *Treponema*. Among these we mention the following:

S. or *T. pitheci*, described by THIROUX and DUFOUGÉRÉ (1910) in the blood of *Cercopitecus patas* in Soudan. Other spirochaetas have been found in the blood of several other species of African and Asiatic monkeys (PLIMMER, 1912; RANKEN, 1912; CASTELLANI and CHALMERS, 1910; BALFOUR, 1911; LEISHMAN, 1910 etc.).

S. or *T. vespertilionis* is the name of a spirochaeta found in the blood of some species of bats by NICOLLE and COMTE (1906); by GONDER (1907); by COLES (1914); in Northern Africa and in England.

S. or *T. canina* is a spirochaeta observed by BOSSELUT (1925), in a dog's blood in Algeria.

S. or *T. raillieti* has been described by MATHIS and LEGER (1911), in a rabbit's blood in Tonkin, *S.* or *T. naganophila* by SAVINI (1923), in the mouse, *S.* or *T. normandi* by NICOLLE and Coll. (1927), in *Meriones shawi* in Tunis, *S.* or *T. gundii* by NICOLLE (1907), in *Ctenodactylus gundii*.

A species apart is *T. hyos*, which is shorter and bigger than the others and has been found in the blood and in the intestinal ulcers of hogs affected by hog cholera (KING and DRAKE, 1915).

S. or *T. theileri* is a spirochaeta seen first by THEILER and described by LA-VERAN (1903), in bovine blood in Transvaal and later found several times in cattle and sheep affected by a sort of relapsing fever (THEILER, 1904, 1905; DODD, 1906).

Very probably *S. equi* described by NOVY and KNAPP (1906), in the horse and *S. ovina* found by BLANCHARD, in sheep's blood, are identical to *T. theileri*.

Another species of dubious systematic position is *T. glossinae* found only in the stomach of the tse-tse fly (*Glossina palpalis*).

Finally a species which has been known a long time and widely studied is *T. (Borrelia) anserinum*, the causative agent of a spirochaetosis in fowls, geese and ducks, carried by various species of ticks.

The following species will be considered from the point of view of experimental infection of laboratory animals:

T. pallidum, T. pertenue, T. carateum, T. cuniculi, T. anserinum, T. theileri, the causative agent of lice-borne relapsing fever (*T. recurrentis*) and the causative agents of tick-borne relapsing fever.

B. Infection with Tissue Spirochaetas

1. Treponema pallidum

Treponema pallidum is the causative agent of syphilis in man. In nature it does not infect other animal species.

Its morphology is the usual one for the genus *Treponema*. Its length is 8 to 15 microns; its transversal diameter is a little more than 0.1 micron.

a) Culture

The culture of *T. pallidum* has been repeatedly attempted with not very satisfactory results. SCHERESCHEWSKY was the first to maintain in 1909 that he was able to culture a strain of spirochaeta which was pathogenic for rabbits and mice and remained so for at least 40 years and after several passages (1954). These results have been questioned by other Authors who tried such cultures without success, among them NOGUCHI (1911, 1912f., 1916), who succeeded in cultiving some strains which, however, proved thoroughly avirulent for animals.

It is impossible to state with certainty that the causative agent of syphilis was obtained in artificial culture and this is also the conclusion of the members of the WHO Scientific Group on Treponematoses Research, who discussed this point widely in 1959.

At present there are a certain number of cultured strains of treponema in laboratories, which are, however, completely avirulent. It is dubious whether they actually are avirulent mutants of *T. pallidum*, or rather saprophytic treponemas occasionally present in syphilitic lesions, cultivated instead of the authentic luetic agent.

It is also interesting to observe how these cultured strains differ from one another in antigenic characters. So EAGLES and GERMUTH (1948) have proved that among the better known strains, the NICHOL's and NOGUCHI's are identical to each other, whereas REITER's and KAZAN's constitute a different antigenic group. KROO's strain, on the contrary, is completely different from any of the previous ones.

These observations, as well as the circumstance that these strains have no very close affinities with *T. pallidum*, favour the hypothesis that these strains may be commensal saprophytic treponemas, occasionally cultured.

There have been many attempts to grow pathogenic treponemas in tissue cultures, either using tissue of the same animal as the spirochaetas were sampled from (SHAFFER, 1926; GAMMEL and ECKER, 1931), or by inoculating treponemas on to established cell cultures (BESSEMANS and DE GEEST, 1934; HAAGEN and SCHLOSSBERGER, 1930; FOLDVARI, 1932; KAST and KOLMER, 1933, 1940, 1943; PERRY, 1948).

The results, however, have been negative. Only in some cases it was possible to observe a probable initial growth which soon stopped. If the spirochaetas did survive in these conditions, they thoroughly lost their virulence.

The attempt to culture spirochaetas in chick-embryos (BESSEMANS and DE MEIRSMAN, 1938; STERZI and STAUDACHER, 1939; CALLAWAY and SHARP, 1941; MASON, 1939; BEARDMORE and DODD, 1950, etc.) have been equally negative.

The only positive result is that reported by HALLAUER and KUHN (1942) who are said to have succeeded in culturing the pathogenic *T. pallidum* strain "Truffi" on the chorionallantoic membrane. It seems that more than 20 successive passages have been effected with this strain, and that the strain was still virulent for the rabbit. These results, however, are still to be confirmed.

The failure of the attempts to culture *in vitro* pathogenic strains of *T. pallidum* was also confirmed recently by the WHO Scientific Group on Treponematoses Research (WHO, 1970).

b) Isolation and Maintenance in Animals

T. pallidum can usually be isolated, though with a certain difficulty, in the rabbit, and maintained in this animal.

For isolation it is necessary to start from a primary or secondary syphilitic lesion, rich in treponemas. The surface of the lesion is carefully washed with distilled or salt water, and then abrased. The serum coming out of it is very rich in spirochaetas. It is drawn out with a Pasteur pipette or a syringe and mixed with salt water with 10% inactivated serum added.

About 0.5 ml of the material thus drawn out is immediately inoculated into a rabbit's testicle or intradermally into the scrotum. The first lesions appear after about 40 days, sometimes even later.

Infection of the rabbit may not always be successful, especially if the material inoculated is very much contaminated by bacteria.

Besides the rabbit, it is possible to use the monkey and the hamster for isolation. In the latter the treponema usually does not produce any overt sign of disease, but it is found in great quantities in the lymph-vessels and lymph-nodes.

The isolated strain is kept in the laboratory by serial passages from rabbit to rabbit, usually by intratesticular injection.

The strains of *T. pallidum* isolated and maintained in the rabbit so far are very numerous. TURNER and HOLLANDER (1957) isolated 47 of them alone in the International Treponematosis Laboratory Center.

The best known of these strains are TRUFFI's, NICHOL's (pathogenic), GAND's, GENT's. The first has been maintained in the rabbit for over 50 years.

These strains have maintained their virulence for man, as shown by the cases of laboratory infection they have provoked from time to time.

c) Experimental Infection of Animals

The first experimental infection of an animal with syphilis was achieved by METCHNIKOFF and ROUX, who in 1903 were able to infect the monkey. A few years later, in 1906, BERTARELLI succeeded in transmitting the infection to the rabbit, this animal still being the one of choice for the experimental study of this disease.

The experimental infection of laboratory animals has some characteristics which are common to all the animal species used. There are, however, remarkable differences in the clinical evidence of the infection. This is very showy in the rabbit and monkey, but only slender or non-existent in the hamster, mouse, rat or guinea pig.

α) Infection of the Monkey

The experimental infection of the monkey has been accurately described by NEISSER (1911), and by TURNER and HOLLANDER (1957), among others.

The monkeys most often used for this purpose have been *Macacus rhesus* and *Cercopithecus aethiopis sabaesis*. The most suitable monkey is however, the chimpanzee (METCHNIKOFF and ROUX, 1903; WILSON and MILES, 1955).

The infection is generally started with a suspension of material drawn out of an infected rabbit's testicle. The infecting material can be inoculated intracutaneously (we advise 0.1 ml containing roughly 5 million spirochaetas), into the preputial sac after scarification or on to the eyebrow by scarification.

The first definite lesions appear after 14–15 days and consist of small reddish or violaceous papules at the site of inoculation. They reach 7–8 mm in diameter and last for a limited length of time.

In fact they begin to subside after 2–3 weeks. It is possible to prove the presence of spirochaetas in these lesions. Three months after inoculation the lesions have usually disappeared. The appearance, in some cases, of evanescent non-infectious skin eruption is dubious. METCHNIKOFF and ROUX (1903, 1904, 1905, 1906) described in the chimpanzee the appearance of a papular skin eruption, palmar psoriasis, oral mucous patches and splenomegalia after 3–9 weeks. In some cases this symptomatology is accompanied by alopecia, emaciation and paresis of the hind limbs. Lesions of tertiary syphilis are always absent.

In infected monkeys, serological tests become positive; tests on the cerebrospinal fluid however remain negative (TURNER and HOLLANDER, 1957).

The internal organs of infected animals do not show any evident lesions; only the limph-nodes appear somewhat enlarged.

The treponemas remain in the organism of at least some of the infected monkeys for some months.

The brief duration of evident lesions, the scarty histopathologic findings in the various organs and the high costs involved in acquiring and maintaining monkeys make them hardly the animal of choice for the study of experimental syphilitic infection.

β) Infection of the Rabbit

The rabbit is the animal of choice for experimental infection with *T. pallidum*.

The methods of inoculation most often used are the intratesticular, the scrotal and the intradermal ones. More rarely infection has been achieved by ocular inoculation or by corneal scarification (BERTARELLI, 1906; HOFFMANN and BRUNING, 1907; GREGORIEW, 1929, etc.) or by intravenous injection (UHLENHUTH and MULZER, 1910, 1911).

The infection of the rabbit has been studied in particular depth by TRUFFI (1909), NICHOLS (1910, 1914), BROWN and PEARCE (1920, 1921, 1924, 1927), TURNER and HOLLANDER (1957), OVCHINNIKOV (1955), MATSUMOTO (1930, 1942).

The intraocular one has been the first method. Experimental infection of the rabbit was first achieved by the intraocular method as early as 1881 (HAENSELL), when the causative agent of disease had not yet been discovered.

UHLENHUTH and MULZER (1913) have observed that the inoculation of infectious material into the anterior chamber of the rabbit's eye produces keratitis, which reaches its peak after 3–6 weeks. The lesion then recedes until healing is apparently complete. However, relapses are frequent. Repeated passages may enhance the virulence of the spirochaeta (WILSON and MILES, 1955).

Following intratesticular inoculation, the first recognisable signs usually appear between the 3rd and 4th week; they come a little later if the spirochaetas used for inoculation have been taken from old, regressing lesions.

Testicular lesions have a cyclic course and can take a rapid acute course, or a slower, chronic one.

In the acute cases swelling of the testicle is the first sign to appear. Swelling persists for about 6 days and is accompanied by scrotal edema. The scrotal sac is filled with a gelatinous exudate, sometimes blood-stained which permeates the testicle also and the scrotum. Starting from the 7th day, the swelling regresses and the oedema subsides until, after about one week, the condition of the organ returns to normal. After 12 days the testicle begins to swell again and continues to do so for another week, when the swelling regresses once more. These cycles may be repeated several times, usually diminuishing in intensity.

In the cases of less acute type, a focus of induration appears in the testicle slowly growing for 2–3 weeks until the whole testicle appears larger, very hard, smooth or slightly nodular. These lesions regress slowly and not completely. In the cases, too, there is alternation of successive cycles of exacerbation and regression of the lesions.

Luetic lesions generally involve the whole testicle and often the scrotum too, but sometimes the reaction involves in a particular way only some portion of the testicle and of the scrotum and may bring about necrosis of the tissues.

Large masses of spirochaetaes are found in testicular and scrotal lesions as well as in the gelatinous exudate. These become immobile and quickly decrease in

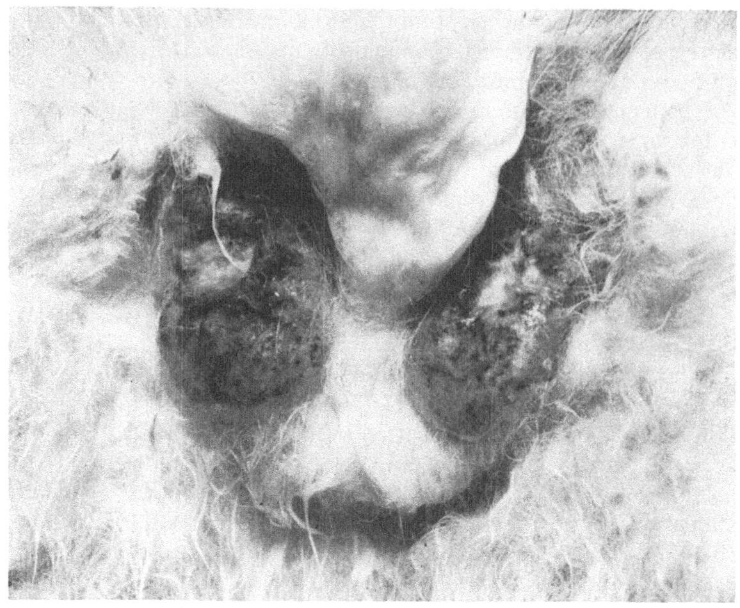

Fig. 1. Syphilitic lesions in rabbit's testicles

number during the regressive phases of the lesions, the increase again in quantity and mobility in the phases of reactivation.

The scrotal injection was first effected by Tomasczewski (1910), and has since been used by Brown and Pearce (1920b, c), McLeod and Arnold (1951), Volosceanu et al. (1955), Wilson and Miles (1955).

In this case, the incubation period lasts two weeks, whereupon a typical primary chancre develops with marked inguinal adenitis. The peak is reached after 30–55 days when the appearance of an ulceration is usually observed. The scrotal lesions may be absent in 10% of cases (Kolle and Evers, 1926), though infection of the popliteal lymphnodes is present.

Numerous secondary lesions appeared which lasted for 1–18 months in some cases.

The rabbit may also be infected by intradermal injection, usually given in the skin of the previously-shaven back. This method of infection has been studied in particular depth by Turner and Hollander (1957).

In this case, after an incubation period that may vary between few days and some weeks, a small papule appears at the site of injection, rapidly increasing in size for about 10 days, it may then measure as much as 10–15 mm diameter. The lesion then becomes indurated and necrosis and ulceration appear.

Subsequently the lesion slowly subsides and generally heals within a month or so, with or without scarring.

In some cases, however, there is no complete recovery and the ulceration torpidly persists for a long time.

The lesions described so far as a results of testicular, scrotal, endoocular or intradermic inoculation, are primary lesions appearing at the sites where the spirochaeta has been inoculated.

From these lesions the syphilis spirochaetas spread all over the organism. Indeed, in some cases (Raiziss and Severac, 1937) the dissemination takes place very early, before the appearance of visible lesions, sometimes already within minutes or hours of inoculation. This dissemination is particularly extensive in the case of intratesticular inoculation (CHESNEY and SCHIPPER, 1950).

After injection into a testicle, the infection usually spreads into the other one, though provoking lesions of minor entity.

Metastatic lesions, more or less generalized, usually occur from 35 to 60 days after inoculation. They are particularly evident on the skin, with the appearance of erythematous spots or of well-developed papular eruption. These are most likely to appear on the lower fore and hind legs, at the base of the ears, around the nose and along the tail.

Skin lesions are often accompanied by bone lesions, mostly in the form of periostitis, more rarely as osteitis with formation of granulomatous lesions which may successively ulcerate and lead to bone fracture. The bones of the forelegs, the metatarsals, the bones of the nose and of the tail are particularly involved (BROWN and PEARCE, 1921; MATSUMOTO, 1930). Similar lesions may also be observed on cartilages.

These cutaneous, cartilagineous, bone metastatic lesions may be accompanied by small secondary nodular lesions of the scrotum around the area of the primary lesions. In some cases, if this one is not healed, secondary lesions mix with the primary one thus forming a single big granuloma. Similar phenomena may also take place in the testicles.

Other metastatic lesions may occur in the eye (keratitis, conjunctivitis, iritis, chorionretinitis, etc.) (BROWN and PEARCE, 1921 b; NICHOLS, 1910; REASONER, 1916).

The frequency of generalized lesions is not only dependent upon the strain employed, but also, according to CHESNEY and SCHIPPER (1950), with the chosen method of inoculation. It is greatest following an intravenous injection of the spirochaeta (bone lesions in 90%, cutaneous lesions 79%, ocular 14%; total 96%), it is least after an intradermic injection (bone lesions 14%, cutaneous 18%, ocular 3.6%; total 52%). The intratesticular injection gives intermediate values (bones 37%, skin 40%, eye 15%; total 52%).

Obvious lesions of internal organs are rare in the rabbit, but WARTHIN (1914, 1916), has described a form of myocarditis. They are more frequent if the inoculated rabbit is kept at 0°–6° C (EAGLE and GERMUTH, 1948).

These secondary lesions, too, have a tendency to regress slowly and the disease becomes latent.

In the rabbit no transplacental diffusion of the infection from mother to fetus has been observed (PAUTRIZEL et al., 1957).

After recovery of the primary and secondary lesions, spirochaetas do not disappear from the infected animal. They persist in it practically for the rest of its life (JORDAN and BURROWS, 1945; OVCHINNIKOV, 1955), without causing any more evident clinical signs. The treponema is chiefly found in the lymphatic vessels and in the lymphnodes, which appear somewhat enlarged. Its virulence is unchanged. From time to time spirochaeta may flow into the blood stream (FRAZIER et al., 1950, 1952).

The lesions in experimental syphilis in rabbit are attributable to three different determining factors.

The first is the spirochaeta, whose accumulation at the site of the lesions is accompanied by the appearance of a particular mucoid substance, which has already been observed by UHLENHUTH and MULZER (1912) and by GRAETZ and DELBANCO (1914). This substance, which is a chondroitin sulfate, is most probably produced by the spirochaeta itself (Turner and Hollander, 1957) and in a way it might be compared to the capsular substance excreted by some bacteria.

The second factor is the immune response of the host. This takes the form of infiltration by cells chiefly of lymphocytic or epitheloid nature, reaching then highest number at the time of the peak of syphilitic lesions.

The third factor is represented by necrotic phenomena and by the consequent recovery-processes. The necroses only appear in extensive lesions and are the consequence of an inadequate oxygen supply to the tissues. Together with them it is possible to find accumulations of pseudo-eosinophil leukocytes which correspond, in the rabbit, to neutrophil leukocytes in man.

In the rabbit there are no lesions of the tertiary gummatous type, which are peculiar to human infection.

γ) Infection of the Guinea Pig

Kolle and Evers (1926) were the first to prove that the guinea pig could be infected by syphilis. Their observations have since been confirmed by Tani et al. (1930), by Kakishita and Saito (1930), and by Kato (1932).

Like the rabbit, the guinea pig is infected by inoculation of the pathologic material intracutaneously on the back, scrotum or prepuce.

The infection is usually completely symptomless and its presence can only be proved by inoculation of lymph into the rabbit or by the observation of spirochaetas under darkfield microscope. However, as observed by Kato (1931), and by Turner and Hollander (1957), in some cases guinea pigs, too, may show evident signs. These are, nevertheless, scarce and consist of short-lasting local induration; only seldom is the formation of a real nodule observed. These lesions and the regional lymph-nodes contain a high number of spirochaetas.

Altogether the inconsistency and scarcity of the lesions appearing in guinea pig make this animal hardly suitable for experimental research on syphilitic infection.

δ) Infection of the Rat and Mouse

Kolle and Schlossberger showed in 1926 that rat and mouse can be infected by *T. pallidum*.

In the infected animals evident lesions are extremely rare (Bessemans and De Potter, 1931); the infection usually has a completely symptomless course. Direct observation of spirochaetas in the tissues of the animals infected is rather difficult and their presence can be more easily revealed by inoculating rabbit with the material suspected. The difficulty of locating the treponema into surely infecting tissues has led some workers (Levaditi et al., 1928) to postulate the existence in the tissues of a granular filtrable phasis of the spirochaeta.

Rosahn et al. (1948) and Rosahn and Rowe (1950) have proved that the adult mouse is as susceptible as the new-born one, and that after subcutaneous or intraperitoneal infection, lymphnodes, blood and various tissues become infectious and remain so for a very long time, even longer than one year (Rosahn, 1952). Though evident lesions are absent, the infected mice show, when checked, a significantly shortened lifespan (Rosahn, 1952).

TPI antibodies are formed in the serum of infected rat and mouse, but cardiolipin type antibodies are not formed.

ε) Infection of the Hamster

The hamster (*Mesocritus auratus*) is also susceptible to infection by *T. pallidum*. The infection usually has a symptomless course, as in mouse and rat. In the hamster, however, the regional lymph-nodes appear enlarged and contain very high quantities of treponemas, which reach the peak 4–6 weeks after infection and decrease in number after 3–4 months.

In some cases of intradermal inoculation TURNER and HOLLANDER (1957) have observed small crusted ulcers appearing at the site of inoculation after about a month and quickly healing. Equally rare is the appearance of only insignificant papules coming out a short time after inoculation, which usually disappear after two weeks. They are relatively more frequent in the animals inoculated with particular strains of *T. pallidum* (strain Baghdad A).

ζ) Infection of Other Animals

Besides those mentioned above, it is probable that many other animals may be receptive to syphilitic infection; however, there has been little research in this field.

BERTARELLI succeeded in infecting the dog as early as 1907, by inoculation both into the anterior chamber of the eye, and into the scrotum, which resulted in local lesions interpreted as syphilomas.

HOFFMANN and BRUNING (1907) also succeeded in infecting the dog.

LEVADITI and YAMANOUCHI (1908) have infected suckling cats with *T. pallidum*, inoculating the infectious material into the corneal tissue and obtaining keratitis.

BÉCLÈRE (1934) was able to infect some calves; BERTARELLI (1907) a pig and a sheep, which developed local lesions.

2. Treponema pertenue

Treponema pertenue, discovered by CASTELLANI in 1905, is the causative agent of yaws. In morphology and biological properties it is very similar to *T. pallidum*.

This treponema has also proved impossible to culture in artificial media, and the strains kept in laboratories are maintained by means of successive passages into animals, especially rabbits. TURNER and HOLLANDER (1957) have kept 20 strains of it.

Experimental Infection of Animals

The methods of experimental infection of laboratory animals and the course the infection takes in them, correspond in the man to what has already been said of *T. pallidum*. Our present purpose is consequently to point out only the most striking differences.

BAERMANN and HALBERSTADTER (1906) were the first to transmit yaws to monkeys. In gibbons and in anthropoid apes the disease appears after an incubation period of 13–14 days. CASTELLANI (1907) observed a generally longer incubation in inferior monkeys up to 90 days.

The infection becomes apparent when a flattened papula forms at the site of inoculation, surrounded by an infiltration zone. The papula enlarges quickly, becomes moist, and covers itself with a thick crust covering a granulating surface.

Infection with *T. pertenue* has been in particular depth studied by SCHÖBL (1928) who found the species *Cynomolgus philippinensis* especially suitable. In this animal the infection causes the appearance of a papula, as described above, which has a tendency to heal within a few weeks. The generalisation of local lesions does not occur, however, following superinfections and reinfections. SCHÖBL (1918) was able to achieve diffusion of the lesions, which are not unlike those found in man when struck by yaws.

The infection of the rabbit with *T. pertenue* was first achieved in 1910 by Nichols using the intratesticular method.

The lesions produced in this animal are very similar to those caused by *T. pallidum*, as described above. Pearce and Brown, however, in 1925, described a typical periorchitis of granular or finely nodular type, with or without involvement of the vaginal tunic in the rabbit infected by *T. pertenue*, which is different from the lesions caused by *T. pallidum* in the testicle.

According to Turner and Hollander (1957) *T. pertenue* causes lesions less evident than *T. pallidum*. These lesions do not usually become generalized. In addition *T. pertenue* produces much less mucoid material than *T. pallidum* in the lesions of the rabbit (Ferris and Turner, 1937, 1938).

In the guinea pig infection with *T. pertenue* has a course very similar to that of infection with *T. pallidum*.

In the hamster, *T. pertenue* causes diffused cutaneous lesions wich ulcerate and have a chronic course, with pronounced involvement of the lymphnodes. At the beginning there is a small zone of slightly indurated erythema at the site of inoculation, which gradually grows and finally ulcerates and covers itself with a crust. The central area of the ulcer shows a tendency to heal, whereas at the margin the lesion expands. These lesions are slow to subside and recovery does not occur for 6 months or longer. The treponemas are found at the margin of these lesions.

Some strains of *T. pertenue* (strains Samoa), studied by Turner and Hollander (1957), cause particularly serious lesions, with wide ulcerations and metastatic lesions, especially on the soles of the feet, in the nares and on the tail. In these cases, however, the fluid in the lymphnodes does not usually contain any spirochaetas, or only very few. The exudate of cutaneous lesions, in contrast is very rich in treponemas.

In the mouse, *T. pertenue* was first inoculated by Schlossberger (1927, 1929). The infection has a completely symptomless course in this animal and in the rat, quite similar to the course of infection with *T. pallidum*. The spirochaeta persists for a long time in the tissues of infected animals.

3. Treponema carateum

This treponema is the causative agent of a human disease present in tropical and sub-tropical America, called "pinta" or "carate". It was discovered in 1938 by Saenz et al.

T. carateum, which has the typical morphology of *Treponema*, has not only never been kept in culture, but it has not even been serially transmitted to laboratory animals.

Leony Blanco and Oteiza (1945) managed to transmit the infection to a rabbit once; Turner and Hollander (1957) succeeded in infecting three hamsters in one experiment, but other attempts at serial transmission have failed completely.

It is necessary, however, to remember that the attempts at infecting animals esperimentally with *T. carateum* have been, so far, rather few in number.

4. Treponema cuniculi

In the rabbit there is a spontaneous treponematosis caused by a spirochaeta: *T. cuniculi*, not morphologically distinguishable from *T. pallidum*, but not naturally pathogenic for other species of animals and harmless to man. It was first seen by Ross (1912). So far, the spirochaeta has not been obtained in culture.

Infection with *T. cuniculi* has been widely studied by Klarenbeek (1921, 1930) and by McLeod and Turner (1946a, b).

Unlike the treponemas discussed so far, *T. cuniculi* only produces local lesions of the epidermis. In spontaneous infection, which usually occurs during coitus, these are generally limited to the perineum, more rarely to the nose and eyelids, and consist of inflammatory processes. The tissues appear swollen and covered with sores. Underneath there is a smooth oedematous surface, liable to bleeding, which exudes a serous liquid rich in spirochaetas. This infection differs from infection with *T. pallidum*, in that these lesions are not indurated.

If inoculated into the testicle, *T. cuniculi* produces scrotal lesions; if into the anterior chamber of the eye, it causes keratitis, followed by the appearance of generalized lesions of the skin.

In intratesticular inoculation we can also observe fine granular nodules scattered throughout the tunica vaginalis. Small nodular lesions are also found in the body of the testicle.

After repeated passages from rabbit to rabbit, the testicular lesions become more evident with induration and enlargement of the organ, which, however, never reach the intensity of the lesions seen in infections with *T. pallidum*. Another feature is the appearance of indurated nodules in the head of the epididymis.

The infection streads from one testicle to the other and, after 2–4 month, often causes extensive cutaneous lesions, flat, with no induration. The lymphnodes will contain virulent spirochaetas for a long time. *T. cuniculi*, like *T. pertenue* produces little mucoid material.

In the experimentally infected monkey, *T. cuniculi* produces small lesions at the site of inoculation, lasting longer than those caused by *T. pallidum* (TURNER and HOLLANDER, 1957). In some cases, however, these are completely absent. In the monkey there are no generalized cutaneous signs, nor are there lesions of the other organs.

According to some other authors (BESSEMANS et al., 1938; SCHERESCHEWSKY, 1920; NOGUCHI, 1921; LEVADITI et al., 1921) monkeys are not at all susceptible to infection with *T. cuniculi*.

Pathogenicity of *T. cuniculi* for the hamster, the mouse and the rat is rare and inconsistent; it is not pathogenic for man (LEVADITI et al., 1921).

On the whole, *T. cuniculi* is very different from the other pathogenic treponemas, both in the characteristics it displays in experimental infection, and in its immunologic characteristics.

5. Factors Affecting Experimental Infection by Treponemas

a) Infecting Agent

The duration of the incubation period is inversely proportional to the infecting dose inoculated. This has been observed by CHESNEY and KEMP (1925), by MAGNUSON et al. (1948), and by others.

According to TURNER and HOLLANDER (1957) this incubation period is not to be considered as a latent period, but rather as the time necessary for the inoculated spirochaetas to increase sufficiently in number to constitute a mass of parasites large enough to produce a lesion. Under favourable conditions the number of the treponemas inoculated increases tenfold every fourth day and clinically evident lesion is produced when the count of treponemas in one area reaches about 10 million organisms. These data, reported by TURNER and HOLLANDER (1957), give us an idea of the relationship between the size of the infecting dose and the length of the incubation period, and enable us to calculate that the longest duration of the incubation, the duration theoretically following the inoculation of a single virulent organism, cannot be much longer than one month.

It has also been observed that when a constant dose of the inoculum is used the infection has a quicker course if effected with material taken from recent lesions. It is probable that in old lesions there may exist a certain number of spirochaetas unable or only hardly able to reproduce themselves.

The serial passage of a treponema into a certain animal species generally enhances its virulence as well as the entity of the lesions it produces.

It has been observed that some types of lesions (e.g. chorionretinitis) are caused with greater frequency by some strains of treponema than by others (Reasoner, 1916).

b) Animal Host

From the research so far, which is hardly voluminous, it does not appear that the breed of the animals used has much influence on the evolution of experimental infection (Turner and Hollander, 1957). Let us only mention Rosahn's statement, 1933, according to which the Havana and Dutch breeds of rabbits are more resistent to infection with *T. pallidum* than the English, Himalayan or Rex breeds.

The animals' age does not seem to be very important, though Chesney (1923), affirms that in young male rabbits inoculated in the testicle, initial lesions are more marked and generalized lesions appear later than in older rabbits.

According to the same authors and to Magnuson et al. (1951), the lesions are more evident and occur sooner in male than in female rabbits.

Regarding the feeding of experimental animals, it is necessary to bear in mind that many kinds of feed previously prepared in pellets contain antibiotics. These may prevent or disturb experimental infection.

According to Otsuji (1938, 1939), diets inducing acidosis increase susceptibility to syphilitic infection in the rabbit, while diets inducing alkalosis delay it.

c) Temperature

Both the environmental and the local tissue temperature of the infected animal, are very important in the evolution of treponematosis in rabbit. In vivo, *T. pallidum* only develops between 30° and 38° C and the optimal growth temperature is 35°–37° C.

It is well-known to anyone working on experimental syphilis that in the winter the animal infected shows worse and more frequent lesions that during the summer. It was believed for some time that this might be due to some particular metabolic deficiency animal might be subject to during the winter (Matsumoto, 1930; Brown and Pearce, 1924, 1927, etc.), but Hollander and Turner (1957) observe that this is not true and that a modification in the local temperature is enough to have an evident influence on the evolution of the infection. The lesions are bad and diffused if the animal is kept in an environment at 18°–21° C; in contrast they are scarce and sometimes absent if the local temperature is kept at 29°–31° C.

Higher temperatures can even cause the disappearance of the spirochaetas. For example, Weichbrodt and Jahnel (1919), were able to cure testicular syphiloma in the rabbit simply by keeping the animal at 41° C for half an hour and Schamberg and Rule (1927, 1928), observed that the infectious animal subjected to daily hot baths recovers from superficial lesions though the treponemas do not disappear from deep-set lymph nodes.

The testicle constitutes the organ of choice for experimental infection, precisely because, owing to its anatomic position, its temperature is inferior to that of the other tissues. In fact the infection does not develop if the testicles are kept in the abdominal cavity for a few hours (BESSEMANS and HAEQUAERT, 1930; HOLLANDER and TURNER, 1954).

A brilliant demonstration of the influence of body temperature over the evolution of syphilitic lesions of the rabbit was given by TURNER and HOLLANDER (1957), who partially shaved two rabbits, taking off all the fur on the fore part of the body of one of them, and all the fur on the hind part of the other. Then the two rabbits were inoculated intravenously with a high dose of treponemas. After about 20 days it was possible to observe a large dissemination of syphilitic lesions, limited to the shaven areas, where the absence of the protection of the fur had led to a decrease in skin temperature.

Let us remember that treponemas can be maintained for years without losing their virulence, if kept at a temperature of $-70°$ C (dry ice) (TURNER, 1938; TURNER and FLEMING, 1939).

To be able to obtain good results, however, it is advisable to freeze the treponemas without drawing them out of the tissues (TURNER and HOLLANDER, 1957), or to add 15% of glycerol to a suspension of them (HOLLANDER and NELL, 1954).

d) Cortisone

The administration of cortisone to animals infected by treponemas, especially to rabbits, greatly modifies the course of the experimental infection. The production of antibodies is arrested, or noticeably limited, the lymphocytal infiltration usually surrounding the lesions is very much reduced; the lesions do not show the peculiar induration of syphilitic lesions, and their tendency to ulcerate is scarce. On the contrary, they take a characteristic globoid aspect, they are pale, soft, and spongy with a sharply circumscribed basis.

The lesions are filled with a thick mucoid gelatinous material, oozing from the cut surface. Enormous quantities of spirochaetas are contained in this material (TURNER and HOLLANDER, 1950, 1954, 1957), so much so that it is advisable to administer cortisone when a large quantity of treponemas is required for research. The usual daily dose of cortisone is 6.0 mg per Kg of body weight for periods of 1–4 weeks, starting on the 25th day after inoculation.

e) Antibodies

In the induction of experimental infections in rabbit it must be borne in mind that the animal may have previously overcome an infection with *T. cuniculi*. In this case the antibodies present in its organism do not only prevent the rooting of an experimental infection with the same treponema, but also make it difficult to achieve further infection with other pathogenic treponemas which have particular antigenic affinities with *T. cuniculi*. According to HARDY and NELL (1955) these rabbits may be singled out by agglutination test (TPA), which is positive in the animals which have overcome an infection with *T. cuniculi*.

Some degree of cross-immunity has also been demonstrated between the syphilis strains and *T. pertenue*.

Another possibility of error to be borne in mind is the possible inoculation of antibodies produced by the donor animal, together with the spirochaetas. This may happen in the cases when the inoculation is permained using abundant material taken from animals already infected for some time and therefore rich in antibodies (BROWN and PEARCE, 1920). In these cases the infection has a difficult rooting and the lesions may be atypical.

6. Confirmation of Infection by Treponema

For the confirmation of an experimental infection with Treponema two methods can be followed: one consists in demonstrating, directly or indirectly, the presence of Treponema in the tissues; the other consists in the application of immunologic tests specific for infections by Treponema.

The direct detection of the Treponema is to be effected in cutaneous, mucous, or testicular lesions; they may appear when the material is taken from the margin

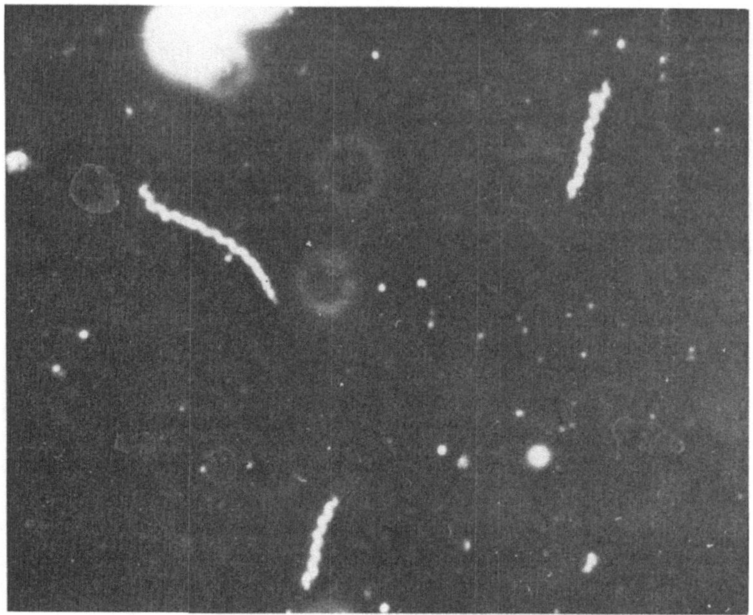

Fig. 2. *T. pallidum*. Dark-field illumination. 2000×

area. If the lesions are healed, the spirochaeta may be sought in the lymphatic system and more particularly in the regional lymph nodes. We have already mentioned, however, that in chronic cases, the Treponema report in the lymphatic tissue is often very difficult.

The suspect material can be examined directly, as soon as drawn out, under dark-field- or phase-contrast microscope (De Lamater et al., 1950, 1952), or after fixation and prolonged staining with Giemsa dye or by silver impregnation (methods used by Levaditi, by Fontana-Tribondeau, or by one of the numerous modifications of these methods).

a) Fontana-Tribondeau Method

The film is made as thin as possible and then washed for one to two minutes in a solution composed of: glacial acetic acid, 1 part; formol, 2 parts; distilled water, 100 parts. The film is then washed in running water for half a minute and afterwards mordanted in the following solution: phenol, 1 part; tannic acid, 5 parts; distilled water 100 parts. This solution is poured on to the film and the slide then warmed over a flame until it steams. It is kept in this mordant for about half a minute, then rinsed in distilled water and ammoniacal silver nitrate poured on to the film. The slide is again warmed for about half a minute, after which the film is washed, dried and mounted in Canada balsam. The ammoniacal silver nitrate is prepared by adding liquid ammonia to a 0.25% solution of silver nitrate in distilled water until the precipitate which first forms is redissolved. Finally, silver nitrate solution is added drop by drop, until the liquid becomes opalescent.

With this method the spirochaetas are coated with a deposit of metallic silver and they stand out very distinctly as dark filaments, which are much thicker than the living organisms.

YAMAMOTO successfully used two new dye-stuffs for treponemas in 1929: Blue BBX acid (BA) (carbolised) and Blue B Alkali (SB) with 5% carbolic acid, added.

If a direct examination should not permit detection of the presence of treponemas, it is advisable to inculate the suspect material into a susceptible animal, such as the rabbit.

b) Dobell's Modification of Levaditi's Silver Impregnation Method

The tissues are fixed in 4% formaldehyde solution for at least 1 to 3 days, but may be kept in this solution indefinitely before being stained. They are then transferred to 95% alcohol for 24 hours, and afterwards through graded alcohols to distilled water until all traces of alcohol are removed. The tissues are then soaked in a 0.25 to 0.5% solution of silver nitrate in distillated water for 18 to 24 hours in the dark at 37° C. They are afterwards in changes of distilled water for an hour until the wash water is free from silver nitrate, and then soaked in a 0.5 to 1% solution of Hydroquinone in 50% alcohol for 18 to 24 hours at room temperature. Finally, the tissues are washed in 70% alcohol, dehydrated and embedded in paraffin in the usual manner. The sections, after having been fixed on slides, are washed with xylol and may then be mounted in Canada balsam or may be counter-stained by any of the ordinary staining methods. The spirochaetas stand out very distinctly as dark filaments, owing to the deposit of silver on their surface, and can usually be readily distinguished from any other structures that may take the stain in a similar manner.

The indirect confirmation of infection by Treponema can be achieved by the usual *serological tests* for the diagnosis of syphilis. Though it is possible to observe remarkable antigenic differences between the various types of pathogenic treponemas, they also possess common antigens permitting the execution of serological cross-tests.

It must be borne in mind, that after experimental infection of laboratory animals, conventional serum reactions to syphilis, based on cardiolipin-type antibodies, remain negative in the mouse and in the guinea pig (BERLINGHOFF, 1957; OVCHINNKOV, 1955). Nor does the golden hamster develop a positive Kahn test for the disease (WILE and JOHNSON, 1945).

On the contrary, the reactions to be used are: Nelson's immobilization test (T.P.I. test) (GASTINEL et al., 1959), which, in the mouse, becomes reactive only after a considerable time, the fluorescence treponemal antibody absorption test (F.T.A-A B S test) or the agglutination one (T.P.A.).

Recently a new serologic test, which is highly specific also in experimentally infected animals, has been developed: this is the *Treponema pallidum* haemo-agglutination test (T.P.H.A. test) (TOMIZAWA and KASAMATSU, 1955). An automated microhaemoagglutination technique, the AMHA-Typ test, has been developed in Atlanta (LOGAN and COX, 1970). In *T. cuniculi* infections in rabbits, the TPHA test has been found to be reactive, whereas both the TPI and the FTA-ABS tests are non-reactive (WHO, 1970).

7. Laboratory Infections

It must be borne in mind that pathogenic Treponema strains, even after several passages into laboratory animals, maintain their virulence for man, as shown by the rather frequent cases of accidental infection in laboratory staff. The spirochaetas do not pass through healthy skin, but can penetrate into the organism through small lesions, especially of mucous membranes. There may be a much greater risk of infection from accidental pricks with a contaminated syringe or with instruments used for post-mortem examination.

Consequently, when working with pathogenic treponemas, scrupulous observation of the rules of good laboratory technique is essential; gloves should be worn and for complicated inoculations rabbits should be anesthetized with Nembutal, hamsters with ether.

When possible, it is preferable to work with *T. cuniculi*, which is not pathogenic for man.

If an accident should occur in spite of all precautions it is advisable to treat the subject at once with penicillin and to continue with it for as long as necessary

C. Infection by Blood (Relapsing-Fever) Spirochaetas

The relapsing-fever Treponemata have many characteristics in common with regard to transmission, clinical pattern of the infection caused by it. The first part of this chapter will therefore deal with the characteristics common to the whole group.

1. Culturing

The blood spirochaetas are more easily cultured than the tissue Treponemata. They are not, however, easy to culture, and in the subcultures the strain may be lost quite easily for causes not always ascertainable. Anyhow in culture the relapsing-fever spirochaetas retain their initial virulence and their morphology is unchanged.

Many kinds of culture media have been suggested. The general conditions required are the following:

1. A limited supply of oxygen obtained by covering the surface of the medium with paraffin oil or vaseline.

2. The presence of albumin: either coagulated (egg-white) or not (rabbit or horse-serum, diluted with saline).

3. The addition of some drops of blood or of pieces of fresh tissue or embryonic tissue.

4. An optimum pH value, varying slightly from strain to strain, but amounting to about 7.4.

The first positive results in this field were obtained by Noguchi (1912d) who used the following medium: A small piece of rabbit-kidney and small amount of citrated blood containing the spirochaetas to be cultured are added to 15 ml of sterile ascitic or hydrocele fluid in a sterile test-tube. The surface of the medium is covered by a layer of sterile paraffin oil. The tubes are incubated at 37° C. The spirochaetas usually attain their maximum growth on the 7th–10th day, after which they sometimes disappear, to appear again towards the 16th day, reaching a new peak between the 20th and 30th day.

Another good culture medium is the following, suggested by Lapidari and Sparrow (1928): One ml of egg-yolk is coagulated by keeping the test tube which contains it slanting whilst rotating in boiling water. Some ml of fresh rabbit serum diluted to one-sixth with either Ringer solution (glucose 1 gm, $NaCl_2$ 9 gm, $CaCl_2$

0.24 gm, $NaHCO_3$ 0.1 gm, distilled water 1 liter) or Hartley's broth are then added and the medium is covered with a layer of sterile paraffin and heated at 56°–58° C for one hour. Several drops of infected blood are then added to the medium. By subcultures it is necessary to add a drop of sterile human, rabbit or mouse blood to the medium.

It is advisable to effect subcultures every seventh day.

A complete list of media used for the culture of these spirochaetas is reported by MUEHLENS (1930).

The relapsing-fever spirochaetas can be stored in a laboratory for a long time at −60° C.

2. Maintenance in Animals

The relapsing-fever spirochaetas can be maintained by repeated passages into the animal which is their usual host, or in many cases, also in laboratory animals of various species, especially mice and rats, with successive transfers of infectious blood. It is necessary, however, to effect the transfer during the viremic phasis of the infection, after ascertaining the presence of spirochaetas by microscopic blood tests.

When the spirochaeta is no longer present in the blood, it may be found in the spleen, or even better, in the brain, where it may last for as long as two months after its disappearance from the blood stream (ADDAMIANO and BABUDIERI, 1957).

The spirochaetas of tick-borne relapsing fevers are usually easily transmitted to the white mouse or rat, and they can generally be maintained in these animals. The spirochaetas of lice-borne relapsing fevers (*T. recurrentis*) are generally transmitted to the mouse only after having passed at least once through the monkey.

When this is possible, it is easier to keep the spirochaetas in the arthropod which is their usual carrier. This is simple enough as far as tick-borne spirochaetas are concerned. In the ticks, in fact, the spirochaeta lasts for very long periods, even for years, as it is usually transmitted from one generation to the next, through the eggs of these arthropods.

Another advantage of this method of maintenance is that many species of ticks can live for a long time, months and years, without needing any food.

To obtain the spirochaetas when required, usually it is not even necessary to kill the tick, but only to feed it on an animal. Spirochaetas are found in great quantities in the coxal fluid emitted by the tick before and after the engorgement.

The problem is much more complex in the case of louse-borne spirochaetas. The life of the louse, in fact, is much shorter than the tick's; besides which lice require frequent nourishment on man, involving the risk that the infection will be transmitted to him. There are, however, some strains of rabbit-adapted lice, which can feed on the rabbit, and therefore relieve the problem of maintaining these spirochaetas, at least to some extent.

3. Experimental Infection of Laboratory Animals

The course of relapsing fevers produced by spirochaeta in laboratory animals has rather uniform characteristics, in spite of the remarkable differences of virulence not only from species to species, but also from strain to strain in the range of the same species. The method of inoculation, too, according to TOMIOKA (1924) is supposed to influence the severity of the infection. According to this author the mice infected percutaneously by spirochaetas causing European relapsing-fever showed a mortality rate of 70%, whilst those inoculated sub-cutaneously or intraperitoneally had a rate of only 42%. The mouse's splenectomy strongly increases its receptiveness to experimental infection (PLAUT, 1928).

The cutaneous infection is effected by leaving a drop of infected blood on the shaven skin of a mouse for about half an hour.

Subcutaneous or intraperitoneal infection is achieved by inoculating subcutis and in peritoneum, respectively, with a small quantity (0.1–0.5 ml) of infectious blood, diluted with saline or not.

The animals of choice for experimental infection with relapsing-fever spirochaetas are the mouse and the rat. The guinea pig and the rabbit are only seldom and inconsistently susceptible to the infection.

The incubation period generally lasts 1–10 days according to the virulence of the strain and to the quantity of the inoculum, after which the appearance of spirochaetas is observed in the blood, accompanied by a sudden rise in temperature. The spirochaetas remain in the blood for two or four days, after which the febrile attack ends by lysis and the spirochaetas disappear from the blood.

In some cases the infection is concluded by this single attack, more often, instead, after few days begins a more or less prolonged succession of relapses, gradually diminishing in severity. At each relapse there is fever and the spirochaetas reappear in the blood.

In fatal cases, the animal's temperature does not fall and the spirochaetas remain in the blood in large quantities. In these cases the body temperature falls to subnormal soon before death.

During each relapse, a spirochaetal population antigenically distinct from the previous one appears. The fluorescin-labeled antibody technique allows detection and direct differentiation of the different serotypes in the infected animal's plasma (Coffey and Eveland, 1967).

For preparing the immune sera, a very pure antigen might be prepared by separating relapsing-fever spirochaetas from blood by DEAE cellulose anion exchange (Ginger and Katz, 1970).

The most common bodily changes in inoculated animals are loss of weight and anemia. Leukocytosis is frequent and reaches its peak when the spirochaetas are about to disappear. The spleen is usually much enlarged and very soft.

In the fatal cases of infection the changes observed in internal organs are the following: spleen and liver are enlarged, with small hemorrhages and small necrotic lesions in longstanding cases. The bone-marrow is dark purple in colour and softened to a semi-fluid consistency (Breinl and Kinghorn, 1906; Bykowa, 1926). The lymphatic vessels are frequently hemorrhagic. Capillaries become obstructed by masses of polymorphonuclear leukocytes. Exudates are present in the peritoneal, pleural, and pericardial cavities. Lungs become edematous and show hemorrhagic infarcts and small subpleural petechiae. In acute cases numerous hemorrhagic infarcts occur throughout the internal organs.

The mechanism by which the relapsing-fever spirochaetas determine these lesions is still unknown. In fact, it has not been possible to observe in them any exo-or endo-toxin.

In the monkey the course of the infection is very similar to that in man. The disease is usually mild and without relapses, except in the case of infections by *T. duttoni*, which may even be fatal.

The spirochaetas are found in all the organs of the infected animal. They live and multiply inside the blood-vessels.

Soon after the final disappearance of the spirochaetas in the blood, they are no longer found even in the organs, except for the brain where they can persist for at least 20 (Tomicka, 1924), or even 50 days (Addamiano and Babudieri, 1957). The duration of this persistence generally varies from strain to strain and shows remarkable differences also between different animals.

In the brain of spirochaeta-carrying animals, no pathologic changes are generally observed, except for the rats which sometimes show some histological changes involving areas into which fibres have entered from posterior nerve-roots (HINDLE, 1931).

As it is generally impossible to ascertain the presence of spirochaetas in the brain, except indirectly by inoculation of a suspension of tissue into another animal, it was suggested that there might exist in this organ (LEVADITI and ANDERSON, 1928, 1929) an invisible filterable phasis of the spirochaetas. This hypothesis, however, has not yet been confirmed.

The brain infection is particularly resistent to the action of chemotherapeutic agents.

The animal which has overcome an infection with relapsing-fever spirochaetas acquires an immunity usually short-lasting, especially if the infection has been mild. The immunity, however, concerns only the species and often only the strain which has provoked the infection (ADDAMIANO and BABUDIERI, 1957).

a) Treponema anserinum

T. anserinum is the causative agent of the spirochaetosis seen in several species of domestic fowls. It was described in 1891 by SAKHAROFF, as occurring in the blood of sick geese in the Caucasus, and it has been discovered, since, by MARCHOUX and SALIMBENI (1903) in diseased fowls in South America. It has since been reported in various countries, and with particular frequency in the countries of Mediterranean Africa. It has at times been given different names, like *T. marchouxi* or *T. gallinarum*, or *T. neveuxi* or *T. nicollei* or *T. granulosum penetrans.* The valid name, however, remains *T. anserinum* (SAKHAROFF, 1891).

Besides the goose this spirochaeta affects in nature, the duck, the chicken and the turkey. It is usually transmitted by ticks *Argas persicus, A. reflexus, A. miniatus.* Its morphology is the typical one of relapsing-fever spirochaetas.

This spirochaeta is associated with a high death rate in the infectious fowl, especially in young birds. In severe cases the blood contains an enormous number of spirochaetas and the animal generally succumbs to the infection after about one week.

There is also a chronic type of infection involving paralysis of the feet and wings, progressive emaciation and death in 8 to 15 days.

This spirochaeta can be transmitted to the mouse and to the rabbit. In these animals it does not cause very severe disease.

Small birds such as canaries can also be experimentally infected.

b) Treponema theileri

This treponema is the cause of relapsing-fever in cattle, and has been reported in several countries. It is transmitted by numerous species of ticks. These can transmit the spirochaeta to their offsprings for many generations.

The disease produces only one attack in cattle, but after apparent recovery the animal's blood may remain infective for a long period.

T. theileri can be experimentally transmitted to the sheep.

c) Lice-borne Relapsing-Fever Spirochaetas

T. recurrentis (*T. obermejeri*), the agent of epidemic relapsing fever, was observed by OBERMEJER in patient's blood as early as 1868. It is transmitted by the louse (*Pediculus hominis*).

We have already mentioned that *T. recurrentis* cannot be transmitted directly from man to mouse or rat except in exceptional cases and with great difficulty. The infection can, in contrast, be easily transmitted to the monkey and then the transfer from this animal to the mouse becomes quite easy. The guinea pig and the rabbit, on the other hand remain not susceptible to the infection.

In the experimentally infected mouse *T. recurrentis* can produce a high death rate. Its virulence varies widely from strain to strain.

T. carteri is another spirochaeta transmitted by the louse and causes the Indian relapsing-fever. Unlike *T. recurrentis*, this spirochaeta can be transmitted, though with a certain amount of difficulty, direct from man to rat, mouse and rabbit. In the monkey it produces a single febrile attack, during which the spirochaetas are very scarce in the blood.

d) Tick-borne Relapsing-Fever Spirochaetas

We have already made out a partial list of the presumed "species" of spirochaetas transmitted by ticks to man. These relapsing fevers, which have an endemic character, are diffused to all countries with a tropical or subtropical climate. The virulence of the single strains varies widely from case to case, and the severity of the disease they precipitate both in man and in experimental animals is equally variable.

We have already mentioned that in the first passage this group of spirochaetas easily infects mouse and rat. Guinea pig and monkey can also be experimentally infected.

The course of the infection and the lesions caused by it are as described above.

e) Confirmation of Infection with Relapsing-Fever Spirochaetas

Infection is confirmed quite simply by observation of fresh specimens of presumably infected blood under a light or dark-field microscope. The presence of spirochaetas is revealed by the movements they transmit to the red blood cells all around.

Blood films fixed with methyl alcohol or May-Gruenwals stain, then stained with Giemsa may also be used.

Leishman (1918) reported good results obtained by dark-field observations of relapsing-fever spirochaetas previously stained with Leishman dye.

If the spirochaetas are supposed to be very scarce in the blood, the thick drop method can be adopted. It consists in laying on a well-cleaned slide a drop of blood and in enlarging it until it has a diameter of about 1–2 cm. Then the drop must be dried in the air and after $^1/_2$–1 hour, without fixation, it is stained for 30 minutes with a solution of 1 drop of Giemsa's stain in 1 ml of distilled water. Finally the slide is gently washed in water and then left to dry. The red blood cells are lysed by this procedure and do not disturb the observation of the rare spirochaetas which may be present.

In particular cases, however, silver impregnation methods may be used (see page 17).

In the tissues, the spirochaetas should be sought either in smears stained with Giemsa or in sections stained by silver impregnation (see page 17).

A negative result of the test for spirochaetas in the blood does not exclude the possibility of a latent infection. Therefore, in such cases, it is necessary to try a transmission of the infection to a healthy mouse, either by inoculating a little blood or a suspension of the suspected animal's spleen, or, even better, by inoculating a small amount of brain triturate.

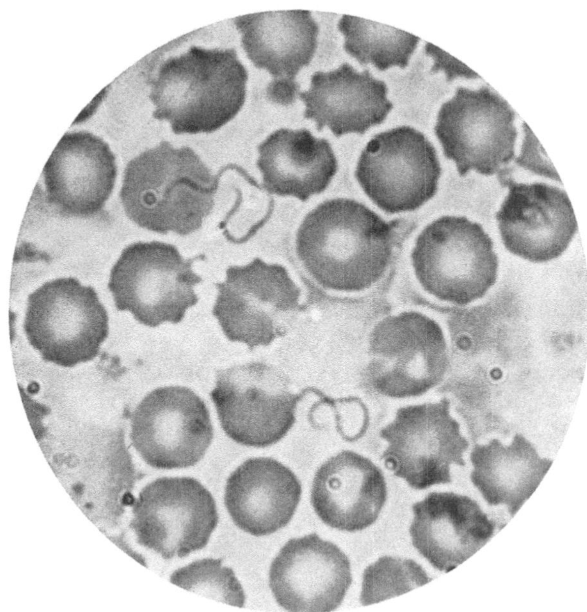

Fig. 3. Relapsing fever spirochaetas in a blood smear, from mouse. Giemsa stain. 2000×

II. Experimental Infection by Leptospira

A. Genus Leptospira Noguchi (1917)

The definition of this genus is the following, proposed by Taxonomic Sub-committee on Leptospira of the International Committee for the Bacterial Nomenclature: "Helicoidal organisms which may be a few microns to 40 microns or more in length, but usually 6 to 20 microns: and not much more than 0.1 micron in diameter. The coils measure about 0.2 to 0.3 microns in overall diameter and about 0.3 to 0.5 microns in wavelength. In liquid media both ends usually hooked; but in some strains only one end is hooked and in other strains the ends are straight and show no hooks. In the living state the organism is not visible with ordinary illumination; it is observed clearly by dark-field and much less clearly by phase-contrast microscopy; not readily stained by aniline dyes but can be demonstrated by silver-impregnation techniques. The structure of Leptospiras as revealed by electron microscopy consists of a protoplasmic cylinder bound by a limiting membrane and helicoidally wound round an axistyle. Both protoplasmic cylinder and axistyle are covered by a common external sheath. The axistyle is apparently a single structure about 0.01 to 0.02 microns in diameter which is inserted in the protoplasmic cylinder subterminally at each end; but there is purported evidence that the axistyle is comprised of two components (axial filaments) each inserted by one end at opposite extremities of the protoplasmic cylinder with their free ends overlapping in the middle region of the organism. There is no free flagellum or undulating membrane. In liquid media the characteristic movements are rapid rotation around the longitudinal axis and translation without polar differentiation; in semi-solid media flexion, vermiform and boring movements also occur. Can usually be grown in artificial media; oxygen is required. This genus includes forms which are parasitic in man and various animals (some forms are pathogenic), as well as free-living forms."

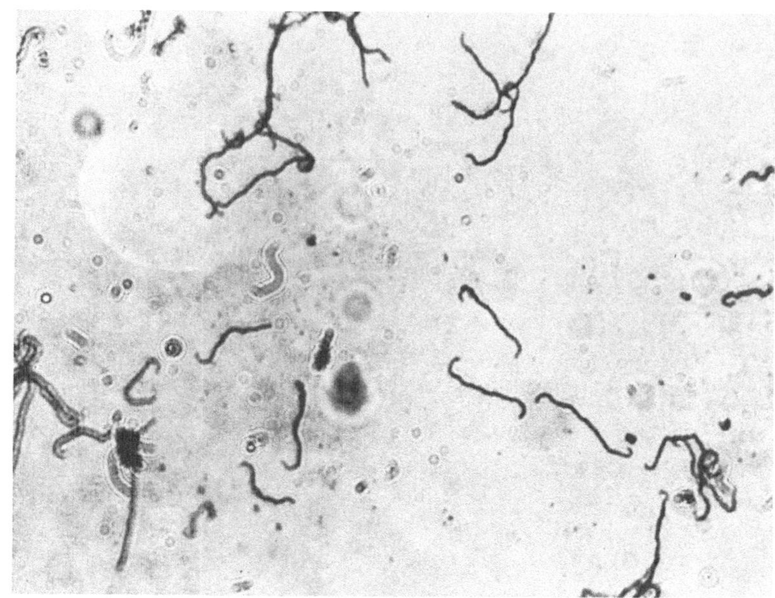

Fig. 4. Leptospira. Silver impregnation. 2000×

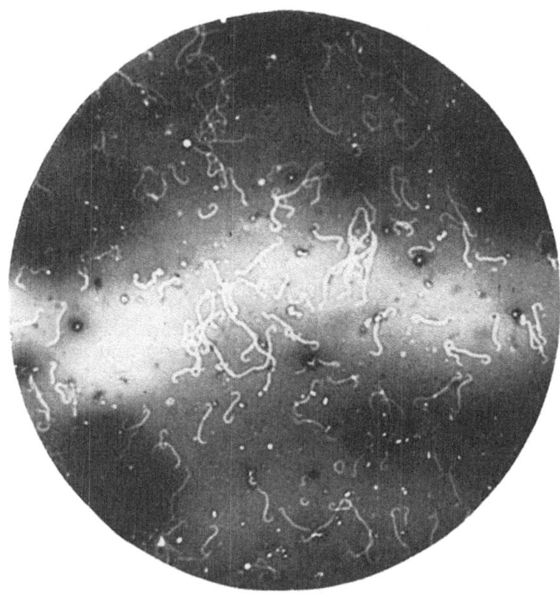

Fig. 5. Leptospira. Negative staining, Congo red. 1000×

The genus *Leptospira* comprehends a single species: *Leptospira interrogans*. Until a short time ago saprophytic leptospira were grouped under the name of species *Leptospira biflexa*, but at present it is believed that there should be no sufficiently reliable elements justifying the maintenance of this species, and we have preferred to group parasitic and saprophytic leptospiras into a single species.

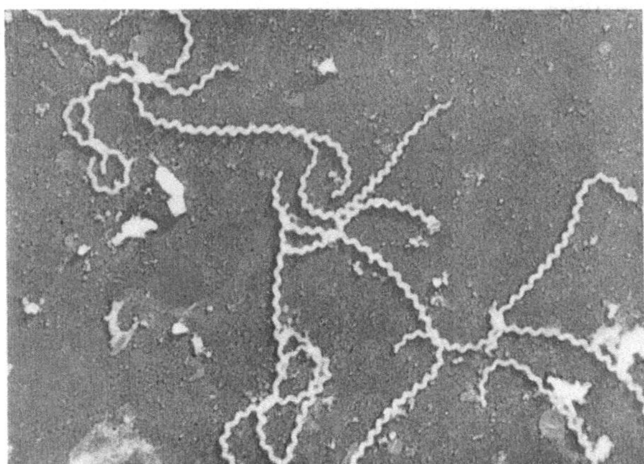

Fig. 6. Leptospira. Electron microscopy. 5000×

The name "biflexa", grouping all the saprophytic strains, is now considered as a "complex", without any taxonomic value.

Leptospiras are subdivided into serogroups, according to the serologic affinities shown by cross-agglutination tests, and in serotypes. The latter are the basic taxa and are represented by recommended type strains. As far as the definition of serotype is concerned, it is based on the antibodies cross-absorption test. More precisely, two strains are considered to belong to different serotypes if, after cross-absorption with adequate amounts of eterologous antigen, 10% or more of the homologous titre regularly remains in at least one of the two antisera in repeated tests. This definition is based on the use of antisera prepared in rabbits.

At present we recognize the following 16 serogroups of parasitic leptospiras and the following 120 serotypes (Report of a WHO Expert Group, 1967):

Serogroup: *icterohaemorrhagiae*
  Serotypes: icterohaemorrhagiae, copenhageni, mankarso, naam, mwgolo, dakota, sarmin, birkini, smithi, ndambari, ndahambukuje, budapest, weaveri, icteroides*
Serogroup: *javanica*
  Serotypes: javanica, poi, sorex-jalna, coxi, sofia
Serogroup: *celledoni*
  Serotypes: celledoni, whitcombi
Serogroup: *canicola*
  Serotypes: canicola, bafani, kamituga, jonsis, sumneri, broomi, bindjei, schueffneri, benjamin, malaya
Serogroup: *ballum*
  Serotypes: ballum, castellonis, arboreae*
Serogroup: *pyrogenes*
  Serotypes: pyrogenes, zanoni, myocastoris, abramis, biggis, hamptoni, alexi, robinsoni, manilae
Serogroup: *cynopteri*
  Serotypes: cynopteri, canalzonae, butembo
Serogroup: *autumnalis*
  Serotypes: autumnalis, rachmati, fort-bragg, sumatrana*, bulgarica, bangkinang, erinacei-auriti, mooris, sentot, louisiana, orleans, djasiman, gurungi

Serogroup: *australis*
  Serotypes: australis, lora, muenchen, jalna, bratislava, fugis, bangkok, peruviana*, pina*, nicaragua*
Serogroup: *pomona*
  Serotypes: pomona, monjakov, mozdok*, tropica, kennewicki*, proechimys*
Serogroup: *grippotyphosa*
  Serotypes: grippotyphosa
Serogroup: *hebdomadis*
  Serotypes: hebdomadis, nona, kambala, kremastos, worsfoldi, jules, maru, borincana, kabura, mini, szwajizak, georgia, parameles, hardjo, medanensis, wolffii, sejroe, balcanica, polonica, saxkoebing, nero, haemolytica, ricardi, recreo*, trinidad*
Serogroup: *bataviae*
  Serotypes: bataviae, paidjan, djatzi, kobbe, balboa, claytoni*, brasiliensis*
Serogroup: *tarassovi* (hyos)
  Serotypes: tarassovi (hyos), bakeri, guidae, atlantae, kisuba, bravo, atchafalaya, chagres*, rama*, gatuni*
Serogroup: *panama*
  Serotype: panama
Serogroup: *shermani**
  Serotype: shermani*

Many more serogroups and serotypes have been reported recently, but their validity has not yet been officially recognized.

They are listed here below:

Serogroup: *icterohaemorrhagiae*
  Serotypes: hualien, gem, monymusk, tonkini, bog-vere, waskurin
Serogroup: *javanica*
  Serotype: ceylonica
Serogroup: *canicola*
  Serotypes: kahendo, portland-vere
Serogroup: *pyrogenes*
  Serotypes: varela, cam-lo
Serogroup: *autumnalis*
  Serotypes: alice, weerasinghe
Serogroup: *australis*
  Serotype: hawain
Serogroup: *pomona*
  Serotype: cornelli
Serogroup: *grippo-typhosa*
  Serotypes: ratnapura, vanderhoedeni
Serogroup: *hebdomadis*
  Serotype: guaicurus
Serogroup: *bataviae*
  Serotype: los bonós
Serogroup: *tarassovi*
  Serotypes: vietnam, langati, darien, vu-ghia
Serogroup: *ranarum*
  Serotype: ranarum
Serogroup: *bufonis*
  Serotype: carlos

* Provisional classification pending further work.

B. Infection by Leptospira

All these serotypes are pathogenic for man and for several other mammals. The differences between the various serotypes are of antigenic in nature; there are also, however, at least in many of them, differences in virulence or in affinities to animal species.

The infection may be in some cases completely symptomless or oligo-symptomatic; in others, in contrast, it may have a serious course with fatal outcome.

Small rodents or insectivora are the most common carriers of leptospiras. However dogs, cattle and swine may also carry the spirochaeta.

Recently pathogenic leptospiras have been isolated also from Reptilia (FERRIS and Coll., 1961) and from Amphibians (DIESCH et al., 1966; BABU-DIERI, CARLOS and CARLOS, 1972).

The leptospira are excreted with the urine and may survive for some days if they come into water or damp ground, with a near-neutral pH.

Man and animals are generally infected by contact with water and mud contaminated in this way, more rarely by direct contact with the carriers.

1. Culture

Leptospiras are easily cultured in liquid media containing serum, e.g., rabbit serum.

The formulas of some of the more frequently used media are given below:

Korthof-Babudieri's medium (BABUDIERI and ZARDI, 1961)

To 1 liter of distilled water add:	
Peptone (possibly Witte)	0.800 g
Natrium chloratum	1.400 g
Natrium bicarbonate	0.020 g
Kalium chloratum	0.040 g
Kalium phosphoricum	0.180 g
Natrium phosphoricum bibasicum	
($Na_2HPO_4 \cdot 2\ H_2O$)	0.960 g
Nicotinic acid	0.001 g
After sterilization (half an hour at 120° C) add	
Vitamin B_{12}	0.001 g
Rabbit serum (haemolyzed)	50 ml
Sterilized separately by filtration	

After distribution in test tubes, add to each of them a little paraffin oil.

The test tubes containing the medium are heated twice, over a water bath at 56° C, each time for one hour.

Vervoort's medium, modified by WOLFF (WOLFF, 1954)

Dissolve 1 g of peptone Witte in one liter of distilled water and bring the solution to the boil.

Add Ringer's solution 200 ml and boil again

(NaCl	8.5 g	
KCl	0.2 g	
$CaCl_2$	0.2 g	
Na_2CO_3	0.01 g	distilled water 1 liter)

Add Sörensen's solution pH = 7.2 100 ml and boil

(KH$_2$PO$_4$	9.078 g per l	28 ml
Na$_2$KPO$_4$	12.28 g per l	72 ml)

Add phosphoric acid 1 N solution: 2 ml.

Boil this mixture for 5 minutes. The addition of phosphoric acid will give a better precipitate and a clearer solution after filtering.

After cooling, filter the solution through paper and heat for 30 minutes at 100° C.

Decant the solution into small sterile bottles or test tubes, 3 ml in each.

Heat the bottles or test tubes for 30 minutes at 100° C.

Add 0.3 ml rabbit serum with a trace of hemoglobin to each bottle or test tube.

Inactivate for 30 minutes over a water bath at 56° C.

Check sterility by placing the bottles or test tubes over-night in the incubator at 37° C.

Stuard's medium (Stuart, 1946)

m/10 d-asparagine	2 ml
m/10 NH$_4$Cl	10 ml
m/10 MgCl$_2$	4 ml
m/10 NaCl	66 ml
glycerol	1 ml
phenol-red (water solution)	10 ml
distilled water	91 ml

Heat the solution for 30 minutes at 100° C.

Add 16 ml of Sorensen's solution (pH = 7.6) sterilized separately

1/15 m KH$_2$PO$_4$	13 ml (9.078 g/l)
1/15 m Na$_2$HPO$_4$ · 2 H$_2$O	8 ml (11.876 g/l)

Heat the solution for one hour at 100° C.

Add 8–10% of rabbit-serum, sterilized by filtration.

Decant the medium into test tubes.

The previous liquid media may be turned into semi-solid ones by the addition of 0.25–0.65% of agar.

The cultures are incubated preferably at 30°, and a good development of leptospiras is generally obtained after 7–10 days.

Leptospiras can also be cultivated in solid media, but with greater difficulty, especially for some strains. In these media, leptospiras develop a little below the surface of the culture medium.

The formula of the Cox and Larson medium (1957) is given below:

Cox and Larson's medium.

0.2 g of tryptose phosphate or tryptose or neopeptone or proteose-peptone No. 3 (Difco) and 1 g agar (Difco) are dissolved in 90 ml distilled water: the pH is set at 7.5 and the solution is sterilized at 120° C for 30 minutes.

10 ml of sterile rabbit-serum and 1 ml of haemoglobin solution (I) are added to the solution after cooling.

The medium is heated over a water bath at 50° for 30 minutes and is decanted into Petri dishes.

(I) The haemoglobin solution is prepared by adding one part of sheep-blood red-cells to 20 parts of distilled water. The mixture is then centrifuged and filtered through a Seitz filter.

A liquid medium containing no rabbit serum, was proposed by ELLINGHAUSEN and McCULLOUGH (1965), for the culture of parasitic leptospiras. The rabbit serum was replaced either by an oleic-bovine albumin complex, or by polysorbate 80.

Oleic Albumin Complex (OAC) Medium (ELLINGHAUSEN and McCULLOUGH)

Substance	Concentration per liter
OAC (20% by volume)[a]	1% albumin
NH_4Cl	214.0 mg
$MgCl_2 \cdot 6_2HO$	152.0 mg
NaCl	1.54 g
KH_2PO_4	69.0 mg
Na_2HPO_4	531.0 mg
$ZnSO_4$	3.2 mg
$CuSO_4 \cdot 5\ H_2O$	2.4 mg
l-cystine	40 mg
Vitamin B_{12}	160 µg
Thiamine-HCl	160 µg

[a] Oleic Albumin Complex, Difco Laboratories, Detroit, Mich., essentially containing 5.0% solution of bovine albumin fraction V and 0.05% alkalinized oleic acid.

To 700 ml of distilled water was added 50 ml of a concentrated salt solution (NH_4Cl 5.35 g; $MgCl_2 \cdot 6H_2O$ 3.72 g and NaCl 38.5 g per liter) 40 ml of buffer solution (Na_2HPO_4 16.6 g; KH_2PO_4 2.172 g per liter), appropriate levels of the 3 trace metals and l-cystine. No attempt was made to achieve complete solution of the l-cystine; the medium was shaken then filtered, vitamin B_{12} and thiamine were added, and the volume was adjusted to 1.000 ml; sterilized for 15 minutes at 121° C and sterile OAC added after cooling.

Synthetic culture media have been proposed. However, these media do not support the growth of all leptospira strains and bring about a very rapid decline in the virulence of the cultures. For these reasons, these media are not suitable for the maintenance of leptospira strains to be used for experimental infection (STALHEIM, 1966).

There are some strains, especially those belonging to the serotype hardjo, which, if recently isolated, may be particularly difficult to culture (difficult strains). The addition of a few drops of guinea-pig blood to the medium, as well as the repeated transfers, may, however, permit a gradual adaptation of the strain to the medium.

All strains have the greatest virulence at the moment of isolation. When cultured in artificial media, they lose their virulence, more or less rapidly. This loss is often accompanied by a lengthening of the leptospira's bodies, by a decrease in their mobility and sometimes by a loss of the terminal hooks.

It must, however, be mentioned that even strains maintained in artificial culture for many years can transmit a serious disease in man, as has been shown by cases of accidental laboratory infection, or else they can kill young guinea-pigs when inoculated into them in high doses.

When the intention is to keep laboratory strains of leptospiras without any more or less complete loss of their virulence, low temperature may be employed. To obtain good results, it is necessary, according to RESSELER and VAN RIEL (1965) to go down to the temperature of liquid azote ($-195°$ C) and to freeze the leptospiras slowly. Thawing, in contrast, should be rapid. TARASEVICH et al. (1963)

have obtained some good results also with less low temperatures ($-78°$ and $-30°$ C).

It is also possible to use lyophilisation, protecting the leptospiras with the addition of 5–10% glycerol or dimethylsulfoxide (Resseler and van Riel, 1965). Results are not always satisfactory.

2. Isolation and Maintenance in Animals

Virulent leptospira strains may be isolated from carrier animals, both directly and indirectly.

Direct isolation is achieved by disseminating small fragments taken under sterile conditions from a carrier animal's kidney into test tubes containing a suitable medium. If in the animal an acute infection is in course, the leptospira may be isolated by inoculating a few drops of blood into the culture medium.

Indirect isolation is usually employed when the material is contaminated by bacteria, or when the carrier animal's sacrifice is to be avoided. The leptospira is usually isolated from urine in such cases.

For this purpose it is necessary to inoculate into a young guinea pig's peritoneum several ml of infectious urine. Five or six days later several drops of blood are drawn the guinea pig by intracardial punction and disseminated into the culture medium.

The best way of maintaining the virulence of a leptospira strain is to transmit it serially from one animal to the next, preferably using for this purpose young guinea pigs with a body weight of 170–250 g. It is advisable in this case to sacrifice the animal as soon as it shows evident signs of disease (loss of weight, ruffled fur, often a raised temperature) or, at latest, when jaundice begins to appear.

A piece of the animal's liver is taken, then triturated and suspended in a little broth or saline; after that it is inoculated into another young healthy guinea pig.

It is also possible to attain good results by alternating passage into a guinea pig with passage into a medium, keeping the spirochaetas in it for as much as one-two months between passage into one animal and another.

To restore the virulence of a strain already kept in culture for a long time, it is advisable to inoculate a strong dose of leptospiras into a young guinea pig's peritoneum, choosing a guinea pig weighing less than 200 g. The animal is to be sacrifice after 5 days, then a piece of liver is taken from it and triturated and inoculated into another guinea pig. This proceeding is to be repeated several times. It is not always possible, however, to restore the virulence of a leptospira which has lost its aggressiveness, by this procedure.

According to Bertok et al. (1964) it is possible to make albino rats more susceptible to infection with less virulent leptospira strains by administering ethiotine (0.4%) with the food.

The administration of cortisone does not remarkably modify the animal's resistence to the infection (Zardi, 1965).

3. Experimental Infection of Animals

Virulent leptospira strains belonging to different serotypes produce practically the same type of disease, varying only in severity, if at all.

Consequently, when we want to obtain in an animal an experimental leptospirosis, usually we have recourse to a virulent strain belonging to the serotype icterohaemorrhagiae or copenhageni, because these two serotypes, very like each other, and until a short time ago included in the single serotype "icterohaemorrhagiae", are particularly pathogenic and may be obtained quite easily by preparing cultures from kidneys of wild rats.

These leptospiras are in fact diffused everywhere and very frequently found in adult rats (*Epimys rattus* and *Epimys decumanus*) which are their usual carriers.

The animal of choice for experimental infection is the guinea pig, preferably with a body weight of 250 g. Inoculation is to be effected intracutaneously or peritoneally.

The first sign of disease is a fever, generally appearing after 3–4 days, and remaining high for a couple of days. This fever, however, may sometimes not appear, even in severe cases with fatal outcome. The animal loses weight, it looks sleepy, its fur is ruffled and, towards the 5th or 7th day, when the temperature falls, subicterus begins, which then develops into frank jaundice. In severe cases the animal dies on the 7th–10th day.

In milder cases the guinea pig may recover, but however it remains for some weeks carrier of leptospiras which it spreads in its urine.

Particularly virulent strains can kill the guinea pig in as little as 4–5 days, sometimes without icterus, but with diffused haemorrhage.

Other strains in contrast, especially those belonging to serotypes different from icterohaemorrhagiae and copenhageni, may kill the guinea pig after relatively long periods, even more than 30 days, as in the case of serotype pomona (BABUDIERI and BIANCHI, 1940).

The infection in monkey, mouse, rat and hamster, has a course very similar to the one described for guinea pig. Mice and rats, however, are more resistent than the other animals and succumb to the infection only rarely and when they are young (less than 4 weeks old) (LARSON, 1941; NICOLAIEW and ANANJIN, 1951). These small rodents, when infected exhibit no overt signs of disease but become carriers and remain such for a long time. Therefore they are suitable for the study of drugs or conditions which may affect the state of the carrier.

Infection is usually achieved by intraperitoneal inoculation, usually with the serotypes icterohaemorrhagiae and copenhageni.

The hamster is susceptible to the infection produced by these two leptospira serotypes, but the infection has a clinical course less typical than that in guinea pig.

The hamster is the most susceptible of all laboratory animals to infection by leptospiras belonging to serotype canicola (MORTON, 1942), which is, in contrast, scarcely pathogenic for guinea pig. Virulent strains, inoculated into the peritoneum, may kill this animal within 5–10 days, mostly with icterus and haemorrhagies.

The hamster is also more susceptible than the guinea pig to infections produced by serotype pomona and grippo-typhosa, especially if the strain has become adapted to this animal by repeated passages (HAMDY and FERGUSON, 1957; BAUER and MORSE, 1958; KMETY et al., 1967).

The adult rabbit is very resistant to leptospirosis and rarely shows signs of disease. Young rabbits about 14–20 days of age, however, are very receptive (WARFOLOMEEVA, 1960) to infection by serotype pomona, which almost always has a total outcome.

Other types of leptospiras may also cause severe and even fatal infections in young rabbits (WARFOLOMEEVA, 1960).

Dogs, especially pups, easily become acutely ill when infected with types icterohaemorrhagiae, copenhageni or canicola. When adults, the disease takes an often chronic course leading to severe kidney lesions, usually causing the animal's death.

Anatomo-pathologic lesions more evident in the animals dying of leptospiras are: diffused and intense icterus, particularly clearly visible on the skin, and only

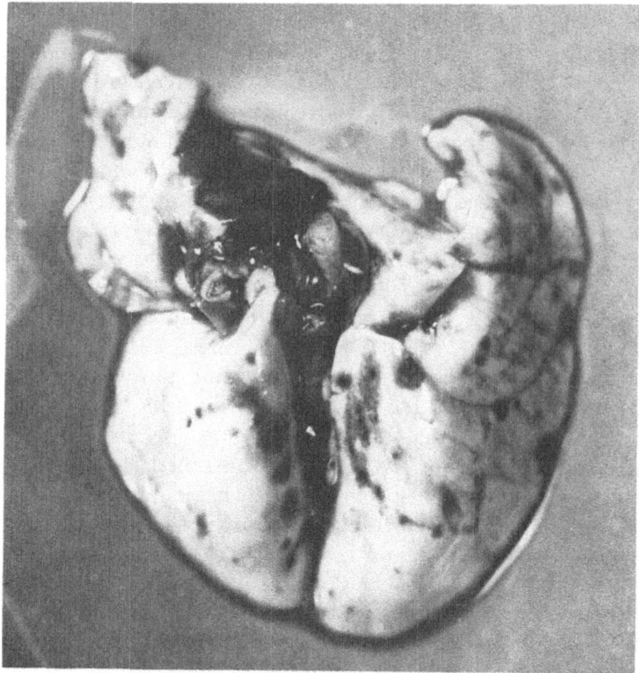

Fig. 7. Guinea-pig lungs in leptospirosis. "Butterfly's wing" aspect

rarely absent, and haemorrhages, usually slight and disseminated. They are most marked under the skin, peritoneum, pericardium and pleura and in the lymphatic glands, brain, kidneys and gastro-intestinal tract. The adrenal glands are often completely haemorrhagic.

Haemorrhages take a very characteristic aspect in the lungs. Here they have different dimensions, often extensive, more or less numerous. On the surface of the organ they assume a roundish shape, with very well-limited margins, so that the lung, disseminated with these roundish dark-red spots on a rosy background, assumes the so called "butterfly's wing" appearance, which permits diagnosis of leptospirosis even in cases where icterus is absent.

The liver does not show any very evident macroscopic lesions; the kidneys are somewhat enlarged; the spleen is enlarged and diffluent.

The most evident and frequent macroscopic lesions apart from those constituted by haemorrhages or depending on those, are:

In the liver we observe at the beginning a serious inflammation with the Disse's spaces filled with sero-sanguineous exudate (Ostertag, 1950). Then comes a dissociation of the cord structure with separation of the hepatic cells when necrotic areas are present around the central veins. Small foci of infiltration of polymorphs and round cells are present, sometimes near the smaller bile ducts. The liver cells may show varying degrees of cloudy swelling. Mitotic figures are not uncommon. The cells around the hepatic veins usually contain large amounts of bile pigment.

The severity of hepatic lesions varies widely from case to case, even if only fatal cases are considered.

In the kidney, in which an interstitial oedema is observed, the main damage is confined to the cells of the tubules, particularly to the epithelium of the convoluted tubules.

The tubules are often dilated and the epithelial cells show changes varying from cloudy swelling to complete necrosis with desquamation of cells into the lumen of the tubules. The tubules are often filled with blood-cells and granular and hematic cylinders.

Haemorrhages, and areas of infiltration of mononuclear cells are scattered in the kidney.

The necrosis of the kidney tubules brings about uremia which is usually fatal.

Lesions of the myocardium and of the voluntary muscles, affecting either single muscle fibres or small groups of adjacent fibres, have also been reported (BEITZKE, 1916; ASHE et al., 1941).

The spleen contains focal haemorrhages into the pulp and a large number of fragmented red-blood cells, many of them undergoing phagocytosis.

Altogether the histological lesions caused by leptospirosis are toxic in nature, but their pathogenesis remains very obscure.

It has never been possible, in fact, to observe in leptospiras or in the culture medium where they develop, a real toxin which might be held responsible for the alterations peculiar to the disease.

Besides, it has been observed that the administration of antibiotics highly active on leptospiras, such as penicillin, does not usually arrest the evolution of the infection, unless it has been effected very early (AUSTONI, 1962, 1966).

These facts led (AREAN, 1964; BABUDIERI, 1966) to suggest that leptospiras, though not in themselves producers of toxins, may cause a sort of chain reaction, with production and release of toxic substances from the cells of the organism invaded. Something of this kind has already been observed in the infection caused by anthrax bacillus (SMITH, 1958, 1960).

Even if this is still to be considered a mere hypothesis, it is necessary, however, to bear the facts in mind, especially in studies on the effectivity of leptospirolytic drugs in animals experimentally infected.

4. Confirmation of Infection by Leptospiras

Infection by leptospiras can be confirmed by haemoculture in the first 5 or 6 days of the infection in animals which are to be kept alive and then by kidney culture. One can also inoculate the suspect material into the guinea pig and start a haemoculture from this after 5 days, bearing in mind that leptospirosis is not always fatal in this animal.

A direct search for leptospira in the blood does not usually yield any concrete result; in contrast positive results may be obtained in a triturate of infected tissues or in urine. The best method in these cases is direct examination of the material under dark-field microscope.

If the leptospiras are scarce, it is also possible to apply the direct or indirect immunofluorescence technique (MOULTON and HOWARD, 1957; COFFIN and MAESTRONE, 1962, 1953; SHELDON, 1953; WHITE and RISTIC, 1959; etc.).

Staining the leptospiras with Giemsa is not very satisfactory. It is preferable, whenever stainings are required, to use Fontana-Tribondeau's method (see page 16), or another method of silver impregnation to test for leptospiras in tissues.

Another effective method of confirming an infection is by testing for agglutinating antibodies which may occur in animal serum. These are specific for the serotype

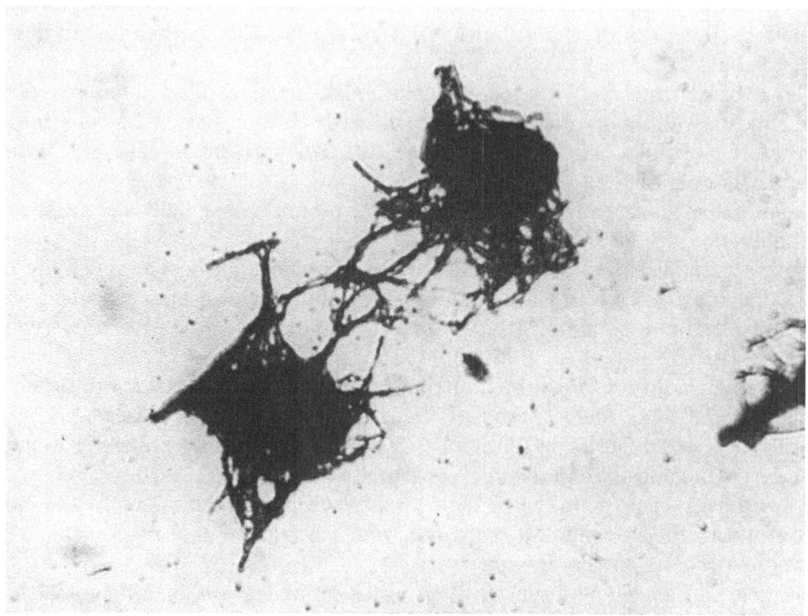

Fig. 8. Agglutinated leptospiras. Silver impregnation. 2000×

and, partially, for the serogroup; they appear 7–10 days after infection and may reach very high levels.

The agglutination test is effected by exposing serial dilutions of serum to an antigen preferably constituted by a culture of living leptospiras, or, if this is not desiderable by a recently-prepared suspension of leptospiras killed with formol. The reading of the agglutination is taken on a mixture drop, under dark-field microscope (Wolff, 1954; Babudieri, 1959).

Many parasitic leptospira serotypes produce enzymes acting on the phospholipids membranes of the red-blood cells, causing haemolysis (Addamiano and Kasarov, 1969).

A cross neutralization was observed between haemolysins from different serotypes both in vitro and in vivo (Kazar and Chorvath, 1962; Alexander et al., 1971). Nevertheless some pathogenic serotypes do not produce haemolysins, and conversely, some saprophytic serotypes do.

The complement fixation test may also be successfully used. It is advisable to use a suspension of leptospiras kept at 100° C for 15 minutes as the antigen (Terzin, 1956).

5. Laboratory Infections

The risk of an accidental infection should not be neglected, during any work with pathogenic leptospira strains or with infectious carrier animals, especially since leptospiras can pass through healthy mucous membranes and perhaps even through skin. It should also be pointed out that even strains almost completely harmless for the guinea pig may be remarkably virulent for man (Van Thiel, 1936). Thus, it is advisable to adopt every possible precaution and to wear gloves whenever possible.

It must be borne in mind that leptospiras are very delicate microorganisms, that they do not resist to drying and are rapidly killed by any kind of disinfectant.

When infection is suspected, it is advisable to take high dosed of an effective antibiotic, such as penicillin for some days, even though this does not always prevent the disease (BROOM and NORRIS, 1957).

We have also observed good results following the administration (BABUDIERI, 1964) of high doses of specific antileptospira gammaglobulins (WARFOLOMEEVA, 1960, 1964).

References

ADDAMIANO, L., BABUDIERI, B.: Research on spirochaetal strains isolated in Jordan. Bull. Wld Hlth Org. 17, 483–485 (1957).

ADDAMIANO, L., KASAROV, L. B.: Metabolism of the lipoproteins of serum by leptospiras: degradation of the triglycerides. J. med. Microbiol. 2, 165–168 (1969a).

ADDAMIANO, L., KASAROV, L. B.: Degradation of the phospholipids of the serum lipoproteins by Leptospirae. J. med. Microbiol. 3, 243–248 (1969b).

ALEXANDER, A. D., WOOD, G., YANCEY, F., BYRNE, R. J., YAGER, R. H.: Cross neutralization of leptospiral haemolysins from different serotypes. Infect. a. Immun. 4, 154–159 (1971).

AREAN, V. M.: Toxin production by Leptospira icterohaemorrhagiae. Am. J. vet. Res. 25, 836–843 (1964).

ASHE, W. F., PRATT THOMAS, H. R., KUMPE, C. W.: Weil's disease: a complete review of american literature and an abstract of world literature. Medicine (Baltimore) 20, 145–210 (1941).

AUSTONI, M.: Problemi attuali in tema di terapia della leptospirosi. Rass. Clin. Ter. 61, 191–207 (1962).

AUSTONI, M.: Therapie der Leptospirosen des Menschen. In: Leptospiren und Leptospirosen; Infektionskrankheiten und ihre Erreger, Bd. 1, S. I, 68–77. Jena: G. Fischer 1966.

BABUDIERI, B.: Proposta di una nuova sistematica dell'ordine delle Spirochaetales. Atti VI. Congr. Internaz. Microbiol. Roma 5, 46–50 (1954).

BABUDIERI, B.: Laboratory diagnosis of leptospirosis. Bull. Wld Hlth Org. 24, 45–58 (1959).

BABUDIERI, B.: Discussions. In: II. Symp. Leptospirae and Leptospirosis in man and animals, Lublin. Pol. Akad. Nauk, Warszawa, 463 (1964).

BABUDIERI, B.: Moderne metodiche per la diagnostica delle leptospirosi. II. Simp. Naz. delle Leptospirosi, Messina 1965. Ann. Sclavo 8, 473–478 (1966).

BABUDIERI, B., BIANCHI, L.: Untersuchungen über ein epidemisches Vorkommen der Reisfelderleptospirosis in der Provinz Pavia. Z. Immun.Forsch. 98, 37–75 (1940).

BABUDIERI, B., BOCCIARELLI, D.: Ricerche di microscopia elettronica. II. Studio morfologico del genere Spironema. R. C. Ist. sup. Sanità 6, 305–314 (1943).

BABUDIERI, B., BOCCIARELLI, D.: Electron microscope studies on relapsing-fever Spirochaetes. J. Hyg. (Lond.) 46, 438–439 (1948).

BABUDIERI, B., CARLOS, E. R., CARLOS, E. T., Jr.: Pathogenic Leptospira isolated from Toad kidneys. In press. (Geogr. a. Trop. Med.)

BABUDIERI, B., ZARDI, O.: Studies on the metabolism of Leptospirae. I. Vitamin B_{12} as a growth factor. Z. Vitamin-, Hormon- u. Fermentforsch. 4, 299–309 (1961).

BAERMANN, G., HALBERSTADTER: Experimentelle Versuche über Framboesia tropica in Affen. Geneesk Tijdschr. Ned.-Ind. 40, 181 (1906).

BALFOUR, A.: Trans. XVII. Int. Congr. Med., London, Sect. 21, Part 2, 275 (1914), quoted by HINLE, E. (1931).

BAUER, D. C., MORSE, E. V.: Variation and hemolysin production in relation to virulence of L. pomona. Proc. Soc. exp. Biol. (N.Y.) 98, 505–508 (1958).

BEARDMORE, W. B., DODD, M. C.: The growth of the Reiter strain of T. pallidum in the chick embryo. J. Bact. 60, 5–7 (1950).

BECLERE, A.: Transmission expérimentale de la syphilis à l'espèce bovine. Ann. Inst. Pasteur 53, 23–42 (1934).

BEITZKE, H.: Über die pathologische Anatomie der ansteckenden Gelbsucht. Berl. klin. Wschr. 1, 188–199 (1916).

BERGEY's Manual of determinative bacteriology, VIII. ed., Baltimore: Williams & Wilkins Co. 1957.

BERLINGHOFF, W.: Die experimentelle Syphilis der weißen Maus. Derm. Wschr. 136, 929–931 (1957).

Bertarelli, E.: Sulla trasmissione della sifilide al coniglio. Riv. Igiene e San. Pubbl. **57**, 646–660 (1906); Zbl. Bakt., I. Abt. Orig. **41**, 320–326 (1906).

Bertarelli, E.: Über die Empfänglichkeit der Fleischfresser (Hund) und der Wiederkäuer für experimentelle Syphilis. Zbl. Bakt., I. Abt. Orig. **43**, 790–793 (1907).

Bertok, L., Kemenes, F., Simon, G.: Fatal leptospirosis icterohaemorrhagica induced by ethionine in albino rats. J. Path. Bact. **88**, 329–331 (1964).

Bessemans, A., Baert, H.: Réceptivité du furet à l'inoculation expérimentale de divers tréponèmes: palldoïdose inapparente chez la souris blanche. Rev. Belge Path. **25**, 488 (1956).

Bessemans, A., Geest, B. de: Essais de culture "in vitro" du Tréponème pâle en symbiose avec du tissu testiculaire de lapin. Rev. Belge Sci. méd. **6**, 28–36 (1934).

Bessemans, A., Haequaert, R.: Quoted by Bessemans, A. Urol. cutan Rev. **34**, 71–91 (1930).

Bessemans, A., Meirsman, E. de: Tentatives de culture de *Treponema pallidum* sur ia membrane chorioallantoïdienne de l'embryon de poulet vivant. C. R. Soc. Biol. (Paris) **127**, 847–848 (1938).

Bessemans, A., Potter, F. de: Manifestation syphilitique primaire et transmissible chez la souris blanche. Syphilis apparente et inapparente. C. R. Soc. Biol. (Paris) **104**, 818–820 (1930).

Bessemans, A., Potter, F. de: Note complémentaire sur la syphilis apparente de la souris. C. R. Soc. Biol. (Paris) **107**, 279–282 (1931).

Bessemans, A., Wilde, H. de, Thielen, E. van: Syphilis inapparente du Macaque et résistance à la pallidoïdose. C. R. Soc. Biol. (Paris) **129**, 373–376 (1938).

Bosselut, R.: Sur un spirochaete sanguicole du chien domestique. Bull. Soc. Path. exot. **18**, 702–704 (1925).

Breinl, A., Kinghorn, A.: An experimental study of the parasite of the african tick-fever. Mem. L.pool Sch. Trop. Med. **21** (1906).

Broom, J. C., Norris, T. St. M.: Failure of prophylactic oral penicillin to inhibit a human laboratory case of leptospirosis. Lancet **1957 I**, 721–722.

Brown, W. H., Pearce, L.: Experimental syphilis in the rabbit. I. Primary infection in the testicle. J. exp. Med. **31**, 475–498 (1920a).

Brown, W. H., Pearce, L.: Experimental syphilis in the rabbit. II. Primary infection in the scrotum. Part I. Reaction to infection. J. exp. Med. **31**, 709–727 (1920b).

Brown, W. H., Pearce, L.: Experimental syphilis in the rabbit. II. Primary infection in the scrotum. Part 2. Scrotal lesions and the character of the scrotal infection. J. exp. Med. **31**, 729–748 (1920c).

Brown, W. H., Pearce, L.: Experimental syphilis in the rabbit. III. Local dissemination, local recurrence, and involvement of regional lymphatics. J. exp. Med. **31**, 749–764 (1920d).

Brown, W. H., Pearce, L.: Experimental syphilis in the rabbit. IV. Cutaneous syphilis. Part I. Affections of the skin and appendages. J. exp. Med. **32**, 445–471 (1920e).

Brown, W. H., Pearce, L.: Experimental syphilis in the rabbit. IV. Cutaneous syphilis. Part 2. Clinical aspects of cutaneous syphilis. J. exp. Med. **32**, 473–495 (1920f).

Brown, W. H., Pearce, L.: Experimental syphilis in the rabbit. V. Syphilitic affections of the mucous membranes and mucocutaneous borders. J. exp. Med. **32**, 497–512 (1920g).

Brown, W. H., Pearce, L.: A note on the dissemination of *Spirochaeta pallida* from the primary focus of infection. Arch. Derm. Syph. (Chic.) **2**, 470–472 (1920h).

Brown, W. H., Pearce, L.: Note on the preservation of stock strains of *Treponema pallidum* and on the demonstration of infection in rabbits. J. exp. Med. **34**, 185–188 (1921a).

Brown, W. H., Pearce, L.: Experimental syphilis in the rabbit. VII. Affections of the eyes. J. exp. Med. **34**, 167–181 (1921b).

Brown, W. H., Pearce, L.: Latent infections, with the demonstration of *Spirochaeta pallida* in lymphoid tissues of the rabbit. Amer. J. Syph. **5**, 1–8 (1921c).

Brown, W. H., Pearce, L.: The influence of light on the reaction to infection in experimental syphilis. J. exp. Med. **45**, 497–518 (1927).

Brown, W. H., Pearce, L., Allen, C. M. van: Solar energy. The animal organism and susceptibility to disease. Trans. Ass. Amer. Physics **39**, 251–355 (1924).

Brown, W. H., Pearce, L., Witherbee, W. D.: Experimental syphilis in the rabbit. VI. Affections of bone, cartilage, tendons and synovial membranes. Part 1. Lesions of the skeletal system. J. exp. Med. **33**, 495–514 (1921a).

Brown, W. H., Pearce, L., Witherbee, W. D.: Experimental syphilis in the rabbit. VI. Affections of bone, cartilage, tendons and synovial membranes. Part 2. Clinical aspects of the skeletal system. Affections of the facial and cranial bones and the bones of the forearm. J. exp. Med. **33**, 512–523 (1921b).

Buchanan, R. E.: Studies on the classification and nomenclature of the bacteria. X. Subgroups and genera of the mixobacteriales and spirochaetales. J. Bact. **3**, 541–545 (1918).

Bykowa, O.: Über die Veränderung einiger blutbildender Organe bei Typhus recurrens. Virchows Arch. path. Anat. **260**, 169–175 (1926).

CALLAWAY, J. L., SHARP, J.: Cultivation of *Spirochaeta pallida* on the chorioallantoic membrane of the developing hen egg. J. Lab. clin. Med. **27**, 232–234 (1941).

CASTELLANI, A.: On the presence of spirochaetes in two cases of ulcerated parangi (yaws). Brit. med. J. **1905** II, 1280.

CASTELLANI, A., CHALMERS, A. J.: Manual of tropical medicine, 1st ed. London: Baillière, Tindall & Cox 1910.

CHESNEY, A. M.: The influence of the factors of sex, age and method of inoculation upon the course of experimental syphilis in the rabbit. J. exp. Med. **38**, 627–643 (1923).

CHESNEY, A. M., KEMP, J. E.: Studies in experimental syphilis. I. The influence of the size of the inoculum on the course of experimental syphilis in the rabbit. J. exp. Med. **41**, 479 (1925).

CHESNEY, A. M., SCHIPPER, G. J.: The effect of the method of inoculation upon the course of experimental syphilis in the rabbit. Amer. J. Syph. **34**, 18–24 (1950).

COFFEY, E. M., EVELAND, W. C.: Experimental relapsing fever initiated by *Borrelia hermsi*. I. Identification of major serotypes by immunofluorescence. J. infect. Dis. **117**, 20 (1967).

COFFIN, D. L., MAESTRONE, D.: Detection of leptospirae by fluorescent antibody. Amer. J. vet. Res. **23**, 159–164 (1962).

COLES, A. C.: Blood parasites found in mammals, birds and fishes in England. Parasitology **7**, 17–61 (1914).

COX, C. D., LARSON, A. D.: Colonial growth of Leptospirae. J. Bact. **73**, 587–589 (1957).

DE LAMATER, E. D.: A study of the life-cycle of spirochaetes and other microorganisms by means of phase contrast and routine microscopy. Trans. N.Y. Acad. Sci. **14**, 199–201 (1952).

DE LAMATER, E. D., NEWCOMER, V. D., HAANES, M., WIGGALL, R. H.: Studies on the life-cycle of spirochaetes. I. The use of phase contrast microscopy. Amer. J. Syph. **34**, 122–125 (1950).

DIESCH, S. L., McCULLOCH, W. F., BRAUN, J. L., ELLINGHAUSEN, H. C., JR.: Leptospires isolated from frog kidneys. Nature (Lond.) **209**, 939 (1966).

DODD, S.: A preliminary note on the identity of the *Spirochaeta* found in the horse, ox and sheep. J. comp. Path. **19**, 318–322 (1906).

EAGLE, H., GERMUTH, F. G.: Serologic relationships between five cultured strains of supposed *T. pallidum* (Noguchi, Kroó, Nichols, Reiter and Kazan) and two strains of mouth treponemata. J. Immunol. **60**, 223–239 (1948).

ELLINGHAUSEN, H. C., JR., McCULLOUGH, W. G.: Nutrition of *Leptospira pomona* and growth of 13 other serotypes: A serum-free medium employing oleic albumin complex. Amer. J. vet. Res. **26**, 39–44 (1965 a).

ELLINGHAUSEN, H. C., JR., McCULLOUGH, W. G.: Nutrition of *Leptospira pomona* and growth of 13 other serotypes: Fractionation of oleic albumin complex and a medium of bovine albumin and polysorbate 80. Amer. J. vet. Res. **26**, 45 (1965b).

FERRIS, D. H., RHOADES, H. E., HANSEN, L. E., GALTON, M., MANSFIELD, M. E.: Research into the nidality of *Leptospira Ballum* in campestral hosts, including the Hog-nosed Snake (*Heterodon platyrhinys*). Cornell Vet. **51**, 405 (1961).

FERRIS, H. W., TURNER, T. B.: Comparative histology of yaws and syphilis in Jamaica. Arch. Path. **24**, 707–737 (1937).

FERRIS, H. W., TURNER, T. B.: Comparison of cutaneous lesions produced in rabbits by intracutaneous inoculation of spirochaetes from yaws and syphilis. Arch. Path. **26**, 491–500 (1938).

FOLDVARI, F.: The conduct of the *Spirochaeta pallida* in tissue explantations. Amer. J. Syph. **16**, 145–154 (1932).

FRAZIER, C. N., BENSEL, A., KEUPER, C. S.: Phenomena of disease in rabbits fed cholesterol and inoculated with *Treponema pallidum*. II. Infectivity of blood. Amer. J. Syph. **34**, 453–459 (1950).

FRAZIER, C. N., BENSEL, A., KEUPER, C. S.: Further observations on the duration of spirochaetemia in rabbits with asymptomatic syphilis. Amer. J. Syph. **36**, 167–173 (1952).

GAMMEL, J. A., ECKER, E. E.: The virulence of *Spirochaeta pallida* in culture. Arch. Derm. Syph. (Chic.) **23**, 439–444 (1931).

GASTINEL, P., COLLART, P., DUNOYER, F.: Étude sur le comportement du tréponème de Reiter en milieu penicilliné. Ann. Inst. Pasteur **96**, 381–401 (1959).

GINGER, C. D., KATZ, F. E.: Separation of relapsing fever spirochaetes from blood by DEAE cellulose anion exchanger. Trans. roy. Soc. trop. Med. Hyg. **64**, 700 (1970).

GONDER, R.: Studien über die Spirochaete aus dem Blute von *Vesperugo Kulii*. Arb. Gesundh.-Amt Berlin **27**, 406–413 (1908).

GRAETZ, F., DELBANCO, E.: Beiträge zum Studium der Histopathologie der experimentellen Kaninchensyphilis. Med. Klin. **10**, 375, 420 (1914).

GRAETZ, F., DELBANCO, E.: Weitere Beiträge zum Studium der Histopathologie der experimentellen Kaninchensyphilis. Derm. Wschr. **58**, 6–28 (1914).

Gregoriew, P. S., Jarisheva, K. G.: The histologic structure of syphilitic lesions of rabbits. Amer. J. Syph. **12**, 67–81 (1928).

Haagen, E., Schlossberger, H.: Über das Verhalten von Spirochäten in der Gewebekultur. 1st Intern. Congr. Microbiol. Rep. **2**, 105, Paris (1930).

Haensell, P.: Vorläufige Mitteilung über Versuche von Impfsyphilis der Iris und Cornea des Kaninchenauges. Albrecht v. Graefes Arch. Ophthal. **27**, 93–100 (1881).

Hallauer, C., Kuhn, H.: Dauerpassagen von *Leptospira icterogenes* und *Spirochaeta pallida* (Truffi) im Hühnerembryo. Z. Hyg. Infekt.-Kr. **124**, 125–130 (1942).

Hamdy, A. H., Ferguson, L. C.: Virulence of *Leptospira pomona* in hamsters and cattle. Amer. J. vet. Res. **18**, 35 (1957).

Hardy, P. M., Nell, E. E.: Specific agglutination of *Treponema pallidum* by sera from rabbits and human beings with treponemal infection. J. exp. Med. **101**, 367–382 (1955).

Hindle, E.: Blood spirochaetes. In: A system of bacteriology in relation to medicine, vol. 8, p. 147–184. London: Med. Res. Council 1931.

Hoffmann, E., Bruning, W.: Gelungene Übertragung der Syphilis auf Hunde. Dtsch. med. Wschr. **33**, 553 (1907).

Hollander, D. H., Nell, E. E.: Improved preservation of *T. pallidum* and other bacteria by freezing with glycerol. Appl. Microbiol. **2**, 164–170 (1954).

Hollander, D. H., Turner, T. B.: The role of temperature in experimental syphilis infection. Amer. J. Syph. **38**, 489–505 (1954).

Jordan, E. O., Burrows, W.: The spirochetes. In: Textbook of bacteriology, 14th ed., p. 671–699. Philadelphia: W. B. Saunders 1945.

Kakishita, Saito: *Spirochaeta pallida*. J. infect. Dis. **19**, 138 (1930).

Kast, C. C., Kolmer, J. A.: On the cultivation of *Spirochaeta pallida* in living tissue media. Amer. J. Syph. **17**, 529–532 (1933).

Kast, C. C., Kolmer, J. A.: One successful cultivation of *Spirochaeta pallida* from syphilitic chancre of the rabbit. Amer. J. Syph. **17**, 533–538 (1933).

Kast, C. C., Kolmer, J. A.: Methods for the isolation and cultivation of treponemes, with special reference to culture media. Amer. J. Syph. **24**, 671–683 (1940).

Kast, C. C., Kolmer, J. A.: A note on the cultivation of *Treponema pallidum* with the preservation of virulence. Amer. J. Syph. **27**, 309–313 (1943).

Kato, N.: Lues 7, 71 (Quoted by Matsumoto, S., 1942).

Kazar, J., Chorvath, B.: Prisperok k studin antigennej struktury hemolyzinie leptospir. Czech. Epidemiol. Microbiol. Immunobiol. **11**, 353 (1962).

Klarenbeek, A.: Recherches expérimentales avec un spirochète se trouvant spontanément chez le lapin et ressemblant au *T. pallidum*. Ann. Inst. Pasteur **35**, 326–331 (1921).

Klarenbeek, A.: Infection oculaire expérimentale du lapin par le *Spirochaeta cuniculi*. Ann. Inst. Pasteur **44**, 201–207 (1930).

Kmety, E., Plesko, I., Bakoss, P.: Leptospirosen im Tierexperiment. In: Leptospiren und Leptospirosen; Infektionskrankheiten und ihre Erreger, Bd. 1, S. I, 426–454. Jena: G. Fischer 1966.

Kolle, W., Evers, E.: Experimentelle Untersuchungen über Syphilis- und Recurrens-Spirochaetose. III. Experimentelles über Syphilisinfektion ohne Symptome. Dtsch. med. Wschr. **52**, 557–559 (1926).

Kolle, W., Schlossberger, H.: Experimentelle Studien über Syphilis- und Recurrens-Spirochaetose. V. Über symptomlose Infektion von Mäusen und Ratten, sowie symptomlose Superinfektionen syphilitischer Kaninchen mit *Spirochaeta pallida*. Dtsch. med. Wschr. **52**, 1245–1247 (1926).

Lapidari, M., Sparrow, H.: Sur la culture des spirochètes des fièvres récurrentes. Arch. Inst. Pasteur Tunis **17**, 191–205 (1928).

Larson, C. L.: Susceptibility of young mice (*Mus musculus*) to *L. icterohaemorrhagiae*. Publ. Hlth Rep. (Wash.) **56**, 1546–1556 (1941).

Laveran, A.: Sur la spirillose de bovide. C. R. Acad. Sci. (Paris) **136**, 939–941 (1903).

Leishman, W. B.: Observations on the mechanism of infection in tick fever and on hereditary transmission of *Spirochaeta duttoni* in the tick. Trans. roy. Soc. trop. Med. Hyg. **3**, 77–106 (1910).

Leishman, W. B.: A note on the "granula clumps" found in African relapsing fever (tick fever). Ann. Inst. Pasteur **32**, 49 (1918).

Leony Blanco, F., Oteiza, A.: Sobre la transmisión experimental de la pinta, mal del pinto o carate al conejo. Rev. méd.-soc. Sanid. **4**, 11–15 (1944).

Leony Blanco, F., Oteiza, A.: The experimental transmission of pinta, mal del pinto or carate, to the rabbit. Science **101**, 309–311 (1945).

Levaditi, C., Anderson, T. E.: Neurotropisme du *Sp. duttoni*. C. R. Acad. Sci. (Paris) **186**, 653 (1928).

LEVADITI, C., ANDERSON, T. E.: L'état du virus de la fièvre récurrente (*Spirochaeta duttoni*) dans l'encèphale de la souris. C. R. Soc. Biol. (Paris) **100**, 1121–1123 (1929).

LEVADITI, C., MARIE, A., ISAICU, L.: Recherches sur la spirochétose spontanée du lapin. C. R. Soc. Biol. (Paris) **85**, 51–54 (1921).

LEVADITI, C., MARIE, A., NICOLAU, S.: Virulence pour l'homme du spirochète de la spirillose spontanée du lapin. C. R. Acad. Sci. (Paris) **172**, 1542–1543 (1921).

LEVADITI, C., VAISMAN, A., SCHOEN, R.: L'état ou se trouve le virus syphilitique dans la névraxe des souris syphilisées, par voie sous-cutanée. C. R. Soc. Biol. (Paris) **112**, 1669–1672 (1933).

LEVADITI, C., YAMANOUCHI, T.: La transmission de la syphilis au chat. C. R. Acad. Sci. (Paris) **146**, 1120–1122 (1908).

LISTGARTEN, M. A., SOCRANSKY, S. S.: Electron microscopy of axial fibrils, outer envelope and cell division of certain oral spirochaetes. J. Bact. **88**, 1087 (1964).

LOGAN, L. C., COX, P. M.: Automated qualitative and quantitative micro-hemoagglutination assay for *Treponema pallidum* antibodies (AMHA-Tp). Provisional technique, modified October 20, 1970. Amer. J. clin. Path. **53**, 163 (1970).

MAGNUSON, H. J., EAGLE, H., FLEISHMAN, R.: The minimal infectious inoculum of *Spirochaeta pallida* (Nichols strain) and a consideration of its rate of multiplication "in vivo". Amer. J. Syph. **32**, 1–18 (1948).

MAGNUSON, H. J., ROSENAU, B. J., GREENBERG, B. C.: The effects of sex, castration and testosterone upon the susceptibility of rabbits to experimental syphilis. Amer. J. Syph. **35**, 146–163 (1951).

MARCHOUX, E., SALIMBENI, A.: La spirillose des poules. Ann. Inst. Pasteur **17**, 569–580 (1903).

MASON, H. C.: Avirulence of cultured *Spirochaeta pallida*. Urol. cutan. Rev. **43**, 733–736 (1939).

MATHIS, C., LEGER, M.: Spirochète du lapin. C. R. Soc. Biol. (Paris) **70**, 212–214 (1919).

MATSUMOTO, S.: Experimental syphilis and framboesia with special reference to the comparative pathology and immunity. Monographiae Actorum Dermatologicorum, Series B, Syphilidologica N° 3, Imperial University, Kyoto (1930).

MATSUMOTO, S.: Experimentelle Syphilis und Framboesia, insbesondere die Frage ihrer Identität oder Dualität. Monographiae Actorum Dermatologicorum, Series B, Syphilidologica N° 10, Imperial University, Kyoto (1942).

McLEOD, C. P., ARNOLD, R. C.: A comparison of two methods of gland transfer in experimental syphilis. J. vener. Dis. Inform. **32**, 96–99 (1951).

McLEOD, C. P., TURNER, T. B.: Studies on the biologic relationship between the causative agents of syphilis, yaws and venereal spirochaetosis of rabbits. I. Observations on *Treponema cuniculi* infection in rabbits. Amer. J. Syph. **30**, 442–454 (1946a).

McLEOD, C. P., TURNER, T. B.: Studies on the biologic relationship between the causative agents of syphilis, yaws and venereal spirochaetosis of rabbits. II. Comparison of the experimental disease produced in rabbits. Amer. J. Syph. **30**, 455–462 (1946b).

METCHNIKOFF, E., ROUX, E.: Etudes expérimentales sur la syphilis. Ann. Inst. Pasteur **17**, 809–821 (1903); **18**, 1–6, 657–671 (1904); **19**, 673–698 (1905); **20**, 785–800 (1906).

MORTON, H.: Susceptibility of Syrian hamsters to leptospirosis. Proc. Soc. exp. Biol. (N.Y.) **49**, 566–568 (1942).

MOULTON, J. C., HOWARD, J. A.: The demonstration of *Leptospira canicola* in hamster kidneys by means of fluorescent antibody. Cornell Vet. **47**, 424–432 (1957).

MUEHLENS, P.: Rückfallfieber. In: KOLLE, KRAUS, UHLENHUTH, Handbuch der pathogenen Mikroorganismen, Bd. 7, S. 383–486. Jena-Berlin-Wien: G. Fischer und U. Schwarzenberg 1930.

NEISSER, A.: Bericht über die unter finanzieller Beihilfe des deutschen Reiches während der Jahre 1905–1909 in Batavia und Breslau ausgeführten Arbeiten zur Erforschung der Syphilis. Berlin: Springer 1911.

NICHOLS, H. J.: Experimental yaws in the monkey and rabbit. J. exp. Med. **12**, 616–622 (1910).

NICHOLS, H. J.: Observations on a strain of *Spirochaeta pallida* isolated from the nervous system. J. exp. Med. **19**, 362–371 (1914).

NICOLLE, C.: Sur une piroplasmose nouvelle d'un ronger. C. R. Soc. Biol. (Paris) **63**, 213–214 (1907).

NICOLLE, C., ANDERSON, C., COLAS-BELCOUR, J.: Sur un noveau spirochaete sanguicole patogene (*Sp. normandi*) trasmis par un Ornithodore (*O. normandi*) hôte des terriers de rongeurs nord africaines. C. R. Acad. Sci. (Paris) **185**, 344–336 (1927).

NICOLLE, C., COMTE, C.: Sur une spirillose d'un cheiroptère (*V. kuhli*). C. R. Soc. Biol. (Paris) **59**, 200 (1905) and Ann. Inst. Pasteur **20**, 311–320 (1906).

NIKOLAIEW, J. J., ANANJIN, V. V.: Leptospiros u miscei. Vopr. Kraevoi obscei experim. parasit. i mediz. zool. **7**, 217–221 (1951).

NOGUCHI, H.: A method for the pure cultivation of pathogenic *Treponema pallidum* (*Spirochaeta pallida*). J. exp. Med. **14**, 99–108 (1911).

Noguchi, H.: Cultural studies in mouth spirochaete (*T. microdentium* and *macrodentium*). J. exp. Med. 15, 81–89 (1912a).

Noguchi, H.: Pure cultivation of *Spirochaeta refringens*. J. exp. Med. 15, 466–469 (1912b).

Noguchi, H.: *Treponema mucosum* (new species). A mucin producing spirochaete from pyorrhoea alveolaris, grown in pure culture. J. exp. Med. 16, 194–198 (1912c).

Noguchi, H.: The pure cultivation of *Spirochaeta duttoni, Spirochaeta Kochi, Spirochaeta Obermeieri*, and *Spirochaeta Novyi*. J. exp. Med. 16, 199–210 (1912d).

Noguchi, H.: Pure cultivation of *Spirochaeta phagedenis* (new species), a spiral organism found in phagedenic lesions on human external genitalia. J. exp. Med. 16, 261–268 (1912e).

Noguchi, H.: A method for cultivating *Treponema pallidum* in fluid media. J. exp. Med. 16, 211–215 (1912f).

Noguchi, H.: Cultivation of *Treponema calligyrum* (new species) from condylomata of man. J. exp. Med. 17, 89–98 (1913).

Noguchi, H.: Certain alterations in biological properties of spirochaetes through artificial cultivation. Ann. Inst. Pasteur 30, 1–4 (1916).

Noguchi, H.: A note on the venereal spirochaetosis of rabbits: a new technique for staining *Treponema pallidum*. J. Amer. med. Ass. 77, 2052 (1921).

Novy, F. G., Knapp, R. E.: Studies on *Spirillum Obermeieri* and related organisms. J. infect. Dis. 3, 291–293 (1906).

Obermeier, O.: Vorkommen feinster, eine Eigenbewegung zeigender Fäden im Blute von Rekurrens-Kranken. Klin. Wschr. 152, 378, 391, 455 (1873).

Ostertag, H.: Leptospirosis icterohaemorrhagica in Bulgarien. Z. Hyg. 131, 482–500 (1950).

Otsuji: Lues 18, 153 (1938) (Quoted by Matsumoto, 1942).

Otsuji: Lues 19, 31 (1939) (Quoted by Matsumoto, 1942).

Otsuji: Lues 20, 71 (1939) (Quoted by Matsumoto, 1942).

Ovchinnikov, H. M.: Experimental syphilis. Moscow: Medgiz [in Russian] 1955.

Pautrizel, R., Mayer, G., Rivasseau-Coutant, A., Szersnovicz, F.: Immunité naturelle du foetus de lapin vis-à-vis de *Treponema pallidum*. Rev. Immunol. (Paris) 21, 383–392 (1957).

Pearce, L., Brown, W. H.: Distinctive characteristics of infections produced by *Treponema pertenue* in the rabbit. J. exp. Med. 41, 673–690 (1925).

Perry, W. L. M.: The cultivation of *Treponema pallidum* in tissue culture. J. Path. Bact. 60, 339–342 (1948).

Plaut, F.: Untersuchungen über die Rolle der Milz für die Aufrechterhaltung der isolierten Gehirnspirochätose bei Recurrensratten. Klin. Wschr. 7, 301–303 (1928).

Plimmer, H. G.: Proc. Zool. Soc. London part 2, 406 (1912) (Quoted by Hindle, E., 1931).

Raiziss, G. W., Severac, M.: Rapidity with which *Spirochaeta pallida* invades the blood stream. Arch. Derm. Syph. (Chic.) 35, 1101–1109 (1937).

Ranken, H. S.: A note on "granule-shedding" in *T. pertenue*. Brit. med. J. 1912 I, 1482.

Reasoner, M. A.: Some phases of experimental syphilis with special reference to the question of strains. J. Amer. med. Ass. 67, 1799–1805 (1916).

Resseler, R., Riel, M. van: Conservation des leptospires après refroidissement ou lyophilization. Intern. Colloq. on Leptospirosis, Antwerpen, 1965. Ann. Soc. Belge Méd. Trop. 46, 213–222 (1966).

Rosahn, P. D.: The reaction of standard breeds of rabbits to experimental syphilis. J. exp. Med. 57, 907–923 (1933).

Rosahn, P. D.: The adverse influence of syphilitic infection on longevity of mice and men. Arch. Derm. Syph. (Chic.) 36, 17–37 (1952).

Rosahn, P. D., Gueft, B., Rowe, C. L.: Experimental mouse syphilis. I. Organ distribution of the infectious agent. Recent Advances in the study of Venereal Diseases; a Symposium, Washington D.C., p. 36–48, VD Education Inst., USPHS, Raleigh N.C. (1948).

Rosahn, P. D., Rowe, C. L.: Experimental mouse syphilis. II. Minimal infectious number of *Treponema pallidum*. Amer. J. Syph. 34, 40–44 (1950).

Ross, E. H.: An intracellular parasite developing into spirochaetes. Brit. med. J. 1912 II, 1651–1654.

Saenz, B., Grau Triana, J., Alfonso Armenteros, J.: Demonstración de un *Treponema* en el borde activo de un caso de pinta de las manos y pies y en la linfa de ganglios superficiales (reporte preliminar). Arch. med. internat. 4, 112–117 (1938).

Sakharoff, M. N.: *Spirochaeta anserina* et septicémie des oies. Ann. Inst. Pasteur 5, 564–566 (1891).

Savini, E.: Infection trypano-spirochetique. C. R. Soc. Biol. (Paris) 88, 956–958 (1923).

Schamberg, J. F., Rule, A. M.: Therapeutic effect of hot baths in experimental syphilis. J. Amer. med. Ass. 88, 1217–1218 (1927).

Schamberg, J. F., Rule, A. M.: The effect of extremely hot baths in experimental syphilis; further studies. Arch. Derm. Syph. (Chic.) 17, 322–331 (1928).

SCHAUDINN, F.: Zur Kenntnis der *Spirochaeta pallida*. Dtsch. med. Wschr. **31**, 1665–1667 and 1728 (1905).

SCHAUDINN, F., HOFFMANN, E.: Vorläufiger Bericht über das Vorkommen von Spirochaeten in syphilitischen Krankheitsproducten und bei Papillomen. Arb. Gesundh.-Amt **22**, 527–534 (1905).

SCHERESCHEWSKY, J.: Züchtung der Spirochaete pallida (Schaudinn). Dtsch. med. Wschr. **35**, 835 (1909).

SCHERESCHEWSKY, J.: Weitere Mitteilung über die Züchtung der *Spirochaeta pallida*. Dtsch. med. Wschr. **35**, 1260–1261 (1909).

SCHERESCHEWSKY, J.: Bisherige Erfahrungen mit der gezüchteten *Spirochaeta pallida*. Dtsch. med. Wschr. **35**, 1652–1654 (1909).

SCHERESCHEWSKY, J.: Geschlechtlich übertragbare originäre Kaninchensyphilis und Chinin-Spirochätotropie. Berl. klin. Wschr. **57**, 1142–1144 (1920).

SCHERESCHEWSKY, J.: Pallidakultur und Immunodiagnostik der Syphilis. Haut. Gesundh. **17**, 233–236 (1954).

SCHLOSSBERGER, H.: Syphilis und Framboesie bei Mäusen. Zbl. Bakt., I. Abt. Orig. **104**, 237–239 (1927).

SCHLOSSBERGER, H.: Über das Verhalten der Syphilisspirochäten im Mäuseorganismus bei Passagen. Med. Klin. **25**, 307–308 (1929).

SCHOEBL, O.: Experimental yaws in Philippine monkeys and a critical consideration of our knowledge concerning framboesia tropica in the light of recent experimental evidence. Philipp. J. Sci. **35**, 209–332 (1928).

Scientific Group on Treponematoses Research, WHO: *Treponema pallidum*. WHO/VDT/Res/8, Geneva (1961).

SHAFFER, L. W.: Cultural methods for increasing the number of *Spirochaeta pallida* in fresh syphilitic tissue. Arch. Path. Lab. Med. **2**, 50–58 (1926).

SHELDON, W. H.: Leptospiral antigen demonstrated by the fluorescent antibody technic in human muscle lesions of Leptospirosis icterohaemorrhagiae. Proc. Soc. exp. Biol. (N.Y.) **84**, 165–167 (1953).

SMITH, H.: The use of bacteria grown in vivo for studies on the basis of their pathogenicity. Amer. Rev. Microb. **12**, 77–102 (1958).

SMITH, H.: Studies on organisms grown in vivo to reveal the bases of microbial pathogenicity. Ann. N.Y. Acad. Sci. **88**, 1213–1226 (1960).

STALHEIM, O. H. V.: Leptospiral selection growth, and virulence in synthetic medium. J. Bact. **92**, 946 (1966).

STERZI, G., STAUDACHER, V.: Tentativi di coltura della spirocheta di Schaudinn sulla membrana chorionallantoidea di embrione di pollo vivente. G. ital. Derm. Sif. **80**, 777–783 (1939).

STUART, R. D.: The preparation and use of a simple culture medium for leptospirae. J. Path. Bact. **58**, 343 (1946).

SWAIN, R. H. A., ANDERSON, N.: The ultrastructure of Treponemas and Borreliae. In: The fine morphology of Spirochaetas, edited by B. BABUDIERI. Roma: Leonardo ediz. scientif. 1972.

TANI, T., KAKISHITA, M., SAITO, K.: Beiträge zur Meerschweinchensyphilis. Zbl. Bakt., I. Orig. **117**, 73–81 (1930).

TARASEVICH, M. N., BULKE, B. F., MUDROVA, P. L.: A method of conservation of pathogenic Leptospira organisms while preserving their virulence. J. Hyg. Epidem. (Praha) **7**, 352–359 (1963).

TERZIN, A. L.: Leptospiral antigens for use in complement fixation. J. Immunol. **76**, 366–372 (1956).

THEILER, A.: Spirillosis of cattle. J. C. Path. a. Ther. **17**, 47–55 (1904) and J. Th. Veter. **1**, 421–431 (1906).

THEILER, A.: Transmission and inoculability of *Sp. theileri*. Proc. roy. Soc. B **76**, 504–506 (1905).

THIEL, P. H. VAN: Immunisatie gegen de ziekte van Weil met levende avirulente leptospirae. Geneesk. T. Ned.-Ind. **78**, 1859–1874 (1938).

THIROUX, A., DUFOUGERE, W.: Persistance de l'infection des mèninges chez un singe guéri, sans médication, d'une infection sanguine à Spirilles naturelle. Bull. Soc. Path. exot. **3**, 23–24 (1910).

TOMASCZEWSKI, E.: Über eine einfache Methode, bei Kaninchen Primäreffekte zu erzeugen. Dtsch. med. Wschr. **36**, 1025 (1910).

TOMIOKA, Y.: Experimenteller Beitrag zur Frage der Immunität bei Recurrens und ihre Beeinflussung durch die Salvarsantherapie. Zbl. Bakt., I. Abt. Orig. **92**, 41 (1924).

TOMIZAWA, T., KASAMATSU, S.: Haemagglutination tests for diagnosis of syphilis. A preliminary report. Jap. J. med. Sci. Biol. **19**, 305 (1966).

Truffi, M.: Über die Übertragung eines menschlichen syphilitischen Primäraffektes auf die Haut des Kaninchens. Zbl. Bakt., I. Abt. Orig. **48**, 597–599 (1909).

Turner, T. B.: The preservation of virulent *T. pallidum* and *T. pertenue* in the frozen state: with a note on the preservation of the filtrable viruses. J. exp. Med. **67**, 61–78 (1938).

Turner, T. B., Fleming, W. J.: Prolonged maintenance of spirochaetes and filtrable viruses in the frozen state. J. exp. Med. **70**, 620–637 (1939).

Turner, T. B., Holander, D. H.: Cortisone in experimental syphilis- a preliminary note. Bull. Johns Hopk. Hosp. **87**, 505–509 (1950).

Turner, T. B., Holander, D. H.: Studies on the mechanism of action of cortisone in experimental syphilis. Amer. J. Syph. **38**, 371–387 (1954).

Turner, T. B., Holander, D. H.: Biology of the treponematoses. Wld Hlth Org. Monogr. Ser. No 35 (1957).

Uhlenhuth, P., Mulzer, P.: Beiträge zur experimentellen Pathologie und Therapie der Syphilis mit besonderer Berücksichtigung der Impf-Syphilis der Kaninchen. Arb. Gesundh.-Amt **44**, 307–530 (1913).

Volosceanu, D. I., Oprescu, C. C., Voiculescu, R.: Contributions to the study of strains of *T. pallidum* isolated in Roumania. Problems in Therapeutica III, 19–29 (1955).

Warfolomeeva, A. A.: Young rabbits as a laboratory model for leptospirosis. In: Leptospirae and leptospirosis in man and animals. Pol. Akad. Nauk, Warsawa 18–21 (1960).

Warfolomeeva, A. A.: Leptospiroses in USSR and their specific prophylaxis and treatment. In: Leptospirae and leptospirosis in man and animals. Pol. Akad. Nauk, Warsawa 197–210 (1960).

Warfolomeeva, A. A.: Specific therapy in leptospirosis. II. Symp. on Leptospirae and leptospiroses in man and animals. Pol. Akad. Nauk, Warsawa, 377–380 (1964).

Warthin, A. S.: Myxoma-like growths in the heart, due to localization of *Spirochaeta pallida*. J. infect. Dis. **19**, 138 (1916).

Weichbrodt, R., Jahnel, F.: Einfluß hoher Körpertemperaturen auf die Spirochaeten und Krankheitserscheinungen der Syphilis im Tierexperiment. Dtsch. med. Wschr. **45**, 483–484 (1919).

White, F. H., Ristic, M.: Detection of *Leptospira pomona* in guinea-pig and bovine urine with fluoresceinlabeled antibody. J. infect. Dis. **105**, 118–123 (1959).

W.H.O. Treponematoses research, techn. Rep. Ser. Geneva (1970).

WHO Expert Group: Current problems in leptospirosis research. Wld Hlth Org. techn. Rep. Ser. No 380 (1967).

Wile, U. J., Johnson, S. A. M.: Experimental syphilis in the golden hamster. Amer. J. Syph. **29**, 418–422 (1945).

Wilson, G. S., Miles, A. A.: The Spirochaetes. In: Topley and Wilson's Principles of bacteriology and immunity, 4th ed. London: E. Arnold, p. 1031–1056, and Syphilis, rabbit syphilis, yaws and pinta, p. 2027–2044 (1955).

Wolff, J. W.: The laboratory diagnosis of leptospirosis. Springfield (Ill.) USA: Ch. C. Thomas 1954.

Yamamoto, T.: Studien über Spirochätenfärbung. I. Untersuchung der pallidafärbenden Farbstoffe. Acta Derm. (Kyoto) **13**, 591 (1929).

Yamamoto, T.: Studien über Spirochätenfärbung. III. Färberische Unterschiede zwischen *Sp. pallida, Sp. pallidula* und *Sp. cuniculi*. Acta derm. (Kyoto) **14**, 145 (1929).

Zardi, O.: Influenza della terapia cortisonica e corticotropa nell'infezione sperimentale da leptospire. R. C. Ist. sup. Sanità **19**, 188–195 (1956).

Experimental Infections by Spirilla

B. Babudieri

With 1 Figure

"Sodoku" or "Rat-Bite-Fever"

The genus *Spirillum* Ehrenberg *1832*, belongs to the *Spirillaceae* family and comprises more or less long spiral microorganisms. They usually contain volutin granules and are mobile through tufts of flagella situated at one or both ends. Multiplication takes the form of binary division; they are aerobic and grow easily in the usual culture media, except for the only pathogenic species: *Spirillum minus*, which has not yet been grown in culture. They are usually found in fresh as well as in salt water, especially if it is rich in putrefying organic substances.

They may be readily observed under dark-field illumination; they are easily stained by common bacteriological dyes or by silver impregnation methods.

A. General Characters

Spirillum minus (Carter, 1887) is the only species pathogenic for man and animals. It causes "sodoku" or "rat-bite fever", an infection well-known since the remotest antiquity. However, it was not until 1915–1916 that Futaki, Takaki, Taiguchi and Osumi proved that the spirillum which Carter had seen years before in the blood of *Epimys decumanus* was the causal organism of the disease.

Sodoku is seen all over the world, but with greater frequency in the countries of the Far East. It is usually transmitted to man by rat bite, more rarely by mouse, cat, dog, ferret and squirrel bite.

In man the disease gives local symptoms at the site of the bite and general, more or less serious, symptoms.

Spirillum minus is a spirillum 0.5 to 5 μ long, about 0.2 μ across.

The pitch of the waves from crest to crest varies between 0.8 and 1 μ. At both ends it has a tuft of flagella, 2–3 μ long, which give it a lively motility. These flagella are hardly visible and may be coloured by means of Fontana-Tribondeau's method.

The microorganism is Gram-negative and facultative aerobic. Unlike most of the other spirilla it appears to contain no volutin granules.

Some of the earliest workers considered *S. minus* a spirochaeta and named it *Spirochaeta morsus muris* (Futaki et al., 1917b).

That it belongs to the spirilla, however, is shown by its rigidity, the fact that its spirals, unlike those of the spirochetas, all lie in one plane and its sensitivity to sulphonamides.

Ruys (1925, 1926, 1927) proposed the existence of two different species of spirilla, similar to each other: one usually having the rat as host and pathogenic for the guinea pig, the other a parasite of the mouse and not pathogenic for the guinea pig. This hypothesis was not confirmed. The species is now considered to be unique and there is only a difference in virulence from strain to strain.

The early reports that this spirillum had been cultured in various media (Futaki et al., 1925 in Shimamina's medium, as well as in 1% glucose broth with an addition of rat blood or even in a mixture of Shimamina's and Vervoort's media; Stretti and Mantovani, 1921, in Reiter-Ramme's medium with guinea pig blood; Robinson, 1922, in agar at 0.2% + 20% of undefibrinated guinea-pig blood, etc.) have not been confirmed (McDermott, 1928; Schockaert, 1928; Knowles and Das Gupta, 1928; etc.). It is possible that the spirillum may be kept alive in the above-mentioned media for some time, without however, multiplying appreciably.

B. Experimental Infection

Experimental sodoku in laboratory animals was studied widely about half a century ago, but there is scarcely any recent work on this subject. In the evaluation of earlier work we must bear in mind that in those days another infection transmitted by rat bite was very little known: the infection due to *Streptobacillus moniliformis* (Schottmüller, 1914; Blake, 1916). This infection and the one by *S. minus* may sometimes coexist, and it is not certain whether some of the symptomats attributed by some authors to spirillar infection were not due rather to *Sreptobacillus*. As no *S. minus* cultures are available in artificial media, experimental infection cannot be performed with strains of known and constant virulence. It is necessary to use the blood of naturally infected rats, or to employ strains kept through repeated passages in the rat, or guinea pig.

As regards the natural infection of the rat, it must be borne in mind that this infection varies in frequency from country to country. E.g. Ishiwara et al. (1917) in two successive investigations of rats in Japan, found respectively 11.2% and 25% were infected; Joekes (1925) found 25% in London; Ruys (1925) a little over 1% in Amsterdam.

As infecting material, it is necessary to use the blood of naturally or experimentally infected animal, after a microscope blood-film examination has confirmed the presence of spirilla.

1. Infection in Man

S. minus inoculation has been used in man for pyretotherapy in cases of paralysis (Kihn, 1927; Solomon et al., 1926; Mooser, 1925b, 1926; Grabow and Kreg, 1929; etc.). The infection has achieved by subcutaneous injection of 0.1–1 ml of blood from infected mouse or guinea pig.

After an incubation period of 14–21 days, the infection is characterized by inflammatory edema, pain at the injection spot, involvement of the regional lymphnodes and a sudden febrile attack precided by shivering. The fever reaches 40–41° C and lasts about 2–3 days, sometimes longer. The fall to normal is abrupt and the fever recurs after an internal of 3–7 days. There may be further febrile periods, often progressively less in intensity and duration. When used for pyretotherapy, the infection was generally broken down after few pyrexial periods by treatment with Salvarsan or its derivates.

With the first febrile attack we observe the appearance of a diffused maculopapular rash, neither itching nor painful, which is found in slightly raised areas of varying size, with welldefined borders, of a characteristic deep purplish-black. The rash disappears when the temperature falls and seldom reappears in subsequent febrile attacks.

Pains in the muscles and around the joints are frequent, the pulse is fast and shallow, and there is leucocytosis.

The spirilla are present in the blood and at the site of injection. Usually the patient's general condition is not very much affected. In order to avoid local involvement, the spirilla have sometimes been inoculated directly into a vein.

2. Infection in the Monkey

FUTAKI et al. (1917b, 1925), KOBAYASHI and KODAMA (1919), ISHIWARA et al. (1917b), RUYS (1925), and others have infected with *S. minus* the macacus monkey. In this animal the disease runs a course very similar to that in man. There are febrile attacks starting a week after infection and relapsing several times. The animal loses weight and, about a month after the infection, alopecia begins in the face and spreads all over the body. The spirilla appears in the blood within 10 days.

If the strain employed is of low virulence, the monkey may have a completely asymptomatic reaction.

3. Infection in the Mouse

The mouse is the animal most susceptible to *S. minus* infection. There are, however, white mice naturally infected by low-virulence strains, so that the animal shows no over symptoms of disease, except for the presence of the spirilla in the blood (1% of cases according WORMS, 1926). Though rare, this possibility must be borne in mind, in order to avoid mistakes in the interpretation of experimental results.

Mice are generally injected subcutaneously with a small quantity of infectious blood. The incubation period is very variable and may last 3 to 15 days, according to the virulence of the strain employed. After repeated passages from mouse to mouse, the incubation period shows a tendency to stabilize in about 8–10 days.

The infection in the mouse generally has no very visible pathologic manifestations. The spirillum appears in the blood at the end of the incubation period and can persist there for a long time, even for over three months (MCDERMOTT, 1928) or for life (WORMS, 1926). The distribution of the spirilla in the blood is not constant but varies considerably from day to day. Sometimes there is a clear prevalence of short shapes, at other times of medium or long ones (ROBERTSON, 1924).

In chronically infected mice there may be hyperplasia of the reticulo-endothelial system, especially of lymphnodes, spleen and liver, also small zones of necrosis.

According to SALIMBENI et al. (1925), spirilla are difficult to identify in the spleen of the infected mouse; this organ, however, is so highly infectious that it was suggested the pathogenic agent might exist there in a particular form, possibly filterable granules.

4. Infection in the Rat

With the rat, as with the mouse, it must be ascertained in advance that the animals to be experimented upon do not have a natural infection.

The infection in the rat, usually effected by intraperitoneal or subcutaneous injection, has a course which resembles syphilis, in man.

According to MCDERMOTT (1928), there is an incubation period, followed after a few days by a period called the "primary stage" during which the spirillum is detectable only in the subcutaneous tissue around the inoculation spot, and in the regional lymphnodes.

After a period of 4–30 days, with non "stabilised" strains, the "secondary period" begins, characterized by the appearance of the spirillum in peripheral blood. The microorganism remains in the blood for some 4–16 weeks, reaching its climax after 3 weeks, then it disappears. There is then a "latent stage"; lasting several weeks, then there is no overt sign of disease, but the microorganism is present in the lymphatic and subcutaneous systems.

Then follows the "tertiary stage", which appears with various symptoms, including conjunctivitis, keratitis, iritis and palpebral edema, with spirilla present in the lachrymal secretion. In the lymphnodes, especially in the mediastinum, and sometimes in the liver and in the spleen, there appear gummatoid lesions. There is hyperplasia and proliferation of the reticulo-endothelial system, followed by diffused necrotic processes, often surrounded by a zone of fibrous tissue (HEITZMANN, 1927). There are numerous spirilla in the necrotic tissue. They are frequent in the subcutaneous and submucous connective tissue and may also be found in the cerebrospinal fluid (ONORATO, 1923). In the tertiary period, however, they disappear from the blood.

Usually, the infection is not lethal in the rat, which, however, loses weight, becomes weak, and shows zones of alopecia.

5. Infection in the Guinea Pig

The virulence of *S. minus* for the guinea pig varies widely from strain to strain (MOOSER, 1925b, 1926; RUYS, 1925, 1926; Row, 1917; PARMANAND, 1952; ROBERTSON, 1931; McDERMOTT, 1928; FUTAKI et al., 1917a, etc.). In some cases the infection is clinically silent and non-febrile; in others, the animal dies after a few weeks. The fever starts 9–20 days after the infection and has a relapsing course.

Repeated passages from guinea pig to guinea pig generally stabilize the virulence of the spirillum for this animal. In strains adapted to guinea pig, the incubation period lasts about 9 days.

Young guinea pigs (250–300 g) inoculated with virulent strains, generally die after 12–15 days, with a septicemic form. The only post-mortem signs are hypertrophy of the liver, and of the adrenal glands and lymph nodes.

In adult guinea pigs (400–500 g) inoculated with virulent strains, the disease is also fatal, but it lasts 2–3 months. In these guinea pigs the disease can assume, according to *Salimbeni* et al. (1925), two different forms: visceral and cutaneous. In the former there is no cutaneous edema and the disease is characterized only by fever and the presence of spirilla in the blood, the latter starting 12–15 days after infection.

In the cutaneous form periocular and perinasal edema, with conjunctivitis, and sometimes keratitis, has been reported, appearing from 7 to 22 days after infection. The edematic fluid contains a few spirilla. After a few days, the rash disappears and edematic zones are characterized by a whitish infiltration. Zones of alopecia are frequent, usually starting from the *3rd week and more evident in young animals*. The post-mortem shows some hypertrophy of the adrenals, whereas the spleen and the liver appear normal. In the visceral form, on the other hand, there is considerable enlargement of the spleen and hyperplasia of the reticulo-endothelial system. Guinea pigs that survive the infection has a good recovery and the spirilla disappear from the organism (RUYS, 1925, 1926).

MOOSER (1925b) and GRABOW et al. (1929) have also infected the guinea pig by intratesticular injections. In this case, after 5 days, tumefaction appears on the inoculated testicle, which then spreads to the collateral one, and is accompanied by swelling of the lymphnodes. Then the testicles show a tendency to atrophy.

In the infected guinea pig the spirilla remain in the blood as long as the disease lasts. There are considerable fluctuations in their numbers, not associated with the presence or absence of fever.

6. Infection of the Rabbit

MATSUMOTO and ADACHI (1923) infected the rabbit by intrascrotal injection, thus obtaining lesions very similar to those produced in the rabbit by the syphilis spirochaeta. After 6–9 days the scrotum becomes inflamed and after 10–14 days the primary black-brown, hemorrhagic infiltrative lesion sets in this is very liable to necrosis. These lesions recede after 3–4 weeks.

Delayed edema of the eyelids and alopecia also occur in the rabbit. The spirilla appear in the blood between the 7th and 21st day after the infection, but there are always few in number and disappear from the blood after a few days.

In the rabbit, unlike the guinea pig, there is no typical febrile reaction.

7. Infection of the Cat

Experimental infection of the cat has been achieved by STRETTI and MANTOVANI (1921) and by MOOSER (1925a), later by others workers. The animals bear the infection well and show hardly any signs of disease. There may be oedema at the site of injection after 3 days, and, occasionally, after three weeks, there may be palpebral oedema followed by keratitis and infection of episcleral vessels. The spirilla appear in the blood after 12 days, but are rather scarce.

8. Infection of the Dog

The dog has been experimentally infected by MOOSER (1925b, 1926). In this animal the disease is clinically evident, with febrile attacks and weakness. After 5 days a strange form of oedema appears at the site of inoculation, with superficial blisters whose liquid contains a few spirilla. These lesions have a tendency to regress and, generally, completely disappear within two weeks.

Palpebral oedema may also appear later. The spirilla appear in the blood after 14 days, but are always few in number.

C. Conclusions

The animal of choice for infection by *S. minus* is the white mouse, which is extremely receptive to the infection and retains the spirillum in its blood for practically the whole of its life.

The mouse, however, does not show any evident morbid symptoms, and the lesions produced by the spirillum are very scarce. Anyone interested in studying the damage effected in the tissues by the infection or in following the cours of fatal infections should use rats or guinea pigs, always bearing in mind the variable severity and course of the disease in these animals, and that it is not always easy to detect the spirillum in the blood.

Spirilla may be detected in the blood with a light microscope or under dark-field illumination. The spirilla are easily traceable due to their lively movements. Blood smears fixed and stained with Giemsa or silver impregnation methods may also be used.

The spirilla may also be found in the edematic fluid, especially at the site of injection, or in the lymph.

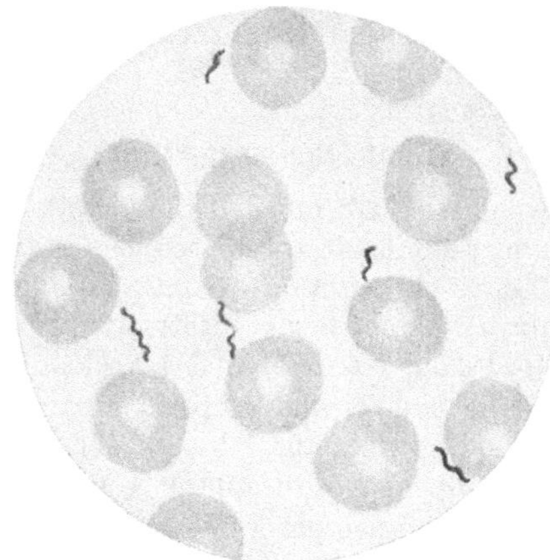

Fig. 1. *S. minus* in a blood smear, from mouse; Silver impregnation. 2000×

Their incidence in urine, feces, lachrymal secretion and saliva is low and irregular, so that at least for diagnostic purposes, it is not advisable to look for spirilla there.

It must be borne in mind that the absence of spirilla in the blood is not enough for absolute exclusion of the possibility that an animal may be immune to infection by *S. minus*. For this purpose the animal's blood must be inoculated to mice and the presence or absence of spirilla in their blood determined.

An animal that has survived infection with *S. minus*, or in which the infection has taken a chronic course, shows in the serum antibodies specific for the spirillum, which is killed or lysed by them. In addition the animal acquires immunity to reinfection (Ruys, 1925, 1926).

S. minus is sensitive to arsenobenzols (Hata, 1912; Surveyor, 1913) to sulphonamides (Nitti et al., 1942) and to many antibiotics including penicillin (Wheeler, 1945; Nitti et al., 1946; Frank and Perlman, 1948; etc.) streptomycin and tetracycline (Sen et al., 1945). For more details on this subject, see Roughgarden's monograph (1965).

References

Blake, F.: The etiology of rat-bite fever. J. exp. Med. **23**, 39 (1916).
Frank, L., Perlman, H. H.: Fever caused by *Spirillum minus* treated with penicillin: case. Arch. Derm. Syph. (Chic.) **57**, 261 (1948).
Futaki, K., Takaki, J., Taniguchi, T., Osumi, S.: Rat-bite disease Spirochaetes inoculated in to Guinea pigs [jap.]. Iji Shimbun **985**, 1513 (1917a).
Futaki, K., Takaki, J., Taniguchi, T., Osumi, S.: *Spirochaeta morsus muris* N. Sp., the cause of rat-bite fever. J. exp. Med. **25**, 33 (1917b).
Futaki, K., Takaki, J., Taniguchi, T., Osumi, S., Ishiwara, K., Otawara, T.: Demonstration of the spirochaeta causing rat-bite fever. Trans. 6th Congr. Far East. Ass. Trop. Med. Tokyo **2**, 133 (1925).
Grabow, C., Kreg, J.: Der Impfrattenbiß in der Behandlung der progressiven Paralyse. Z. ges. Neurol. Psychiat. **121**, 621 (1929).
Hata, S.: Salvarsantherapie der Rattenbißkrankheit in Japan. Münch. med. Wschr. **59**, 854 (1912).
Heitzmann, O.: Vergleichende pathologische Anatomie der experimentellen Rattenbißkrankheit und der Infektion mit Mäusespirillen. Arch. Derm. Syph. (Berl.) **153**, 399 (1927).
Ishiwara, K., Otawara, T., Tamura, K.: Spirochaetes in rats [jap.]. Jap. J. Derm. Urol. [jap.] **17**, 87 (1917a).

ISHIWARA, K., OTAWARA, T., TAMURA, K.: Experimental rat-bite fever. First report. J. exp. Med. **25**, 33 (1917b).

JOEKES, T.: Cultivation of the spirillum of rat-bite fever. Lancet **1925 II**, 1225.

KIHN, B.: Einige Neuerungen auf dem Gebiete der Infektionsbehandlung der Paralyse. Münch. med. Wschr. **1927**, 1390.

KNOWLES, R., DAS GUPTA, B. M.: Rat-bite fever an Indian disease. Indian med. Gaz. **63**, 493 (1928).

KOBAYASHI, R., KODAMA, M.: Contribution to the study of *Spirochaeta morsus muris* in the Nippon field vole (*Microtus montebelli*). Kitasato Arch. exp. Med. **63**, 199 (1919).

MANTOVANI, M.: Virus del sodoku. 1° nota, Pathologica **15**, 197 (1923).

MATSUMOTO, SH., ADACHI, Y.: Primary sclerosis in rat-bite fever in the rabbit. Acta derm. (Kyoto) **1**, 403 (1923).

McDERMOTT, E. N.: Rat-bite fever; study of experimental disease, with critical review of literature. Quart. J. Med. **21**, 433 (1928).

MOOSER, H.: Die Katze als Überträgerin von Sodoku. Arch. Schiffs- u. Tropenhyg. **29**, Beih. 1, 253 (1925a).

MOOSER, H.: Etudes expérimentales sur le sodoku. Schweiz. med. Wschr. **57**, 1154 (1925b).

MOOSER, H.: La enfermedad producida por mordedura de rata. Gac. Med. de México. Conferencia 17 nov. 1926.

NITTI, F., BOYER, F., CONGE, M.: Action du p-amino-phényl-sulfamide dans le sodoku expérimental du cobaye. Ann. Inst. Pasteur **68**, 497 (1942).

NITTI, F., CONGE, M., KAUFFMANN, G.: Traitement du sodoku expérimental du cobaye par de penicilline. Ann. Inst. Pasteur **72**, 294 (1946).

ONORATO, R.: Sodoku in Tripolitania. Arch. ital. Sci. med. colon. **4**, 156, 162, 193, 221 (1923).

PARMANAND, M. J.: Rat-bite fever with special reference to its etiological agent. Indian J. med. Res. **11**, 181 (1923) and **12**, 669 (1952).

ROBERTSON, A.: Observations on causal organism of rat-bite fever in man. Ann. Trop. Med. Parasit. **18**, 157 (1924).

ROBERTSON, A.: Rat-bite fever or sodoku. A system of bacteriology in relation to medicine. Med. Res. Counc. (Lond.) **8**, 286 (1931).

ROBINSON, G. H.: Some observations on a case of rat-bite fever. Amer. J. Hyg. **2**, 324 (1922).

ROUGHGARDEN, J. W.: Antimicrobial therapy of rat-bite fever. A review. Arch. intern. Med. **116**, 39 (1965).

ROW, R.: A new species of spirochaete, isolated from a case of rat-bite fever in Bombay. Indian J. med. Res. **5**, 386 (1917).

RUYS, A. CH.: De verwekker der rattebeetziekte. Thèse Amsterdam 1925.

RUYS, A. CH.: Der Erreger der Rattenbißkrankheit. Arch. Schiffs- u. Tropenhyg. **30**, 112 (1926).

RUYS, A. CH.: Klassifikation des Erregers der Rattenbißkrankheit. Zbl. Bakt., I. Abt. Orig. **103**, 258 (1927).

SALIMBENI, A. T., KERMORGANT, Y., GARCIA, R.: L'existence de formes filtrables du parasite du sodoku dans la rate des souris expérimentalement infectées. C. R. Soc. Biol. (Paris) **93**, 229 (1925).

SALIMBENI, A. T., KERMORGANT, Y., GARCIA, R.: L'infection expérimentale du cobaye, provoquée par le parasite du sodoku. C. R. Soc. Biol. (Paris) **93**, 335 (1925).

SCHOCKAERT, J.: Contribution à l'étude de sodoku. Arch. intern. Méd. expér. **4**, 133 (1928).

SCHOTTMUELLER: Zur Ätiologie und Klinik der Bißkrankheit (Ratten-, Katzen- und Eichhörnchen-Bißkrankheit. Derm. Wschr., Ergänzungsheft (Festschrift) **58**, 77 (1914).

SEN, S., BASU, B. C., BANERJEE, D.: Streptomycin and terramycin (oxytetracycline) in fever due to *Spirillum minus*. Indian med. Gaz. **89**, 3 (1954).

SOLOMON, H. C., BERK, A., THEILER, M., CLAY, C. L.: Use of sodoku in the treatment of general paralysis. Arch. intern. Med. **38**, 391 (1926).

STRETTI, G. B., MANTOVANI, M.: Contributo all'eziologia del Sodoku. Policlin. **28**, 875 (1921).

SURVEYOR, N. F.: A case of rat-bite fever treated with neosalvarsan. Lancet **1913 II**, 1764.

WHEELER, W. E.: Penicillin treatment of fevers due to *Streptobacillus moniliformis* and *Spirillum minus* respectively. Amer. J. Dis. Child. **69**, 215 (1945).

WORMS, W.: Vergleichende experimentelle Untersuchungen mit dem Erreger der Rattenbißkrankheit und der Mäusespirille. Zbl. Bakt., I. Abt. Orig. **98**, 195 (1926).

A Study of the Chemotherapeutics Active on Syphilis

B. BABUDIERI

The chemotherapeutics active on *T. pallidum* can also be studied "in vitro", as NELSON (1948–1949), WEBER (1953) and others have been able to maintain the motility and virulence of the spirochaetas for several days, in particular media.

Below we give the formulae of the two media most commonly used for this purpose:

	Nelson's medium (1948–1949)	Weber's medium (1953)
Bovine serum fraction V or crystalline bovine albumin	2.0%	2.0%
Na_2HPO_4	0.36%	0.4%
KH_2PO_4	0.05%	0.05%
Sodium thioglycolate	0.03%	0.05%
Cysteine L (+) HCl	0.03%	0.02%
Glutathione	0.02%	0.06%
Sodium pyruvate	0.01%	0.025%
Sodium chloride	0.255%	0.255%
Human serum ultrafiltrate	5.0%	10.0%
Vitamin[a]	0	5.0%
Sodium bicarbonate	0.06%	0
Dist. water	100 ml	100 ml

[a] This mixture contains 14 different vitamins. In addition it has to contain traces of sodium citrate, tyrosine, tryptophane, gelatin hydrolysate, calcium chloride and indigo disulfonate as indicator of a satisfactory reduction level.

Individual test tubes are used, in which the medium is layered with paraffin oil containing 2.6-di-tert-butyl p-cresol as a powerful anti-oxidant.

For the preparation of the inoculum a suspension of treponemas developed in the rabbit's testicle is prepared. The suspension is centrifuged at low speed in order to eliminate gross tissue debris, spermatozoa and red blood cells. The treponemas are eventually resuspended in the preserving medium, to give a concentration of between 5×10^5 and 10×10^6 per ml.

The addition of graded doses of the chemotherapeutic being studied to a series of these test tubes permits quantitative determination of its activity.

During the test, the tubes should be kept at a constant temperature, preferably 35° C. At lower temperatures the efficiency of the chemotherapeutics is less evident (NELL, 1954).

The percentage of spirochaetes which have not yet lost their motility should be calculated and recorded after 12, 18, and 24 hours.

These tests are very sensitive and the use of appropriate controls for detection of non-specific effects on the motility of *T. pallidum* is essential.

Particular attention must be paid to the so-called "sensitization" phenomenon: the presence of a small quantity of antibodies and of complement deriving from the rabbit donor of treponema in the preserving medium, can quickly immobilize it (KAHN et al., 1951).

The use of *Treponema* strains grown in culture, for example Reiter's, for these in vitro tests is not advisable. In fact, EAGLE (1946) has proved in his studies on antitreponemic effect of penicillin that the results obtained in vitro with Reiter's strain do not correspond to those obtained in vivo with pathogenic *Treponema* strains.

Consequently, the assay of drugs in "in vivo" is preferable, though this too, is a delicate procedure requiring the use of a large number of animals.

One method was proposed by EAGLE and FLEISCHMANN (1948); according to their method a certain number of rabbits is inoculated intradermally with 2000 *T. pallidum*. After 4 days the animals are treated with graded doses of the chemotherapeutic being tested. The efficacy of the drug is determined by the appearence of a syphiloma at the site of inoculation. The observation period is 3–4 months.

Another method is the one elaborated by TURNER, CUMBERLAND and LI (1947). It consists in inoculating the rabbit with treponemas several times by intraderma. injection, so as to cause the appearence of numerous syphilomas. When these are well-developed, a count of the treponemas present in two of these lesions is made in each of the rabbits.

The count is made by grasping the base of the syphilitic nodule with a hemostat to fix the lesion. Then the syphiloma is sectioned with a razor-blade and 0.05 ml of serum are collected on each of 2 slides. The number of the treponemas is counted in 100 microscopic fields (oil immersion) per slide.

The number of the spirochaetas is usually 600–1200 per 200 fields. If the number is inferior to 200, the animal is not used for the tests.

Graded doses of the chemotherapeutic are administered to the rabbits by injection after the count. Over the next few days the spirochaetas are counted at intervals of 24 hours. Therapeutics doses usually reduce the number of the treponemas by 99% in 48 hours.

This method allows a result in only 48 hours, or in about three weeks if the time elapsing between the inoculation of the treponemas and the appearence of the syphilomas is also taken into account.

These methods have permitted a satisfactory study of the action of the various fractions of penicillin on syphilis and it has been shown that fraction G is by far the most active, with a therapeutic activity superior to that of the other most commonly used antibiotics (derivatives of tetracycline, chloromycetin, erythromycin, magnamycin, etc.).

Other treponemicidal substances, such as gold compounds and iodides, have also been studied by these methods (TURNER and SCHAEFFER, 1954).

Most of the studies on arsenobenzenes and bismuth, which date back many years, have been performed in contrast, using mice infected with relapsing fever spirochaetas, and it is on tests of this type that the official methods for control of these drugs have been based in various countries.

All laboratory tests, confirmed by clinical experience, have proved that penicillins, more particularly of type G, are very effective in syphilis, much so that this antibiotic has now replaced all the chemotherapeutics formerly used in the treatment of this disease. We do not know of any case of penicillin-resistent syphilis, nor have we been able to make any pathogenic *Treponema* strain penicillin-resistent in laboratory tests (TURNER and HOLLANDER, 1959; PROBEY, 1953; HOLLANDER, TURNER and NELL, 1952).

The possibility that this may happen in the future nonetheless justifies the request for the study of other antiluetic drugs.

References

EAGLE, H.: The relative activity of penicillin F, G, K and X against spirochetes and streptococci in vitro. J. Bact. **52**, 81 (1946).

EAGLE, H., FLEISCHMAN, R.: The relative anti-syphilitic activity of penicillin F, G, K and X, and of bacitracin, based on the amounts required to abort early syphilitic infections in rabbits. J. Bact. **55**, 341 (1948).

HOLLANDER, D. H., TURNER, T. B., NELL, E. E.: The effect of long continued subcurative doses of penicillin during the incubation period of experimental syphilis. Bull. Johns Hopk. Hosp. **90**, 105 (1952).

KHAN, A. S.: Immunological relationship between species and strains of virulent treponemes. Baltimore Md. Thèse Johns Hopkins University (1950).

KHAN, A. S., NELSON, R. A., JR., TURNER, T. B.: Immunological relationships among species and strains of virulent treponemes as determined with the treponemal immobilization test. Amer. J. Hyg. **53**, 296 (1951).

NELL, E. E.: Comparative sensitivity of Treponemes of syphilis, yaws and bejel to penicillin in vitro, with observations on factors affecting its treponemicidal action. Amer. J. Syph. **38**, 92 (1954).

NELSON, R. A., JR.: Factors affecting the survival of *Treponema pallidum* in vitro. Amer. J. Hyg. **48**, 120 (1948).

NELSON, R. A., JR., MAYER, M. M.: Immobilization of *Treponema pallidum* in vitro by antibody produced in syphilitic infection. J. exp. Med. **89**, 369 (1949).

PROBEY, T. F.: Attempt to produce a penicillin-resistant strain of *Treponema pallidum* in experimental syphilis. Amer. J. Syph. **37**, 369 (1953).

TURNER, T. B., CUMBERLAND, M. C., LI, H. Y.: Comparative effectiveness of penicillin G, F, K and X in experimental syphilis as determined by a short in vivo method. Amer. J. Syph. **31**, 476 (1947).

TURNER, T. B., HOLLANDER, D. H.: Biologie des Tréponématoses, OMS, Genève (1955).

TURNER, T. B., SCHAEFFER, K.: The comparative effect of various antibiotics in experimental syphilis. Amer. J. Syph. **38**, 81 (1954).

WEBER, M. M.: Factors influencing the in vitro survival of the virulent Nichols strain of *Treponema pallidum*. Baltimore Md. Thèse, Johns Hopkins University (1953).

Experimentelle Infektionen durch Vibrionen

Hildegard Winkler und Uwe Ullmann

Mit 6 Abbildungen

I. Grundlagen

1. Systematik und Definition der Gattung Vibrio

Vibrionen werden beim Menschen, bei Tieren und im Wasser als frei lebende Mikroorganismen angetroffen. Neben den Choleravibrionen, die bei natürlichem Infektionsmodus nur für den Menschen pathogen sind, gibt es einige Species, die

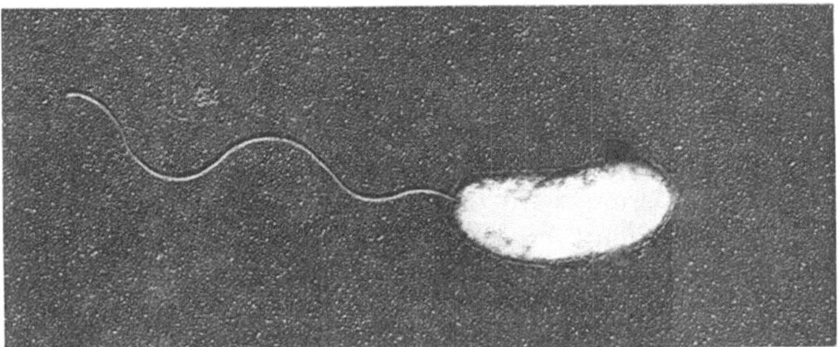

Abb. 1. V. cholerae. Vergr. 12 500fach

bei Rindern, Schafen, Schweinen, Hühnern und Fischen nachgewiesen werden und deren Pathogenität für einige Tiere bekannt ist. Alle diese Mikroorganismen werden in der Familie VII Spirillaceae der Ordnung I Pseudomonadales und der Klasse Schizomycetes zusammengefaßt (Bergey, 1957). Vibrionen sind gram-negative, kurze, leicht gebogene, kommaförmige Mikroorganismen, deren Länge mit 1,5—5,0 µ und deren Breite mit 0,2—0,5 µ angegeben wird. Die einzeln liegenden oder zu einer Wendelform vereinigten Bakterien sind beweglich und zeigen gewöhnlich eine einzelne, polar angeordnete, relativ kurze Geißel. Das Sauerstoffbedürfnis der Vibrionen gestattet eine grobe Einteilung in aerobe, mikroaerophile und anaerobe Arten (Bergey, 1957). Die aeroben Vertreter stellen in der Regel keine besonderen Ansprüche an ihr Nährmedium, während mikro-aerophile und anaerobe Arten für ihre Vermehrung spezielle Zusätze zum Nähr-substrat benötigen, wie Blut, Serum oder Ascitesflüssigkeit. Zur weiteren Ein-teilung der Vibrionen wird die Überprüfung der Stoffwechselleistungen, die Unter-suchung serologischer Eigenschaften und das Verhalten im Tierexperiment heran-gezogen. Die Einordnung aller für tierexperimentelle Untersuchungen verwendeten Arten in die bei Bergey (1957) angegebene Systematik ist nicht möglich. Bei Bergey (1957) sind nur 34 Arten aufgeführt, während die Zahl der anerkannten Species im Index Bergeyana (1966) bereits 170 beträgt. Die Systematisierung der verschiedenen Vibrionen stößt noch immer auf erhebliche Schwierigkeiten, da

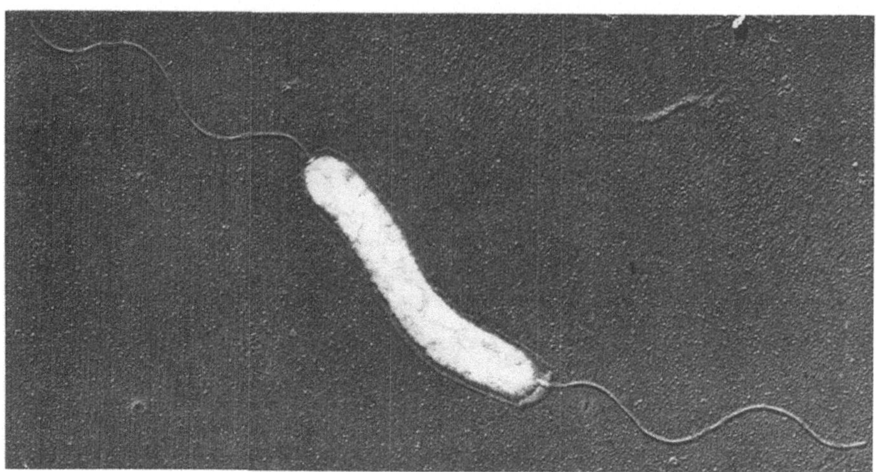

Abb. 2. V. cholerae. Vergr. 15000fach

es trotz zahlreicher Untersuchungen bisher nicht gelungen ist, einen exakten differentialdiagnostischen Schlüssel aufzustellen. Es besteht keine einheitliche Meinung darüber, welche biochemischen und serologischen Kriterien hierfür anzuwenden sind. Die Gliederung wird dadurch weiter kompliziert, daß die Arten teilweise nach ihrer Herkunft bezeichnet werden, wobei jedoch das natürliche Wirtsspektrum und der natürliche Standort mancher Vibrionenspecies noch nicht ausreichend erforscht sind.

2. Morphologische Eigenschaften

Die Feststellung der polaren, monotrichen Begeißelung ist neben der Kommaform ein unerläßliches morphologisches Kriterium für die Zuordnung eines Bacteriums zur Gattung Vibrio. Eine Unterscheidung zwischen Angehörigen der Gattung Vibrio und der Gattungen Plesiomonas, Aeromonas und Pseudomonas ist auf Grund dieses Merkmals jedoch mitunter schwierig (s. Tabelle 1). Dies trifft besonders für Vibrionen zu, die aus Wasser isoliert werden, da hier zuweilen gestreckte Formen gefunden werden. Andererseits liegen manche Pseudomonaden als leicht gebogene Stäbchenbakterien vor (Rucker, 1959; Park, 1962). Morphologische Veränderungen treten insbesondere bei älteren Kulturen auf. Hier imponieren die Vibrionen als wendelförmige Gebilde, die mit Spirillen verwechselt werden können. Von diesen lassen sich Vibrionen jedoch durch die andersartige Begeißelung unterscheiden (Löffler, 1889). Wendelformen von V. cholerae wurden bereits von Koch (1884) beschrieben. In jungen, bis 72 Std alten Kulturen von V. fetus überwiegt die kurze, kommaförmige Gestalt und die fischzugartige Anordnung, während in älteren Kulturen überwiegend Wendelformen zu sehen sind (Smith, 1918). Die bisweilen festgestellten Granula werden als Degenerationsprodukte aufgefaßt. Wendelformen sind auch in Fetalflüssigkeiten zu beobachten (Smith und Taylor, 1919).

Morphologische Varianten treten auch in Kulturen von V. anguillarum auf, wenn bei höherer Temperatur bebrütet wird. Dann werden Mikroorganismen gefunden, deren Soma nur lückenhaft angefärbt ist, sowie annähernd kugelförmige Bakterien oder fadenförmige Verbände fast gestreckter Individuen (Bergman, 1909). Von Schäperclaus (1927) wurde mitgeteilt, daß V. anguillarum in älteren

Tabelle 1. Differentialdiagnostische Merkmale verschiedener Gattungen (nach BADER 1972)

	Vibrio	Aeromonas	Plesiomonas	Pseudomonas
Glucose	$+^1$/−	$+^1$/d	$+^1$/−	$+^1$/−
Glucose, anaerob	+	+	+	−
Lactose	−	d	d	−
Mannit	+	+	−	
Inosit	−	−	+	
Gelatine	+	+	−	d
Lysin	+	d	+	
Ornithin	+	−	+	
Arginin	−	+	+	+
Begeißelung	polar monotrich	polar monotrich	polar lophotrich	polar monotrich oder lophotrich

$+^1$/− positiver Ausfall der Reaktion nach 1 Tag, keine Gasbildung; − negativer Ausfall der Reaktion; d verschiedene Reaktionen möglich. Ausnahmen sind nicht berücksichtigt.

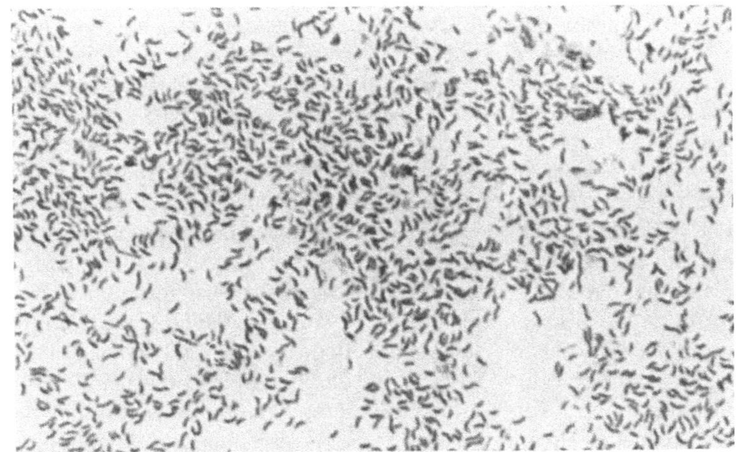

Abb. 3. V. fetus, teils in fischzugartiger Anordnung (aus 24 Std alter, flüssiger Kultur). Vergr. 800fach

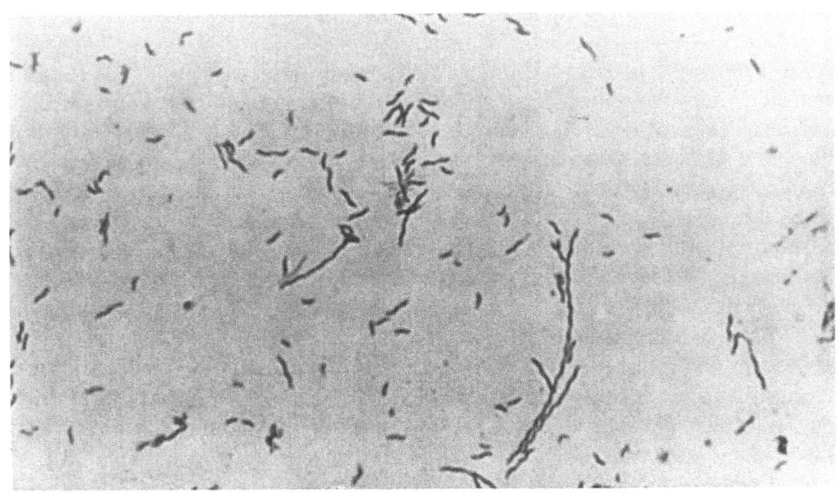

Abb. 4. V. fetus, teils wendelförmig (aus 72 Std alter, flüssiger Kultur). Vergr. 800fach

Kulturen oder bei ungeeigneten Nähr- und Vermehrungsbedingungen zur Bildung von Involutionsformen neigt. Dabei treten neben punktförmigen, kugeligen und sporenähnlichen Formen sehr langgestreckte S-förmige Gebilde auf.

3. Aerobe Vibrionen

a) Aus Menschen isolierte Vibrionen

Der bekannteste und für den Menschen bedeutsamste Vertreter ist V. cholerae, der bei Bergey (1957) als Vibrio comma bezeichnet wird. Er wurde 1883 von Koch (1884) als Erreger der Cholera des Menschen erkannt und in Reinkultur gezüchtet. Spätere Untersuchungen ergaben, daß es sich bei V. cholerae um eine serologisch nicht einheitliche Art handelt, sondern daß die beiden serologischen Typen Ogawa und Inaba nebeneinander auftreten, die als klassische Choleravibrionen bezeichnet werden; diesen beiden zuzurechnen ist der Biotyp El Tor.

Bei diagnostischen und experimentellen Arbeiten mit Cholerabakterien sind in der BRD die Vorschriften des Bundesseuchengesetzes (1961) zu beachten. Die Züchtung von Choleravibrionen ist einfach, da sie keine besonderen Ansprüche an das Nährsubstrat stellen. Für die Vermehrung günstig ist ein alkalisches Milieu von pH 8,0. Als fester Nährboden ist ein bei 37° C bebrüteter Nähragar der von Koch (1884) benutzten Nährgelatine überlegen. Dieudonné (1909) vereinfachte die Erstisolierung entscheidend durch die Einführung eines alkalisierten Blutnähragars, der die Entwicklung von Colibakterien unterdrückt. In den Stuhlproben von Cholerakranken sind die Mikroorganismen im allgemeinen so reichlich vorhanden, daß der Nachweis auf festen Nährböden primär gelingt. Werden wenige Vibrionen im Untersuchungsmaterial vermutet, so sind flüssige Medien zur Anreicherung der Erreger vorzuziehen. In ihnen vermehrt sich V. cholerae als sauerstoffhungriger Mikroorganismus nahe der Oberfläche (Schottelius, 1885). Ganz besonders hat sich das alkalische Peptonwasser (Bujwid, 1888) als Anreicherungsmedium bewährt. Nach 3—4stündiger Bebrütung bei 37° C bilden die Choleravibrionen eine Kahmhaut, so daß bereits zu diesem Zeitpunkt die Aussaat auf feste Nährböden Erfolg verspricht. Eine eingehende Darstellung von Isolierungsmethoden und Nährbodenrezepten geben Pollitzer (1959), Caselitz (1960), Felsenfeld (1966) und Bockemühl (1971). Gelegentlich finden sich in der Literatur Hinweise auf die Züchtung von Choleravibrionen unter anaeroben Bedingungen. Diese Bakterienstämme werden als besonders virulent angesehen (s. S. 70).

NAG-Vibrionen (in Choleraseren nicht agglutinierbare Vibrionen) werden gelegentlich als Erreger von sporadisch auftretenden Darmerkrankungen isoliert. Aus dem älteren Schrifttum am besten bekannt ist V. proteus (Kommabacillus der Cholera nostras, Finkler, 1884). Über die Isolierung von NAG-Vibrionen bei zum Teil schweren Darmerkrankungen aus Stuhlproben berichteten Baerthlein (1913) sowie Greig (1915, 1917). Bei epidemisch auftretenden Gastroenteritiden mit mildem Verlauf wurden sie von Gupta et al. (1956) nachgewiesen. Die Nährsubstrate für Cholerabakterien sind in gleichem Maße für die Isolierung von NAG-Vibrionen geeignet. Da diese jedoch im Untersuchungsmaterial meist in geringer Zahl vorhanden sind, ist eine Isolierung in der Regel nur mit Hilfe eines Anreicherungsmediums möglich. Es sei darauf hingewiesen, daß die Anreicherung keine quantitative Aussage über die Zahl der im Untersuchungsmaterial vorhandenen Vibrionen erlaubt. V. massauah nimmt eine Sonderstellung ein. Pfeiffer (1892) hatte V. massauah für seine „Untersuchungen über das Choleragift" verwendet. Der Stamm war in Massauah, Erythrea, isoliert worden. Dieser Mikroorganismus ist insofern bemerkenswert, weil er 1. als besonders virulent galt,

2. für eine Reihe von tierexperimentellen Untersuchungen als „Choleravibrio" herangezogen wurde, und 3. die damit erzielten Ergebnisse als „typisch für Cholera" beschrieben wurden. Da sich in späteren Untersuchungen herausstellte, daß das Bacterium 4 Geißeln besitzt, war eine Zugehörigkeit zur Gattung Vibrio auszuschließen. Obschon die damit erzielten Ergebnisse für die experimentelle Vibrioneninfektion bedeutungslos sind, werden sie doch mit angeführt, um auf die Problematik der Spezifität der mit Vibrionen erhaltenen Versuchsdaten hinzuweisen (s. S. 169).

Im Speichel der Mundhöhle des Menschen wurden Mikroorganismen gefunden, die die gleiche Form und Größe besaßen wie V. cholerae (LEWIS, 1884), aber auch Bakterien, die morphologisch mehr V. proteus ähnelten (HÜPPE, 1884). Als aerobe Vibrionenarten der Mundhöhle führt BERGEY (1957) V. sputigenus und V. tonsillaris an. *V. sputigenus* wurde neben Fränkelschen Diplokokken bereits bei der mikroskopischen Untersuchung des Auswurfes eines Patienten beobachtet, der an Pneumonie erkrankt war (BRIX, 1894). *V. tonsillaris* ist ein von STEPHENS et al. (1896) aus der Mundhöhle isolierter Mikroorganismus. *V. parahaemolyticus* wurde bei Menschen isoliert, die an einer Enteritis erkrankt waren (SAKAZAKI et al., 1963). Sie trat häufig nach dem Genuß von „Shirasuboshi" (halbgetrocknete, junge Sardinen) und „Sushi" (gekochter Reis mit rohem Fisch oder Schellfisch) auf. Die Untersuchung gesunder Kontrollpersonen, welche in den Sommermonaten Fische verzehrten, erbrachte den Nachweis des Bacteriums in 0,8% des Kollektivs (ZEN-YOJI et al., 1965).

Für die Praxis der Choleradiagnostik wichtig ist die Unterscheidung zwischen V. cholerae und anderen Vibrionen, die Identifizierung der Typen Ogawa und Inaba sowie die Abgrenzung des Biotyps El Tor und die Klassifizierung der NAG-Vibrionen. Die Abgrenzung der NAG-Vibrionen von den Choleravibrionen erfolgt auf Grund biochemischer und serologischer Untersuchungen (HEIBERG, 1934; GARDNER und VENKATRAMAN, 1935). Nach HEIBERG (1934) lassen sich Choleravibrionen von anderen Vibrionenarten durch die unterschiedliche Vergärung von Saccharose, Arabinose und Mannose trennen (s. Tabelle 2). Sie gehören der Gruppe I an; die anderen Vibrionen finden sich in den Gruppen II—VI. Eine serologische Einteilung ist mit Hilfe der Agglutinationsreaktion möglich (GARDNER und VENKATRAMAN, 1935). Die „klassischen" Choleravibrionen sowie die Mehrzahl der hämolysierenden El-Tor-Stämme sind Angehörige der Untergruppe 1. In den Untergruppen 2—4 sind unter anderem aus Wasser isolierte Vibrionen, in den Untergruppen 5 und 6 auch einzelne El-Tor-Stämme angeführt. Eine zusammenfassende Darstellung der Stoffwechseluntersuchungen (BOCKEMÜHL, 1971) und serologischen Verfahren für die Identifizierung von Vibrionen geben POLLITZER (1959) und FELSENFELD (1966).

Tabelle 2. Einteilung der Vibrionen nach HEIBERG (1936) und SMITH et al. (1965). (Zusammenstellung nach BADER, 1972)

Gruppe	Saccharose	Arabinose	Mannose	Agglutinabilität in Ogawa- oder Inabaserum	Zahl der Stämme	
					nach HEIBERG (1936)[a]	nach SMITH et al. (1965)[b]
I	+	Ø	+	+ seltener Ø	287	47
II	+	Ø	Ø	Ø	75	140
III	+	+	+	Ø	12	13
IV	+	+	Ø	Ø	3	1
V	Ø	Ø	+	Ø	2	13
VI	Ø	Ø	Ø	Ø	5	3
VII	Ø	+	+	Ø	0	22
VIII	Ø	+	Ø	Ø	0	0

[a] Stämme verschiedener Herkunft.
[b] "Noncholera vibrios from diarrheal disease".

b) Aus Wasser und Kaltblütern isolierte Vibrionen

Zum Nachweis von Vibrionen aus Wasser ist in der Regel die Pepton-anreicherung anzuwenden, da auf festen Nährböden die vorhandene Begleitflora ihre Entwicklung unterdrückt. Ob die einzelnen Artbezeichnungen ihre Berechtigung haben, oder ob mitunter einige Arten identisch sind, muß dahingestellt bleiben. Eine biochemische oder serologische Überprüfung der Stämme ist heute zum Teil nicht mehr möglich, da sie nicht mehr zur Verfügung stehen.

V. berolinensis wurde von Pfeiffer (1889) als neue, aus Wasser isolierte Vibrionenart beschrieben. *V. aquatilis* isolierte Günther (1892, 1893) aus unfiltriertem Spreewasser. *V. albensis* ist eine aus der Elbe gezüchtete Art (Dunbar, 1896). *V. parahaemolyticus* konnte aus Meer- und Brackwasser sowie aus der Einmündung von Abwasserkanälen in das Meer isoliert werden (Sakazaki et al., 1963; Barros und Liston, 1970; Aldová et al., 1971). Der Mikroorganismus war im küstenfernen Seewasser nicht mehr zu finden (Zen-Yoji et al., 1965). *V. anguillarum* wurde von Bergman (1909) bei einer Krankheit des Aales isoliert und damit erstmals als Erreger einer Fischseuche verifiziert. Schäperclaus (1927) konnte V. anguillarum ebenfalls bei einer Aalkrankheit in der Ostsee züchten. In neuerer Zeit berichten Lagarde und Chakroun (1965) über eine durch V. anguillarum hervorgerufene Epizootie bei Aalen, Bagge und Bagge (1956) über eine Infektion bei Dorschen, während Smith (1961) eine Infektion von Bachforellen in Schottland beobachtete.

Für eine ansteckende Keratomalazie bei Dorschen an der Südküste Schwedens wurden ebenfalls Vibrionen verantwortlich gemacht, die allerdings nicht näher benannt worden sind (Bergman, 1912).

David (1927) isolierte bei einer Karpfenseuche *V. piscium.* Dieser Erreger wurde von V. anguillarum mit dem Hinweis unterschieden, daß letzterer aus Meerwasser isoliert worden war. *V. piscium var. japonicus* ist als Erreger einer infektiösen Erkrankung der Regenbogenforelle ermittelt worden (Hoshina, 1956, 1957).

V. ichthyodermis wurde von Wells und ZoBell (1934) als Erreger einer infektiösen Dermatitis bei Seefischen erkannt und zunächst in die Gattung Pseudomonas eingeordnet. Spätere Untersuchungen ergaben, daß er der Gattung Vibrio zuzuordnen ist (Shewan et al., 1960). *V. alginolyticus* wies Sakazaki (1965) in etwa 80% bei 336 Untersuchungsproben aus Seewasser, Seefischen und Fischprodukten nach. Dieses Bacterium konnte auch aus menschlichem Untersuchungsmaterial bei Enteritiden isoliert werden. V. parahaemolyticus wurde ebenfalls aus Seefischen, vor allem in Sommermonaten (Zen-Yoji et al., 1965; Nakanishi et al., 1968), gezüchtet.

Manche Vibrionen erhielten keine Artbezeichnung, so die als Krankheitserreger bei 5 verschiedenen Lachsspecies im Pazifik nachgewiesenen Mikroorganismen (Rucker et al., 1954). Vor kurzem wurde vorgeschlagen, die Species V. anguillarum (Bergman, 1909), V. piscium (David, 1927) und V. ichthyodermis (Wells und ZoBell, 1934; Shewan et al., 1960) in einer einzigen Species zusammenzufassen, die die Bezeichnung V. anguillarum tragen soll (Hendrie et al., 1971).

Aus Muscheln wurden *V. cardii* (Klein, 1905) und *V. toulonensis* (Defressine und Cazeneuve, 1919) gezüchtet. V. parahaemolyticus konnte ebenfalls aus Krabben (Krantz et al., 1969) und Austern (Bartley und Slanetz, 1971) isoliert werden.

Falls die im Wasser vorkommenden Vibrionen von Warmblütern stammen, gelingt ihr Nachweis auf den für V. cholerae angegebenen Nährmedien. Bei der

Isolierung von fischpathogenen Vibrionen und Seewasservibrionen ist zu beachten, daß sie ein niedriges Temperaturoptimum besitzen und zumeist halophil sind. Fischpathogene Vibrionen gedeihen aerob auf Agar und Gelatinenährböden; V. anguillarum vermehrt sich jedoch auch in anaerobem Milieu (BERGMAN, 1909; SMITH, 1961). Bei Zimmertemperatur benötigt V. piscium 3—4 Tage, bevor eine makroskopisch sichtbare Kolonie auf dem Nährmedium festgestellt werden kann. Nach einigen Kulturpassagen verkürzt sich die Generationszeit, so daß die Kolonien innerhalb 24 Std zu beobachten sind (DAVID, 1927). Eine Vermehrung von V. anguillarum findet bei Temperaturen zwischen 5 und 38° C statt; das Optimum beträgt 30° C (BERGMAN, 1909). Bei 37° C auf festen und flüssigen Nährmedien bebrütete Kulturen sterben nach wenigen Tagen ab (SCHÄPERCLAUS, 1927; SMITH, 1961). Im Gegensatz hierzu gibt SAKAZAKI (1965) an, daß der von ihm isolierte V. parahaemolyticus noch bei 42° C Vermehrung zeigt. Der optimale Salzgehalt des Nährmediums für aus Seewasser isolierte Vibrionen beträgt 1,5—2% (SCHÄPERCLAUS, 1927; BAGGE und BAGGE, 1956; SMITH, 1961; LAGARDE und CHAKROUN, 1965). Ein NaCl-Gehalt von 3% wirkt bereits hemmend auf diese Mikroorganismen. V. anguillarum vermehrt sich in geringem Umfang noch bei einer Salzkonzentration von 7% (BERGMAN, 1909). Zur biochemischen Identifizierung der fischpathogenen Vibrionen werden die Kohlenhydratvergärung, Indolbildung, Nitratreduktion, Gelatineverflüssigung und Ammoniakproduktion herangezogen (SMITH, 1961).

c) Aus Großtieren isolierte Vibrionen

In der Veterinärmedizin spielen aerobe Vibrionen eine untergeordnete Rolle im Gegensatz zu mikroaerophilen Vibrionen, die aus Rindern, Schafen und Schweinen isoliert werden. SMITH (1891) berichtete über einen aeroben, Gelatine nicht verflüssigenden Vibrio, den er aus dem Dickdarm von Schweinen züchten konnte. Er war bereits bakterioskopisch im nekrotischen Gewebe kleiner Geschwüre zu finden. Aus Schweinen und Großtieren isolierte FLORENT (1957) ebenfalls aerobe Vibrionen, die den von SMITH (1891) erwähnten Mikroorganismen entsprechen dürften.

d) Aus Vögeln isolierte Vibrionen

Die bekannteste Art ist *V. metschnikovii*, der als Erreger einer Infektionskrankheit von Hühnern erstmals in der Gegend von Odessa erkannt wurde (GAMALEIA, 1888a). Auch bei 500 importierten Sonnenvögeln (Leiothrix luteus L.) wurden aerobe Vibrionen als Ursache eines seuchenhaften Sterbens nachgewiesen; alle Tiere waren auf dem Transport oder bald nach der Ankunft am Bestimmungsort zugrundegegangen. Der Erreger wurde als sehr nahe verwandt, wenn nicht identisch mit V. metschnikovii angesehen (KRAUSE und WINDRATH, 1919). Möglicherweise ebenfalls identisch mit diesem Krankheitserreger sind auch die von KUMJUMGIEV (1957) aus Hühnern und Fasanen isolierten Vibrionen. V. metschnikovii vermehrt sich aerob auf Nähragar und Gelatinemedium bei Zimmertemperatur. Zur Anreicherung hat sich eine leicht alkalische Kalbsbouillon mit und ohne Peptonzusatz bewährt. Bereits nach 6—7 Std zeigt dieses flüssige Medium eine gleichmäßige Trübung und nach 24 Std ein allmählich dichter werdendes Oberflächenhäutchen. Das Bacterium vermehrt sich auch unter mikroaerophilen und anaeroben Bedingungen (GAMALEIA, 1888a; PFEIFFER, 1889). Daß manche dieser aeroben Vibrionen unter mikroaerophilen bzw. anaeroben Bedingungen gedeihen, macht es erforderlich, das Sauerstoffbedürfnis der Vibrionen in jedem Fall zu ermitteln.

e) Aus anderen Tieren und Untersuchungsmaterial isolierte Vibrionen

Die im folgenden aufgeführten Mikroorganismen wurden selten, zumeist nur einmal nachgewiesen; manche besitzen 2—3 polare Geißeln, werden jedoch von Bergey (1957) den Vibrionen zugerechnet. *V. xenopus* konnte aus dem Absceß eines afrikanischen Frosches (Xenopus laevis) isoliert werden. Da hierbei noch 2 weitere Bakterienarten gezüchtet wurden, ist seine pathogene Bedeutung fraglich (Schrire und Greenfield, 1930). *V. extorquens* wurde aus den Exkrementen von Regenwürmern gezüchtet (Bhat und Barker, 1948) und *V. leonardi* aus Raupen der Gattung Pyrausta (Métalnikov und Chorine, 1928). Dieser Mikroorganismus wurde als pathogen für Insekten angesehen. Bei *V. tyrogenus* (Deneke, 1885) handelt es sich um ein aus Käse isoliertes Bacterium. *V. percolans* (Mudd und Warren, 1923) konnte aus Heuinfus gezüchtet werden.

4. Mikroaerophile Vibrionen

Züchtungsbedingungen und Identifizierung. Mikroaerophile Vibrionen haben ihren Standort beim Tier. Die bedeutendste pathogene Art ist *V. fetus*, der bei Rind und Schaf zu Aborten und Sterilität führt. *V. jejuni* verursacht Darmerkrankungen bei Rind und Kalb, *V. coli* ruft eine Enteritis beim Schwein hervor. Hinzu kommen weitere pathogene und apathogene Vibrionen mit vorläufigen Sammel- und Gruppenbezeichnungen, die aus Großtieren und Vögeln isoliert wurden. Infektionen des Menschen mit mikroaerophilen Vibrionen wurden bisher nur vereinzelt mitgeteilt.

Mikroaerophilen Vibrionen ist gemeinsam, daß für ihre Vermehrung komplizierte Züchtungsbedingungen erforderlich sind. Als festes Nährmedium wird häufig ein Nähragar verwendet, dem 10% Blut zugegeben ist. Eine Erhöhung der CO_2-Spannung fördert die Vermehrung. Da im Untersuchungsmaterial von Rindern, Schafen, Schweinen und Hühnern meist eine Mischflora vorliegt, empfiehlt sich für die Isolierung der Vibrionen die Verwendung von Selektivnährböden. Mit einer mehr oder weniger starken Begleitflora ist bei Untersuchungsproben aus Genitalsekreten (Praeputialspülproben, Vaginalschleim), bei der Untersuchung von Feten, Nachgeburten und bei Fäkalproben zu rechnen. Als Selektivmedien sind geeignet ein Rinderherzbouillonagar mit Brillantgrün-Lösung (Florent, 1956) sowie antibioticahaltige Nährsubstrate (s. Bisping et al., 1964; Maciak und Winkenwerder, 1964). Zur Isolierung von Hühnervibrionen aus Leber- und Galleproben wird das bebrütete Hühnerei bevorzugt (Peckham, 1958; Vielitz et al., 1965). Seit einiger Zeit werden auch Membranfilter zur Selektion der Vibrionen von Begleitbakterien benützt (Loesche et al., 1965; Smibert, 1965; Dufty, 1967). In Subkulturen vermehren sich mikroaerophile Vibrionen auch auf Nährmedien ohne Serumzusatz, so auf einem Kligler-Nähragar (Bader et al., 1966). Ausführliche Zusammenstellungen über geeignete Nährsubstrate geben Kamel (1960), Laing (1960), Bisping et al. (1964). Als wesentlichste Kriterien für die Artbestimmung der Vibrionen gelten die Überprüfung der Katalase- und Schwefelwasserstoffbildung. Stämme, die Katalase bilden, aber keinen Schwefelwasserstoff, werden im allgemeinen der Species V. fetus zugerechnet. Eine Reihe der vom Rind und Schaf isolierten apathogenen Vibrionen zeigen keine Katalase, dagegen reichlich Schwefelwasserstoffbildung und sind zur Vermehrung in einem Milieu fähig, das 3,5% NaCl enthält. Hierzu gehören unter anderen die Vibrionen der Gruppe 2 von Bryner und Frank (1955) sowie andere, vorläufige Bezeichnungen tragende Vibrionen. Zur Sicherung der Artdiagnose sind weiter serologische Verfahren, wie die Agglutination, die Komplementbindung und indirekte Hämagglutination anzuwenden (MITSCHERLICH und LIESS, 1958a—c; BADER et al., 1966; BERG et al., 1971).

a) Aus Großtieren isolierte Vibrionen

α) *Rind*. Der überwiegende Teil der tierexperimentellen Untersuchungen wurde mit V. fetus durchgeführt. SMITH (1918) hatte diese Bakterienspecies beim seuchenhaften Verwerfen des Rindes isoliert. Von 109 Aborten waren nach SMITH 57% durch Brucella abortus, 24% durch V. fetus und die restlichen durch andere Mikroorganismen oder aus unbekannter Ursache verursacht. Im allgemeinen sind Rinder ab der 2. oder späteren Trächtigkeit betroffen, jedoch können auch Aborte bei Jungkühen auf V. fetus-Infektionen zurückgeführt werden (SMITH, 1918, 1919b). Neben der morphologischen, serologischen und biochemischen Charakterisierung ist es das Verdienst dieses Autors, den Kausalzusammenhang zwischen tierischer Infektion und Abort aufgezeigt zu haben. SMITH (1918) vertrat die Ansicht, daß der von McFADYEAN und STOCKMAN (1913) aus Rinder- und Schaffeten isolierte Mikroorganismus mit dem von ihm beschriebenen V. fetus identisch sei. In Deutschland gelang GMINDER (1922) zuerst der kulturelle Nachweis von „Spirillen" in abortierten Rinderfeten. V. fetus ist nicht nur Ursache von Aborten, sondern führt auch zur Sterilität. Er liegt in 2 Varianten vor, deren Reaktionsverhalten sich biochemisch und serologisch unterscheidet. Die wesentlichen klinischen Unterschiede zwischen den von beiden Erregern verursachten Genitalvibriosen sind folgende (FLORENT, 1959):

1. V. fetus var. venerealis (Typ A) ruft eine venerische Infektion hervor, deren Folge Abort oder enzootische Sterilität sein kann.

2. V. fetus var. intestinalis (Typ B) führt zum seuchenhaften Verwerfen; eine Fertilitätsstörung wird nicht beobachtet.

Demnach wäre V. fetus var. intestinalis nicht der Erreger einer venerischen Infektion. PARK et al. (1962) berichten jedoch, daß auch der von ihnen isolierte Typ B im Genitaltrakt des Schafes bis zu 12 Monate überleben und eine Genitalvibriosis verursachen kann. BRYNER und FRANK (1955) sowie TERPSTRA (1956) geben den bei Feten, Rindern und Bullen nachgewiesenen Vibrionen Gruppenbezeichnungen. Dabei wird V. fetus var. venerealis der Gruppe I und V. fetus var. intestinalis der Gruppe III zugeordnet. Weiterführende Darstellungen finden sich im Veter. Record (anonym, 1958) und bei LAING (1960). Während ursprünglich noch keine Beziehung zum Bullen als möglichem Überträger der Vibriosis genitalis vermutet wurde (SMITH, 1918), haben neuere Forschungen ergeben, daß der Verbreitung durch den Deckakt große Bedeutung zukommt. V. fetus var. venerealis hat seinen Sitz im Praeputialsack des Bullen. Bei der Untersuchung von 795 Bullen wurden 114mal apathogene Vibrionen und bei 8 Tieren V. fetus var. venerealis nachgewiesen (s. BISPING et al., 1964).

Aus Bullensperma und der Vagina gedeckter Färsen isolierte FLORENT (1953) einen Mikroorganismus, der die Bezeichnung *V. bubulus* erhielt. Er besitzt keine Antigengemeinschaft mit V. fetus und gilt als Saprophyt (FLORENT, 1953; THOUVENOT und FLORENT, 1954). V. bubulus wird von V. fetus durch eine ausgeprägtere Anaerobiose, die Produktion von Schwefelwasserstoff und fehlende Katalasebildung unterschieden. *V. jejuni* wird dagegen als ein rinderpathogener Vertreter erachtet. Er ist aus dem Darminhalt bei Dysenterie von Rindern und Kälbern zu isolieren und als Ursache einer vornehmlich in den Wintermonaten auftretenden blutig-schleimigen Enteritis anzusehen (JONES und LITTLE, 1931a, b). Bei einer Synopsis der bisher isolierten und als V. jejuni bezeichneten Bakterienstämme ist hervorzuheben, daß sie sehr unterschiedliche biochemische Merkmale aufweisen

(Maciak et al., 1966), die berechtigte Zweifel an der Einheitlichkeit dieser Bakterienspecies aufkommen lassen.

β) Schaf. McFadyean und Stockman (1913) waren die ersten, die über infektiöse Aborte beim Schaf berichteten. Die kontagiöse V. fetus-Infektion ist durch einen Abort im fortgeschrittenen Stadium der Trächtigkeit charakterisiert. Der noch nicht völlig aufgeklärte Infektionsmodus scheint anders zu verlaufen als beim Vibrionenabort des Rindes. Dem männlichen Tier wird hier keine oder nur untergeordnete Bedeutung für die Übertragung der Krankheit zugemessen (Firehammer et al., 1956).

γ) Schwein. Bei diesem Tier werden Vibrionen aus dem Verdauungstrakt gesunder und kranker Tiere gezüchtet. Die während einer Dysenterie der Schweine gefundenen Vibrionen erhielten die Artbezeichnung *V. coli* (Doyle, 1944, 1948). Auch sie sind, wie die Überprüfung der Stoffwechselleistungen zeigt, nicht einheitlich (Roberts, 1956 b; Maciak und Winkenwerder, 1964; Söderlind, 1965).

b) Aus Vögeln isolierte Vibrionen

Zahlreiche Untersuchungen liegen über die Verbreitung von Vibrionen bei Hühnern vor. Sie werden häufig aus dem Intestinaltrakt gesunder und kranker Tiere isoliert. Von besonderem Interesse für tierexperimentelle Arbeiten sind jene Vibrionen, die als Ursache krankhafter Leberveränderungen bei diesen Tieren gelten. In verschiedenen Ländern gelang bei Hepatitiden die Züchtung aus Lebergewebe und Gallenflüssigkeit. Aus den USA liegen darüber Untersuchungen vor von Hofstad et al. (1958) und Peckham (1958), aus Holland von Voute und Grimbergen (1959), aus Österreich von Grünberg und Otte (1963) sowie Kölbl (1964), aus Deutschland von Bisping et al. (1963) und Vielitz et al. (1965). Die Beurteilung der hepatopathogenen Bedeutung der vom Huhn isolierten Vibrionen ist mitunter schwierig, da bei den erkrankten Tieren nicht selten neben Leberschäden auch andere Organveränderungen festzustellen sind. Wahrscheinlich sind die Vibrionen nur eine Ursache der bei Hühnern vorkommenden Hepatitis, zumal dieses Krankheitsbild auch ohne Vibrionennachweis beschrieben wurde (Beaudette und Hudson, 1954; Tudor, 1954). Noch nicht hinreichend untersucht ist die Frage, ob Hühner diese Vibrionen auch als Saprophyten beherbergen. Ihre Übertragung auf das Huhn durch Wildvögel wird von Grünberg und Otte (1963) angenommen. Bei dem in der Umgebung von Hühnerbeständen weitverbreiteten Haussperling (Passer domesticus L.) wurden bei 20% der Tiere Vibrionen im Darmkanal bzw. in den inneren Organen nachgewiesen (Abdallah und Winkenwerder, 1966).

Offenbar gehören auch die aus Hühnern isolierten mikroaerophilen Vibrionen, besonders diejenigen, welche für das als infektiöse Hepatitis bezeichnete Krankheitsbild verantwortlich sind, mehreren Arten an, deren biochemische und serologische Merkmale sich beträchtlich unterscheiden (Peckham, 1958; Whenham et al., 1961). Nach Einteilung zahlreicher, von Hühnern isolierter Vibrionen in zwei morphologisch verschiedene Gruppen zeigten die Stämme der beiden Gruppen ein unterschiedliches biochemisches Verhalten (Bisping et al., 1963). Auch eine serologische Klassifizierung biochemisch unterschiedlicher Hühnervibrionen ist noch nicht eindeutig gelungen. Eine Antigengemeinschaft mit V. fetus O-Antigen 1 und O-Antigen 2 scheint zu bestehen (Winkenwerder und Bisping, 1964; Abdallah und Winkenwerder, 1966).

c) Aus Menschen isolierte Vibrionen

Veröffentlichungen über die Infektion des Menschen mit Vibrionen, die ihren Standort bei Rind und Schaf haben, sind selten. In der Weltliteratur wurden bisher über 80 derartige Erkrankungen beschrieben (ULLMANN, 1969). Meist handelt es sich um eine Infektion mit V. fetus der serologischen Gruppe 1 oder 2 nach MITSCHERLICH und LIESS (1958a—c). Die Isolierung der Erreger bei septischem Abort wurde selten beschrieben, bei den meisten Erkrankten bestand eine Septicämie oder Meningitis. Ein von KING (1957) als „*related vibrio*" bezeichnetes Bacterium, das sich serologisch und biochemisch von V. fetus differenzieren läßt, wurde gelegentlich aus Darminhalt bei Gastroenteritis, aber auch aus Blut bei Bakteriämien gezüchtet. Eine Übersicht der bekannt gewordenen V. fetus-Infektionen des Menschen geben BADER et al. (1966), WINKENWERDER (1966a), STILLE und HELM (1969) und ULLMANN (1969).

d) Aus anderen Tieren isolierte Vibrionen

Mikroaerophile Vibrionen wurden bei Antilopen und Ziegen (TRUEBLOOD und POST, 1959) und bei Pferden (WINKENWERDER und BÖTTCHER, 1965) nachgewiesen. Aus dem Uterus einer Katze, die an einer chronischen Endometritis litt, konnte ebenfalls ein Vibrio isoliert werden, dessen biochemische Eigenschaften mit denen von V. fetus identisch waren (VALLEE et al., 1961). Die Untersuchung des Darminhaltes (Jejunum, Colon und Rectum) von 100 klinisch gesunden Hunden und 8 Katzen erbrachte in 15,7% den Nachweis von mikroaerophilen Vibrionen. Ob diesen eine pathogene Bedeutung zukommt, ist nicht bekannt (WINKENWERDER, 1966b).

5. Anaerobe Vibrionen

Züchtungsbedingungen. Die Züchtung anaerober Vibrionen gelingt in der Regel auf blut- oder serumhaltigen Nährmedien. Als ein optimales, flüssiges Nährsubstrat bietet sich die Thioclykolat-Bouillon mit 10% Serumzusatz an (MOORE, 1954). Nach 2 Tagen wird in diesem Medium eine diffuse Trübung bis 0,5 cm unterhalb der Oberfläche festgestellt. Die Bebrütung erfolgt im allgemeinen im Zeisslertopf bei 37° C unter Zugabe von 90% H_2 und 10% CO_2. Nach den Untersuchungen von MOORE (1954) waren alle Stämme bei der Erstisolierung strikt anaerob, nach mehreren Subkulturen vermehrten sie sich jedoch mäßig gut auch ohne Zusatz von CO_2. Auf serumfreien und bei 22°C bebrüteten Nährmedien entwickelten sie sich nicht. *V. sputorum* wird bei BERGEY (1957) als strikt anaerober Mikroorganismus aufgeführt. Nach den Untersuchungen von LOESCHE et al. (1965) scheint es indessen, daß eine strenge Unterscheidung zwischen mikroaerophilen und anaeroben Vibrionen bei manchen Arten nicht mehr aufrechterhalten werden kann. So gedeiht V. sputorum auch mikroaerophil, wenngleich weniger gut als beispielsweise V. fetus. Die Autoren untersuchten eingehend die biochemischen Merkmale von V. sputorum und empfahlen, diesen Mikroorganismus als V. sputorum var. bubulus zu bezeichnen. Hier muß allerdings angefügt werden, daß V. sputorum im Gegensatz zu V. bubulus nicht in der Lage ist, H_2S zu bilden oder sich in einem Medium mit 3,5% NaCl zu entwickeln. Eine Klassifizierung anaerober Vibrionen ist von PRÉVOT (1940, 1955) erarbeitet worden.

a) Aus Menschen isolierte Vibrionen

Für den Menschen ist die pathogene Bedeutung anaerober Vibrionen nicht gesichert. PRÉVOT (1955) ist der Ansicht, daß sie nicht in der Lage sind, charakteristische Erkrankungen hervorzurufen. In Verbindung mit anderen Bakterien können sie insbesondere in Körperhöhlen eine pathogene Wirkung entfalten. Für Krankheitsbilder dieser Art wird die Bezeichnung „anaerobe Vibriose" vorgeschlagen (PRÉVOT, 1955). Nach ihrem Standort können unterschieden werden:

Vibrionen, die bei mischinfizierten putriden Prozessen in Kavitäten gefunden werden, Vibrionen der Mundhöhle und Vibrionen im Genitaltrakt der Frau bei pathologischen Prozessen.

V. niger wird als Ursache gangränöser fötider Eiterungen angesehen (Rist, 1901). *V. tenuis* konnte aus superinfizierten tuberkulösen Kavernen isoliert werden (Veillon und Repaci, 1912). Bei derartigen putriden und gangränösen Prozessen mit fötiden Sputen können stets anaerobe Bakterien gezüchtet werden. *V. sputorum* fand Tunnicliff (1914) bei einem Patienten mit akuter Bronchitis. Bevor die Pathogenität dieses Bacteriums im Tierversuch überprüft werden konnte, war der Mikroorganismus jedoch abgestorben. Curtis (1913) isolierte aus dem Uterus und Vaginalsekret einer Patientin mit Puerperalinfektion einen anaeroben, kommaförmigen Mikroorganismus, während Smith (1930) auch bei einer Angina Plaut-Vincenti Vibrionen nachweisen konnte. Anaerobe Vibrionen wurden schließlich auch bei Frauen isoliert, die wegen Infertilität in Behandlung waren (Moore, 1954).

b) Aus Tieren isolierte Vibrionen

Fraser (1961) züchtete einen strikt anaeroben Vibrio aus einem Königspinguin (Aptenodytes longirostris). Er wurde als nahe verwandt mit V. bubulus angesehen, jedoch waren die Untersuchungsergebnisse begrenzt, da es nicht gelungen war, ihn über einige Subkulturen hinaus vermehrungsfähig zu halten. Obwohl Vibrio bubulus auch unter anaeroben Bedingungen gedeiht, wird er in Übereinstimmung mit der Ansicht anderer Autoren (s. Maciak et al., 1966) bei den mikroaerophilen Vibrionen besprochen.

II. Versuchstiere, Infektionsmethoden und Verlauf des Tierexperiments

Tierexperimentelle Untersuchungen mit Krankheitserregern dienen der Entwicklung von Modellvorstellungen über ein Krankheitsgeschehen, um daraus Methoden der Verhütung und Heilung der Erkrankung des Menschen abzuleiten. Beim Umgang mit Versuchstieren sind die entsprechenden gesetzlichen Bestimmungen einzuhalten. Während früher hauptsächlich mit vermehrungsfähigen Choleravibrionen experimentiert wurde, arbeiten die Untersucher in jüngerer Zeit überwiegend mit abgetöteten Choleravibrionen, Kulturfiltraten und Zellextrakten. Über Tierversuche mit anderen Vibrionen wird in dem Abschnitt C berichtet.

A. Infektion mit vermehrungsfähigen Choleravibrionen

Ein „choleraähnliches Krankheitsbild" im Tierversuch hervorzurufen schien zunächst schwierig, da es keine Tierspecies gibt, die unter natürlichen Bedingungen an Cholera erkrankt (Koch, 1884). Dies erklärt die Suche nach geeigneten Methoden, um beim Tier möglichst die gleichen Krankheitssymptome auslösen zu können, wie sie bei der Cholera des Menschen beobachtet werden. Die Infektion mit Cholerabakterien ist dadurch ausgezeichnet, daß diese nicht in das Gewebe oder die Blutbahn eindringen, sondern sich im Darmkanal ansiedeln, vermehren und dabei profuse Diarrhoen hervorrufen. Tierexperimentelle Arbeiten dienten zum großen Teil zur Klärung der Frage, wodurch die charakteristischen Symptome hervorgerufen werden. Nach neueren Forschungsergebnissen sind die Diarrhoen begründet durch eine Hemmung des aktiven Natriumtransports vom Darmlumen in das Plasma. Die Blockade der „Natriumpumpe" führt zu einer Wasser- und Natriumverarmung des Plasmas, als deren unmittelbare Folge

Oligurie oder Anurie auftreten, die Nierenschädigungen und Kreislaufkollaps mit sich bringen. Die auf unterschiedliche Weise und an verschiedenen Tierspecies vorgenommenen Untersuchungen haben zu meist wenig übereinstimmenden und auch einander widersprechenden Ergebnissen geführt. Dies beruht vor allem auf der unterschiedlichen Methodik der Vorbehandlung der Tiere und der differierenden Virulenz der benutzten Bakterienstämme, so daß es erforderlich erscheint, einige allgemeine Bemerkungen vorauszuschicken über: 1. Maßnahmen, um Tiere für eine Infektion empfänglich zu machen, 2. die Gewinnung von virulenten Choleravibrionen sowie 3. über Tierversuche mit infektiösem Patienten- bzw. Tiermaterial anstelle von Reinkulturen.

1. Maßnahmen, um Tiere für eine Infektion empfänglich zu machen

Da *Unterernährung* und gastrointestinale Störungen den Menschen für eine Choleraerkrankung prädisponieren, wurde versucht, Tiere durch Hungernlassen empfänglicher zu machen. Im allgemeinen wird Meerschweinchen und Kaninchen, aber auch Affen, 24—48 Std vor der Infektion unter Weitergabe von Wasser, das Futter entzogen. Um bei oraler Applikation eine bessere Aufnahme der Mikroorganismen oder der Toxindosis zu erreichen, wurde häufig vor Versuchsbeginn eine Magenspülung vorgenommen (Tizzoni und Cattani, 1888; Koch, 1885; Issaeff und Kolle, 1894; Cohendy und Wollman, 1922). Mit dieser Maßnahme gelingt es jedoch nicht, den Magen von Meerschweinchen vollständig zu entleeren (Koch, 1885). In einer anderen Versuchsanordnung wurde vor oraler Infektion nach Alkalisierung des Magens entweder eine Ruhigstellung des Darmes durch Opium angestrebt oder der Darm durch Alkohol in Reizzustand versetzt. Koch (1885), der die verschiedensten Reizmittel auf ihre Tauglichkeit erprobte, vermerkt, daß Alkohol davon die sicherste Wirkung erbrachte, doch eine Ruhigstellung des Darmes durch Opium allen anderen Maßnahmen vorzuziehen ist.

Eine präzise quantitative Angabe der Alkoholdosis gibt Doyen (1885), der vor der Applikation von Choleravibrionen in den Magen 1,6—1,8 ml 40%igen Äthylalkohol pro 100 g Körpergewicht des Versuchstieres instillierte.

Durch orale Verabfolgung von absolutem Alkohol an 2 aufeinanderfolgenden Tagen gelang es Thomas (1893), die Empfänglichkeit von Kaninchen für Choleravibrionen nach intravenöser Infektion um etwa das 6fache zu steigern (s. S. 92). Thomas glaubte, damit eine Bestätigung für die Beobachtung gefunden zu haben, daß Alkoholiker besonders häufig an Cholera erkranken. Von anderer Seite wurde gegen diese Methodik eingewandt, daß Alkohol in der verwendeten Dosierung bereits eine stark toxische Wirkung besitzt (Issaeff und Kolle, 1894). Laxantien auf saliner Basis — im allgemeinen 10 g Natriumsulfat — verabreichten Pottevin und Violle (1913a) zusammen mit den Erregern bei Tierexperimenten mit Affen. Als Voraussetzung für eine erfolgreiche Infektion des Meerschweinchens wurde die intraperitoneale Injektion von 0,01—0,02 g Podophyllin erachtet (Cantacuzene und Marie, 1914). Die damit erzielten Ergebnisse sind zurückhaltend zu bewerten, da die angegebene Podophyllinmenge allein toxisch wirkte. Bei Verwendung kleinerer Dosen kam es zu keiner erfolgreichen Infektion (Freter, 1955). Untersuchungen an Affen ergaben, daß Abführmittel allein eine Diarrhoe hervorrufen, an der die Tiere zugrunde gehen können (Hasan et al., 1965).

Die Gabe von *Gallenflüssigkeit* wurde ebenfalls angewandt, um Tiere für Choleravibrionen empfänglich zu machen. Dabei erlagen die Versuchstiere der Infektion mit Erregerdosen, die ohne Gallevorbehandlung nicht tödlich waren. So injizierte Bezzola (1912) Kaninchengalle mit Choleravibrionen vermischt Meerschweinchen und Kaninchen intraperitoneal, Masaki (1922) gab erwachsenen

Kaninchen Galle oral, während GOLOVANOFF (1923) 10 ml Ochsengalle gemischt mit Lakritzenpulver am Tag davor und 4 Std vor der intravenösen Infektion per os verabfolgte.

Die Verwendung von *Mucin* erleichtert gleichfalls die Infektion des Versuchstiers. Durch den Zusatz von 5% Mucin zu niedrigen Erregerdosen gelang es GRIFFITS (1942a), die Todesrate intraperitoneal infizierter weißer *Mäuse* zu steigern, allerdings nur bei Verwendung frisch isolierter Bakterienstämme. Zu einem ähnlichen Ergebnis kamen DUTTA und HABBU (1955), die bei intraintestinaler Infektion saugende Kaninchen zusammen mit der Erregerdosis teilweise 5% Mucin verabfolgten. Eine DL 100 war jedoch nur zu erreichen mit einem Bakterienstamm, der über das Tier passagiert worden war.

Als weitere Maßnahme zur Herabsetzung der Widerstandskraft der Tiere sei noch die *Röntgenbestrahlung* erwähnt. Meerschweinchen, die am Tag vor oraler Infektion mit 100—200 r bestrahlt werden, sind im Gegensatz zu bestrahlten Ratten sehr empfänglich. Die DL 50 für Meerschweinchen beträgt 170—180 r, für Ratten 700—800 r (BURROWS et al., 1950).

Einen Einfluß auf den Ablauf der experimentellen Choleraerkrankung besitzt offensichtlich auch die *Darmflora* der Versuchstiere, da eine Störung ihres Gleichgewichtes die Infektion begünstigen kann. METCHNIKOFF (1894) räumte der Beschaffenheit der Darmflora einen entscheidenden Einfluß ein. Er begründete die hohe Empfänglichkeit junger saugender Kaninchen damit, daß der Darm dieser Tiere, solange sie sich nur von Muttermilch ernähren, sehr keimarm sei, während junge Meerschweinchen, die bereits 2—3 Tage nach der Geburt Grünfutter fressen, eine mannigfaltige Darmflora besitzen und dadurch nicht in dem Maße wie junge Kaninchen für die Infektion empfänglich sind. METCHNIKOFF glaubte auch aus Choleradejekten Bakterienarten isoliert zu haben, die teils einen begünstigenden, teils einen hemmenden Einfluß auf die Entwicklung von Choleravibrionen in Kultur und Tierversuch besitzen. Gegenteiliger Ansicht ist SCHOFFER (1895), der zur Erzeugung einer typischen Choleraerkrankung beim saugenden Kaninchen den Einfluß anderer Mikroorganismen für nicht erforderlich hielt. Der Zusatz von Colibakterien kann nach WIENER (1896b) die Erkrankung des Kaninchens fördern. Auch bei Anwendung wenig virulenter Cholerastämme, die in höherer Dosierung kein eindeutiges Ergebnis brachten, war „der unterstützende Einfluß von Bact. coli in der Auslösung der Erkrankung unverkennbar". Zusammen mit Colibakterien gelang es SANARELLI (1916), die Erkrankung erwachsener Kaninchen hervorzurufen. Ohne ihre fördernde Mitwirkung konnten die Versuchstiere nur bis zum 10. Lebenstag erfolgreich infiziert werden. Diese Untersuchungsergebnisse wurden von SDRODOWSKI und BRENN (1924) im wesentlichen bestätigt; von diesen Autoren wird jedoch einschränkend bemerkt, daß auch eine Injektion von Colibakterien allein zu einer tödlichen Erkrankung des Kaninchens führen kann. Eine regelmäßig erfolgreiche Infektion von Meerschweinchen erreichte FRETER (1955) mit streptomycinresistenten Choleravibrionen, indem er die Tiere zuvor hungern ließ und die Darmflora gleichzeitig durch Streptomycin schädigte.

Weitere Untersuchungen befassen sich mit der Verfütterung einer *Mangeldiät* oder sterilisierten Futtermitteln, wodurch die Widerstandskraft gegenüber einer Infektion herabgesetzt werden soll. Nach METCHNIKOFF (1894) führt die Aufzucht von Tieren mit sterilem Futter zu keinem befriedigenden Ergebnis. Von anderer Seite wurde betont (SCHOFFER, 1895), daß beim Kaninchen das Alter des Tieres größeren Einfluß auf die Erzeugung der Erkrankung besitze. Verabfolgte er 6 Monate alten, 1 200—1 500 g schweren Kaninchen 10 Tage lang als Diät nur sterilisierte Milch, um die Darmflora möglichst einförmig zu gestalten, so magerten die Tiere zwar ziemlich stark ab, erkrankten jedoch nicht, wenn sie anschließend täglich zusammen mit alkalisierter Milch teils Bouillon-, teils Agarkulturen virulenter Choleravibrionen über einen Zeitraum von 14 Tagen erhielten. COHENDY und WOLLMAN (1922) hielten eine Fütterung von Meerschweinchen mit sterilisierten Nahrungsmitteln als Bahnungsmethode für die Erzeugung einer tödlichen Choleraerkrankung für ungeeignet; dagegen gelang ihnen die Infektion 10 bis 15 Tage alter Meerschweinchen, die unter sterilen Bedingungen aufgezogen waren. Um die Widerstandskraft herabzusetzen, wurde in neuerer Zeit eine skorbuterzeugende Diät (bestehend aus autoklaviertem Hafer, Nüssen und Heu sowie 1 Eßlöffel Fleischpulver/die) für einen Zeitraum von 45—55 Tagen an Meerschweinchen verfüttert. Zusätzlich war der verwendete Stamm 71mal über Meerschweinchen geführt worden. Die DL 100 für die Versuchstiere betrug ursprünglich $3,2 \times 10^{10}$ Vibrionen. Unter den angegebenen Versuchsbedingungen reduzierte sie sich auf 10^9. Nach annähernd dreijähriger Kultivierung dieses Stammes auf künstlichen Nährböden zeigte es sich, daß kaum ein Virulenzverlust eingetreten war. Die DL 100 betrug jetzt noch 4×10^9 Choleravibrionen (KOTLYAROVA und LEDOWSKAJA, 1961).

Eine andere Möglichkeit, Versuchstiere für die Infektion empfänglich zu machen, besteht darin, die Wirkung der *Sekrete von Galle und/oder Pankreas auszuschalten*. NICATI und RIETSCH (1884a) waren die ersten, die nach Unterbindung des Ductus choledochus bei Hunden und nachfolgender intraduodenaler Infektion eine tödliche Erkrankung hervorrufen konnten. Die Untersucher waren der Ansicht, daß intraduodenal injizierte Vibrionen sich nur bei fehlendem Gallefluß ungehindert vermehren, da sie beobachtet hatten, daß die Stühle bei menschlicher Choleraerkrankung entfärbt sind. Kritisch zu dieser Feststellung äußerte sich HÜPPE (1887b), der nachwies, daß auch gallig gefärbte Stühle reichlich Vibrionen enthalten. Eine Choledochusunterbindung mit nachfolgender intraduodenaler, gelegentlich auch oraler Infektion wurde später bei verschiedenen Tierspecies vorgenommen, so bei Meerschweinchen von NICATI und RIETSCH (1884a), KOCH (1885), bei erwachsenen Kaninchen, Affen und Hunden von VIOLLE (1912, 1914b) und ebenfalls bei Affen von HASAN et al. (1965). Nach Zerstörung des Pankreas konnte VIOLLE (1914b) durch intraintestinale Infektion des erwachsenen Kaninchens keine Erkrankung auslösen. In anderen Untersuchungen, die sich auf die Befunde von DUTTA und OZA (1963) stützen, wonach das Fehlen von Lipase und Phosphorylase für die Empfänglichkeit saugender Kaninchen verantwortlich ist, konnten die charakteristischen Symptome nach Unterbindung des D. choledochus und/oder des D. pancreaticus provoziert werden (HASAN et al., 1965).

2. Gewinnung von virulenten Choleravibrionen

Für die Gewinnung virulenter Bakterien ist das Alter der Kultur und die Art des Nährbodens von entscheidendem Einfluß. Es besteht schon bei den älteren Autoren weitgehend Übereinstimmung darüber, für tierexperimentelle Arbeiten mit lebenden Choleravibrionen 18—24 Std alte Kulturen zu verwenden.

Nach GRUBER und WIENER (1892a) hatten nur 15—30 Std bebrütete Agarkulturen ihre „volle Infektionstüchtigkeit". Zwei Tage alte und ältere Kulturen führten in Mengen, die bei jungen Kulturen tödlich waren, nur noch zur Erkrankung der Tiere. Je älter die Bakterienkultur, um so geringer ist ihre Virulenz. Für eine erfolgreiche Infektion benötigte SOBERNHEIM (1893a) bei Applikation einer 5 Tage alten Cholerakultur die doppelte Dosis gegenüber einer 24 Std bebrüteten Kultur. Diese Ergebnisse werden von CANTACUZENE und MARIE (1914), die 18—20 Std bebrütete Kulturen bevorzugten, bestätigt. Bei Untersuchungen „über die Beziehungen zwischen Virulenz und Individuenzahl einer Cholerakultur" wurde festgestellt, daß nach 18stündiger Bebrütung die Zahl der vermehrungsfähigen Mikroorganismen in der Kultur sehr rasch abnahm. In 2 Tage alten Kulturen waren nur noch 10% der Vibrionen einer 12—16 Std alten Kultur vermehrungsfähig (Gotschlich und Weigand, 1895). Auch in neueren Arbeiten wird in der Regel eine 18, höchstens jedoch 24 Std alte Kultur für die Infektion verwendet (Oza und Dutta, 1963; Hasan et al., 1965).

Besonders für die orale Infektion wurden früher den Versuchstieren Agar- oder Bouillonkulturen verabfolgt. Die Erregerdosen von festen Nährböden wurden meist in Ösen berechnet, von denen dann eine oder mehrere oder nur Bruchteile in physiologischer Kochsalzlösung, Bouillon oder Aqua dest. suspendiert wurden. Manche Untersucher verwendeten alkalische Pufferlösungen, so Arnold und Shapiro (1930) für die intraduodenale Infektion von Kaninchen und Burrows et al. (1947) für die orale Applikation an Meerschweinchen. Die Angaben über Größe der Ösen und Bakteriengehalt sind unterschiedlich, meist wurde die Erregerdosis nur als „groß" oder „klein" bezeichnet. In neuerer Zeit wird die Zahl der Mikroorganismen im allgemeinen mit Hilfe von Zählkammern (Steiner, 1929), elektronischer Teilchenzählung (Kubitschek, 1958), oder die Bakterienmasse durch photometrische Verfahren bestimmt (Monod, 1949; Koch und Kaplan, 1964; Ullmann, 1971).

Den Vermehrungs- und Züchtungsbedingungen wird ebenfalls ein Einfluß auf das Ergebnis der tierexperimentellen Infektion zugeschrieben. Während im allgemeinen die Züchtung unter aeroben Bedingungen vorgenommen wird, gab Pfeiffer (1892) den Hinweis, daß an mikroaerophiles Milieu adaptierte Choleravibrionenstämme in besonderem Maße virulent sein können. Wurden Meerschweinchen oral mit Choleravibrionen infiziert und der vibrionenhaltige Darminhalt wiederholt von Tier zu Tier übertragen, so genügten bei jeder neuen Passage geringere Mengen des Darminhaltes, um die Krankheit zu erzeugen. Gleichzeitig änderte sich aber auch das Aussehen der flüssigen Medien. Während die Ausgangskultur nach kurzer Bebrütungszeit ein dichtes Oberflächenhäutchen bildete, das auf dem sonst klaren Nährmedium schwamm, trübte sich nach der 5. Tierpassage die Flüssigkeit unter Beibehaltung einer Kahmhaut. Nach der 10. Passage war unter den gleichen Züchtungsbedingungen bei gleichmäßiger Trübung der Bouillon kein Häutchen mehr zu sehen. Das Ausbleiben einer Vermehrung an der Oberfläche führte Pfeiffer (1892) auf ein geringeres Sauerstoffbedürfnis und eine Gewöhnung der Vibrionen an „anaerobes" Milieu zurück.

a) Virulenzsteigerung von V. cholerae

Die Virulenz ist eine stammgebundene Eigenschaft (s. Bader, 1965), die bei verschiedenen Stämmen beträchtliche Unterschiede aufweisen kann. Aber auch ein und derselbe Bakterienstamm zeigt erhebliche Virulenzschwankungen. Insbesondere führen wiederholte Kulturpassagen zu einer Abschwächung dieses Merkmals. Bei Erkrankungen des Menschen wurde festgestellt, daß der Erreger in verschiedenen Stadien der Erkrankung eine unterschiedliche Virulenz aufweisen kann. Gallut (1953) fand, daß etwa 60 Std nach Beginn der Erkrankung isolierte Vibrionen die größte Virulenz besitzen. Ähnlich ist die Beobachtung von De et al. (1962) zu werten, die angeben, die Toxicität der Vibrionen sei zu Beginn einer Epidemie größer als an ihrem Ende.

Keinen Unterschied der Dosis letalis beobachtete Pfeiffer (1894a) bei der Überprüfung von Stämmen, die aus tödlich oder leicht verlaufenen Choleraerkrankungen isoliert worden waren, im Meerschweinchenversuch nach intraperitonealer Infektion. Die DL 100 betrug in beiden Fällen $^1/_6$—$^1/_8$ Öse Kulturmaterial. Die Eigenschaft „sehr virulent" oder „wenig virulent" wurde in früheren Untersuchungen durch die intraperitoneale Injektion im Meerschweinchenversuch ermittelt. Auf diese Weise ließ sich feststellen, ob ältere Laboratoriumsstämme durch Kulturpassagen einen Virulenzverlust erlitten hatten (PFEIFFER und ISSAEFF, 1894; SCHOFFER, 1895; HAHN, 1926). Da diese häufig an Virulenz einbüßen, werden für tierexperimentelle Untersuchungen überwiegend frisch isolierte Bakterien verwendet. Die Aufbewahrung dieser Stämme in lyophilisiertem Zustand ist anzustreben (DUTTA und HABBU, 1955).

Zur Steigerung der Virulenz ist die wiederholte Tierpassage der Erreger geeignet. Es genügen dann mitunter Bruchteile der ursprünglichen Dosis, um den Tod der Versuchstiere herbeizuführen. Als solche dienten hauptsächlich Meerschweinchen. PFEIFFER und NOCHT (1889) gaben den Tieren von 10 Generationen jeweils Darminhalt von zugrunde gegangenen Tieren. Es genügten schließlich 0,25—0,5 ml, um Meerschweinchen mit Sicherheit in 18—20 Std zu töten. Eine Virulenzsteigerung durch Tierpassagen beobachteten auch GRUBER und WIENER (1892a). Sie stellten jedoch eine ab der 7.—8. Passage auftretende Virulenzminderung fest: die Tiere erkrankten dann nur noch leicht oder zeigten keine Krankheitszeichen mehr, obschon noch massenhaft Vibrionen in den Faeces nachzuweisen waren. Nach Zwischenschaltung eines aeroben Kulturverfahrens erlangten die Vibrionen wieder ihre frühere Virulenz. Eine Steigerung der Giftigkeit durch Meerschweinchenpassagen erreichten ebenfalls SALUS (1893) sowie ISSAEFF und KOLLE (1894). Gelegentlich wurden Choleravibrionen auch über andere Tiere weitergeführt, so von GAMALEIA (1892) über das Rippenfell von Ratten, während ROTKY (1913) eine Virulenzsteigerung von El-Tor-Vibrionen durch Mäusepassagen erzielte.

SCHÖBL (1916b) führte einen V. cholerae-Stamm wiederholt über die Gallenblase von Meerschweinchen; die anschließend mit diesem Stamm infizierten Versuchstiere gingen meist zugrunde. Mit einem Stamm, der keine Tierpassage erfahren hatte, konnten diese Ergebnisse nicht erzielt werden (SCHÖBL, 1916a). Die Passage eines El-Tor-Stammes über 45 Meerschweinchen ergab, daß schließlich im günstigsten Fall 1 ng ausreichte, um 175 g schwere Meerschweinchen innerhalb 12 Std zu töten. Diese Menge entsprach etwa 628—900 Vibrionen (KABESHIMA, 1918a). Beim saugenden Kaninchen konnten DUTTA und HABBU (1955) eine DL 100 nach intestinaler Infektion nur mit einem Stamm erreichen, der vom Herzblut eines an der Infektion zugrunde gegangenen Tieres isoliert worden war und dessen Virulenz durch eine alle 6 Monate wiederholte Tierpassage aufrechterhalten wurde. Teilweise wurde eine Methode zur Virulenzsteigerung mit einem Verfahren zur Erhöhung der Empfänglichkeit der Versuchstiere kombiniert, wie die Verabfolgung von Mucin (OZA und DUTTA, 1965), oder die Erzeugung eines Meerschweinchenskorbuts (KOTLYAROVA und LADOVSKAYA, 1961) und Gabe von Vibrionen, die über Tiere geführt worden waren. Daß nicht nur die Virulenz eines Stammes, sondern auch die Rasse der Versuchstiere das Ergebnis beeinflussen, zeigen die Untersuchungen von FRETER (1955), der bei oraler Infektion die Empfänglichkeit zweier verschiedener Meerschweinchenrassen testete. Die DL 50 betrug für die eine Rasse ungefähr 10^5, für die andere etwa 10^{12} Mikroorganismen.

Ein hohes Maß an Virulenz besitzen bei 18° C bebrütete Kulturen. Die Bebrütung bei höheren Temperaturen führt zu einem Virulenzverlust, der mit der Zahl der Kulturpassagen zunimmt. Er ist bei höheren Bebrütungstemperaturen nur bedingt reversibel (JUDE und GALLUT, 1955).

b) Infektiöses Untersuchungsmaterial

Bevor es möglich war, Choleravibrionen in Reinkultur zu züchten, wurden Tierversuche mit Untersuchungsmaterial durchgeführt, das von Cholerakranken und -verstorbenen entnommen worden war. Die damit erzielten Ergebnisse waren widersprechend, da nicht nur mit Stuhlproben und bei Sektionen gewonnenem Darmgewebe gearbeitet wurde, sondern auch mit ungeeigneten Proben, wie Blut (s. Nicati und Rietsch, 1885a; Wyssokowitsch, 1886; Thomas, 1893). Auf verschiedenen Infektionswegen hatten Nicati und Rietsch (1885a) bei Meerschweinchen und Ratten mit Darminhalt und vibrionenhaltiger Gallenflüssigkeit von Cholerakranken tödlich verlaufende Infektionen gesetzt. Koch (1885) stellte fest, daß sich eine Choleraerkrankung übertragen läßt, wenn anstelle der Kulturvibrionen kleine Mengen des Darminhalts eines an der Infektion zugrunde gegangenen Meerschweinchens anderen Tieren inkorporiert wird. Mit Darminhalt eines Tieres, das kurz zuvor der Erkrankung erlegen war, infizierten Pottevin und Violle (1913b) oral Affen, während Hasan et al. (1965) diesen Tieren frischen Reiswasserstuhl von cholerakranken Menschen verabfolgten.

Auf eine Fehlerquelle bei derartigen Untersuchungen wies Smith (1918) hin, als er zu Recht folgerte, daß bei der Übertragung tierischen Materials auf Versuchstiere gleichzeitig auch andere Krankheitserreger weitergegeben werden können, die das Tierexperiment verfälschen.

c) Vibrionennachweis in infizierten Tieren

Eine erfolgreiche Cholerainfektion über den Magen-Darm-Kanal führt beim Versuchstier — wie bei der Erkrankung des Menschen — zu einer Vermehrung der Vibrionen im Darm. Die frühere Streitfrage, ob die oral verabfolgten Vibrionen vom Darmtrakt in die Blutbahn und andere Organe einwandern, und ob bei parenteraler Infektion die Vibrionen in den Darm gelangen, dürfte dahin entschieden sein, daß dies weitgehend eine Frage der Dosierung ist. Nur bei besonders hohen Erregerdosen kommt es zur Bakteriämie der Versuchstiere.

Der überwiegende Teil der tierexperimentellen Arbeiten galt dem Studium der Veränderungen am Verdauungskanal. Aus diesem Grunde kommt der bakteriologischen Untersuchung von Faeces und Darminhalt besondere Bedeutung zu. Geeignet ist die Anreicherung in Peptonwasser und die Züchtung auf festen Nährböden. Diese müssen dann verwendet werden, wenn die Vibrionen quantitativ bestimmt werden sollen. Die Peptonanreicherung ist zu bevorzugen, wenn im Untersuchungsmaterial nur wenige Vibrionen vermutet werden, wie in Organen und Geweben. In jedem Fall muß aus dem infizierten Versuchstier der Nachweis vermehrungsfähiger Vibrionen geführt werden. Von entscheidender Bedeutung ist die bakteriologische Untersuchung unmittelbar nach dem Tod der Versuchstiere, um eine postmortale Einwanderung anderer Mikroorganismen auszuschließen und die Überwucherung der Vibrionen durch andere Bakterien zu verhindern. Der direkte mikroskopische Nachweis der Vibrionen kann nur Anhaltspunkte geben und ist weniger ergiebig als das Kulturverfahren. Häufig werden die Vibrionen bakterioskopisch vermißt, besonders wenn der Erregernachweis aus Organen oder Blut geführt werden soll (Pfeiffer, 1889; Kolle, 1894).

3. Meerschweinchen

a) Infektion über den Magen-Darm-Kanal

α) Die *orale Infektion* im Tierexperiment entspricht dem Infektionsweg beim Menschen. Das Mißlingen der Fütterungsversuche an Meerschweinchen führte Koch (1884) darauf zurück, daß die Choleravibrionen durch den sauren Magensaft abgetötet werden. Durch Gabe von 5 ml einer 5%igen Sodalösung mit der Schlundsonde wurde eine bis zu 3 Std andauernde alkalische Reaktion des Magensaftes erzeugt. Obwohl jetzt die Vibrionen den Magen vermehrungsfähig passierten und aus dem Darm wieder isoliert werden konnten, erkrankten die Tiere in der Regel nicht. Die Beobachtung, daß von 19 Meerschweinchen dasjenige Tier erkrankte, welches kurz zuvor abortiert hatte, wurde auf die dadurch bedingte zeitweilige Erschlaffung des Darmes und die damit verbundene längere Verweildauer der Vibrionen im Darm zurückgeführt. Diese Überlegung war der Anlaß, nach geeigneten Mitteln zu suchen, mit deren Hilfe eine Ruhigstellung des Darmes erreicht werden kann. Als besonders vorteilhaft erwies sich die intraperitoneale Injektion von Opiumtinktur. KOCH (1885) erarbeitete schließlich folgende Methode:

1. Gabe von 5 ml einer 5%igen Sodalösung zur Neutralisierung des Magensaftes.

2. Wenig später Applikation der Erreger.

3. Unmittelbar danach intraperitoneale Injektion von 1 ml Opiumtinktur/ 200 g Körpergewicht.

Die von KOCH (1884) vorgeschlagene Opiumdosis veranlaßte BÜRGERS (1911) zu dem Einwand, daß nach Gabe einer nur wenig größeren Menge, nämlich 1,5—2 ml, ein 250 g schweres Meerschweinchen 1—2 Std später verendet. Für die erfolgreiche orale Infektion wird in neuerer Zeit Opium ebenfalls niedriger dosiert. Eine Modifikation der Kochschen Technik geben BURROWS et al. (1947): 400—500 g schweren Meerschweinchen wird 24 Std vor der Infektion das Futter entzogen; einige Minuten vor Gabe der Erreger erhalten die Versuchstiere 0,2 ml Opiumtinktur intraperitoneal; anschließend werden mit einer Magensonde maximal 2 ml einer phosphatgepufferten Vibrionensuspension (pH 8) appliziert, welche von 24 Std bebrüteten, festen Nährböden abgeschwemmt wurden. In späteren Untersuchungen geben die Autoren (BURROWS et al., 1950) anstelle von Opiumtinktur kurz vor der Infektion 2 mg Morphiumsulfat intraperitoneal. Mit Morphiumsulfat arbeitete auch FRETER (1955), während LABREC et al. (1965) wiederum 1 ml Opiumtinktur intraperitoneal injizierten.

Anstelle von Opium gab DOYEN (1885) Äthylalkohol. Nach Opiumbehandlung erlagen wesentlich mehr Tiere der Infektion als dies nach Alkoholinjektion der Fall ist (TIZZONI und CATTANI, 1888). Gelegentlich gelang es auch, eine tödliche Erkrankung ohne Vorbehandlung zu provozieren. NICATI und RIETSCH (1885a) fütterten 7 junge Meerschweinchen durch die Schlundsonde mit einer größeren Menge Darminhalt von Cholerapatienten. Dabei gingen 2 der Tiere bereits nach 10 bzw. 28 Std zugrunde, die übrigen 5 nach 3 und 4 Tagen. Der Tod der nach kurzer Zeit verstorbenen Tiere wurde als Intoxikation, der der übrigen als Infektion interpretiert.

Versuchstieren, die 24 Std gehungert hatten, applizierten CANTACUZENE und MARIE (1914) 0,01—0,02 g Podophyllin. Als wenige Stunden danach Diarrhoen auftraten, erhielten sie als Erregerdosis jeweils $^1/_3$ der Vibrionenkolonien, die sich auf einer 24 Std bebrüteten Agarkultur entwickelt hatten. Die Paralleluntersuchung von hungernden und ernährten Tieren ergab, daß nach vorheriger Alkalisierung des Magens und Gabe von Podophyllin 83% der hungernden und nur 30% der gefütterten Tiere starben. Wurde Podophyllin nicht gegeben, sank die Sterblichkeit bei hungernden Meerschweinchen auf 12%, während keines der gefütterten Tiere der Infektion erlag.

Für die Infektion der Meerschweinchen entwickelte FRETER (1955, 1956) 2 Methoden, die durch Hungern und durch Antibioticumgabe die Widerstandskraft der Tiere herabsetzten. Voraussetzung für das zweite Verfahren ist die Verwendung antibioticumresistenter Choleravibrionen. Bei dem ersten Verfahren ist folgendermaßen vorzugehen (Freter, 1955):

1. 350—500 g schweren Meerschweinchen wird 4 Tage lang das Futter unter Beibehaltung von Wasser entzogen.

2. Am Tag der Infektion sind 250 mg $CaCO_3$ in 10 ml Aqua dest. gelöst durch die Magensonde zu geben.

3. 3 Std danach werden streptomycinresistente Vibrionen in 15 ml Kalbfleischinfusionsbouillon (1:1 mit Wasser verdünnt) zusammen mit 250 mg $NaHCO_3$ und 5 mg Streptomycinsulfat durch die Magensonde verabfolgt.

4. 30 min später sind 8 mg Morphiumsulfat intraperitoneal zu injizieren.

Die auf solche Weise infizierten Tiere sterben meist nach 18—24 Std.

Wird den Meerschweinchen oral zusätzlich ein streptomycinresistenter E.-coli-Stamm verfüttert, so führt dies zu einer zunehmenden Resistenz der Tiere gegenüber einer Cholerainfektion. Bei der 2. Methode ist folgender Verfahrensgang einzuhalten (Freter, 1956):

Die über 350 g schweren Versuchstiere erhalten 2 Tage vor der Infektion 100 mg Streptomycin und 10 mg Erythromycin in 10 ml Aqua dest. gelöst durch die Magensonde. An diesem Tag wird kein Futter gegeben; abgekochtes Wasser, das 4 mg Streptomycin, 0,1 mg Erythromycin und 400 Einheiten Nystatin/ml enthält, steht ad libitum zur Verfügung.

2. Am Tag vor der Infektion bekommen die Tiere wieder Futter.

3. Nach weiteren 24 Std sind 750 mg $CaCO_3$ in 10 ml Wasser durch die Magensonde zu applizieren.

4. 3 Std danach werden 15 ml Kalbfleischinfusionsbouillon, die die Choleravibrionenabschwemmung einer 24 Std bebrüteten Agarkultur, 50 mg Streptomycin und 250 mg $CaCO_3$ enthält, durch die Sonde verabfolgt.

Der dadurch gesetzten „latenten" Cholerainfektion erliegen die Versuchstiere nur sehr selten.

Als Vorbehandlungsmethode ebenfalls geeignet ist die Anwendung von Röntgenstrahlen (Burrows et al., 1950). Die 300—400 g schweren Meerschweinchen wurden 24 Std vor der Infektion mit 100—200 r bestrahlt. Kurz vor Applikation der Choleravibrionen erhielten die Tiere 2 mg Morphiumsulfat intraperitoneal. Erregerdosis waren 2 ml in isotonischem Phosphatpuffer (pH 8) suspendierte Bakterien, die von einem 18 Std bebrüteten Nährboden abgeschwemmt wurden. Die Menge der Vibrionen in 2 ml entsprach einem Trockengewicht der Bakterien von 20 mg.

Das Ziel, nach entsprechender Vorbehandlung beim Meerschweinchen durch orale Infektion eine „Erkrankung durch Choleravibrionen" hervorzurufen, wurde nicht immer erreicht. Nur ein wechselnder Prozentsatz der Tiere erlag der Erkrankung, die anderen Tiere erkrankten zwar, überlebten jedoch. In Abhängigkeit von der Vorbehandlung und der Erregerdosis verendeten zwischen 30 und 70% der Tiere. Bei einer Verringerung der Erregerdosis nahm die Zahl der überlebenden Tiere zu (Koch, 1885; Burrows et al., 1947). Als klassisches Beispiel für die Beschreibung einer tödlich verlaufenden Erkrankung des Meerschweinchens ohne Opiumvorbehandlung (s. S. 73) sei die von Koch (1884) angeführt:

Das Tier wurde an den beiden nach der Infektion folgenden Tagen sehr krank, sah struppig aus und fraß nicht. Eine lähmungsartige Schwäche der hinteren Extremitäten trat auf. Schließlich starb es. Diarrhoe hat nicht bestanden. Bei der Sektion fand sich ein stark geröteter Dünndarm, schwappend gefüllt mit einer wäßrigen, flockigen, farblosen Flüssigkeit. Auch Magen und Coecum enthielten eine große Menge Flüssigkeit. Sowohl mikroskopisch als auch in der Kultur ließen sich massenhaft Choleravibrionen nachweisen.

Das Krankheitsbild alkali-, opium- oder morphiumvorbehandelter Tiere wies folgende Symptomatik auf (KOLLE, 1894; BURROWS et al., 1947):

Bereits nach 12—24 Std, bei niedrigen Dosen nach etwa 2 Tagen, waren die ersten Krankheitserscheinungen zu beobachten. Die Tiere wurden matt und gleichgültig, fraßen nicht und verloren an Gewicht. Es bestand zum Teil eine erhebliche Hypothermie. An den hinteren Extremitäten trat eine lähmungsartige Schwäche auf. Nach 1—2 weiteren Tagen, mitunter auch später, starben die Tiere unter den Zeichen eines Kreislaufkollapses.

Das Krankheitsbild der tödlich infizierten Tiere ähnelte dem Stadium algidum der Cholerainfektion des Menschen (KOLLE, 1894). Obschon von älteren Autoren angegeben wird, daß die Tiere unter den für Cholera charakteristischen Krankheitserscheinungen zugrunde gehen, fehlt doch zumeist das Hauptsymptom, die Diarrhoe. HÜPPE (1887a) verglich deshalb die Infektion des Meerschweinchens mit einer Cholera sicca, bei welcher ebenfalls kein Darminhalt abgeht. Diarrhoen, bei denen massenhaft Vibrionen nachzuweisen waren, traten dann auf, wenn zur Schwächung der Tiere Abführmittel appliziert wurden (CANTACUZENE und MARIE, 1914).

Bei der Sektion verendeter Meerschweinchen ist makroskopisch eine starke Flüssigkeitsansammlung im Darmtrakt auffällig. Der Dünndarm ist stark gerötet und schwappend gefüllt mit 50—60 ml Flüssigkeit, in der zahlreiche Schleimflocken und Epithelfetzen schwimmen und die Choleravibrionen annähernd in Reinkultur vorliegen (FRETER, 1955, 1956). Ferner wird eine vermehrte Gefäßzeichnung des Darmes beobachtet.

Die ursprünglich erhobenen histologischen Befunde des Dünndarmes nach oraler Infektion wurden als Nekrose des Darmepithels gedeutet. Daraus entwickelte sich die Ansicht, daß durch Läsionen der Epithelschicht eine rasche Resorption der von vermehrungsfähigen Choleravibrionen gebildeten Giftstoffe in den Organismus erfolgt. Bei unverletzter Epithelschicht sollte es nicht zum Stadium algidum kommen, selbst wenn Choleravibrionen in „ungeheurer Menge, fast in Reinkultur" im Darm vorhanden sind (PFEIFFER, 1894). Diese Anschauung hält neueren Untersuchungsergebnissen nicht stand. Die Epithelläsionen erwiesen sich als Veränderungen, die postmortal aufgetreten waren. Nach den experimentellen Ergebnissen von LABREC et al. (1965) ist das Darmepithel — wie bei der Choleraerkrankung des Menschen — intakt und bildet eine Barriere, die von den Vibrionen nicht durchbrochen wird. Selbst wenn sich eine große Zahl von Vibrionen im Darm ansiedelt und das Mucosaepithel bedeckt, werden in der Lamina propria der Villi keine Mikroorganismen gefunden.

Das mikroskopische Präparat der Darmflüssigkeit zeigt bei erfolgreicher Infektion das uniforme Bild der kommaförmigen Mikroorganismen (KOCH, 1885; KOLLE und PRIGGE, 1928). Die Bestimmung der Gesamtbakterienzahl der Stuhlflora ergab, daß in den ersten 2—4 Tagen nach der Infektion 40—90% der Darmbakterien Vibrionen sind (BURROWS et al., 1947). Die Ermittlung der vermehrungsfähigen Cholerabakterien in einem Abschnitt des terminalen Ileums zu verschiedenen Zeiten ($^1/_2$, 1, 2, 4, 8, 12, 16 und 24 Std post infectionem) ließ erkennen, daß die meisten Mikroorganismen 16 Std post infectionem anzutreffen sind. Mit Hilfe fluorescierender Antikörper konnte durch Untersuchung einzelner Abschnitte des Ileums, die zu verschiedenen Zeitpunkten den getöteten Tieren entnommen wurden, ein bestimmtes Verteilungsmuster der Vibrionen festgestellt werden: 1, 2 und 4 Std nach oraler Infektion waren im terminalen Ileum vereinzelt, 6 Std später mäßig viel und nach 8—12 Std massenhaft Vibrionen vorhanden. Die Lage der Mikroorganismen erweckte den Eindruck, als ob sie auf dem intakten Epithel der Villi hafteten. Im Lumen von Ileumproben, die 16—24 Std nach der Infektion von getöteten moribunden oder kranken Tieren gewonnen wurden, waren Vibrionen zum Teil massenhaft nachzuweisen. Große Zusammenballungen von Mikroorganismen bedeckten auch das Mucosaepithel und lagen eingeschlossen zwischen den Villi an der Basis der Villi-Krypten (Labrec et al., 1965). Im Coecum und Colon waren 1, 2, 4 und 6 Std nach der Infektion vereinzelt Choleravibrionen zu sehen, nach 8 und 12 Std dagegen zahlreiche Exemplare. Bei kranken und moribunden Tieren wurden dann auch in diesen Darmabschnitten massenhaft Vibrionen angetroffen. Eine Anlagerung der Mikroorganismen auf die Epithel-oberfläche wurde hier jedoch nicht registriert. Die Durchwanderung des Mucosa-epithels mit Vibrionen war in keinem Darmabschnitt zu sehen (Labrec et al., 1965).

Bei infizierten Meerschweinchen, die steril aufgezogen worden waren, wurden die Mikroorganismen reichlich aus dem Darminhalt isoliert; bei Tieren jedoch, die sterilisierte Nahrung erhielten, ließen sich die Vibrionen bereits 1—2 Tage post infectionem nicht mehr nachweisen (Cohendy und Wollman, 1922). Ebenfalls negativ waren die Kulturverfahren bei solchen Tieren, die wenige Tage nach der Infektion starben, nachdem zuvor ein experimenteller Skorbut erzeugt worden war. Ein rasches Verschwinden der Choleravibrionen aus dem Stuhl war auch dann festzustellen, wenn die Meerschweinchen mit einem streptomycinresistenten Vibrionen- und E.-coli-Stamm infiziert wurden (Freter, 1956).

Von der Regel, daß Choleravibrionen ausschließlich im Darm nachzuweisen sind, gibt es Ausnahmen, wenn mit sehr großen Erregerdosen infiziert wird und die Tiere einer Vorbehandlung unterzogen werden, die den Organismus zusätzlich stark belastet. In derartigen Fällen konnten die Vibrionen als Folge einer Bakteriämie auch aus anderen Organen isoliert werden (Tizzoni und Cattani, 1888). Vereinzelt wurden Vibrionen von Gruber (1892 b) und Kolle (1894) im Peritoneal-exsudat, Blut und in anderen Organen festgestellt. Auf die Dosisabhängigkeit wies Sewastianoff (1910) hin. Die Gabe von 5—10 ml einer 24 Std bebrüteten Bouillonkultur führte nach 3 Std zu einem Übertritt der Erreger ins Blut und in andere Organe, während die inneren Organe von solchen Meerschweinchen, die mit wenigen Tropfen dieser Kultur infiziert worden waren, steril blieben. Über eine Isolierung der Choleravibrionen aus Gallenflüssigkeit berichteten Cantacuzene und Marie (1914), Schöbl (1916a) und Horowitz-Wlassowa und Pirojnikowa (1926). Zu einer Überschwemmung des Tierkörpers mit Choleravibrionen führte die Behandlung mit Röntgenstrahlen. Die Mehrzahl der von Burrows et al. (1950) infizierten Tiere starb an einer generalisierten bakteriellen Infektion, die bei unbehandelten infizierten Tieren nicht auftrat. Die Bakteriämie war allerdings nur bei 50% der Tiere durch Choleravibrionen, beim Rest durch andere Mikroorganismen verursacht.

β) Intranasale Infektion. Nach Sanarelli (1923a) ist die naso-pharyngeale Mucosa des Meerschweinchens für Choleravibrionen durchlässig. Bereits 15 min nach der nasalen Infektion ließen sich die Erreger im Blut nachweisen. Als Folge trat eine chronische Erkrankung mit Gewichtsverlust und Läsionen an Darm und Nieren auf, die tödlich enden konnte.

γ) Rectale Infektion. Um die bactericide Wirkung des sauren Magensaftes zu umgehen, wurden Meerschweinchen, allerdings äußerst selten, rectal infiziert; Sewastianoff (1910) infizierte neben Kaninchen auch Meerschweinchen mit der von Nasaroff und Jurgelunas (1910) ausgearbeiteten Methode, bei welcher der Anus nach der Erregergabe mit Collodium verklebt wird. Auf diese Art der Infektion reagierten nur wenige Tiere mit einer tödlichen Erkrankung.

δ) Injektion in Magen, Duodenum und Dünndarm. Eine Injektion der Vibrionen in den Magen wurde von Schöbl (1916a) vorgenommen. Nach Magnesiumoxyd-gabe und Laparotomie wurde die Bakterienaufschwemmung in den Magen der

Versuchstiere eingebracht. Die Tiere wurden nach 3, 7 und 8 Tagen getötet. Die Choleravibrionen konnten in der Regel aus Gallenblase, Magen und verschiedenen Darmabschnitten isoliert werden.

Durch die Injektion von Choleravibrionen oder infektiösem Darmmaterial in das Duodenum der Meerschweinchen gelingt es, auch mit niedrigen Erregerdosen eine Erkrankung hervorzurufen. Der operative Eingriff bedeutet dann allerdings eine erhebliche zusätzliche Belastung für das Tier, insbesondere wenn gleichzeitig der Gallengang unterbunden wird. NICATI und RIETSCH (1884a) merkten an, daß bisweilen derart operierte Tiere auch ohne Infektion nach einigen Tagen abmagerten und nach 3—28 Tagen den Operationsfolgen erlagen. Der größere Teil der auf diese Weise infizierten Tiere starb an einer Choleraerkrankung, die anderen Tiere hingegen wiesen keinerlei Krankheitssymptome auf (NICATI und RIETSCH, 1885a). Zu ähnlichen Ergebnissen gelangte auch KOCH (1885). Von 10 infizierten Meerschweinchen verendeten 6 Tiere nach 48 Std unter Cholerasymptomen, die übrigen 4 Tiere erlagen den Folgen der Unterbindung des Ductus choledochus. Dabei war eine starke Ausdehnung der Gallenblase und des Gallengangs oberhalb der Unterbindungsstelle auffällig sowie teilweise eine Ruptur der Gallenblase oder Knickung und Darmverschluß infolge entzündlicher Verklebungen in nächster Umgebung der Ligatur. Unterblieb die Unterbindung des Gallengangs, so überlebten alle Tiere die Folgen der Operation; von 18 infizierten Tieren gingen dann 13 unter den Zeichen der Cholera zugrunde (KOCH, 1885).

Im Gegensatz zu dem Befund nach intraduodenaler Infektion ist die Injektion von cholerahaltigem Material in den unteren Teil des Dünndarms nahe des Coecums wenig erfolgreich. Die Tiere erholen sich entweder oder sterben, jedoch ohne die Symptome einer Choleraerkrankung zu zeigen (KOCH, 1885; NICATI und RIETSCH, 1885a).

Bei den erkrankten Tieren konstatierten NICATI und RIETSCH (1885a) sowohl Diarrhoen als auch Krämpfe der Skeletmuskulatur. Bemerkenswert war auch eine Hypothermie bis etwa 34° C, in einem Fall bis 24° C. Durch die intraduodenale Infektion kann „ein der Cholera des Menschen analoger Prozeß in den Verdauungswegen erzeugt werden" (KOCH, 1885). Ähnlich äußerten sich auch v. ERMENGEM (1884) sowie FINKLER und PRIOR (1885). Der Dünndarm enthielt eine breiige Masse, leicht gelblicher Farbe, und der Dickdarm war angefüllt mit einer weißlichgrünen Flüssigkeit. Die pathologisch-anatomischen Veränderungen des Darmes waren denen des Stadium algidum beim Menschen ähnlich (NICATI und RIETSCH, 1885a). Choleravibrionen wurden sowohl aus den diarrhoischen Entleerungen als auch aus dem Dünndarm isoliert (v. ERMENGEM, 1884; NICATI und RIETSCH, 1885a).

ε) *Injektion in das abgebundene Darmsegment.* SAYAMOV (1963a) injizierte nach einer 24stündigen Futterpause 51 erwachsenen, 600—700 g schweren Meerschweinchen 10^7 bis $2{,}5 \times 10^7$ Choleravibrionen in das Lumen eines abgebundenen Darmsegments von 5—7 cm Länge. 31 weitere Tiere erhielten El-Tor- und Makassar-Vibrionen (nach SAYAMOV sind Makassar-, wie El-Tor-Vibrionen, eine Variante der Choleravibrionen). Nach 24 Std bzw. 48 Std wurden die Meerschweinchen getötet. Bei 88,5% der Tiere fiel eine starke Hyperämie und Erweiterung des abgebundenen Darmstücks auf. Der Darminhalt bestand aus einer trüben, flockigen Flüssigkeit, die häufig Spuren von Blut enthielt und an den Stuhl von Cholerapatienten erinnerte. An der Schleimhaut war eine hämorrhagische Infarzierung auffällig. Auf der Serosa des isolierten Segments fand sich bei den meisten Tieren ein Eiterfilm, der zu Adhäsionen mit benachbarten Dünndarmschlingen geführt hatte. Die Injektion von El-Tor- und Makassarvibrionen erbrachte ähnliche Ergebnisse; bei 3 von 15 mit El-Tor-Vibrionen infizierten Tieren war jedoch das abgebundene Darmstück kollabiert, leicht hyperämisch und beherbergte eine dick-flockige, graue Substanz, der Blut beigemengt war. Das abgebundene Darm-segment von Kontrolltieren, denen physiologische Kochsalzlösung injiziert worden war, wurde stets kollabiert vorgefunden. Der Darminhalt dieser Tiere bestand aus einer geringen Menge halbflüssiger, bräunlicher Masse.

Die histologische Untersuchung der unterbundenen Darmwandabschnitte er-brachte nach Injektion von Choleravibrionen Zeichen der Entzündung, be-gleitet von Kongestion, Hämorrhagien, Destruktion von Bezirken der Schleim-haut, fokaler Epitheldesquamation und Leukocyteninfiltration. El-Tor- und Makassarvibrionen verursachen wie Choleravibrionen einen akuten sero-hämor-rhagischen Katarrh mit zirkulatorischen Störungen, Ödem der Mucosa, Epithel-desquamation, Bildung von Leukocyten- und Erythrocytenzusammenballungen und teilweise veränderten Epithelzellen in verschiedenen Degenerationsstadien Sayamov, 1963a).

Die Vibrionen vermehrten sich bei erfolgreicher Infektion innerhalb des ab-gebundenen Darmstücks außerordentlich rasch, selbst dann, wenn als Erreger-dosis nur 10 Vibrionen injiziert wurden. Die zwischen 10 und $2,5 \times 10^6$ Bakterien variierte Erregerdosis führte in dem abgebundenen Darmsegment zu einem Bak-teriengehalt von $1,1 \times 10^7$ bis $2,7 \times 10^9$ Vibrionen/ml Darminhalt. Auch die Injek-tion von El-Tor- und Makassarvibrionen erbrachte eine starke Vermehrung der Mikroorganismen, die bei den El-Tor-Vibrionen zwischen $3,5 \times 10^8$ und 7×10^9 Mi-kroorganismen/ml Darminhalt lag. In einer weiteren Untersuchung applizierte Sayamov (1963b) 10^2—10^3 Choleravibrionen. Nach 24 Std wurden in der unter-bundenen Darmschlinge 10^8 bis über 10^9 Vibrionen/ml Inhalt nachgewiesen. Bei einigen Tieren waren die Mikroorganismen auch oberhalb und unterhalb der Unterbindungsstelle sowie in Blut, Leber und Gallenblase zu finden.

ζ) Infektion der Gallenblase. Hauptsächlich in der älteren Literatur gibt es Angaben darüber, daß Choleravibrionen gelegentlich auch in der Gallenblase des Menschen gefunden werden (Nicati und Rietsch, 1885b; Tizzoni und Cattani, 1886). Es wurde die Ansicht vertreten (Bezzola, 1912), daß die Gallenblase ein Organ sei, in dem Choleravibrionen bevorzugt persistieren und über lange Zeit mit Faeces ausgeschieden werden. Bei 10 von 235 Obduktionen von Menschen, die an Cholera gestorben waren, zeigte die Gallenblase bereits makroskopisch erkennbare, entzündliche Veränderungen. Die histologische Untersuchung erbrachte aus-gedehnte strukturelle Veränderungen der Gallenblasenwand mit massenhaft daran haftenden Vibrionen (Greig, 1914). Diese Befunde veranlaßten Schöbl (1916a), die Gallenblase von Meerschweinchen experimentell zu infizieren, um die Dauer-ausscheidung von Choleravibrionen zu studieren. In einer ersten Untersuchungs-reihe (Schöbl, 1916a) blieben die Tiere nach der Infektion bei guter Gesundheit. Die Sektion ergab keine Veränderungen der inneren Organe, die Gallenblase war normal groß, die Gallenflüssigkeit unauffällig. Mit demselben, jedoch mehrfach über Kaninchen geführten Cholerastamm wurden später andere Ergebnisse erzielt (Schöbl, 1916b). Die meisten Meerschweinchen erkrankten unter Cholera-symptomen und gingen 3—4 Tage nach der Infektion zugrunde. Bei der Sektion wurden mitunter Leberveränderungen konstatiert und aus diesen Vibrionen isoliert. Ihre ursächliche Rolle ist jedoch zweifelhaft, da entsprechende Kon-trollen fehlten.

Als nach einem Vorversuch mit 4 Meerschweinchen (Schöbl, 1916a) aus Gallenflüssigkeit und verschiedenen Abschnitten des Dünndarms der am 1., 2., 4. und 7. Tage post infectionem getöteten Tiere die Mikroorganismen in Peptonwasser isoliert werden konnten, wurde eine größere Versuchsreihe mit 33 Tieren angeschlossen. Zwischen dem 1. und 30. Tag nach der Infektion waren bei 31 Meerschweinchen Choleravibrionen aus Galle zu züchten (2 Proben vom 16. bzw. 30. Tag waren negativ). Ferner wurden Vibrionen aus dem Magen (1mal), Duodenum (28mal), Ileum (31mal), Coecum (26mal) und Rectum (2mal) isoliert. Die unmittelbar nach der Sektion angelegten Kulturen aus dem Duodenum und dem Ileum ergaben in diesem proximalen Teil des Darmkanals fast ausschließlich Choleravibrionen. Die Differenz ihrer Zahl in der Gallenflüssigkeit und im Darm führte SCHÖBL (1916b) auf individuelle Faktoren der Versuchstiere zurück. Die zum Teil negativen Ergebnisse der Untersuchung von Faecesproben könnten auch durch die antagonistische Wirkung der natürlichen Darmbakterien erklärt werden. Auch HASAN et al. (1965) isolierten nach oraler Infektion von Rhesusaffen aus Rectalabstrichen die Erreger häufig nicht, obwohl sie aus den oberen Darmabschnitten und aus Gallenflüssigkeit gezüchtet werden konnten.

b) Parenterale Infektion

Diese Infektionstechniken haben heute kaum mehr Bedeutung. Anders als bei der oralen Infektion ist es jedoch mit solchen Verfahren teilweise möglich, bei Versuchstieren ohne Vorbehandlung mit niedrigen Erregerdosen eine tödliche Erkrankung hervorzurufen.

α) *Intravenöse Infektion.* TIZZONI und CATTANI (1888) injizierten Meerschweinchen in steigender Menge 0,7—2,75 ml Bouillonkultur. Eine Erkrankung der Versuchstiere konnte damit nicht hervorgerufen werden. Wesentlich gesteigert wurde die Empfänglichkeit der Versuchstiere durch intraperitoneale Injektion von Opium. Von 7 Meerschweinchen, die mit $^2/_5$ Tropfen bis 1,5 ml Bouillonkultur infiziert wurden, gingen 5 Tiere zugrunde; den beiden überlebenden Tieren war weniger als 1 Tropfen injiziert worden.

Bereits nach 1 Std lagen die Tiere schwerkrank danieder, mit kalten Extremitäten, Muskelzucken, starker Prostration und erniedrigter Körpertemperatur; einige Stunden später trat der Tod ein (KOLLE, 1894). Dieser foudroyante Krankheitsverlauf wird als Intoxikation durch die Resorption freiwerdender giftiger Substanzen interpretiert. Die für das Meerschweinchen tödliche Minimaldosis beträgt $^1/_2$ Öse Kulturmaterial (KOLLE, 1894; PFEIFFER und WASSERMANN, 1893). Nach den Untersuchungen von SCHÖBL (1916a) erlagen die Tiere innerhalb 24 Std der Infektion, wenn mit $^1/_{10}$ der auf einer Schrägagarkultur gezüchteten Bakterien infiziert wurde. Derartige Mengenangaben sind wenig exakt und erlauben keine vergleichende Wertung der Untersuchungsergebnisse.

Bereits nach wenigen Minuten waren die in die Blutbahn injizierten Vibrionen nicht mehr nachweisbar. Bei Injektion sehr großer Mengen, die die tödliche Minimaldosis um das 4—8fache überstiegen, konnten 3 Std nach der Infektion keine vermehrungsfähigen Vibrionen aus Blut und Organen nachgewiesen werden (KOLLE, 1894; PFEIFFER und WASSERMANN, 1893). Zu ähnlichen Ergebnissen kam auch SCHÖBL (1916a), der nach Injektion kleinster Erregermengen die Mikroorganismen weder aus Darm, Gallenblase noch Faeces züchten konnte. Bei Gabe größerer Erregermengen gelang ihm jedoch die Isolierung der Vibrionen aus Leber, Gallenblase, Ileum und Coecum.

β) *Intraperitoneale Infektion.* Diese Methode fand früher häufig Anwendung zur Bestimmung des Virulenzgrades eines Vibrionenstammes. Als eine serologische Untersuchung der Mikroorganismen noch nicht möglich war, diente diese Technik auch im „Pfeifferschen Versuch" (PFEIFFER, 1894b) zur Differentialdiagnose zwischen Vibrio cholerae und anderen Vibrionen. Die Identifizierung beruht auf dem immunologischen Phänomen, daß nach gleichzeitiger Injektion von Vibrionen und hochtitrigem Choleraserum in die Peritonealhöhle eines Meerschweinchens die

Choleravibrionen innerhalb kurzer Zeit zunächst unbeweglich und dann lysiert werden. Diese Reaktion wird nach Injektion anderer Vibrionenarten vermißt.

Erhalten die Versuchstiere vor der intraperitonealen Infektion 1 ml Opiumtinktur, so genügt 1 ml Bouillonkultur, um innerhalb 24 Std regelmäßig ihren Tod herbeizuführen (Hüppe, 1887 b). Ohne Vorbehandlung gelang es Vincenzi (1887) nicht, nach Gabe von 10—20 Tropfen einer 48 Std bebrüteten virulenten Bakterienaufschwemmung Krankheitszeichen beim Tier auszulösen. Selbst die Gabe von 3 ml dieser Suspension nach Laparotomie in die Bauchhöhle überstanden die Tiere. Ohne Vorbehandlung führten 1—2 ml aus Eikulturen gewonnene Bakterienaufschwemmung zum Tod der Meerschweinchen, während ein Zusatz von 1—3% Pepton zu 5 ml dieser Suspension ihr Wohlbefinden nicht beeinträchtigte (Gruber und Wiener, 1892 b). Als tödliche Minimaldosis gab Sobernheim (1893 a) 1 ml einer 24 Std bebrüteten Agarkultur-Abschwemmung an. Die Abhängigkeit der Dosis letalis von der Virulenz der Choleravibrionen untersuchte Bezzola (1912). Bei Stämmen, die als „avirulent" eingestuft wurden, war die Injektion von 5 Ösen Kulturmaterial erforderlich, um eine tödlich verlaufende Erkrankung auszulösen, während bei anderen eine Dosis von 1 und 2 Ösen ausreichend war. Die Diskrepanzen in den Mengenangaben, die für eine erfolgreiche Erkrankung als notwendig erachtet wurden, beruhen teils auf der unterschiedlichen Vorbehandlung der Versuchstiere, teils auf der Verwendung von Vibrionenstämmen, deren Virulenz durch einen vorausgegangenen Tierversuch nicht definiert war.

Bereits 2 Std nach Injektion traten Symptome einer schweren Allgemeinerkrankung auf: die Tiere wurden in zunehmendem Maße hinfällig, die Temperatur sank innerhalb 2—3 Std um 6—8° C, der Tod trat nach 12—18 Std ein (Gruber und Wiener, 1892 a; Sobernheim, 1893 a).

Bei der Sektion fand Hüppe (1887 b) in der Peritonealhöhle etwas seröse, klare Flüssigkeit, wie dies häufig auch nach oraler Infektion zu beobachten war. Das Peritoneum wies in der Regel keine Alterationen auf. Nur gelegentlich wurden einige kleine Hämorrhagien beobachtet. Seröse Exsudate in Bauchhöhle und Brusthöhle in Mengen von 12—15 ml sowie kleine Blutungen, besonders im Zwerchfell, wurden von Gruber und Wiener (1892 a) festgestellt. Am Darm waren ähnliche Veränderungen wie nach intraduodenaler Infektion zu registrieren: die Darmschleimhaut war diffus rosig verfärbt mit kleinen Hämorrhagien, die Dünndarmschlingen schwappend mit flüssigem Inhalt gefüllt, der meist noch leicht gallig und mit feinen weißen Flöckchen oder Blut durchsetzt war. Aufgrund des Nachweises von Vibrionen in Peritonealexsudat, an Bauchwand, Zwerchfell und Leber glaubten die Autoren an eine Infektionskrankheit, während Pfeiffer (1892) die Symptome als Intoxikation interpretierte, weil die injizierten Vibrionen nach seinen Untersuchungen in der Peritonealhöhle schnell zugrunde gingen. Dieser von Pfeiffer und Wassermann (1893) weiter untersuchte Vorgang war jedoch dosisabhängig. Sie unterschieden 4 Infektionsstadien:

1. Minimale Erregerdosen erzeugen eine wenige Stunden anhaltende Temperaturerhöhung ohne sichtbare Störung des allgemeinen Befindens.

2. „Etwas höhere Dosen" bewirken nach einem kurzen, fieberhaften Intervall ein starkes Absinken der Körpertemperatur und ausgesprochene Symptome der Choleraintoxikation, wie Muskelschwäche, fibrilläre Muskelzuckungen und allgemeine Prostration; die Versuchstiere überleben.

3. Die Injektion der Dosis letalis minima bewirkt den Tod der Tiere „mit allen Erscheinungen der Choleraintoxikation". Das Peritoneum erweist sich als steril oder es lassen sich nur vereinzelt Choleravibrionen nachweisen. Im Peritonealexsudat werden zahlreiche Leukocyten gefunden, auf der Leber eitrig-fibrinöse

Beläge; Eiterflocken bedecken auch die Oberfläche des Mesenteriums und den Darm.

4. Nach der Gabe massiver Erregerdosen enthält das Peritoneum massenhaft vermehrungsfähige Choleravibrionen. In dem fast klaren Peritonealexsudat, das mehrere Milliliter beträgt, werden vereinzelt Erythrocyten und polynucleäre Zellen nachgewiesen.

In der Peritonealflüssigkeit nahm nach HÜPPE (1887b) die Zahl der injizierten Vibrionen rasch ab. Nach 16—24 Std wurden sie nur noch vereinzelt angetroffen. Dagegen waren die Erreger regelmäßig aus dem Darmlumen zu isolieren, wo nach Auffassung von HÜPPE eine intensive Vermehrung stattgefunden hatte. Hinsichtlich des Krankheitsverlaufes und des Sektionsbefundes wurden von GRUBER und WIENER (1892a) sowie PFEIFFER (1894) gleiche Resultate erhoben; die andersartigen bakteriologischen Ergebnisse wurden bereits erwähnt. In Übereinstimmung mit den erstgenannten Autoren befindet sich auch SOBERNHEIM (1893a), der die Vibrionen im Peritonealexsudat meist in solcher Menge fand, daß eine Untersuchung im hängenden Tropfen je Gesichtsfeld viele hundert Exemplare erkennen ließ. Bei den meisten von SOBERNHEIM untersuchten Tieren wurden die Mikroorganismen auch aus Darminhalt isoliert. Die vorherrschende Meinung, daß der Darm nach intraperitonealer Injektion frei von Mikroorganismen bleibe, stützte KOLLE (1894) mit seinen Ergebnissen. Choleravibrionen wurden nur dann aus dem Darm gezüchtet, wenn dieser durch fehlerhafte Injektionstechnik verletzt worden war.

γ) Intrapleurale Infektion. Mit den für die intraperitoneale Infektion verwendeten Erregerdosen erreichte KOLLE (1894) nach intrapleuraler Injektion ähnliche Ergebnisse. Bei 6 Meerschweinchen, denen jeweils $^1/_2$ Öse Kulturabschwemmung injiziert worden war, konnten bei der Sektion die Vibrionen sehr reichlich aus der Pleurahöhle isoliert werden, aus Blut und Darm dagegen nur bei 2 Tieren. Den 10. Teil einer Schrägagarkultur inoculierte SCHÖBL (1916a) 3 Meerschweinchen in die Pleurahöhle. Bei einem Tier, das 24 Std nach der Infektion ante finem getötet worden war, erbrachte die Peptonkultur den Nachweis der Vibrionen aus Pleura, Peritoneum, Blut, Lunge, Leber und Milz. Bei den am 2. und 5. Tag untersuchten Tieren gelang er nicht mehr.

δ) Die nach *subcutaner Infektion* erzielten Ergebnisse sind sehr divergierend. HÜPPE (1887b) hielt die subcutane Infektion für ungeeignet, da nach seiner Ansicht die Tiere an einer Intoxikation zugrunde gehen. Von besonderem Einfluß auf das Resultat sind, wie schon mehrfach betont, die Virulenz des verwendeten Bakterienstammes, die Dosierung und die Vorbehandlung der Tiere. Die mit besonders virulenten Choleravibrionen an der Bauchhaut subcutan infizierten Meerschweinchen verendeten nach wenigen Stunden (KOCH, 1885). Ähnliche Befunde erhoben auch CUNNINGHAM (1886) und WYSSOKOWITSCH (1886). Durch intraperitoneale Vorbehandlung mit 1 ml Opiumtinktur und anschließende subcutane Injektion von $^1/_{10}$ Tropfen bis 3 ml Cholera-Bouillon-Kultur erreichten TIZZONI und CATTANI (1888), daß von 11 Meerschweinchen 8 innerhalb von 2 Tagen zugrunde gingen. Nach Injektion einer Erregerdosis von 1—5 ml und nach Gabe von 40%igem Alkohol durch die Magensonde (1,7 ml/100 g Körpergewicht) starben die meisten Tiere ebenfalls innerhalb 48 Std. Ohne Vorbehandlung und nach Injektion von $^1/_2$ Tropfen bis 7,5 ml erkrankten sie nicht, abgesehen von einer geringen, vorübergehenden Hypothermie. Nach Injektion von 2—4 ml einer Aufschwemmung virulenter Vibrionen starben die Tiere 10—72 Std später, während Meerschweinchen, die mit etwa der gleichen Menge eines weniger virulenten Stammes infiziert worden waren, überlebten (KRAUS und RUSS, 1908; HAHN, 1926).

Die Krankheitserscheinungen nach subcutaner, oraler oder intravenöser Infektion werden von Tizzoni und Cattani (1888) als identisch angesehen. Die Tiere sind wenig lebhaft, freßunlustig, kauern sich mit gesträubtem Fell zusammen und werden mitunter von Krämpfen geschüttelt. Bei der Sektion wurde etwas gelatinöses Bindegewebe an der Injektionsstelle, aber keine entzündliche Reaktion beobachtet. Der pathologisch-anatomische Befund der Bauchorgane glich dem nach oraler Infektion. Von anderer Seite wurden Infiltrate und Abscesse an der Injektionsstelle beschrieben (Masaki, 1922). Wurden die Versuchstiere nach 4—6 Std post infectionem getötet, so war eine starke Hyperämie der Darmwände auffällig (Hahn, 1926).

Die Vibrionen können bereits mikroskopisch an der Inoculationsstelle nachgewiesen werden. Bei 9 von 11 der Infektion erlegenen Meerschweinchen konnten Vibrionen aus Blut, und bei 3 Tieren aus Peritonealflüssigkeit isoliert werden (Tizzoni und Cattani, 1888). Deshalb wurde die Ansicht vertreten, daß es beim Meerschweinchen nach subcutaner Injektion zu einer tödlich verlaufenden septicämischen Erkrankung komme (Wyssokowitsch, 1886; Masaki, 1922; Hahn, 1926). Dagegen kam Gruber (1892) zu dem Ergebnis, daß die Vibrionen nicht über die Injektionsstelle und das benachbarte subcutane Bindegewebe hinausgelangten. Ähnliche Feststellungen traf auch Kolle (1894). Er beobachtete, daß nach subcutaner oder intraperitonealer Injektion die Choleravibrionen im Blut von Meerschweinchen nur dann zu finden waren, wenn die Sektion nicht sofort nach dem Tod der Tiere vorgenommen wurde.

ε) Die *intramuskuläre Infektion* wurde kaum angewandt. Gruber (1892) erwähnt, daß 1 von 3 intramuskulär infizierten Meerschweinchen unter Cholerasymptomen verendete; die anderen Tiere überlebten, jedoch war an der Injektionsstelle eine ausgedehnte Nekrose der Haut und der Muskulatur festzustellen, die eine bleibende Kontraktur der Extremität zur Folge hatte.

ζ) Intracutane Infektion. Diese Technik wird hauptsächlich zur Untersuchung von Choleratoxinen vorwiegend beim Kaninchen angewandt (s. S. 123). Experimentelle Ergebnisse beim Meerschweinchen liegen von Matsumoto et al. (1927) vor. Sie injizierten in Wasser oder Peptonlösung suspendierte Choleravibrionen teils in die rasierte, teils in die nicht rasierte Haut von Meerschweinchen. Im ersten Falle wurden bei 4 von 10 Tieren, die 15—27 Std nach der Infektion getötet waren, die Erreger von der Injektionsstelle, aus Herzblut und verschiedenen Organen, wie Knochenmark und Darm isoliert. Von den 27 Tieren, denen V. cholerae in die nichtrasierte Haut injiziert worden war, wurden in keinem Falle Vibrionen aus Blut oder anderen Organen isoliert; die Erreger waren lediglich an der Injektionsstelle nachzuweisen.

4. Kaninchen

Im Gegensatz zu Meerschweinchen sind junge Kaninchen auch ohne Ruhigstellung des Darmes oder die Anwendung den Darm reizender Mittel für eine experimentelle Cholera auf intestinalem Weg empfänglich. Da das Alter der Tiere von ausschlaggebender Bedeutung ist, ergaben sich zum Teil widersprüchliche Befunde bei gleichen Infektionsmethoden. Für Versuche, die mit operativen Eingriffen verbunden sind, sollten 10—12 Tage alte Kaninchen verwendet werden (Dutta und Habbu, 1955). Empfänglich sind saugende Kaninchen bis höchstens zum 16. Lebenstag. Bei experimentellen Untersuchungen an erwachsenen Kaninchen wurde versucht, mit besonderen Maßnahmen die Widerstandskraft der Tiere gegenüber einer oralen Infektion herabzusetzen, oder es wurden andere Infektionsmethoden gewählt, z.B. die intravenöse Injektion oder die Injektion der Erregerdosis in ein abgebundenes Darmsegment.

a) Infektion über den Magen-Darm-Kanal

α) *Orale Infektion.* Mit einer Bouillonaufschwemmung von 24 Std bebrüteten, virulenten Cholerakulturen bestrich SCHOFFER (1895) die Saugwarzen des Muttertieres und infizierte auf diese Weise 7 Tage alte, 80—90 g schwere Kaninchen. Sämtliche Tiere gingen nach 4—5 Tagen zugrunde. Wurden jedoch auf diese Weise 5 Tage alte Kaninchen von 80—90 g mit einem $1^1/_2$ Jahre alten Laboratoriumsstamm infiziert, erkrankten sie nicht. Auch 2 Kaninchen, die anschließend nochmals die Abschwemmung von 2 bzw. 3 Agarkulturen per os erhalten hatten, blieben gesund. Das Ausbleiben der Infektion wurde mit dem Virulenzverlust dieses Stammes begründet. Der Beweis hierfür wurde dadurch erbracht, daß dieselben Tiere im Alter von 11 Tagen nach Infektion mit dem zuerst benutzten Stamm der Krankheit erlagen. METCHNIKOFF (1894) infizierte 4—7 Tage alte Kaninchen, die alle starben; ähnliche Ergebnisse erzielte auch WIENER (1896 b). Die Erzeugung einer Cholerainfektion bei neugeborenen Kaninchen wurde von BÜRGERS (1911) angezweifelt. Ihm schien es notwendig, die Tiere in irgendeiner Weise vorzubehandeln. Auch VIOLLE (1914 b) hielt diese Art der Infektion für ungeeignet. Er war der Ansicht, eine Vermehrung der Erreger könne im Darm nur unterhalb des Ductus pancreaticus stattfinden. Der Autor bezweifelte nicht zu unrecht, daß die Erreger in ausreichender Menge dorthin gelangten, selbst bei Verwendung massiver Dosen oder von dünndarmlöslichen Gluten-Kapseln. Nach Angaben von CANO (1914) führte dagegen die orale Gabe von 5 ml einer 24 Std bebrüteten Bouillonkultur an 9—18 Tage alte Kaninchen zum Tod nach 38 Std. SANARELLI (1916, 1921) hielt neugeborene Kaninchen ebenfalls für geeignet, erwachsene Tiere für resistent. Die Widerstandskraft dieser Tiere konnte überwunden werden, wenn in das Lymphgewebe von Appendix oder Sacculus rotundus Colibakterien injiziert und einige Stunden später die in Milch aufgeschwemmten Choleravibrionen per os gegeben wurden. Die Kaninchen erlagen dann der Infektion. Zum gleichen Ergebnis kam SANARELLI (1916), wenn er einige Stunden vor der Infektion 1—2 ml des Filtrates einer 48 Std bebrüteten Colibakterienkultur intravenös injizierte. Erkrankung und Tod bei erwachsenen Kaninchen von 2000 g verursachte MASAKI (1922), indem er die Tiere 1—2 Wochen hungern ließ und vor der Infektion an zwei aufeinanderfolgenden Tagen je 10 ml Galle, vermischt mit Lakritzenpulver, an die Tiere verfütterte. Als Dosis letalis gab er die Choleravibrionen-Abschwemmung von 2 Roux-Flaschen an; die Abschwemmung einer Kultur führte nur zu vorübergehender Erkrankung und die Bakteriensuspension einer halben Kultur blieb ohne Wirkung auf die Versuchstiere. Die orale Infektion junger Kaninchen selbst mit erheblichen Erregerdosen glückte HAHN und HIRSCH (1928) in keinem Fall. Während nach intraintestinaler Injektion lebender Choleravibrionen beim saugenden Kaninchen bis zu 100% der Tiere zugrunde gingen, gelang dies DUTTA und HABBU (1955) auf oralem Weg nicht; nach Verabfolgung von 10^8 Vibrionen/100 g Körpergewicht an 100—200 g schwere Kaninchen verendete nur 1 von 8 Tieren innerhalb 48 Std. Dagegen konnte FEELEY (1965) im Rahmen seiner Immunisierungsversuche bei 9 Kaninchen, die 10—12 Tage alt waren, eine tödlich verlaufende Choleraerkrankung hervorrufen. Eine Minute vor der Infektion hatten die Tiere pro 100 g Gewicht 1 ml einer 1%igen Na_2CO_3-Lösung mit der Magensonde erhalten. Erregerdosis war 1 ml der 10^{-4}-verdünnten Abschwemmung einer 18 Std bebrüteten Schrägagarkultur (entspricht etwa $1,5 \times 10^5$ vermehrungsfähigen Bakterien/ml). Diese Menge, die bei oraler Infektion regelmäßig zu einer Choleraerkrankung führte, lag damit erheblich über der für eine intestinale Infektion erforderlichen Dosis von 10 vermehrungsfähigen Choleravibrionen (McINTYRE und FEELEY, 1964). Wurde oral eine 10^{-5} verdünnte Abschwemmung zugeführt, starben von 9 Kaninchen nur 3. Eine sichere Erkrankung der Versuchstiere war mit dieser Erregerdosis nicht mehr möglich.

Im saugenden Kaninchen war damit ein Versuchstier gefunden, das oral meist leicht infiziert werden kann und Krankheitserscheinungen sowie Sektionsbefunde aufweist, die der menschlichen Cholera in hohem Maße ähnlich sind (Issaeff und Kolle, 1894; Metchnikoff, 1894; Schoffer, 1895; Sanarelli, 1916). Im Vordergrund des klinischen Bildes stehen die Darmsymptome. Anders als beim Meerschweinchen, treten beim Kaninchen in der Regel sehr heftige Diarrhoen auf. Manche Tiere sind „über und über beschmiert und wie in Jauche getaucht" (Wiener, 1896b). Bei der tödlich verlaufenden Infektion ist das Krankheitsbild um so charakteristischer, in je kürzerer Zeit der Tod des Tieres eintritt.

Auch vorbehandelte, erwachsene Kaninchen zeigten Symptome, die dem klinischen Bild einer Cholera entsprachen und an der die Versuchstiere gelegentlich zugrunde gingen (Sanarelli, 1916). Daneben wurden ein Absinken der Körpertemperatur unter 30° C, Cyanose, Gewichtsverlust und generalisierte Krämpfe der Skeletmuskulatur ante finem registriert (Issaeff und Kolle, 1894; Metchnikoff, 1894). Eine Schilderung tödlich verlaufender Erkrankungen bei erwachsenen Kaninchen teilte Masaki (1922) mit:

Nach dem 2.—4. Tag verweigerten die Tiere die Nahrungsaufnahme, nahmen an Gewicht ab und verhielten sich tagelang unbeweglich in einer Ecke ihres Käfigs. Die Körpertemperatur stieg auf 40—41° C. Es traten Diarrhoen auf, die zunehmend profuser wurden; eine Woche nach der Infektion sistierten die Diarrhoen und die Körpertemperatur normalisierte sich; die Tiere fraßen jedoch weiterhin nicht oder nur außerordentlich wenig und nahmen permanent an Gewicht ab. Etwa 2—3 Wochen nach der Infektion gingen sie in einem kachektischen Zustand bei einem Gewichtsverlust von 400—500 g zugrunde.

Im Vergleich zur experimentellen Infektion des saugenden Kaninchens muß der chronische Verlauf und die Erhöhung der Körpertemperatur hervorgehoben werden.

Bei der Sektion verendeter saugender Kaninchen findet man den Dünndarm erweitert und vor allem in seinem oberen Abschnitt eine starke Flüssigkeitsansammlung; die Darmwand ist entzündet und erscheint tiefdunkel- bis rotviolett. Der Dickdarm ist fast nie hyperämisch, Coecum und Colon sind meist stark erweitert; das Coecum ist ebenfalls mit einer großen Menge alkalisch reagierender Flüssigkeit gefüllt, in der Schleimflocken und Epithelzellen schwimmen, vergleichbar den reiswasserähnlichen Stühlen bei der Cholera des Menschen (Metchnikoff, 1894; Wiener, 1896b). Von 32 infizierten Tieren zeigten in den Untersuchungen von Issaeff und Kolle (1894) 9 diesen typischen Befund. Die Tiere, bei denen die Todesursache nicht geklärt werden konnte, wiesen eine deutliche, hauptsächlich durch Verfettung verursachte Gelbfärbung der Leber auf, wie sie von den Autoren auch bei einer Choleraerkrankung nach intravenöser Infektion beobachtet worden war. Daß die bei den überlebenden Tieren vorübergehend aufgetretene Diarrhoe auf eine Infektion mit Choleraerregern zurückzuführen war, bewiesen Issaeff und Kolle (1894) mit der protektiven Wirkung des Serums dieser Tiere im Pfeifferschen Versuch.

Besonders die erwachsenen Kaninchen, denen Colibakterien in den Sacculus rotundus injiziert worden waren, hatten ausgeprägte Läsionen der Darmwände; bei chronischem Verlauf wurden zum Teil schwere Ulcerationen am Darmtrakt und Nierenschädigungen konstatiert. Aufgrund dieser Befunde, die wenig Ähnlichkeit mit einer Choleraerkrankung besaßen, wurde das Krankheitsbild von Sanarelli (1923a) bei chronischem Verlauf als „choleriforme Enterocolitis" bezeichnet.

Die Krankheitserreger werden beim saugenden Kaninchen massenhaft, in der Regel in Reinkultur im Dünndarm angetroffen; das Coecum beherbergt neben anderen Bakterienarten ebenfalls große Mengen Choleravibrionen (ISSAEFF und KOLLE, 1894; METCHNIKOFF, 1894; SCHOFFER, 1895; WIENER, 1896b; CANO, 1914). In besonders foudroyant verlaufenden Krankheitsfällen ist der gesamte Darmtrakt mit Choleravibrionen überschwemmt. Im Coecum werden die Mikroorganismen dicht gedrängt in weißlichen Flocken gefunden; die Vermehrung anderer Bakterienarten ist unterdrückt, so daß diese bakterioskopisch nicht nachweisbar sind. Je länger sich jedoch die Erkrankung hinzieht, um so mehr treten Beimengungen anderer Bakterienspecies auf. Der Magen enthält nur selten Choleravibrionen (METCHNIKOFF, 1894; WIENER, 1896b). Entgegen der allgemeinen Auffassung, wonach Choleravibrionen über den Magen in den Darm gelangen, vertritt SANARELLI (1916, 1923a) den Standpunkt, daß die Mikroorganismen beim saugenden und erwachsenen Kaninchen durch die buccale Mucosa über den Lymphweg oder Blutkreislauf in den Darm eingeschleust werden; die Bakterien sollen beim erwachsenen Kaninchen in Höhe der Ileocöcalklappe in den Darm (Ileum, Coecum) ausgeschieden werden, von wo sie mitunter darmaufwärts gelangen. Das Duodenum erreichen sie jedoch selten, denn Magen und Duodenum waren in der Regel frei von Vibrionen (SANARELLI, 1916). Die beim älteren jungen Kaninchen und beim erwachsenen Tier beobachtete Resistenz gegenüber der Infektion führte SANARELLI (1921, 1923a) hauptsächlich auf eine geringere Durchlässigkeit der buccalen Mucosa für Vibrionen und eine abgeschwächte Sensibilität der Intestinalschleimhaut zurück. SANARELLI (1923a) wies nach, daß die Vibrionen beim erwachsenen Kaninchen 24 Std post infectionem die Darmwand erreichten. Aus Tieren, die nach 2—3 Wochen in kachektischem Zustand zugrunde gingen, konnten keine Vibrionen mehr isoliert werden. Dieser Befund wurde unabhängig davon erhoben, ob oral, intraperitoneal, intranasal oder intratracheal infiziert war. Nicht immer ist der Nachweis von Vibrionen im Darm mit dem Auftreten von Krankheitserscheinungen verbunden. Bei mehreren Kaninchen, die im Alter von 25—28 Tagen infiziert worden waren, konnten sie 24 Std später aus Kotpartikeln gezüchtet werden, obwohl es zu keinen Cholerasymptomen gekommen war (SCHOFFER, 1895). Ob die von MASAKI (1922) mitgeteilten tödlichen Erkrankungen der erwachsenen Kaninchen tatsächlich durch Choleravibrionen ausgelöst wurden, muß dahingestellt bleiben, zumal ein Erregernachweis aus dem Darm nicht gelang. Über die Einschwemmung von Vibrionen in andere Organe liegen unterschiedliche Angaben vor. Bei 20 infizierten jungen, saugenden Kaninchen isolierte SCHOFFER (1895) 10mal Choleravibrionen aus dem Herzblut, 1mal in Verbindung mit anderen Darmbakterien; bei allen Tieren wurden sie aus Leberblut nachgewiesen, in 9 Proben waren allerdings noch E. coli und andere Darmbewohner vorhanden. In $^2/_3$ der Tierexperimente konnte WIENER (1896b) Vibrionen aus Herz und Leber züchten, selten aus Niere und Milz. Ähnliche Befunde teilte CANO (1914) mit. In den von SANARELLI (1916) durchgeführten Untersuchungen dagegen waren Blut- und Organproben erwachsener Kaninchen stets steril.

β) Rectale Infektion. Wie bei Meerschweinchen und Affen wurde auch bei Kaninchen versucht, mit dieser Infektionsmethode die Wirkung des sauren Magensaftes zu umgehen. Die Einführung großer Erregerdosen durch den Anus verursachte bei Kaninchen eine tödlich verlaufende Mischinfektion. Choleravibrionen und Darmbakterien gelangten in sämtliche inneren Organe; die Tiere starben innerhalb 1—2 Std. Wurde der After nicht mit Collodium verschlossen, so war es unmöglich, eine Infektion zu erzeugen (SEWASTIANOFF, 1910; CRENDIROPOULO, 1921; SANARELLI, 1921).

γ) Injektion in Magen und Duodenum. Da der Magen des Kaninchens wie der des Meerschweinchens stark sauer reagiert, scheint die Injektion der säureempfindlichen Choleravibrionen in dieses Organ wenig Erfolg versprechend. Nach Gastrostomie direkt in den Magen eingeführte Choleravibrionen konnten 6 Std später aus dem Darm isoliert werden; Blutkulturen dagegen, die 2—4 Std nach der Infektion angelegt wurden, blieben steril (Solarino, 1939).

Die Rolle, welche Verdauungssekreten von Pankreas und Leber bei einer Choleraerkrankung zukommt, wurde von Violle (1914b) eingehend bei 2—3 kg schweren Kaninchen untersucht. Das Kaninchen schien ihm als Versuchstier besonders geeignet, da bei diesem der D. pancreaticus etwa 20—30 cm unterhalb des D. choledochus in den Darm mündet. Die Wirkung des Pankreassekretes wurde ausgeschaltet durch Hitzecoagulation des Organs oder durch Injektion von geschmolzenem Talg in die Pankreaskanäle. Die Injektion der Choleravibrionen in Höhe der Einmündungsstelle des D. pancreaticus oder oberhalb und unterhalb des Ostiums führte in allen Untersuchungen zu keinen Ergebnissen. Der Gallenfluß wurde durch eine Ligatur des D. choledochus unterbrochen, ein Vorgehen, das nicht ohne Operationsrisiko ist. Durch eine Injektion der Choleravibrionen wenige Zentimeter unterhalb des Pylorus konnte keine Erkrankung ausgelöst werden. Erst die Injektion der Erregerdosis 1—2 cm unterhalb des D. pancreaticus rief eine tödliche Choleraerkrankung hervor. Von 9 Tieren erlagen 8 innerhalb 24 Std unter typischen Symptomen der Infektion. Die benutzte Erregerdosis betrug 0,25—3 ml einer 18 Std bebrüteten Bouillonkultur/kg Körpergewicht. Aus den Untersuchungsergebnissen von Violle (1914b) ist zu entnehmen, daß Pankreasenzym und Gallenflüssigkeit keinen Einfluß auf die Cholerainfektion beim Kaninchen haben (s. hierzu S. 119).

Arnold und Shapiro (1930) suspendierten die Erreger in 0,15 M Dinatriumphosphatlösung. Innerhalb 48 Std starben 7 von 12 Kaninchen, 2 weitere verendeten 72 und 96 Std post infectionem. Erhielten die Tiere die Choleravibrionen dagegen in Kochsalzlösung aufgeschwemmt, so kam es zu keinerlei Krankheitserscheinungen.

Nach Violle (1914b) vermehren sich die injizierten Vibrionen im Darm lebhaft und führen innerhalb weniger Stunden zu einer mehr oder weniger ausgeprägten „Enteritis". Bei der Sektion wurde im gesamten Darm reichlich zähflüssige oder reiswasserähnliche Flüssigkeit weißlicher oder schmutzig-weißgelber Farbe angetroffen. Der Dünndarm einschließlich Coecum schien mehr oder weniger gestaut, rosa bis dunkelweinrot oder leuchtendrot verfärbt. Nahe des Pylorus und der Mündung des D. pancreaticus fanden sich meist ausgeprägte petechiale Blutungen. In 1 Tropfen dieser Darmflüssigkeit konnten bereits mikroskopisch massenhaft kommaförmige Mikroorganismen gesehen werden. Die reisförmigen Körnchen, welche in der Darmflüssigkeit schwammen, enthielten außer Vibrionen desquamierte Epithelzellen, Leukocyten und Schleim. In den daraus angelegten Kulturen wurde V. cholerae gezüchtet.

δ) *Injektion in den Dünndarm.* Nach Injektion von Choleravibrionen in den Dünndarm gelang es den Untersuchern zum Teil nicht, eine Erkrankung hervorzurufen (Koch, 1885; Violle und Crendiropoulo, 1915; Hahn und Hirsch, 1928). Durch Applikation bis zu 2 Ösen Kulturmaterial dagegen konnten Issaeff und Kolle (1894) bei 4 von 11 Kaninchen, die 240—470 g schwer waren, eine tödlich verlaufende Choleraerkrankung auslösen. In neuerer Zeit infizierten Dutta und Habbu (1955) 10 Tage alte, 100—200 g schwere Kaninchen beiderlei Geschlechts. Die Erregerdosis wurde folgendermaßen gewonnen: lyophilisierte Vibrionen werden in einem flüssigen Nährmedium über Nacht zur Vermehrung gebracht; anschließend werden die Mikroorganismen auf Schrägagar überimpft und 18 Std bebrütet. Von den Kolonien wird 1 Öse (Durchmesser 1 mm) Bakterienmaterial entnommen und in 10 ml Nährbouillon eingerieben, die 3 Std bei 37° inkubiert wird. Nach dieser Zeit sind in dem Nährsubstrat annähernd 10^{10} Vibrionen/ml enthalten. Diese Bakterienaufschwemmung kann für Tierexperimente entsprechend verdünnt werden. Die Autoren infizierten bei ihren Untersuchungen:

1. 8 Tiere mit 10^9 Vibrionen/100 g Körpergewicht; von diesen erlagen 3 der Infektion nach 3—4 Tagen;

2. 25 Kaninchen mit 5×10^7 Vibrionen, denen 5% Mucin zugesetzt war; von ihnen gingen 11 Tiere zugrunde;

3. 111 Kaninchen, mit dem zuvor über Tiere geführten Vibrionenstamm; alle Tiere starben, auch wenn die Erregerdosis nur 10^4 oder 10^3 Vibrionen/ml betrug.

Auf diese Arbeit von DUTTA und HABBU (1955) wird in der Literatur wiederholt Bezug genommen. Es sollte allerdings bei der als „Dutta's Methode" bezeichneten Infektionsweise an jungen, saugenden Kaninchen beachtet werden, daß die Autoren die intraintestinale Infektion nur für das Experimentieren mit vermehrungsfähigen Choleravibrionen anwenden, während sie in Übereinstimmung mit anderen Untersuchern beim Arbeiten mit Choleratoxinen die orale Applikation als geeignet ansehen. Eine Resistenz 10 Tage alter Kaninchen gegenüber einer intraintestinalen Infektion mit Choleravibrionen scheint kaum vorzukommen; von 144 infizierten Tieren erkrankte nur 1 Kaninchen nicht, das 10^8 Vibrionen eines nicht über Tiere geführten Stammes/100 g Körpergewicht erhalten hatte (DUTTA und HABBU, 1955). JENKIN und ROWLEY (1960) injizierten 8 Kaninchen, die 7 Tage alt und 68—132 g schwer waren, 0,25 ml einer Vibrionensuspension, welche 10^8 Bakterien/ml enthielt. Innerhalb von 72 Std trat bei allen Tieren der Tod ein. Saugende Kaninchen, denen DUTTA und PANSE (1963) 10^4 Vibrionen/ 100 g Körpergewicht applizierten, erlagen ebenfalls der Infektion.

Die intraintestinale Infektion junger, saugender Kaninchen ist eine besonders empfindliche Methode, mit der auch bei sehr geringen Erregerdosen regelmäßig Krankheitserscheinungen und Tod der Versuchstiere erzielt werden können. Dies gelingt auch noch mit 10 vermehrungsfähigen Choleravibrionen (MCINTYRE und FEELEY, 1964) und, wie GILLMORE (1965) zeigte, durch die Injektion von nur 2—3 Choleravibrionen in das Jejunum 12 Tage alter Kaninchen. Den typischen Krankheitsverlauf beim saugenden Tier beschrieben DUTTA und HABBU (1955): etwa 16—24 Std nach Infektion mit 10^4 Vibrionen wurden die ersten dünnflüssigen Stühle bei den Kaninchen beobachtet. Schwere Diarrhoen traten im Durchschnitt 22 Std post infectionem auf. Die Tiere erlagen frühestens 22 Std, spätestens nach 52 Std der Infektion. Nach den ersten flüssigen Stühlen lebten die Tiere noch durchschnittlich 10 Std. Ante finem lagen die Tiere erschöpft und bewegungslos da; die Haut war kalt, das Fell rauh und glanzlos; gelegentlich wurden kurz vor dem Tod generalisierte Krämpfe beobachtet. Die toten Tiere waren abgemagert und ihre Bauchseite mit flüssigen Ausscheidungen beschmutzt.

Bei Kaninchen, die nicht über Tiere geführte Stämme, sondern als Erregerdosis 5×10^7—10^8 mit Mucin versetzte Vibrionen erhielten, wurden nur zum Teil starke Diarrhoen registriert. Diejenigen Versuchstiere, welche charakteristische Symptome der experimentellen Cholera aufwiesen, hatten einen signifikant erhöhten Hämatokritwert, ebenso waren der Reststickstoff und Harnstoff im Serum erhöht (DUTTA und HABBU, 1955). In den Dejekten der Kaninchen, die Dehydration zeigten, wurde eine Elektrolytkonzentration festgestellt, welche der Konzentration in den Ausscheidungen cholerakranker Menschen ähnlich war (GILLMORE, 1965).

Nach Untersuchungen von ISSAEFF und KOLLE (1894) wiesen nur 4 von 11 Tieren bei der Sektion einen ausgeprägten Cholerabefund auf, bei 3 anderen

Tieren, die 6—15 Tage nach der Infektion gestorben waren, war lediglich eine Rötung des Dünndarms und Leberverfettung auffällig. Dieser pathologisch-anatomische Befund wurde als Zeichen einer abgelaufenen Choleraerkrankung gewertet.

Bei der Obduktion gestorbener saugender Kaninchen war der Dickdarm erweitert, blaß und mit einer wäßrigen Flüssigkeit gefüllt, in der Schleimhautfetzen schwammen. Der Dünndarm zeigte Gefäßstauung und enthielt eine viscöse Flüssigkeit; Teile der Schleimhaut waren zerstört. Der untere Teil des Ileums war nicht so stark erweitert wie der obere des Dickdarms. Leber, Milz und Nieren wurden als normal oder leicht gestaut beurteilt (Dutta und Habbu, 1955). Eine reiswasserähnliche Flüssigkeit im unteren Teil von Ileum und Coecum und des Colon ascendens beobachteten Jenkin und Rowley (1959).

Die Choleravibrionen wurden meist aus dem Dünndarm und aus den wäßrigen Darmentleerungen isoliert (Issaeff und Kolle, 1894; Dutta und Habbu, 1955). Diesen Befunden stehen andere Untersuchungsergebnisse gegenüber; so war es Violle und Crendiropoulo (1915) nicht möglich, 24 Std nach der Gabe großer Mengen Choleravibrionen die Erreger im Dünndarm nachzuweisen. Auch Hahn und Hirsch (1928) gelang bei keinem ihrer Experimente die Isolierung aus dem Kot der Kaninchen. Kurz nach dem Tod von 50 Tieren entnommene Blut- und Organproben erbrachten 3mal den Erregernachweis aus Herzblut und 1mal aus Lebergewebe (Dutta und Habbu, 1955).

ε) *Injektion in das abgebundene Dünndarmsegment.* Violle und Crendiropoulo (1915) konnten am Darm des erwachsenen Kaninchens die Zeichen einer Choleraerkrankung hervorrufen, wenn die Erregerdosis in ein durch 2 Ligaturen abgebundenes Darmsegment injiziert wurde. Die dadurch erzeugten Darmläsionen waren variabel und hingen insbesondere von der Länge des Segments, seiner Lage und der Virulenz der injizierten Bakterien ab. Als geeignet erwies sich ein Teilstück von ca. 10 cm Länge, das dicht unterhalb des D. choledochus abgeschnürt war. Wurde das Segment einige Dezimeter tiefer angelegt oder war es mehrere Dezimeter lang, so waren die pathologisch-anatomischen Veränderungen weniger ausgeprägt. Ein besonderes Operationsrisiko war die pylorusnahe Unterbindung. Denn Kontrolltiere, denen keine Vibrionen injiziert worden waren, starben allein durch diese Art der Ligatur. Ähnliche Beobachtungen teilten Nicati und Rietsch (1884a) sowie Koch (1885) beim Meerschweinchen nach Unterbindung des D. choledochus mit. In den Untersuchungen von De und Chatterje (1953) wurden zehn 1 200—1 500 g schweren Kaninchen 24 Std vor dem Eingriff Futter und Wasser entzogen. Unter lokaler Procainanaesthesie und aseptischen Kautelen wurde 5 cm lang bis kurz unterhalb Abdomenmitte incidiert. Nach Durchtrennung der Muskulatur und Eröffnung des Peritoneums wurde in der Mitte des Dünndarms die Ligatur mit 2 Seidenfäden gelegt und die Unterbindung von Blutgefäßen sorgfältig vermieden. Als Erregerdosis diente die Suspension einer Öse Bakterien aus einer 24 Std bebrüteten flüssigen Cholerakultur in 1 ml Durhams Peptonwasser. Nach diesem Eingriff erhielten die Versuchstiere weder Wasser noch Futter. Weiteren 3 Tieren wurden 4 Std nach der Infektion 4 ml 2%ige Evansblau-Lösung intravenös injiziert. Spätere Untersuchungen beziehen sich meist auf diese Technik, die durch das Anlegen von 3 Segmenten an einem Tier modifiziert wurde (Ghosh und Mukerjee, 1959; Jenkin und Rowley, 1960). Als Erregerdosis wurden teils 0,5 ml Bouillonkultur mit 10^9 Vibrionen verwendet (Ghosh und Mukerjee, 1959), teils 1 ml mit 5×10^8 (Jenkin und Rowley, 1960) oder 5×10^7 bis $1,5 \times 10^8$ Mikroorganismen, die in 0,25 ml Gehirn-Herz-Infusionsbouillon aufgeschwemmt waren (Formal et al., 1961). Bei Experimenten, die Sayamov (1963a) mit 23 Kaninchen durchführte, welche 1 300 bis

1900 g wogen, wurden 0,5 ml der Abschwemmung einer 24 Std alten Agarkultur gegeben, die 2×10^5 bis 5×10^6 Cholera-, El-Tor- oder Makassarvibrionen/ml enthielt.

Die Versuchstiere wurden mitunter nach 48 Std (SAYAMOV, 1963a), im allgemeinen jedoch nach 24 Std getötet (DE und CHATTERJE, 1953; SAYAMOV, 1963a).

Das Ergebnis des Versuchs ist als positiv zu interpretieren, wenn durch die Wirkung der injizierten Choleravibrionen das Lumen des abgebundenen Darmsegments infolge Flüssigkeitsansammlung erweitert ist (VIOLLE und CRENDIROPOULO, 1915; DE und CHATTERJE, 1953; FORMAL et al., 1961; SAYAMOV, 1963a). Kontrollsegmente, in die Kochsalz- oder Nährlösung injiziert wird, sollen kollabiert bleiben und keine Flüssigkeit enthalten.

Die Schleimhaut von Darmsegmenten, die dicht unterhalb des D. choledochus angelegt waren, wurde weinrot verfärbt angetroffen. Eine leichte Desquamation des Mucosa-Epithels konnte in solchen Darmsegmenten beobachtet werden, die weiter caudal abgebunden worden waren und deren Länge mehrere Dezimeter betrug. War dagegen nach einer Ligatur die Erregerdosis intraintestinal oder intravenös injiziert worden, so fanden sich im Bereich der Unterbindungsstelle keine Veränderungen der Darmwand (VIOLLE und CRENDIROPOULO, 1915). Positive Befunde wurden auch am Jejunum und Ileum erhoben. Aus den infizierten Darmsegmenten konnten DE und CHATTERJE (1953) jeweils 14—20 ml einer reiswasserähnlichen, rosagefärbten Flüssigkeit entnehmen, die zahlreiche Schleimhautfetzen, desquamierte Epithelzellen und vereinzelt auch Leukocyten enthielt. Der Albumingehalt dieser Flüssigkeit lag zwischen 1,0—3,8%. Dies deutet darauf hin, daß Plasmaproteine über das Intestinalgewebe und die Capillaren das Lumen des abgebundenen Darmsegments erreichen. Gestützt wird dieser Befund durch die Beobachtung, daß die Flüssigkeit im abgebundenen Darmsegment durch intravenös injizierte Evansblau-Lösung verfärbt wird. Der Nachweis des Farbstoffes in den verschiedenen Wandabschnitten des Dünndarms und im Segmentlumen gelingt 24 Std nach der Injektion. Proximal des infizierten Segments enthielt der erweiterte Dünndarm bei Versuchs- und Kontrolltieren eine gelbliche Flüssigkeit mit einem Albumingehalt von 0,4—0,5%. Distal war der Darm kollabiert und ohne Flüssigkeit. Die histologische Untersuchung des isolierten Darmstückes ergab ein ausgeprägtes Gewebsödem mit entsprechender Erweiterung der Submucosa, der Gewebsspalten und der lymphatischen Kanäle. Die größeren Blutgefäße waren prall gefüllt, während die Capillaren aufgrund des Druckes der Ödemflüssigkeit kollabiert und kaum zu sehen waren. Die Epithelzellen der Zottenspitzen hatten pyknotische Kerne und waren meist nekrotisch. Manche Stromazellen der Mucosa wiesen hydropische Veränderungen auf, die in der Epithelschicht nicht zu beobachten waren. Die Darmwandmuskulatur war unauffällig. Unter der Serosa wurden Fibrinablagerungen beobachtet. Eine celluläre Infiltration konnte in keinem Abschnitt der Darmwand festgestellt werden. Aus diesen Befunden schließen DE und CHATTERJE (1953), daß V. cholerae oder seine toxischen Produkte die Permeabilität der Intestinalcapillaren erhöhen. Dabei treten Plasmaproteine in das Gewebe über, steigern den osmotischen Druck und fixieren die Gewebeflüssigkeit in der Submucosa. FORMAL et al. (1961) konstatierten neben diesem Flüssigkeitsaustritt beim erwachsenen Kaninchen Zeichen einer akuten Entzündung. Im frühen Stadium der Infektion wurden keine Vibrionen in der unversehrten Epithelschicht gefunden; sobald jedoch Epithelzellen innerhalb des abgebundenen Darmsegments nekrotisch wurden, konnten sie auch in der Lamina propria nachgewiesen werden. Aufgrund der pathologisch-histologischen Veränderungen des Darmsegments teilten FORMAL et al. (1961) das Krankheitsgeschehen an dem unterbundenen Darmstück in folgende Stadien ein: 1. akute Entzündung, 2. akute Entzündung mit fokaler Nekrose, 3. Entzündung mit starker Nekrose.

Eine ausgeprägte Entzündung nach Injektion von Choleravibrionen in ein Darmsegment des erwachsenen Kaninchens schildert Sayamov (1963a); dabei wurden Kongestion, Hämorrhagien, Destruktion von Bezirken der Schleimhaut, fokale Desquamation des Epithels und Leukocyteninfiltration in die Darmwand des isolierten Segments protokolliert. Ähnliche Veränderungen zeigten sich nach Injektion von El-Tor- und Makassarvibrionen. Die Läsionen an der Darmwand innerhalb des abgebundenen Segments korrespondieren nach der Ansicht von De und Chatterje (1953) mit den Befunden bei der Cholerainfektion des Menschen; auch der Darminhalt ist makroskopisch und mikroskopisch ähnlich dem Cholerastuhl des Menschen.

Formal et al. (1961) verglichen die pathologisch-anatomischen Veränderungen bei diesem Modellversuch mit den frühen Stadien der Cholerainfektion des Menschen. Da derartige Ergebnisse in der Regel nur nach oraler und intestinaler Infektion des jungen saugenden Kaninchens erzielt werden (Schoffer, 1895; Dutta und Habbu, 1955), vermutet Finkelstein (1965) beim erwachsenen Kaninchen Enzymaktivitäten, die beim saugenden Kaninchen noch nicht ausgebildet sind. Die Spezifität der beschriebenen Läsionen für Choleravibrionen ist fraglich, da diese Veränderungen auch durch andere Vibrionen und gelegentlich auch durch andere Bakterienspecies verursacht werden (Taylor et al., 1961).

Die Vibrionen konnten nach Untersuchungen von Violle und Crendiropoulo (1915) meist in Reinkultur und massenhaft aus dem dicht unterhalb des D. choledochus angelegten Darmstück isoliert werden. Eine geringfügige Vermehrung wurde in Segmenten des distalen Dünndarmabschnittes und in mehreren Dezimeter langen Segmenten festgestellt. Bei einer Ligatur ließen sich die Vibrionen nach 24 Std nicht mehr nachweisen. Die Choleravibrionen konnten von De und Chatterje (1953) stets im unterbundenen Darmsegment, jedoch nie in den übrigen Teilen des Dünndarmes nachgewiesen werden. Hämorrhagische Nekrosen und Flüssigkeitsansammlung wurden von Jenkin und Rowley (1959, 1960) nur dann beobachtet, wenn die injizierten Vibrionen sich vermehrt hatten. Der Bakteriengehalt betrug etwa 2×10^{11}/ml Darminhalt. In einigen Experimenten wurden die Choleravibrionen auch aus Blut und Galle isoliert (Sayamov, 1963a). Nach den Untersuchungen dieses Autors enthielt die Darmflüssigkeit 3×10^7 bis 8×10^8 Choleravibrionen/ml. Neben V. cholerae wurde in dem isolierten Darmsegment auch häufig Darmflora angetroffen, die die Vermehrungstätigkeit der Vibrionen beeinträchtigen kann.

ζ) Infektion der Gallenblase. Die intravesiculäre Infektion wurde 1. zur Erzeugung von Gallenblasenläsionen, 2. zum Studium der Verweildauer der Choleravibrionen in diesem Organ und 3. zur Klärung der Frage einer Ausscheidung von Choleravibrionen über die Gallenwege angewandt. Methodisch ging man so vor, daß die Mikroorganismen ohne (Violle, 1912; Nichols, 1916; Schöbl, 1916b; Calvano, 1933; Sayamov, 1963a) oder nach Unterbindung des D. choledochus und/oder des D. cysticus (Violle, 1912) in die Gallenblase injiziert wurden.

Bei seinen umfangreichen Untersuchungen kam Violle (1912) zu unterschiedlichen Ergebnissen, die im wesentlichen davon abhingen, ob der D. cysticus unterbunden, die Gallenflüssigkeit abgesaugt und die Gallenblase gespült wurden. Nach Unterbindung des D. cysticus ist die Gallenblase ein abgeschlossenes Säckchen, das nach Absaugen der Gallenflüssigkeit mit leicht alkalisch reagierendem Wasser gespült wurde. Anschließend wurde z.B. die Hälfte einer 24 Std bebrüteten Agarkultur in 1 ml physiologischer Kochsalzlösung aufgeschwemmt und in den Pol der Gallenblase injiziert. Das Kaninchen reagierte mit einer vorübergehenden, leichten Temperaturerhöhung ohne weitere Krankheitszeichen. Bei der Sektion des nach 15 Tagen getöteten Tieres war die Gallenblase nicht mit ihrer Umgebung verwachsen, eine Verdickung der Wand wurde nicht festgestellt, lediglich die Schleimhaut zeigte eine leichte Kongestion. Mit Hilfe der Peptonanreicherung konnten Choleravibrionen aus der Gallenblase isoliert werden. Eine mit Herzblut angelegte Peptonkultur blieb steril. Wenn bei diesem Infektionsmodus eine sehr geringe Erregerdosis appliziert wurde, trat eine Rötung der Gallenblasenschleimhaut auf, welcher eine Epithelzelldesquamation folgte; die Einwanderung von Leukocyten führte später zur Vernichtung der Vibrionen, die nach 2—3 Wochen nicht mehr nachzuweisen waren. Die Wand der Gallenblase wurde jetzt hypertrophiert vorgefunden. Bei einem Leerversuch dagegen — nach Aspiration der Gallenflüssigkeit und Unterbindung des D. cysticus — stellte sich nach einigen Wochen die Gallenblase wie eine ausgetrocknete und mit Falten durchfurchte Membran dar. VIOLLE (1912) hielt es für erforderlich, die Gallenblase vor der Infektion zu entleeren, um dadurch die zu injizierenden Choleravibrionen besser auf ihrer Schleimhaut zum Haften zu bringen. Unterblieb diese Manipulation, so vermehrten sie sich sehr rasch, was eine generalisierte Aussaat begünstigte. So ging 1 Kaninchen bereits 12 Std nach der Injektion eines Tropfens einer 18 Std bebrüteten Cholerakultur zugrunde. Die Autopsie erbrachte geringfügige Organveränderungen; die Peritonealflüssigkeit war kaum vermehrt, enthielt jedoch massenhaft Choleravibrionen. Die Gallenblase war geschrumpft und schlaff; ihre Flüssigkeit beherbergte reichlich Mucosazellen, in denen Vibrionen eingeschlossen waren (VIOLLE, 1912). Der entzündliche Prozeß der Gallenblase ist beim Kaninchen nach den Untersuchungen von SCHÖBL (1916b) ausgeprägter als beim Meerschweinchen. Bei den meisten Tieren war es zu Verklebungen des D. cysticus und damit zum Verschluß der Gallenblase gekommen. Wegen dieser Abflußbehinderungen konnten die Choleravibrionen nicht in den Darm gelangen. Die entzündlichen Veränderungen waren unterschiedlich in Ausdehnung und Intensität; sie konnten auf die Gallenblase beschränkt bleiben oder auf die Leber übergreifen. Sie zeigten jedoch eine ausgesprochene Tendenz zur Heilung, so daß die Kaninchen in der Regel überlebten. Im Gegensatz zu VIOLLE konnte SCHÖBL die Mikroorganismen in Blut-, Lungen- und Milzproben nicht mehr nachweisen. Er schloß deshalb einen septicämischen Charakter der Infektion aus. Während NICHOLS (1916) diese Ergebnisse bei intravesiculär infizierten Kaninchen bestätigte, beurteilte CALVANO (1933) die Injektion von kleinen Erregerdosen in die Gallenblase als die geeignetste Methode, um beim Kaninchen eine „choleraähnliche" Erkrankung hervorzurufen. Die von SAYAMOV (1963a) mit Cholera-, El-Tor- und Makassarvibrionen infizierten Kaninchen waren klinisch unauffällig. Bei der Sektion der 1—2 Tage nach der Infektion getöteten Versuchstiere enthielt die Gallenblase eine dicke, mit Schleim angereicherte Flüssigkeit. An der Mucosa waren leichte katarrhalische Entzündungserscheinungen zu registrieren. Bei 1—2 Wochen post infectionem getöteten Kaninchen waren, wie bei den Untersuchungen von VIOLLE (1912), die Gallenblasenmucosa und die Gallenflüssigkeit unverändert, bei den meisten Tieren die Wand der Gallenblase jedoch leicht hypertrophiert.

Zur Überlebensdauer der in die Gallenblase injizierten Choleravibrionen findet sich bei VIOLLE (1912) der Hinweis, daß sie noch 3 Monate nach der Infektion isoliert werden konnten. Aus der Tabelle 3 ist zu entnehmen, daß SAYAMOV (1963a) Choleravibrionen bei 2 von 4 Versuchstieren noch nach 76 bzw. 96 Tagen aus der Gallenblase züchten konnte. Die Isolierung von El-Tor- und Makassarvibrionen gelang zu einem noch späteren Zeitpunkt.

Tabelle 3. Adaptation von Vibrionen an die Galle von Kaninchen; Zahl der Kaninchen, aus denen Vibrionen isoliert wurden/Zahl der Untersuchten. (Nach Sayamov 1963a)

Kaninchen infi-ziert mit	Tage nach Infektion der Gallenblase						
	1—7	8—14	15—41	42—56	57—75	76—96	97—108
El-Tor-Vibrionen	6/6	4/4	3/3	1/1	3/5	5/7	8/10
Makassarvibrionen	3/4	3/3	2/2	1/1	2/4	7/8	2/3
Choleravibrionen	1/1	4/4	2/2	3/3	17/18	2/4	—
Wasservibrionen	8/8	5/6	3/9	4/10	1/6	—	—

Obschon bei nicht unterbundenem D. choledochus die Vibrionen zusammen mit der Galle in den Darm gelangen können, beobachtete Violle (1912) beim erwachsenen Kaninchen keine Krankheitszeichen. Nach den Experimenten von Schöbl (1916b) ist dies auf die entzündlichen Veränderungen der Gallenblase zurückzuführen, die einen Übertritt der Mikroorganismen verhindern. Wertet man diese Befunde kritisch, so zeigt sich, daß die Zahl der aus der Gallenblase in den Darm übertretenden Vibrionen sicherlich zu gering ist, um Krankheitserscheinungen auszulösen. Es sei hier auch auf die umfangreichen bakteriologischen Untersuchungen bei Rhesusaffen hingewiesen, die Choleravibrionen im oberen Darmtrakt und der Gallenblase beherbergen können, ohne daß sie aus Rectalabstrichen nachzuweisen sind (Hasan et al., 1965; s. S. 99).

b) Parenterale Infektion

α) Intravenöse Infektion. Mit dieser Infektionstechnik gelang es Koch (1884) sowie Koch und Gaffky (1887) bei Kaninchen nicht, eine tödliche Erkrankung hervorzurufen. Einige Versuchstiere waren zwar „sehr krank", erholten sich jedoch nach einigen Tagen. Auch Gamaleia (1890) hielt Kaninchen bei intravenöser Applikation der Choleraerreger für nicht empfänglich. Erst durch die intravenöse Injektion von Papain, Pankreatin, Methämoglobin, Natriumnitrat und abgetöteten Pseudomonas-aeruginosa-Bakterien kann es zu einer „Enteritis" mit Vermehrung der Vibrionen im Darm oder zu einer Vibrionenseptikämie kommen. Über tödlich verlaufende Infektionen bei etwa 3 kg schweren Kaninchen mit Vibrionenkulturen, deren Dosis letalis 5 ml betrug, berichtete Thomas (1893). Die Mehrzahl ging nach 18—36 Std, einige wenige Tiere noch nach 3 bzw. 4 Tagen zugrunde. Die zusätzliche Gabe von Äthylalkohol an zwei aufeinanderfolgenden Tagen (am 1. Tag 6—8 ml und am 2. Tag 10—12 ml absoluter Alkohol auf das 4—5fache mit Wasser verdünnt) steigerte die Empfänglichkeit von 11 Kaninchen derart, daß sie der Infektion mit sonst nicht letalen Dosen erlagen, während Kontrolltiere überlebten, die die gleiche oder eine höhere Erregerdosis erhalten hatten. Die tödlich verlaufende intravenöse Infektion des Kaninchens wurde durch die Untersuchungen von Sobernheim (1893a) sowie Issaeff und Kolle (1894) bestätigt, die 35 Kaninchen im Gewicht von 330—2700 g mit Erregerdosen von Bruchteilen einer Öse bis zu 10 Ösen Kulturmaterial erfolgreich infizierten, von Klemperer (1894a), von Baroni und Ceaparu (1912) und von Violle (1914b). Junge, 300 g schwere Kaninchen, denen 2 ml einer 24 Std alten Bouillonkultur injiziert wurden, gingen 8—18 Std nach der Infektion zugrunde (Cano, 1914). Eine wesentlich höhere Erregerdosis, nämlich die Abschwemmung einer halben Roux-Flasche benötigte Masaki (1922), um den Tod eines 260 g schweren Kaninchens innerhalb 10 Std herbeizuführen. Erwachsenen Kaninchen verfütterte Golovanoff (1923) an zwei aufeinanderfolgenden Tagen vor der Infektion je 10 ml mit Lakritzenpulver vermischte Gallenflüssigkeit. 4 Std danach wurden

0,1 ml Agar-Kulturabschwemmung injiziert, eine Menge, die einem Drittel der Dosis letalis entsprach. Die Kaninchen starben innerhalb 24—48 Std; Kontrolltiere, welche ohne Vorbehandlung die gleiche Erregerdosis erhalten hatten, erkrankten nicht. Eine Vorbehandlung der Tiere hielten auch ARNOLD und SHAPIRO (1930) für notwendig. Es gelang ihnen nicht, bei Kaninchen mit einer halben, aus einer 24 Std bebrüteten Bouillonkultur gewonnenen DLM Krankheitssymptome auszulösen. Wurde jedoch gleichzeitig mit der intravenösen Injektion der Erregerdosis intraduodenal Phosphatpufferlösung gegeben, so entwickelten alle 12 Tiere Diarrhoen, an deren Folgen 8 starben. Auch wenn die Pufferlösung bis zu 18 Std nach der Infektion intraduodenal injiziert wurde, traten bei den Tieren noch Durchfälle und Tod innerhalb 24—48 Std auf.

Nach den Untersuchungen von THOMAS (1893) können Choleravibrionen beim Kaninchen nach intravenöser Infektion eine „typische Cholera" mit Durchfällen, Krämpfen und Kälte erzeugen. Gingen die Tiere vor Ablauf von 24 Std zugrunde, so fehlten gewöhnlich die Durchfälle, jedoch nie Darmläsionen. Im Gegensatz dazu sah KLEMPERER (1894a) die „tödliche Erkrankung" als Vergiftung an, da die Symptome sehr schnell eintraten und ihre Intensität offensichtlich von der Erregerdosis abhängig war. Bald nach der Injektion saßen die Kaninchen zusammengekauert und schnell atmend da. Durchfälle traten $^1/_2$—2 Std nach der Infektion auf; der Stuhl war bräunlich, häufig auch leicht rötlich und roch fäkulent. Die Stuhlentleerungen wiederholten sich öfter, wäßrige oder reiswasserähnliche Beschaffenheit wurde nicht beobachtet. Nach 2—3 Std fielen absinkende Körpertemperatur und zitternde Bewegungen der Skeletmuskulatur auf. Schließlich stellte sich eine Lähmung der hinteren Extremitäten ein, die Atmung wurde flacher und der Tod erfolgte 6—24 Std später. Wenn eine kleine Erregerdosis injiziert wurde, kam es zu Temperatursteigerung, nur geringen Durchfällen und weniger ausgeprägten Vergiftungserscheinungen (KLEMPERER, 1894a). Auf die Abhängigkeit der Krankheitssymptome von der Erregerdosis und dem Alter der Versuchstiere wiesen ISSAEFF und KOLLE (1894) hin. Es zeigte sich, daß junge Kaninchen kleinen Erregermengen erlagen, während die älteren erst nach Applikation großer Dosen zugrunde gingen. Je jünger die Versuchstiere waren, desto ausgeprägter waren die Darmsymptome. Bei 500 g schweren Kaninchen gelang es sicher, profuse Diarrhoen auszulösen und die Tiere zu töten. Versuchstiere mit einem Gewicht von mehr als 2 kg erkrankten selbst nach Injektion hoher Dosen nicht. Dagegen berichteten DIATROPTOFF (1894), VIOLLE und CRENDIROPOULO (1915), GOLOVANOFF (1923) sowie ARNOLD und SHAPIRO (1930) über zum Teil heftige Diarrhoen und „choleraähnliche" Krankheitsbilder bei ihren Versuchstieren.

Bei der Sektion wurden im Dünndarm eine mehlsuppen- oder reiswasserähnliche Flüssigkeit, Ekchymosen der Schleimhaut und vermehrte Gefäßzeichnungen der Serosa vorgefunden (THOMAS, 1893). Bereits 10 min nach der Infektion stellten BARONI und CEAPARU (1912) eine starke Anschwellung des Dünndarms mit massiver Exsudation fest. Besonders 20—30 cm unterhalb des Pylorus im Bereich des Wirsungschen Kanals bis zum Coecum zeigte die Mucosa Kongestion, während der obere Dünndarmabschnitt weniger in Mitleidenschaft gezogen war (VIOLLE, 1914b; MASAKI, 1922). Die bei dieser Infektionstechnik selten angefertigten histologischen Schnitte der Darmwand ergaben, daß das Epithel abgestoßen war und die Choleravibrionen tief in die Lieberkühnschen Krypten und die Schichten der Mucosa eingedrungen waren (ISSAEFF und KOLLE, 1894).

Die Anwendung von tödlichen Erregerdosen führt zu einer Bakteriämie. Die Choleravibrionen können aus Blut und Gallenflüssigkeit noch nach dem Tod der Kaninchen isoliert werden, wenn diese innerhalb 1—2 Tagen zugrunde gehen. Die

Infektion mit kleinen Erregerdosen oder mit Vibrionen, deren Virulenz so geschwächt war, daß die Versuchstiere erst nach 5 oder mehr Tagen verendeten, erbrachte keinen Erregernachweis aus Blut und Organen (Thomas, 1893; Diatroptoff, 1894). Jedoch ließen sich die Vibrionen bereits 30 min nach der Infektion mit großen Erregermengen aus der Gallenblase nachweisen (Baroni und Ceaparu, 1912). In mikroskopischen Präparaten, die von Darmmaterial oberhalb des Wirsungschen Kanals angefertigt worden waren, konnten wenige, unterhalb davon sowie in Blut und Dünndarm zahlreiche kommaförmige Mikroorganismen gesehen werden (Violle, 1914b). Ihre Darstellung aus Blut und verschiedenen inneren Organen gelang auch Golovanoff (1923) sowie Arnold und Shapiro (1930). Andere Untersucher verwendeten möglichst geringe Erregerdosen, um eine Septicämie zu vermeiden, doch wurden auch danach die Mikroorganismen aus Blut isoliert (Issaeff und Kolle, 1894; Sanarelli, 1921; Masaki, 1922).

Andere bakteriologische Untersuchungen galten der Frage, ob intravenös injizierte Vibrionen in den Darm gelangen und dort nachzuweisen sind. Wyssokowitsch (1886) verneinte einen Übertritt der im Blut kreisenden Vibrionen in das Darmlumen. Nach seinen Überlegungen sind hierfür schwere Gewebsschädigungen und Blutergüsse Vorbedingung. Jedoch wurden die Erreger von vielen Untersuchern nach dem Tod der Tiere aus Dünndarminhalt isoliert (Issaeff und Kolle, 1894; Diatroptoff, 1894; Cano, 1914; Violle und Crendiropoulo, 1915). Bei den Experimenten von Baroni und Ceaparu (1912) waren sie nach Applikation großer Mengen bereits 30 min später in der Appendix zu finden. Arnold und Shapiro (1930) gelang der Vibrionennachweis aus den Faeces intravenös infizierter Kaninchen.

Der Übertritt von Choleravibrionen in die Gallenblase der Versuchstiere nach intravenöser Injektion wurde vor allem von Greig (1914) untersucht. Sie waren aus dem Stuhl oder aus Gallenflüssigkeit von cholerakranken Menschen isoliert worden. Als Dosis wurden die Kolonien von 0,05—2 Agarkulturen, die 24 Std bebrütet worden waren, den 1,2 kg schweren Kaninchen injiziert. In Abhängigkeit von der Menge und Virulenz der Erreger blieben die Tiere entweder ohne Symptome oder sie erkrankten und wurden 24 Std nach der Infektion getötet, oder aber die Kaninchen starben innerhalb von 24 Std. Die Symptome waren retardierte Motilität, dünnflüssiger Stuhl und mitunter Diarrhoe. Nach dem Tod wurden die Mikroorganismen bei einem Teil der Versuchstiere aus Gallenflüssigkeit, Herzblut und Darminhalt isoliert; Urinkulturen waren stets frei von Vibrionen. Es ist jedoch bemerkenswert, daß mit dem gleichen Erregerstamm und gleicher Dosis 2 Kaninchen verschieden reagierten. Das eine Tier erkrankte schwer mit Cholerasymptomen; die Bakterien wurden 24 Std später in Reinkultur aus Gallenflüssigkeit, Herzblut und Darminhalt gezüchtet. Das 2. Versuchstier erholte sich vollkommen, nachdem vorübergehend dünnflüssiger Stuhl aufgetreten war, aus dem die Erreger allerdings nicht isoliert werden konnten.

Nach erfolgreicher Infektion fand sich bei der Sektion die Epithelschicht der Gallenblase destruiert und die Submucosa zeigte Leukocyteninfiltrationen (Greig, 1914); die Capillaren waren stark erweitert und zwischen den Erythrocyten ließen sich bei mikroskopischer Untersuchung kommaförmige Mikroorganismen nachweisen. Am Darm wurden Hämorrhagien in der Mucosa, bei zum Teil flächenhaft abgehobener Epithelschicht beobachtet; die Villi wiesen Leukocyteninfiltrate auf, die Blutgefäße waren erweitert und mit Erregern durchsetzt. In einer weiteren Untersuchung (Greig, 1916) wurden die Choleravibrionen bei 9 von 18 Kaninchen in der Gallenblase angetroffen. Zusätzlich hatten die Tiere Gallensteine. Nach Anfertigung mikroskopischer Präparate wurden die Bakterien zweimal auch innerhalb der Steine nachgewiesen.

Die Injektion von 1 ml einer 24 Std bebrüteten Bouillonkultur in die Ohrvene verursachte keine Läsionen der Gallenblase, wie 1 Woche später bei der Sektion festgestellt wurde (Nichols, 1916). Die gleiche Dosis in eine Mesenterialvene injiziert, bewirkte bei einem von 3 Tieren eine blutige Gallenflüssigkeit, in der die Mikroorganismen allerdings nicht mehr zu finden waren.

Um nach intravenöser Infektion die Choleravibrionen aus Gallenproben nachweisen zu können, legte Thomas (1893) bei einem Teil der Kaninchen eine D.-choledochus-Fistel an. Nach der Gabe von subletalen Dosen war bei den Tieren ohne Choledochusfistel kein Nachweis der Erreger in der Gallenflüssigkeit möglich, während bei angelegter Fistel die Mikroorganismen bereits nach einer halben Stunde in der Galle gefunden wurden. Die intravenöse Injektion von tödlichen Erregerdosen hatte mit und ohne Fistel einen Übertritt der Vibrionen in die Galle zur Folge. Ferner konnten bei der Sektion der Versuchstiere mit Fistel, trotz kompletten Verschlusses des D. choledochus und bei Ausschluß eines zweiten D. choledochus, aus dem Darminhalt Choleravibrionen isoliert werden. Thomas (1893) glaubte dadurch gesichert zu haben, daß die Mikroorganismen durch die Darmwand in das Lumen des Verdauungskanals gelangen können.

Die Fistelgalle wurde von Nichols (1916) nur über einen Zeitraum von einer Stunde post infectionem gesammelt, da in seinen Versuchen die später untersuchten Proben fast stets steril geblieben waren. Mashimo (1923) verwendete für seine Experimente einen Cholerastamm, dessen DL 8 mg/kg Körpergewicht betrug. Einem Kaninchen von 2250 g wurden 24 Std nach der Fisteloperation 11,25 mg Choleravibrionen intravenös injiziert. Bereits 2 min nach der Injektion waren sie in der Gallenflüssigkeit, aus der sie im Gegensatz zu den Befunden von Nichols (1916) 24 Std später noch in großer Menge gezüchtet werden konnten.

β) Intraperitoneale Infektion. Untersuchungen mit dieser Methode wurden selten durchgeführt. Anstelle von Meerschweinchen wurden mitunter Kaninchen zur Überprüfung der Virulenz eines Cholerastammes intraperitoneal infiziert. Die Experimente von Issaeff und Kolle (1894) bestätigen, daß junge Kaninchen bedeutend empfänglicher sind und der Infektion leichter erliegen als unter gleichen Bedingungen infizierte erwachsene Tiere. Die intraperitoneale Injektion einer Aufschwemmung von $^1/_5$ Öse vermehrungsfähiger Vibrionen genügte, um 6 junge 290—415 g schwere Kaninchen innerhalb 1—3 Tagen zu töten. Dagegen erlagen von acht 1350—2540 g schweren, erwachsenen Kaninchen nur 2 der Infektion. Wurde die Erregerdosis allerdings erhöht, so starben auch diese Tiere. Die intraperitoneale Injektion muß vorsichtig vorgenommen werden, um eine Verletzung des bei Kaninchen stark mit Gasen gefüllten Coecum, das zudem der vorderen Bauchwand dicht anliegt, zu vermeiden.

Ebenso wie Meerschweinchen gehen Kaninchen nach intraperitonealer Infektion unter den Zeichen einer akuten Intoxikation zugrunde (Issaeff und Kolle, 1894). Im Gegensatz dazu gelangte Sanarelli (1921) nach intraperitonealer Infektion junger, saugender Kaninchen zu dem gleichen Ergebnis wie nach intravenöser Infektion. Er bezeichnete das Krankheitsbild als „Vibrionen-Entero-Colitis".

Der Übertritt intraperitoneal injizierter Choleravibrionen in das Blut und damit in andere Organe ist abhängig von der Erregerdosis (Issaeff und Kolle, 1894). Bei Kaninchen, die 2 Ösen und mehr Kulturmaterial erhalten hatten, ließen sich massenhaft Vibrionen im Peritonealexsudat und vereinzelt im Blut und in anderen Organen nachweisen. Nach Applikation kleinerer Mengen erwiesen sich Peritoneal- und Blutproben als steril. Der Übertritt intraperitoneal injizierter Choleravibrionen in den Darm setzte nach Sanarelli (1923a) bereits wenige

Minuten nach der Infektion ein, dauerte in der Regel bis 12 Std und nur selten mehrere Tage. Sie wurden im Peritonealraum und Blut bis zu 2 Std nach der Infektion gefunden.

γ) Eine *intrapleurale Infektion* wurde beim Kaninchen kaum angewendet. Die von Sluyts (1893) derart infizierten Kaninchen gingen einige Stunden später zugrunde. Die Vibrionen konnten post mortem aus Blut und Pleurahöhle gezüchtet werden.

δ) Durch *intrameningeale Infektion* des 8000sten bis 12000sten Teils einer Choleravibrionenkultur verendeten Kaninchen unter den Symptomen einer schweren Meningoencephalitis (Urbain, 1929). Bei der 24 Std später durchgeführten Obduktion zeigten Gehirn, Medulla oblongata und Spinalmark Stauungszeichen. Die Mikroorganismen wurden aus diesen Organen und Herzblut isoliert.

ε) Subcutane Infektion. Eine erste Mitteilung über die subcutane Infektion stammt von Koch und Gaffky (1887). Sie injizierten eine junge Choleramilchkultur in Mengen von 4—5 Pravazsche Spritzen Kaninchen unter die Bauchhaut. Diese starben 1—2 Tage später an einem malignen Ödem. Nur bei einem Tier ließen sich Choleravibrionen an der Inoculationsstelle nachweisen. Blut und innere Organe waren steril. Der Erfolg dieser Infektionstechnik ist ebenfalls dosisabhängig. Die Injektion von etwa $^1/_4$ Öse Kulturmaterial wird von jungen Kaninchen reaktionslos vertragen; 24 Std später waren an der Injektionsstelle keine Mikroorganismen mehr nachzuweisen (Issaeff und Kolle, 1894). Eine Lokalreaktion entsteht nach der Injektion größerer Vibrionenmengen. Nach einigen Tagen bildet sich ein Absceß, der vermehrungsfähige Erreger enthält. Die Versuchstiere können zugrunde gehen, ohne daß im Blut und in anderen Organen Choleravibrionen nachweisbar sind. Issaeff und Kolle (1894) gelang es nicht, vom subcutanen Gewebe aus Darmsymptome zu erzeugen. Dem widersprechen die Ergebnisse von Sanarelli (1916, 1921), dem es stets gelungen war, beim saugenden Kaninchen nach subcutaner Infektion eine typische Cholera zu erzeugen. Zur Septicämie führte die Injektion von $^1/_4$ Öse frisch isolierter Choleravibrionen nach Untersuchungen von Hahn (1905), was von Crendiropoulo (1921) verneint wurde. Die Ergebnisse von Hahn (1905) wurden von Panja und Paul (1943) bestätigt, die nach subcutaner Injektion die Mikroorganismen sehr rasch in der Blutbahn feststellten. Die Todesrate der Kaninchen betrug 50%. Bei der Autopsie waren die Därme mit einer weißlichen, zähen Flüssigkeit angefüllt. Die Vibrionen konnten aus Blut, Peritonealhöhle und Gallenblase gezüchtet werden.

ζ) Die *intracutane Injektion* wird als Kontrollversuch bei Experimenten mit hitzeabgetöteten und ultrafiltrierten Vibrionenkulturen herangezogen (Ghosh und Mukerjee, 1959; Burrows, 1965).

c) Seltene Infektionsmethoden

Intranasale Infektion. In den Nasenöffnungen von 12 Kaninchen verrieb Diatroptoff (1894) je 2 Ösen einer Cholerakultur. Es stellten sich Durchfälle und Gewichtsverlust ein; 5—20 Tage später waren sie tot. Nach der Sektion konnten die Erreger bei 8 Versuchstieren aus dem flüssigen Darminhalt isoliert werden. Starben sie nach dem 10. Tag, so waren die Mikroorganismen nicht mehr zu züchten. Die naso-pharyngeale Mucosa des erwachsenen Kaninchens ist nach den Untersuchungen von Sanarelli (1923a) für Choleravibrionen durchlässiger als die buccale Mucosa. Nach dem Einblasen der Vibrionen in die Nase ließen sich die Erreger im Blut bereits nach 15 min nachweisen. Diese Art der Infektion führte unter Gewichtsabnahme mitunter zum Tod der Versuchstiere. Die Möglichkeit einer Sekundärinfektion mit anderen Mikroorganismen ist jedoch zu erwägen.

Intratracheale Infektion. In die durch Tracheotomie eröffnete Luftröhre instillierte DIATROPTOFF (1894) 2—3 Ösen einer Cholerakultur. Die Kaninchen starben 3 oder 4 Tage später; bei der Sektion gelang der Erregernachweis aus Blut und Dünndarm. Lebten die Versuchstiere einige Tage länger, so waren, wie nach intravenöser Infektion, Blut- und Organproben steril; lediglich im Darminhalt fanden sich noch Choleravibrionen. Nach 15—20 Tagen allerdings waren die Erreger aus den Organen nicht mehr zu isolieren. SANARELLI (1923a) teilte mit, daß sie 15 min nach endotrachealer Infektion in die Blutbahn übertraten und aus den Atmungsorganen 12 Std später eliminiert waren.

Die conjunctivale Infektion mit Choleravibrionen löste bei Kaninchen keine Erkrankung aus (KOCH und GAFFKY, 1887).

5. Feld-, Haus- und weiße Maus
a) Infektion über den Magen-Darm-Kanal

α) Bei *oraler Gabe* wird Mäusen die Erregerdosis durch eine Sonde oder zusammen mit der Nahrung gegeben. Die Untersuchungsergebnisse von THIERSCH (1854), der 104 Tiere mit auf Filterpapier angetrockneten Choleradejekten zum Teil erfolgreich infiziert hatte, konnten in einer Nachuntersuchung von KOCH (1884) nicht bestätigt werden. An einer „enteritischen Infektion" starben die von KAMEN (1895) infizierten Hausmäuse. KARLINSKI (1896) infizierte Haus-, Feld- und weiße Mäuse mit dem von KAMEN verwendeten Vibrionenstamm. Er teilte mit, daß Hausmäuse 24—36 Std post infectionem zugrunde gingen. Mit Feld- und weißen Mäusen konnte dieses Ergebnis nicht erzielt werden. Bei der Sektion waren im Darm der Hausmäuse massenhaft Vibrionen nachweisbar. Nach Gabe von Choleravibrionen erkrankte keines dieser Versuchstiere.

β) Durch *intraintestinale Injektion* von Choleravibrionen gelang es nicht, bei weißen Mäusen Krankheitszeichen hervorzurufen (DUTTA und HABBU, 1955).

b) Parenterale Infektion

α) *Intraperitoneale Infektion.* Der größte Teil der grauen Hausmäuse, die KOCH und GAFFKY (1887) infizierten, starb innerhalb 24 Std. Dies wurde von LOEWENTHAL (1889) und BAUMGARTEN (1921) bestätigt. GRIFFITS (1942a) applizierte 5×10^8 in 0,5 ml physiologischer Kochsalzlösung suspendierte Choleravibrionen. Während nach Verabfolgung dieser Dosis alle Tiere starben, führten 5×10^7 Vibrionen zum Tod von 2 Mäusen aus einem Kollektiv von 60 Tieren. Bei Zugabe von 5% Mucin starben nach Injektion von 5×10^5 Vibrionen 90% und von 5×10^3 Vibrionen 80% der Versuchstiere innerhalb 24—72 Std. Diese Ergebnisse konnten jedoch nur bei Verwendung frisch isolierter Cholerastämme erreicht werden (GRIFFITS, 1942a).

Die ersten Krankheitszeichen beobachtete GRIFFITS (1942a) 2 Std nach Injektion von mehreren 100 Mio. Vibrionen. Die apathisch wirkenden Mäuse hatten ein gesträubtes Fell und hockten dicht zusammen. Ein extremer Flüssigkeitsverlust wurde nicht festgestellt; die Defäkation war zwar gesteigert, die Ausscheidungen blieben jedoch geformt. Bei der Sektion wurde eine eitrige, blutig tingierte Flüssigkeit im Peritoneum angetroffen. In ihr waren mikroskopisch viele intra- und extracellulär gelegene Vibrionen zu sehen (KOCH und GAFFKY, 1887; GRIFFITS, 1942a). Sie konnten aus Herzblut (KOCH und GAFFKY, 1887; GRIFFITS, 1942a), Milz, Leber, Lunge und Gehirn isoliert werden (GRIFFITS, 1942a). Der Tod der weißen Mäuse, bei denen es zur Bakteriämie kommt, wird auf die Toxinwirkung der Choleravibrionen zurückgeführt (GRIFFITS, 1942a; GAULD et al., 1949; BURROWS, 1956).

β) Nach *subcutaner Infektion* mit einer halben Pravazschen Spritze Cholera-vibrionen verendeten die Mäuse innerhalb 1—4 Tagen, nach Injektion in den Schwanz wurden keine Krankheitszeichen beobachtet (Koch und Gaffky, 1887). Eine viertel Öse El-Tor-Vibrionen war nach den Untersuchungen von Kraus und Russ (1908) die Dosis letalis für weiße Mäuse; nach der Applikation von $^1/_{10}$ Öse Kulturmaterial trat eine vorübergehende Erkrankung auf, und nach $^1/_{50}$ wurde keine Wirkung mehr beobachtet. Rotky (1913) verwendete offensichtlich einen sehr virulenten Stamm, da die Injektion von 0,01 Öse Vibrionen innerhalb 6 Std zum Tod der Mäuse führte. An der Injektionsstelle und im Herzblut fanden sie sich massenhaft. Diese Untersuchungsergebnisse wurden von Kabeshima (1918a) bestätigt.

6. Zieselmaus

a) Orale Infektion

Sabolotny (1894) fand in der Zieselmaus (Spermophilus guttatus), einer in Rußland verbreiteten Nagetierart, ein Versuchstier, das per os erfolgreich mit Choleravibrionen zu infizieren war. Durch Alkalisieren des Magensaftes und Opiumvorbehandlung konnte die Erkrankungsrate verbessert werden. Den Mäu-sen wurden je einige Tropfen einer 1 Tag alten Kultur in das Maul gegeben oder mit infiziertem Futter verabfolgt. Die Hälfte der Tiere erlag der Infektion. Von den übrigen Mäusen war ein Teil vorübergehend schwer krank, der andere wies keine Krankheitszeichen auf. Die erkrankten Tiere verweigerten Futter und Wasser; die Körpertemperatur sank von 38° C auf 35—32° C; es stellten sich Cyanose, Krämpfe und häufig auch Diarrhoen ein. Bei der Sektion war eine starke Gefäßzeichnung der meist dilatierten Därme auffällig, der Darminhalt war stets flüssig, mitunter hämorrhagisch und mit weißlichen Flocken durchsetzt. Mikro-skopisch wurden die kommaförmigen Mikroorganismen in Magen- und Darminhalt, oft in der Leber und der Bauchhöhle und nicht selten auch im Blut nachgewiesen.

b) Intraperitoneale und subcutane Infektion

Für die intraperitoneale Infektion der Zieselmaus betrug die kleinste tödliche Dosis 0,1—0,2 ml einer 24 Std bebrüteten Peptonkultur. Die Autopsie erbrachte gelegentlich eine hämorrhagische Peritonitis. Vibrionen ließen sich aus dem Blut züchten. Die gleiche Dosis war auch bei subcutaner Injektion für die Versuchstiere tödlich. Danach kam es zur Bakteriämie, denn in Blut, Leber, Milz und Peritoneum konnten in jedem Falle die Erreger nachgewiesen werden.

7. Ratte

Die Injektion von Darminhalt eines Cholerakranken in das Duodenum der Ratte erzeugte bei diesem Tier keine Krankheitszeichen (Nicati und Rietsch, 1885a). Zum gleichen Ergebnis kamen Koch und Gaffky (1887).

In abgebundene Dünndarmsegmente von insgesamt 15 Ratten injizierten De und Chatterje (1953) je 1 ml Durhams Peptonwasser, in dem 1 Öse einer 24 Std bebrüteten flüssigen Cholerakultur suspendiert war. Danach erhielten die Tiere weder Futter noch Wasser. Bei der Autopsie der nach 24 Std getöteten Tiere war innerhalb des abgebundenen Darmsegments keine Flüssigkeitsansammlung fest-zustellen, der Darminhalt betrug nicht mehr als 0,5 ml. Eine Isolierung von Vibrionen aus dem Segment gelang nur bei einem der Tiere. Die histologische Untersuchung erbrachte eine hämorrhagische und nekrotische Darmwand. Durch intraintestinale Inoculation von Choleravibrionen war es auch Dutta und Habbu (1955) nicht möglich, Ratten zu infizieren.

8. Affe

a) Infektion über den Magen-Darm-Kanal

α) *Orale Infektion.* Eine tödlich verlaufende Erkrankung bei Menschenaffen konnte MENDOZA (1913) durch orale Infektion hervorrufen. Nach Neutralisation des Magensaftes mit Natriumbicarbonat wurden den Tieren 8—10 ml einer 24 Std bebrüteten Bouillonkultur durch die Schlundsonde gegeben. Über eine tödlich verlaufende Infektion bei Affen (Cynomolgus) berichteten POTTEVIN und VIOLLE (1913a). 24 Std vor der Infektion war das Futter entzogen worden. Als Laxans wurden 10 g Natriumsulfat in 20 ml Wasser aufgelöst verabfolgt. 8 Std nachdem die abführende Wirkung eingetreten war, wurden jedem Tier 0,4 g in 20 ml Wasser gelöstes Natriumbicarbonat und als Erregerdosis eine in 20 ml Bouillon suspendierte 18 Std bebrütete Petrischalenkultur gegeben. Innerhalb von 12—24 Std gingen die Affen zugrunde. Nach Applikation von ca. $^1/_5$—$^1/_{10}$ Kulturabschwemmung trat der Tod der Tiere 2—4 Tage post infectionem ein. Umfangreiche Untersuchungen an Rhesusaffen führten HASAN et al. (1965) durch: 97 Tiere, die zwischen 1,5 bis 4 kg schwer waren, wurden 137mal oral infiziert. Erregerdosis waren im allgemeinen 25 ml einer 24 Std bebrüteten Bouillonkultur, die 10^6—10^{11} Choleravibrionen/ml enthielt. Es handelte sich teils um frisch aus Reiswasserstühlen Cholerakranker, teils aus Untersuchungsproben zugrunde gegangener Affen gezüchtete Vibrionen. Vor der Infektion wurden die Tiere einer unterschiedlichen Behandlung unterworfen:

1. wurden sie auf eine unterschiedliche Kost eingestellt, welche entweder vitaminfreies Casein oder Reis und kein Salz enthielt; nach unterschiedlich langer Diätdauer erfolgte die Infektion;

2. erhielten sie 10%iges Natriumsulfat durch die Magensonde; nach Eintritt der abführenden Wirkung wurden die Erreger verabfolgt;

3. war dem Natriumsulfat Kaliumsulfat zugefügt, um dem Kaliumverlust während der Infektion vorzubeugen;

4. wurde anstelle von Trinkwasser 1—2 Tage vor und nach der Infektion eine 3%ige Natriumbicarbonatlösung gegeben;

5. wurde wie unter 4. angegeben behandelt, später zusätzlich Natriumsulfat verabfolgt und nach Auftreten der Diarrhoe infiziert;

6. erhielten die Versuchstiere 3—10 Tage vor der Infektion jeweils 0,1 ml DOCA, um einen Kaliumverlust hervorzurufen;

7. schließlich wurden entweder der D. choledochus und/oder der D. pancreaticus entfernt oder unterbunden. Die Affen wurden 1—4 Wochen nach der Operation infiziert.

Mit keiner der Vorbehandlungen gelang es den Autoren, Affen für die Infektion so empfänglich zu machen, daß regelmäßig eine der Cholera des Menschen entsprechende Erkrankung aufgetreten wäre. In den meisten Infektionsgruppen wurden lediglich sporadisch auftretende akute Diarrhoen beobachtet. Mehrere Tage nach der Infektion wurden Choleravibrionen aus Rectalabstrichen isoliert. Einige Tiere jedoch beherbergten die Vibrionen im oberen Dünndarm und in der Galle, ohne daß sie aus Rectalabstrichen gezüchtet werden konnten. Aufgrund dieses Befundes vermuteten die Autoren dort ein Reservoir für die Erreger, zumal die Bakterien bei den meisten Tieren 15 Tage nach dem letzten Nachweis weder aus Rectalabstrichen noch aus Dünndarm und Galle gezüchtet werden konnten. Da trotz unterbundenem D. choledochus eine Leber- und Galleninfektion bestand, wurde eine Portalblut- oder Lymphinfektion diskutiert. Bei 39 von 69 Affen, die entweder eingegangen oder 61 Tage nach der Infektion getötet waren, wurden die Choleravibrionen aus dem Duodenum und übrigen Dünndarm isoliert, dagegen

nur selten aus dem Colon und dem Rectum. Aus 5 von 20 untersuchten Leberproben, die innerhalb 8 Tagen nach der Infektion entnommen waren, ließen sich
die Choleravibrionen züchten. Vier dieser Organproben stammten von Affen,
denen 1—4 Wochen vor der Infektion der Gallengang unterbunden worden war.

Mendoza (1913) sowie Pottevin und Violle (1913a) berichten über „choleraähnliche" Krankheitsbilder. Bei den erkrankten Affen stellte sich zunächst eine
Diarrhoe mit gelblich verfärbtem Stuhl ein, einige Zeit später traten auch wäßrige
Darmentleerungen auf, die den reiswasserähnlichen Ausscheidungen beim Menschen ähnelten. Die Körpertemperatur war 12—24 Std nach der Infektion auf
34° C abgesunken; unter fortschreitendem Kräfteverfall starben die Tiere innerhalb 2—3 Tagen. Der Temperatursturz konnte sehr erheblich sein; so sank bei
einem Affen die Rectaltemperatur einige Stunden vor dem Tode auf 24° C (Pottevin und Violle, 1913a).

Bei der Autopsie der von Mendoza (1913) infizierten Affen zeigte sich der
Dünndarm stark gestaut und mit einer zähflüssigen Masse gefüllt, die zahlreiche
Schleimflocken enthielt. Der Dickdarm war äußerlich unauffällig, enthielt jedoch
eine ähnliche Flüssigkeit.

Im trübflüssigen Dünndarminhalt waren mikroskopisch kommaförmige Mikroorganismen in Fischzuglagerung zu sehen (Mendoza, 1913; Pottevin und Violle,
1913b), die gezüchtet werden konnten, während Untersuchungsproben von Galle
und Herzblut steril blieben.

β) Die rectale Infektion war nach Untersuchungen von Koch (1884) erfolglos.
Dabei waren den Tieren nach Gabe von Abführmitteln Choleradejekte durch
einen langen, möglichst hoch in den Darm geschobenen Katheter instilliert worden.

γ) Intraduodenale Infektion. Aus einer Anmerkung von Violle (1914b) geht
hervor, daß er nach Unterbindung des D. choledochus und Injektion der Vibrionen
in das Duodenum bei Affen eine Choleraerkrankung auslösen konnte. Aus dem
Jahresbericht des King Institute in Guindy/Madras (Report, 1946) dagegen ist
zu entnehmen, daß dies nach Laparotomie und Injektion der Vibrionen in den
Dünndarm nicht gelang. Die Darmwand war entweder zuvor durch Injektion von
20 ml 56° C heißen Wassers oder durch eine Röntgenbestrahlung geschädigt
worden. Bei 5 von 6 Affen, die diese Bestrahlung überlebten, wurden zwar nach
48 Std Diarrhoen beobachtet, ein spontaner Tod trat jedoch nicht ein. Die
getöteten und sezierten Tiere hatten eine leichte Kongestion des Omentum, histologisch war am Dünndarm eine geringe Epitheldesquamation auffällig.

Im Rahmen von Immunisierungsversuchen infizierten Greer et al. (1968)
16 3,6—6,3 kg schwere Husarenaffen beiderlei Geschlechts. Sie wurden in
4 Gruppen eingeteilt, von denen die 1. als Kontrolle diente. Das 2. Kollektiv
wurde anaesthesiert und die Gallenblase nach Eröffnung des Abdomen mit den
Händen massiert; den Tieren der 3. Gruppe wurden unter aseptischen Bedingungen
Bimssteinchen in die Gallenblase implantiert; bei der 4. Gruppe wurden Teile der
Gallenblasenschleimhaut von 1 × 1 cm Größe mit einer heißen Pinzette ver-
schorft. In der diesen Eingriffen folgenden Woche waren die Tiere klinisch unauffällig. Vier Wochen nach einer Immunisierung wurde den Versuchstieren einschließlich denen der Kontrollgruppe, mit einer Duodenalsonde 2 ml einer Suspension (1,3—1,8 × 10^9 Mikroorganismen) des Biotyps El Tor zugeführt. Danach
traten bei 4 von 16 Tieren Diarrhoen auf, die 36 Std später ohne Behandlung
sistierten. Die Durchfälle wurden auch bei oral, jedoch nicht bei parenteral immunisierten Affen beobachtet. Weitere 4 Wochen später wurde eine Cholecyst-
ektomie vorgenommen, die alle Tiere überstanden. In der Mucosa der Gallenblase waren hauptsächlich nach vorangegangener manueller Reizung, histologisch
ein Ödem und Infiltrate mit Lymphocyten, Plasmazellen und Histiocyten fest-

zustellen. Die Gallenblase eines nicht immunisierten Tieres mit Bimssteinchen zeigte nekrotische Areale. Die nicht immunisierten Affen wiesen 5mal häufiger pathologische Veränderungen an der Gallenblase auf, als immunisierte. Aus Rectalabstrichen, die in 1—2tägigem Abstand untersucht wurden, konnte 15 bis 18 Tage und bei einem Tier auch 27 Tage nach der Infektion V. cholerae gezüchtet werden. Die operierten Tiere schieden die Vibrionen über einen längeren Zeitraum aus als die infizierten Kontrolltiere. Aus der Gallenblase wurden die Vibrionen in keinem Fall isoliert. Da auch die nicht vorbehandelten Affen eine Cholecystitis zeigten, kamen GREER et al. (1968) zu dem Schluß, daß V. cholerae Biotyp El Tor in der Lage ist, bei Husarenaffen pathologisch-anatomische Veränderungen an der Gallenblase hervorzurufen.

b) Parenterale Infektion

Die intravenöse und subcutane Injektion vermehrungsfähiger Choleravibrionen rief bei Affen keine Erkrankung hervor (POTTEVIN und VIOLLE, 1913b).

9. Hund

Hauptsächlich in älteren Arbeiten wird über experimentelle Untersuchungen mit Hunden berichtet. Die Versuche ergaben, daß sie, mitunter nach Vorbehandlung, Cholerasymptome mit Erbrechen und Diarrhoe entwickeln.

a) Infektion über den Magen-Darm-Kanal

α) *Orale Infektion.* NICATI und RIETSCH (1885a) gelang es nicht, durch Verfütterung von Darmmaterial Cholerakranker beim Hund, auch nach Hungernlassen und Alkalisierung des infektiösen Materials, eine Erkrankung auszulösen. Zum gleichen Ergebnis kamen KOCH und GAFFKY (1887).

VIOLLE (1914b) verabreichte einem 3 kg schweren Foxterrier innerhalb 48 Std 1 l Choleravibrionen-Bouillon, ohne mit dieser großen Erregerdosis eine Erkrankung hervorrufen zu können. Bei sehr jungen, wenige Stunden bis 2 Tage alten Hunden, die mit verdünnter Kuhmilch ernährt wurden, der Choleravibrionen zugesetzt waren, führte diese Art der oralen Infektion teils zur Erkrankung und bei einigen Tieren zum Tod (KARLINSKI, 1896). Die Untersuchungen von SANARELLI (1922) erbrachten, daß Hunde nur in den ersten 24 Std nach der Geburt, wenn sie noch keine Muttermilch gesaugt haben, für Choleravibrionen empfänglich sind.

Nach Hungern, Blutentnahme, Alkoholgabe und Neutralisation des Magensaftes infizierte KLEMPERER (1894a) 25 Hunde mit 50—100 ml Choleravibrionen-Bouillon; 4 starben nach 4—12 Std, 8 bekamen Durchfälle, die übrigen 13 erkrankten nicht. Nach diesen Beobachtungen waren die tödlich erkrankten Hunde 3—4 Std nach der Infektion äußerst schwach und lagen kraftlos auf der Seite; ihr Körper wurde von krampfhaften Zuckungen geschüttelt; während die Temperaturen auf 34—32° C sanken, trat 4—12 Std nach der Infektion der Tod unter den Zeichen des Kollapses ein. Neben Erbrechen wurden profuse, in kurzen Zeitabständen aufeinanderfolgende Diarrhoen gesehen. Wasser wurde jedoch nicht so reichlich entleert, daß sich dadurch allein der schwere Krankheitszustand der Hunde ableiten ließ. Aus diesem Grunde diskutierte KLEMPERER (1894a) die Wirkung eines Choleratoxins. Bei der Obduktion imponierte eine hämorrhagisch infarzierte Darmschleimhaut; der schleimige Inhalt beherbergte massenhaft Epithelien. Im histologischen Präparat wurde ein hochgradiger Epithelverlust der Darmzotten festgestellt. Neben anderen Darmbakterien enthielten die diarrhoischen Ausscheidungen massenhaft Choleravibrionen, ebenso das Erbrochene

(Klemperer, 1894a; Karlinski, 1896). In den Exkrementen von Hunden, die als einziges Krankheitssymptom Diarrhoen hatten, wurden ebenfalls Choleravibrionen gefunden (Klemperer, 1894a).

β) Intraduodenale Infektion. Trotz der wenigen vorliegenden Veröffentlichungen scheint diese Methode geeignet zu sein, bei Hunden eine tödliche Choleraerkrankung auszulösen. Nicati und Rietsch (1884a) injizierten erstmals intraduodenal nach Unterbindung des D. choledochus Darmmaterial von Cholerapatienten oder vibrionenhaltige Gallenflüssigkeit von Verstorbenen. Der Tod der Hunde trat 1—2 Tage später ein. Die Infektion verlief auch dann erfolgreich, wenn das infektiöse Material in den nicht unterbundenen D. choledochus injiziert wurde (Nicati und Rietsch, 1885a). Der von Violle (1914b) oral infizierte Hund, der die Applikation von 1 l Cholera-Bouillonkultur schadlos überstanden hatte, ging an einer Choleraerkrankung zugrunde, als ihm 1 ml Cholerabouillon nach Ligatur des D. choledochus intraduodenal injiziert worden war.

Die Hunde reagierten mit Durchfall, Erbrechen, Cyanose und Absinken der Körpertemperatur. Bei der Autopsie war der Darmtrakt bis auf den Dickdarm mit einer an Epithelien außerordentlich reichen, breiigen Masse gefüllt. Die Gallenblase war dilatiert, die Leber sah anämisch aus und hatte auf ihrer Oberfläche weißliche Flecken. Aus dem Darminhalt konnten die Choleravibrionen stets isoliert werden (Nicati und Rietsch, 1885a).

γ) Injektion in das abgebundene Dünndarmsegment. Nach Klemperer (1894b) wandten als erste Denys und Sluyts diese Art der Infektion beim Hund an. Die 6 Std in den Darmabschnitt eingeschlossenen Choleravibrionen führten zu keiner Beeinträchtigung der Gesundheit der Versuchstiere. Das gleiche Ergebnis erzielten Nicati und Rietsch (1885a) auch dann, wenn gleichzeitig mit den Choleravibrionen Luft in den Darm injiziert wurde, um dadurch ihre Vermehrung zu fördern.

b) Parenterale Infektion

α) Nach *intravenöser Injektion* von Choleravibrionen, die aus Kulturmaterial oder Untersuchungsproben des Menschen stammten, starben die Versuchstiere meist sehr rasch. Überlebten bei den Experimenten einige Hunde, so war dies entweder auf eine zu geringe Erregerdosis oder wenig virulente Mikroorganismen zurückzuführen (Nicati und Rietsch, 1885a; Wyssokowitsch, 1886; Gamaleia, 1892; Klemperer, 1894a).

Die Choleraerkrankung nach intravenöser Infektion weist manche gemeinsame Symptome mit der des Menschen auf (Gamaleia, 1892). Sie ist charakterisiert durch eine reiswasserartige oder sanguinolente Diarrhoe und durch Erbrechen, das mehrere Stunden anhalten kann. Ante finem treten generalisierte Krämpfe auf. Nach der Meinung von Klemperer (1894a) starben die Hunde an der Wirkung der „Choleragifte". Er hielt die Toxinbildung jedoch nicht für eine spezifische Eigenschaft vermehrungsfähiger Choleravibrionen, da die gleichen Symptome mit abgetöteten Vibrionen und mit anderen Mikroorganismen, z.B. E. coli, hervorgerufen werden konnten. Für eine Intoxikation des tierischen Organismus sprach ferner, daß nach Injektion einer großen Menge Blut eines Cholerakranken die Hunde mit Cyanose, Stadium algidum und Tod reagierten (Nicati und Rietsch, 1885a). Bei der Sektion zeigte der Verdauungstrakt vom Magen bis einschließlich Rectum pathologische Veränderungen; die gastrointestinale Schleimhaut war sanguinolent, ebenso die darin enthaltene Flüssigkeit, der reichlich desquamierte Epithelzellen beigemengt waren. Das Protoplasma war granuliert und geschrumpft. Über die ganze Epithelschicht verteilt fanden sich hämorrhagische Infarzierungen und leukocytäre Infiltrate. Choleravibrionen konnten nach intravenöser Injektion, zum Teil mit anderen Bakterien, aus dem Blut der Versuchstiere isoliert werden (NICATI und RIETSCH, 1885a). Von SANARELLI (1922) wurde die Ansicht vertreten, daß sie über den Blutkreislauf in den Darm gelangen und dort eine „Gastroenteritis" erzeugen.

β) Intraperitoneale Infektion. Nach der Mitteilung von KLEMPERER (1894a) erbrachten die Versuche von DENYS und SLUYTS, daß Hunde nach intraperitonealer Injektion von Choleravibrionen verenden. Die Autoren unterschieden dabei je nach Erregerdosis 3 Krankheitsstadien: 2—3 Std nach Injektion von 1—2 ml Bouillonkultur in die seröse Höhle, erhöhte sich die Körpertemperatur auf 40—41,2° C; die Tiere waren verlangsamt, fraßen nicht, hatten mitunter Erbrechen und einige diarrhoische Stühle, erholten sich jedoch 2 Tage später wieder. Nach Injektion von 5—20 ml Bouillonkultur trat das 2. Krankheitsstadium ein: die Hunde zeigten Prostration, winselten und hatten profuses Erbrechen mit häufigen Stuhlentleerungen, die zunächst fäkal, dann schleimigwäßrig und blutuntermischt waren. Ein Teil der Tiere überstand die Infektion, andere starben wenige Tage später. Bei der Autopsie waren keine Darmveränderungen festzustellen. Nach der Gabe von mehr als 20 ml Bouillonkultur gingen die Hunde meist ein, teils mit, teils ohne stürmisches Erbrechen und Diarrhoe. In jedem Fall waren Veränderungen an der Darmschleimhaut vorhanden. Über ähnliche Untersuchungsergebnisse wurde von NICATI und RIETSCH (1884), CANTANI (1886) und BEZZOLA (1912) berichtet.

γ) Nach *subcutaner Infektion* starben die Hunde ebenfalls; jedoch waren weder Cholerasymptome noch bei der Autopsie Darmläsionen zu erkennen. Mitunter konnten die Mikroorganismen aus Herzblut isoliert werden (NICATI und RIETSCH, 1885a; CANTANI, 1886; SANARELLI, 1922).

10. Katze

Bei jungen Katzen war es NICATI und RIETSCH (1885a) nicht gelungen, eine Erkrankung herbeizuführen. KARLINSKI (1896), der saugende, 2 Tage alte Katzen mit einer Vibrionen-Milchkultur infizierte, konnte beim überwiegenden Teil Diarrhoen und Tod hervorrufen. Dieses Ergebnis steht mit den von WIENER (1896a) erhobenen Befunden in Einklang. GOHAR und MAKKAWI (1948) erzielten durch die Infektion der Zitzen des Muttertieres bei 2 Tage alten, 150 g schweren saugenden Katzen eine tödlich verlaufende Erkrankung.

Im Vordergrund der klinischen Erscheinungen standen profuse Durchfälle und generalisierte Krämpfe (KARLINSKI, 1896; WIENER, 1896a). Bei den saugenden Katzen traten die Diarrhoen nach einer Inkubationszeit von 7 Tagen auf; in den folgenden 2 Tagen verendeten die Tiere. Als Obduktionsbefund wurde eine starke Kongestion des ganzen Gastrointestinaltraktes festgestellt (WIENER, 1896a); außerdem waren bisweilen bronchopneumonische Infiltrate zu sehen (GOHAR und MAKKAWI, 1948). Die Choleravibrionen konnten zum Teil im Darminhalt der zugrunde gegangenen Tiere nachgewiesen werden (KARLINSKI, 1896; GOHAR und MAKKAWI, 1948), aus Blut, Leber und Nieren (WIENER, 1896a) und auch aus der Lunge (GOHAR und MAKKAWI, 1948). Andere Infektionsmethoden waren bei Katzen äußerst selten; VIOLLE (1914a) erwähnte eine intraduodenale Injektion der Erreger.

11. Schwein

Auf die Verfütterung von vibrionenhaltigem Darminhalt Cholerakranker reagierte ein Schwein mit generalisierten Krämpfen und Tod (RICHARDS, 1884). Es ist fraglich, ob er durch die Vibrionen verursacht wurde, da eine Übertragung durch Verfütterung des Darminhaltes eines verendeten Schweines auf ein weiteres Tier mißlang. Auch Nicati und Rietsch (1885a) war es trotz Vorbehandlung nicht möglich, Schweine zu infizieren.

12. Taube

a) Orale Infektion

Die oralen Infektionsversuche von Pfeiffer und Nocht (1889) glückten trotz Gabe von Opiumtinktur bei Tauben nicht. Es gelang den Erregern anscheinend nicht, den Magen der Taube zu passieren, da sie weder mikroskopisch noch mit Hilfe des Kulturverfahrens aus dem Magen-Darm-Kanal nachgewiesen werden konnten.

b) Parenterale Infektion

Intrapleurale, intraperitoneale, intramuskuläre und subcutane Infektion. Nach intraperitonealer und intrapleuraler Injektion gelang es Pfeiffer und Nocht (1889), Tauben mit einiger Sicherheit zu töten. Die Vibrionen konnten mikroskopisch und mit dem Kulturverfahren im Blut nachgewiesen werden. Sie nahmen an, daß aus Peritoneum und Pleurahöhle mit dem Lymphstrom kontinuierlich Bakterien in die Blutbahn eingeschleppt werden; bei Erschöpfung des Nachschubes verschwinden die Vibrionen dann sehr rasch aus dem Blut.

Die übliche Infektionsmethode der Tauben ist die intramuskuläre und subcutane Injektion. Die Experimente von Gamaleia (1888a) erbrachten, daß Tauben nicht nur für V. metschnikovii, sondern auch für V. cholerae empfänglich sind. Nach wenigen Passagen durch den Taubenkörper konnte er die Virulenz der von ihm benutzten Choleravibrionen so steigern, daß die Injektion von 1—2 Tropfen erregerhaltigen Blutes mit Sicherheit Tauben innerhalb 8—10 Std tötete. Salus (1893) fand, daß intramuskulär verabfolgte Choleravibrionen zu einer septicämischen Erkrankung der Tauben und zur Vermehrung in ihrem Blut führen können. Diese Beobachtung muß mit Skepsis betrachtet werden, da von den meisten Autoren auch bei anderen Versuchstieren zwar die Möglichkeit einer Bakteriämie eingeräumt wird, jedoch mit dem Hinweis, daß die Mikroorganismen im zirkulierenden Blut rasch zugrunde gehen. Diesen Untersuchungen widersprachen entschieden Pfeiffer und Nocht (1889), die Tauben für wenig empfänglich für Choleravibrionen hielten. Auch die Injektion frisch isolierter Choleravibrionen führte zu keinem Ergebnis, wie Pfeiffer (1894) in einer weiterführenden Arbeit feststellte. Bestätigt wurden diese Befunde von Friedrich (1893) und Rindfleisch (1896). Der Tod von Tauben konnte nach diesen Untersuchungen erst dann herbeigeführt werden, wenn zusammen mit den Choleravibrionen eine größere Menge Bouillon intramuskulär injiziert wurde. Durch die Bouilloneinspritzung sollte das Muskelgewebe geschädigt und ein Locus minoris resistentiae geschaffen werden (Rindfleisch, 1896).

13. Huhn und bebrütetes Hühnerei

a) Infektion von Hühnern

Die Infektion von Hühnern führte nach Koch (1884) zu keinem Resultat.

b) Infektion des bebrüteten Hühnereis

Hühnerembryonen sind gegenüber Choleravibrionen außerordentlich empfindlich (Wilson, 1946; Finkelstein und Ransom, 1960; Gardner et al., 1964). Nach den Untersuchungen von Wilson (1946) eignen sich am besten 7 Tage alte, bebrütete Hühnereier, in deren Allantoissack die Mikroorganismen injiziert werden. Dosen von 10^4 bis 5×10^4 Vibrionen lassen die Embryonen innerhalb 48 Std sterben. Wird dagegen die gleiche Dosis in 15 Tage alte Bruteier injiziert, so stirbt ein Teil der Embryonen in kurzer Zeit ab. Aus der Allantoisflüssigkeit von Embryonen, die 5 Tage überlebten, können Mikroorganismen nicht mehr isoliert werden. Nach der Injektion setzen sie sich an der Chorio-Allantois-Membran fest und vermehren sich dort rasch. Die Membran wird trübe und ödematös; sterben die Embryonen nicht gleich ab, so schwillt sie zu beträchtlicher Dicke an. Die Mikroorganismen dringen dann auch in andere Regionen des Eies vor und können kurz vor dem Tod des Embryos aus Allantoisflüssigkeit und Eidotter isoliert werden. Beim Embryo und an den Membranen sind pathologisch-anatomisch keine charakteristischen Veränderungen zu finden. Meist wird eine ausgedehnte Thrombose der Chorio-Allantois-Gefäße beobachtet. FINKELSTEIN und RANSOM (1960) prüften den Einfluß von Colibakterien auf die Vermehrungstätigkeit der Vibrionen im Hühnerembryo. Mit Hilfe von Bakterienzählungen wurde ermittelt, daß die Choleravibrionen sich in bis zu 11 Tage alten Hühnerembryonen stärker vermehren als in 15 Tage bebrüteten. Die Injektion von nicht enteropathogenen E.-coli-Stämmen vor der Injektion von annähernd 10^5 Choleravibrionen in 11 Tage alte Hühnerembryonen hat eine gewisse schützende Wirkung auf den Embryo. Er stirbt dann meist innerhalb 24 Std ab. Wie Bakterienzählungen ergaben, trat die exponentielle Vermehrungsphase der Choleravibrionen bei E.-coli-Injektion erst nach etwa 20 Std ein, während Choleravibrionen allein in Hühnerembryonen injiziert, bereits nach 4 Std in der logarithmischen Vermehrungsphase waren. Colibakterien bewirkten demnach anfänglich eine Vibriostase. Dieser protektive Effekt konnte verdoppelt werden, wenn abgetötete Colibakterien oder ihr Endotoxin appliziert wurden. Abgetötete grampositive Mikroorganismen entwickelten keine derartige „Schutzwirkung".

14. Fische

Infektion von Goldfischen, Karpfen und Seefischen

Da Choleraepidemien häufig an Küstengebieten oder Flußrandzonen auftreten, war es naheliegend, Fische auf ihre mögliche Bedeutung als Träger von Choleravibrionen zu untersuchen. Die mit diesen Tieren durchgeführten experimentellen Arbeiten zielen im wesentlichen auf die Beantwortung der Frage nach einer eventuellen Vermehrung und nach der Überlebensdauer der Vibrionen im Fischorganismus. Neben REMLINGER und NOURI (1908a) arbeiteten CANO und MARTINEZ (1913) mit Goldfischen. Die Tiere waren in Gefäße mit 5 l Wasser eingesetzt, dem jeweils 30 ml einer 24 Std bebrüteten Bouillonkultur zugefügt worden war. Nach 2—4 Tagen konnten die Choleravibrionen im Wasser und im Darm der Goldfische nicht mehr nachgewiesen werden. Bakteriologische Untersuchungen von infizierten Fischen, die gekocht oder gegrillt wurden, erbrachten immer ein negatives Kulturergebnis.

Karpfen, die eine größere Erregerdosis von Cholera- und El-Tor-Vibrionen erhalten hatten, verendeten nach 4—8 Tagen und zeigten die gleichen Symptome wie Fische, die mit V. piscium infiziert worden waren (DAVID, 1927; s. S. 164). Durch eine Magensonde gaben SCHÖBL und NUKADA (1935) 8 jungen 50 g schweren Karpfen jeweils 2,5 ml einer V.-cholerae-Peptonwasserkultur. Bei 5 Karpfen, die innerhalb der ersten 6 Tage post infectionem getötet wurden, konnten Choleravibrionen stets aus Magen und Darminhalt, in einem Fall auch aus Gallenflüssigkeit gezüchtet werden. Positive Kulturergebnisse aus Faeces wurden nur bei 2 am 7. bzw. 19. Tag getöteten Karpfen erhalten.

Mit Seefischen unterschiedlicher Species experimentierte Kabeshima (1918 b), indem er sie in einem Seewassertank hielt und jeweils 50 mg Choleravibrionen (Naßgewicht) zufügte, die aus einer 18 Std bebrüteten Agarkultur gewonnen waren. Die Fische blieben zwischen 5 min und 5 Std im kontaminierten Wasser. Anschließend wurden sie durch 10—15minütiges Eintauchen in $2^0/_{00}$ Quecksilber-chloridlösung getötet. Nach Reinigung mit Äthanol wurden sie seziert und die Innereien in Peptonwasser übertragen, das 15 Std bebrütet wurde. Auf diese Weise konnte Kabeshima aus nahezu 77% der Fische V. cholerae isolieren. In einem weiteren Versuch beließ er tote Fische für 1—5 Std in dem kontaminierten Wasser und konnte anschließend bei 17 von 37 Exemplaren Choleravibrionen aus dem Intestinaltrakt nachweisen. Als Eintrittspforte für die Erreger wurde der After angesehen.

Die Untersucher leiteten aus ihren Ergebnissen ab, daß Fische als Cholera-vibrionenträger in Frage kommen können. Dem muß entgegen gehalten werden, daß die von ihnen verwendete Vibrionenmasse nicht den natürlichen Bedingungen entspricht.

Eine ausführliche Darstellung des Themas geben Sticker (1912) und Pol-litzer (1959). Letzterer weist darauf hin, daß Choleravibrionen von Fischen durch kontaminiertes Wasser aufgenommen werden können. Der Verzehr von rohem Fischfleisch könnte daher eine Infektionsquelle darstellen.

15. Frosch

Infektion in den dorsalen Lymphsack, intramuskuläre Infektion

In seiner Untersuchung „Über eine durch choleraähnliche Vibrionen hervor-gerufene Fischseuche" infizierte David (1927) Frösche mit V. cholerae durch In-jektion in den dorsalen Lymphsack. Erregerdosis war $^1/_4$ Öse Kulturmaterial einer 48 Std bebrüteten Agarkultur. 24 Std nach der Infektion wurde eine Gasansamm-lung im Lymphsack beobachtet, die Frösche schienen immens aufgetrieben und starben mitunter „apoplektiform" innerhalb 4—10 Tagen. Pathologisch-anato-misch wurden Zeichen einer Gastroenteritis und Blutungen in die inneren Organe festgestellt. Durch intramuskuläre Injektion von 2×10^8 Choleravibrionen infi-zierten Gohar und Makkawi (1948) 20 g schwere Frösche. Die bei 18° C Um-gebungstemperatur gehaltenen Tiere starben innerhalb 24 Std, die bei 37° C gehaltenen innerhalb 12 Std. Bei der Sektion waren an den inneren Organen Stauungszeichen zu sehen; die Vibrionen konnten aus dem Blut isoliert werden.

16. Eidechse

Goere (1913) verabfolgte 4 grünen Eidechsen je 0,5 ml 24 Std bebrütete Choleravibrionen, die aus menschlichem Untersuchungsmaterial isoliert worden waren. Eines der Tiere bekam Durchfälle und verendete nach 30 Std. Bei einem zweiten dauerten die Diarrhoen 2 Tage, dann normalisierte sich der Stuhl, das Tier starb jedoch in kachektischem Zustand einen Monat später. Aus den diar-rhoischen Dejekten konnten die Choleravibrionen isoliert werden. Bei den übrigen beiden Tieren hatte 24 Std nach der Infektion Diarrhoe bestanden; sie schieden die Vibrionen 2 bzw. 5 Tage lang mit den Faeces aus. Aus Darminhalt eines dieser Tiere, das 3 Monate später zugrunde ging, konnten die Choleravibrionen ge-züchtet werden.

17. Muschel

Abraham (1954) infizierte im Meeresgebiet von Madras vorkommende Venus-Muscheln (Meretrix casta), um die Lebensfähigkeit der Choleravibrionen in diesen Tieren zu ermitteln. Er wählte Muscheln von 18—30 mm Länge. Er ging von

8 Std bebrüteten Peptonwasserkulturen frisch isolierter Choleravibrionen aus, deren Sediment er nach Zentrifugieren in 2 ml Kochsalzlösung suspendierte. 1 ml enthielt etwa $1,4 \times 10^{10}$ Vibrionen, die teils dem Wasser zugesetzt wurden, in dem sich die Muscheln befanden, teils wurden 0,05—0,1 ml der Aufschwemmung in den Fuß injiziert. Durch tägliche Probenentnahme und quantitative Bestimmung der Choleravibrionen konnte festgestellt werden, daß sie in der Muschel 3 Tage lebensfähig blieben, sich jedoch nicht vermehrten.

18. Fliege und andere Insekten

Bereits vor der Isolierung und Züchtung des V. cholerae wurde vermutet, daß Fliegen, deren Körperoberfläche Vibrionen anhaften, bei der Übertragung der Cholera eine Rolle spielen könnten. Um die Überlebensfähigkeit der Choleravibrionen zu ermitteln, wurde den Darmentleerungen besondere Beachtung geschenkt.

Maddox (1885) gelang es, aus Faeces von Fliegen, die mit Vibrionen kontaminierte Zuckerlösung gefressen hatten, diese Mikroorganismen zu isolieren. Tizzoni und Cattani (1886, 1888) sammelten in Krankenhäusern mit Cholerapatienten Fliegen ein, deren Körper sie nach Dekapitation in flüssigen Nährmedien kultivierten. Aus mehreren Kulturen ließen sich Choleravibrionen isolieren. Sawtschenko (1892) infizierte die Insekten mit Choleravibrionen und konnte 1 bis 2 Tage danach unter sterilen Kautelen aus Darmmaterial die Erreger darstellen. Zu ähnlichen Ergebnissen kam Craig (1894), der an Hausfliegen 3 Tage lang ein mit Cholerabouillon durchtränktes Stück Brot verfütterte. Aus den Faeces eines dieser Tiere gelang die Isolierung des Erregers. Untersuchungen von Passek (1911) erbrachten den Nachweis von Choleravibrionen im Fliegendarm 12 Std nach der Infektion, während er 72 Std später nicht mehr gelang.

Diese Ergebnisse wurden von Gill und Lal (1931) in weiterführenden Untersuchungen bestätigt. Sie fütterten Fliegen mit Cholera-Milchemulsionen, setzten sie danach 5 min auf sterilisiertes Fleisch und brachten ihren Rüssel mit sterilisierter Milch in Kontakt. Anschließend sammelten sie Faeces in sterilen Gefäßen. Die Fliegen wurden chloroformiert, zerrieben und ihre Därme unter sterilen Kautelen entnommen. Die bakteriologische Untersuchung ergab, daß die Mikroorganismen mindestens 5 Tage in dem Insekt überleben. In Fliegenfaeces waren 24 Std nach der Infektion keine Vibrionen über das kontaminierte Fleischstück nachzuweisen, während 5 Tage später die Erreger wieder aus den Faeces isoliert werden konnten. Eine Infektion der sterilisierten Milch über den Rüssel der Fliegen gelang nur bis zu 24 Std nach Kontamination des Insekts mit Choleravibrionen.

Neben Fliegen wurden sehr selten auch andere Insekten zu experimentellen Tierversuchen herangezogen, so Bienen, Wespen und Käfer (Maddox, 1885), Schaben (Cao, 1898) und Raupen (Metalnikow und Gaschen, 1921). Übersichtsarbeiten zu dieser Fragestellung finden sich bei Sticker (1912), Schuckmann (1926) und Pollitzer (1959).

B. Die Wirkung von abgetöteten Choleravibrionen, bakterienfreien Filtraten und Zellextrakten auf Versuchstiere

1. Allgemeines

Tierexperimentelle Untersuchungen mit Choleratoxinpräparationen sollen die Frage klären, ob sie für die Schädigungen verantwortlich sind, die durch die Infektionskrankheit verursacht werden. Zunächst ist zu prüfen, ob und in welchem

Umfang der Vibrionenstamm Toxin bildet und ob durch die Toxinwirkung Organe geschädigt werden. Für die Vibrionen selbst sind diejenigen Bedingungen zu finden, die zu guter Toxinausbeute führen. Hierzu sind geeignete Stämme und Nährmedien erforderlich. Zur Überprüfung der Giftwirkung sind empfängliche Versuchstiere zu ermitteln. Auch muß der Tatsache Rechnung getragen werden, daß Toxine, obwohl sie als Virulenzfaktoren meist mit der Virulenz eines Bakterienstammes korreliert sind, mitunter von virulenten Mikroorganismen in geringem Maße gebildet werden und umgekehrt.

Die Wirkung von Choleratoxin ist noch nicht vollständig geklärt. Über die konventionelle Einteilung in Endo- und Exotoxine hinaus werden Toxine angeführt, die eine besondere Bezeichnung tragen. Soweit jedoch eine Kennzeichnung für die gewonnenen toxischen Produkte nicht gewählt wurde, werden sie bei tierexperimentellen Untersuchungen unter dem Sammelbegriff Choleratoxin geführt, so auch die durch Hitze abgetöteten Vibrionen.

Eine Einteilung der für tierexperimentelle Untersuchungen verwendeten Toxinpräparationen, die vergleichende Aussagen ermöglicht, kann derzeit noch nicht gegeben werden.

2. Toxine

a) Endotoxine

Bei Untersuchungen mit Choleratoxin handelt es sich hauptsächlich um Endotoxin, das nach Lyse der Bakterienzelle freigesetzt wird.

Schon Cantani (1886) äußerte, daß das Toxin der Choleravibrionen nach Absterben der Mikroorganismen im Darm entsteht und resorbiert wird. Boivin et al. (1934) vertraten die Ansicht, es handle sich um Endotoxine, deren Wirkung ähnlich der anderer gramnegativer Stäbchenbakterien sei.

Mitunter werden die Begriffe Endotoxin und Antigen irrtümlich synonym verwendet. Endotoxine sind in der Bakterienzellwand fixiert und bestehen aus Proteinen, Polysacchariden und Lipoiden. Dabei terminiert das Protein den Grad der Antigenität, das Polysaccharid die immunologische Spezifität, während die Lipoide für die Toxicität verantwortlich gemacht werden (van Heyningen und Mellanby, 1969). Endotoxin von Cholerabakterien macht etwa 10% des Trockengewichts der Bakterienzellwand aus, hat eine durchschnittliche Größe von 100 mμ und ist nicht dialysierbar (Gallut, 1965). Die Analyse von aufgearbeiteten Vibrionenextrakten ergab, daß die Zellwand ein typenspezifisches, thermostabiles Polysaccharid enthält, neben einem Protein, das „vibrionen-spezifisch" ist und hämagglutinierende Eigenschaften besitzt (Günther, 1969).

Aus dem Cytoplasma der Zellen isolierte Gallut (1965) zwei Polysaccharid- und Proteinfraktionen, die auch in der Zellwand vorkommen. Die wichtige Frage, ob bei der Cholera des Menschen das Toxin als ganzer Komplex wirksam wird, oder nach enzymatischer Hydrolyse im Gastrointestinaltrakt kleinere Bruchstücke resorbiert werden, ist noch nicht beantwortet (Dutta und Oza, 1963). Einen Überblick über dieses Gebiet geben Pollitzer (1959), die Beiträge des Cholera-Symposions (Proceedings, 1965) und Felsenfeld (1966).

b) Exotoxine

Exotoxine werden, von Ausnahmen abgesehen, durch grampositive Bakterien gebildet. Sie werden in der logarithmischen oder stationären Vermehrungsphase, aber auch bei Autolyse der Zellen frei. Chemisch handelt es sich dabei um Proteine, die weniger hitzestabil sind als die im Bakteriensoma fixierten Eiweißkörper. Exotoxine bewirken die Bildung neutralisierender Antikörper. Die ursprüngliche

Annahme, Choleravibrionen bildeten Exotoxin, das spezifische Antitoxine stimuliere, die für Therapie und Prophylaxe der Infektionskrankheit eingesetzt werden können, hat sich nicht bestätigt (METCHNIKOFF et al., 1896).

Sofern über Exotoxine berichtet wurde, wurden sie in mehrere Tage bis mehrere Wochen alten Kulturen beobachtet. Es ist jedoch nicht auszuschließen, daß es sich bei derartigen „Exotoxinen" teilweise um Endotoxine gehandelt hat, die bei Autolyse frei wurden. Die Frage, ob Exotoxine bei der Cholera von Bedeutung sind, könnte deshalb nur noch von historischem Interesse sein, wenn nicht in neuerer Zeit die Ansicht vertreten würde, sie seien doch relevant. Als Beispiel sei das „Syncasecholeragen" angeführt, das aus Nährmedien isoliert wurde, welche bestimmte Zusätze enthielten (FINKELSTEIN, 1965; s. S. 111).

c) Andere Toxine

α) *Inhibitor der Natriumpumpe und Cholera-Haut-Toxin.* Einige Toxine bzw. Toxinfraktionen, die im Tierversuch unterschiedliche Eigenschaften besitzen, können nicht den Endo- oder Exotoxinen zugeordnet werden. Sie tragen besondere Bezeichnungen. Als Beispiel kann das Toxin gelten, welches als Ursache für die Blockade der Natriumpumpe im Darm angesehen wird und die Bezeichnung „natriumpump-inhibitor" trägt. Er wird von PHILLIPS (1963) als thermolabil und dialysierbar beschrieben. Seine Wirksamkeit zeigt sich an der Froschhaut (s. S. 130). FUHRMAN und FUHRMAN (1960) erzielten mit dem von ihnen isolierten Inhibitor die gleichen Ergebnisse an der Froschhaut, beschrieben ihn jedoch als ein niedermolekulares, dialysierbares, hitze-, säure- und alkali-resistentes Anion.

Aus Sterilfiltraten von Peptonwasserkulturen und Reiswasserstühlen von Cholerakranken isolierte CRAIG (1965a, b) einen hitzelabilen, nicht dialysierbaren, vasculär wirksamen Permeabilitätsfaktor (PF), den er später als „Cholera-Haut-Toxin" bezeichnete (CRAIG, 1966). Seine Wirkung wird an der Kaninchen- oder Meerschweinchenhaut getestet (s. S. 123). Einen mit FAF bezeichneten Faktor (fluid accumulation factor) isolierten AZIZ et al. (1968) aus Kulturfiltraten von V. cholerae. Sein Effekt wird an abgebundenen Darmstücken von Ratten überprüft.

β) *Hämolysin.* Beim Biotyp El Tor kann ein thermolabiles Hämolysin nachgewiesen werden. v. LOGHEM (1911, 1913) unterschied bei V. cholerae und El-Tor-Vibrionen mit Hilfe spektroskopischer Untersuchungen zwischen Hämolyse und Hämodigestion. Durch Hämolyse tritt der Blutfarbstoff unverändert aus dem Erythrocyten aus, während bei der Hämodigestion das Hämoglobin peptisch verdaut wird. Nach den Untersuchungen dieses Autors wirken V. cholerae Biotyp El Tor und V. cholerae mehr oder weniger hämodigestiv, ersterer verursachte stets Hämolyse, letzterer dagegen nie. Deshalb hämolysieren El-Tor-Vibrionen in peptonhaltigen Fleischwasserkulturen rote Ziegenblutkörperchen, V. cholerae dagegen nicht. Für diese Untersuchungen waren nach v. LOGHEM (1911) nur frisch isolierte Stämme geeignet. Dagegen berichteten KOLLE und SCHÜRMANN (1912), daß bei V. cholerae die Eigenschaft, Hämolysine zu bilden, stimuliert werden kann, die dann allerdings quantitativen Schwankungen unterliegt. Spätere Untersuchungen bestätigten diesen Befund, wobei es sich als wichtig erwies, einheitliche Untersuchungskriterien zu erarbeiten. DE et al. (1954) fanden, daß V. cholerae menschliche rote Blutkörperchen in Peptonwasser lysierte, diese Reaktion in einer Nährbouillon jedoch nicht eintrat. El-Tor- und NAG-Vibrionen lysierten menschliche und Schafblut-Erythrocyten in beiden Kulturmedien. Für die hämolysierende Aktivität von V. cholerae war die Anwesenheit von Calcium erforderlich, während die biologische Aktivität des Hämolysins von El-Tor- und NAG-Vibrionen durch Calcium gehemmt wurde.

Das Hämolysin aller Vibrionen ist thermolabil, dialysierbar und kann an Asbestfilter adsorbiert werden.

Finkelstein (1966) wies ebenfalls auf die unterschiedliche hämolysierende Aktivität von V. cholerae und V. cholerae Biotyp El Tor hin und führte den Verlust der hämolysierenden Eigenschaft von Choleravibrionen auf das Alter der untersuchten Bakterienstämme und die Verwendung unterschiedlicher Nährsubstrate zurück. Er forderte nachdrücklich, nur frisch isolierte Kulturen zu verwenden und die Stämme sofort zu lyophilisieren, um reproduzierbare Ergebnisse zu erzielen.

3. Toxingewinnung

Die mit Choleratoxinen angestellten Tierversuche führten zu sehr verschiedenen Ergebnissen. Dies ist in der unterschiedlichen Präparationsweise und den differenten Applikationsverfahren bei den einzelnen Tierspecies begründet. Das Toxin wird hauptsächlich durch Erhitzen, Filtration, Ultraschallbehandlung, Dialyse und Extraktion der Vibrionen mit chemischen und physikalischen Methoden gewonnen. Gelegentlich werden auch zwei oder mehrere Methoden kombiniert angewandt, etwa Erhitzen der Kultur und anschließende Ultrafiltration, oder chemische Extraktion mit folgender Dialyse.

a) Nährsubstrate

Einen nicht geringen Einfluß auf die Untersuchungsergebnisse haben die verwendeten Nährmedien und das Alter der Bakterienkultur. Aus diesem Grunde sollen zunächst einige Angaben über die Zusammensetzung der für die Toxingewinnung verwendeten Nährsubstrate gemacht werden. Früher wurden für die Toxinaufbereitungen mehrere Tage bis einige Wochen alte Bouillon- oder Peptonkulturen verwendet. Heute bedient man sich sehr junger Vibrionenkulturen, deren Virulenz zuvor häufig durch Tierpassagen gesteigert wurde. Alle Toxine sind auf Sterilität zu überprüfen, um sicherzustellen, daß es sich nach der Aufarbeitung um bakterienfreie Präparate handelt.

Bereits Cantani (1886) stellte fest, daß bei Verwendung von durch Erhitzen abgetöteten Vibrionen, die in Fleischbrühe mit Peptonzusatz gezüchtet worden waren, regelmäßig im Tierversuch eine Intoxikation gelang, während in Fleischbrühe ohne Peptonzusatz gezüchtete zu einer nur schwachen Reaktion führten. De et al. (1960) verwendeten für die Kultivierung teils einen halbfesten 1%igen Nähragar, teils Nährbouillon (pH 7,6) oder 1- und 5%iges Peptonwasser. Das Peptonwasser wurde in Portionen von 200 ml in Roux-Flaschen abgefüllt. Für die Toxinpräparation wurde von der Agarkultur auf das flüssige Medium überimpft und 18 Std bebrütet. Anschließend erfolgte die Aussaat auf flüssige und halbfeste Nährsubstrate, die 18 Std bei 37,5° C bebrütet wurden. Die Untersuchung von bakterienfreien Filtraten aus Peptonwasser, Nährbouillon und halbfestem Agar im Tierversuch am Kaninchen zeitigte ein positives Ergebnis, doch waren die Resultate, die mit Ultrafiltraten aus 5%igem Peptonwasser erhalten wurden, stets konstanter und eindeutiger in ihrer Aussage (s. S. 120).

Für die Gewinnung des filtrierbaren Hauttoxins von Craig (1966) war ein Medium mit 2% Peptonzusatz besser geeignet als ein solches mit 5%. Wie er weiter ermittelte, konnte die beste Ausbeute bei 30° C erzielt werden. Für die Toxingewinnung war nach Burrows (1965) eine 3%ige Bactopeptonlösung (pH 8,0) geeignet, die 18 Std bei maximaler Belüftung bebrütet wurde. Die Bakterien wurden anschließend zentrifugiert und lysiert (s. S. 123). Für die Injektion in abgebundene Darmstücke bevorzugten Schafer und Lewis (1965) das Ultrafiltrat von Choleravibrionen, die 18 Std in 5%igem Peptonwasser bebrütet wurden. OZA und DUTTA (1963) verwendeten ein Cholera-Agar-Medium (pH 8,0), das 3% Pepton, 0,5% Natriumchlorid und 3% Fadenagar enthielt. Das Medium wurde in Roux-Flaschen abgefüllt und nach Beimpfen 24 Std bei 37° C bebrütet. Für die Toxingewinnung wurden die geernteten Vibrionen nach der Methode von GALLUT behandelt (s. u.).

α) *Zuckerhaltige Nährmedien.* Über eine Steigerung der Toxinausbeute bei Verwendung zuckerhaltiger Medien berichtete HOROWITZ (1913). Sie verwendete 1%ige Glucosebouillon und beobachtete, daß die Toxicität der Filtrate nicht von der Vitalität der Kultur, sondern von der Lyse der Choleravibrionen abhing. Aus 10^2 Mikroorganismen/ml hatten sich nach 10 Std bei 37° C bereits 2×10^6 Vibrionen entwickelt. Durch die eintretende Säuerung des Mediums begann die Absterbephase nach 24 Std und nach 3 Tagen konnten aus dem Substrat keine vermehrungsfähigen Choleravibrionen mehr gezüchtet werden. Die sterilen Filtrate von 2—3 Tage alten Kulturen erwiesen sich als so giftig, daß 1 ml, einem Meerschweinchen intraperitoneal injiziert, den Tod innerhalb 12—18 Std herbeiführte. Um eine starke Säuerung und damit ein vorzeitiges Absterben der Mikroorganismen zu vermeiden, setzten andere Untersucher den Glucose-Nährmedien Pufferlösungen zu. Dadurch wurden die Vibrionen zu starker Vermehrung angeregt (HAHN und HIRSCH, 1926). Nach 6—10stündiger Bebrütung wurden 2 bis 4×10^9 Mikroorganismen/ml gezählt. Neben Phosphatpuffer fügten ANDU und NIEKERK (1929) dem Nährmedium 2% Kreide zu, da nach ihrer Ansicht ein konstanter pH-Wert von 7,6 durch 10%ige Pufferlösung allein nicht gehalten werden konnte. BERNARD und GALLUT (1943a, b) dagegen verwendeten eine Nährbouillon (pH 8) aus peptisch verdautem Kalbfleisch mit 0,5% Glucosezusatz. Die von Roux-Flaschen abgeschwemmten Choleravibrionen wurden in Portionen von 8—10 mg in 1 ml Nährbouillon aufgeschwemmt und bei 37° C inkubiert. Die toxische Substanz erschien nach 3 Std. Ihre Menge erreichte ein Maximum nach 4 und verminderte sich nach 5 Std rasch. In einer weiteren Untersuchung (GALLUT, 1954) wurden die abgeschwemmten Vibrionen mit 0,85%iger NaCl gewaschen, das Bakteriensediment in 5 ml Glucose-Salz-Lösung aufgenommen (NaCl 8,5 g, Glucose 5 g/1000 ml Aqua dest.) und 4 Std bei 37° C bebrütet. Die Glucose war nach 4 Std vollständig fermentiert, der pH-Wert auf 5,8 abgesunken und die Vibrionen weitgehend lysiert. Im Überstand der 25 min bei 5000 U/min zentrifugierten Suspension war anschließend fast das gesamte Toxin angereichert. Mit dieser auch als „Gallut-Toxin" bezeichneten Aufbereitung experimentierten auch DUTTA et al. (1959), sowie DUTTA und OZA (1963).

Die bessere Eignung, zuckerhaltiger nicht gepufferter oder gepufferter Nährmedien für die Toxinbildung ist eine Frage der Wasserstoffionenkonzentration und daneben ein quantitatives Problem. Während in nicht gepufferten Medien durch Säuerung rasch eine Lyse der Bakterienzelle und damit die Freisetzung zellwandgebundener und möglicherweise auch anderer Toxine eintritt, ist dies in gepufferter Lösung anfänglich nicht der Fall. Hier vermehren sich die Bakterien, ohne daß es zunächst zu einer Lyse kommt. Erst nach mehrtägigem Alter der Kultur sterben sie durch spontane Lyse ab. Hinsichtlich der Autolyse sind beide Verfahren gleichwertig. Allerdings ist es denkbar, daß bei der letztgenannten Methode die Wirksamkeit der Toxine durch die lange Bebrütung leidet.

β) *Besondere Zusätze zum Nährmedium.* Wird einem einfach zusammengesetzten Nährsubstrat ein Aminosäurengemisch (1%ig) als Wachstumsstimulans zugegeben, so kann aus den Filtraten ein Faktor isoliert werden, der von FINKELSTEIN (1965) als „Syncase choleragen" bezeichnet wurde (*synthetic medium supplemented with casamino acids*). Er wird von ihm als nicht identisch mit

Choleraendotoxin angesehen. Ohne Zusatz des Aminosäurengemisches wurde zwar eine gute Vermehrung der Vibrionen beobachtet, jedoch ließ sich der Faktor im Filtrat nicht nachweisen. Mit ihm gelang es, bei Tieren und Menschen in Abwesenheit vermehrungsfähiger Choleravibrionen eine experimentelle Cholera zu erzeugen (Finkelstein, 1965; Wirkung s. S. 121).

Im allgemeinen werden die zur Toxinbildung vorgesehenen Bakterienkulturen aerob bei 37° C bebrütet. Schütteln oder Belüften der Medien führt nach Untersuchungen von De (1959), De et al. (1960) und Burrows (1965) zu einer Steigerung der Toxinbildung. Offen bleibt allerdings, ob die Produktion der Giftstoffe von der Belüftung abhängig oder lediglich eine Folge der größeren Bakterienmasse ist, die unter diesen Bedingungen erhalten wird (Finkelstein, 1965).

Hüppe (1887b) fand, daß die Vibrionen sich auch in Anwesenheit von Wasserstoff vermehren und zur „fakultativen Anaerobiose" fähig sind: „gerade unter diesen Umständen kultivierte Bouillon gibt aber in kürzerer Zeit schon Erscheinungen, wie man sie bei Kulturen mit unbeschränktem Luftzutritt erst nach 8 Tagen erhält". Die anaerobe Vermehrung der Vibrionen im Hühnerei hielt Scholl (1892) für die geeignetste Methode zur Gewinnung von Choleratoxin.

b) Hitzeeinwirkung

Das Abtöten der Vibrionen durch Hitze mit anschließender Filtration ist ein vor allem in der älteren Literatur häufig beschriebenes Verfahren zur Toxingewinnung. Angaben über die Höhe der Temperatur und die Dauer der Abtötungszeit variieren beträchtlich. Daraus resultieren unterschiedliche Angaben über die Wirkung der Toxine. Überzeugende Ergebnisse wurden im Tierversuch mit 5 bis 14 Tage alten Bouillonkulturen erhalten, die 20 min bis 1 Std bei etwa 100° C erhitzt und anschließend filtriert worden waren (Cantani, 1886; Tizzoni und Cattani, 1888; Gamaleia, 1889; Löwenthal, 1889; Ransom, 1895 und Ghosh, 1933). Geringere Krankheitszeichen im Vergleich zur Gabe vermehrungsfähiger Mikroorganismen beobachteten nach Abtötung der Bakterien zwischen 60 und 80° C Sobernheim (1893a), Gruber (1896), Horowitz (1913), Demetrescu (1915) und Sdrodowski und Brenn (1925), während Hahn und Hirsch (1926, 1929) feststellten, daß durch eine Erhitzung auf 70° C während 30 min keine Symptome mehr ausgelöst werden konnten. Nach Angaben von Bürgers (1911) wurde das Toxin durch 30 min langes Erhitzen auf 56° C, 62° C, 70° C und 10 min auf 100° C nicht zerstört. Längere Hitzeeinwirkung verminderte die Giftwirkung. Eine schonende Art der Toxingewinnung beschrieb Kitasato (1889), der Choleravibrionen für 15 min bei 56° C inkubierte. Fujii (1924) schwemmte die Vibrionen von 18 Std bei 37° C bebrüteten Agarkulturen ab, wog sie, suspendierte 1 mg in 1 ml 0,85%iger physiologischer Kochsalzlösung und erhitzte sie 30 min bei 58 bis 60° C. Auf dieses schonende Verfahren (15 min 56° C) griffen in neuerer Zeit De et al. (1951) sowie Ghosh und Mukerjee (1959) zurück.

c) Trocknung

Für die Toxingewinnung aus V. massauah wendete wohl erstmals Pfeiffer (1892) die Trocknung der Bakterien an. Er beließ die abgeschwemmten Vibrionen 6 Tage im Brutschrank bei 37° C. Sobernheim (1893a) tötete die Vibrionen einer 24 Std bebrüteten Agarkultur in einem sterilen Schälchen durch 48stündige Trocknung bei 37° C. Durch diese Maßnahme erzielte er eine Abschwächung der Giftwirkung. Pfeiffer (1894) führte aus, daß die Giftwirkung mit der Verlängerung und Intensivierung des Trocknungsprozesses abnähme.

d) Filtration

In der Regel zeigten nur Sterilfiltrate von älteren Kulturen toxische Wirkung im Tierversuch, Filtrate junger Bakterienkulturen dagegen nicht (NICATI und RIETSCH, 1884b; SCHURUPOW, 1909; HOROWITZ, 1913; HAHN und HIRSCH, 1926). Bei Verwendung von Zusätzen zum Nährmedium werden in neuerer Zeit auch aus Filtraten junger Kulturen Toxine isoliert (s. S. 111). DE et al. (1960) schwemmten das bewachsene Agarmedium mit 10 ml steriler physiologischer Kochsalzlösung ab und filtrierten die Suspension unter Sog durch Whatman-Filterpapier (Nr. 41), um Agarpartikel zu entfernen. Die Vibrionen wurden anschließend in einer Kühlzentrifuge niedergeschlagen, der weitgehend klare Überstand erneut 20 min bei 14000 U/min zentrifugiert, und, um eventuell noch darin enthaltene Vibrionen zu entfernen, durch bakteriendichte Membranfilter gepreßt. Mit ähnlich hergestellten Filtraten experimentierten auch FUHRMAN und FUHRMAN (1960) sowie LYNG (1964).

e) Dialyse

Diese Methode wird zur Anreicherung von Toxinen, zu ihrer Isolierung aus einem Substanzgemisch und zur Prüfung ihrer Membrangängigkeit angewendet. Die Anreicherung von Choleratoxin versuchten METCHNIKOFF et al. (1896), indem sie vermehrungsfähige Vibrionen in ein Collodiumsäckchen gaben und dieses mehrere Tage in der Bauchhöhle eines Meerschweinchens beließen.

Bei der Dialyse von Choleravibrionenaufschwemmungen gegen physiologische Kochsalzlösung wurde das Toxin zurückgehalten, während unwirksame Bestand-teile in die Dialyseflüssigkeit übergingen. Auf diese Weise konnte die Giftigkeit des Präparates erheblich gesteigert werden (HAHN und HIRSCH, 1929; ANDU und NIEKERK, 1929). Im Gegensatz dazu fanden GALLUT und GRABAR (1945) nach Dialyse 2 Toxine, von denen das eine dialysierbare, mit niedrigerem Molekulargewicht ein Glucolipoid, das andere, nicht dialysierbare ein Protein war. Die Dialyse des Ultrafiltrates von Choleravibrionenkulturen in Cellophanfolien erbrachte im Dialysat den Nachweis einer aktiven Substanz, die durch einstündiges Erhitzen auf 80° C keinen merkbaren Aktivitätsverlust erlitt. Sie wurde von FUHRMAN und FUHRMAN (1960) als Inhibitor des aktiven Natriumtransports angesehen. Aus ultraschallbehandelten Choleravibrionen konnten weder im Dialysat noch im Dialysanden Faktoren gewonnen werden, die eine „choleragene" Wirkung besaßen (FINKELSTEIN, 1965). Wurden jedoch beide Fraktionen rekombiniert, so resultierte eine „choleragene" Mischung. Der nicht dialysierbare und der dialysierbare, niedermolekulare Anteil wurden als Procholeragen A und B bezeichnet. FINKELSTEIN (1965) teilte mit, Procholeragen A sei thermolabil, Procholeragen B thermostabil, und Choleraendotoxin sei nicht mit ihnen identisch. Es sei jedoch nicht auszuschließen, daß die „choleragene" Wirkung des Endotoxins erst durch Zugabe von Procholeragen A entstehe. Als Erklärung hierfür wurde angegeben, daß nach Gelfiltration an Sephadex Procholeragen A und Endotoxin mehr oder weniger gut voneinander abzutrennen sind und dabei die „choleragene" Wirkung des Komplexes verlorengeht. Procholeragen A wird von FINKELSTEIN (1965) als ein Substanzgemisch beschrieben, das in der entsprechenden Eluatportion nach Lyophilisierung in einer Menge von 0,05 g/100 ml Elutionsflüssigkeit vorliegt. Außer mit Dialysaten aus ultraschallbehandelten Vibrionen arbeitete er mit Toxinen, die er aus Ultrafiltraten von Choleravibrionen gewonnen hatte, welche in einem Aminosäurengemisch gezüchtet wurden (s. S. 111). Nach Dialyse des als Syncasecholeragen bezeichneten Toxins wurde die „choleragene" Substanz im Dialysanden zurückgehalten.

Die toxische Eigenschaft von Zellwandlysat und intracellulärer Substanz vor und nach Erhitzen untersuchte Leitch (1965). Die Giftwirkung der Intracellularfraktion wurde durch Erhitzen auf 60° C zerstört. Nach Trennung dieser Fraktion durch Dialyse zeigte lediglich der Dialysand eine toxische Wirkung.

f) Chemische Verfahren

Zur Abtötung von Choleravibrionen verwendeten Pfeiffer und Wassermann (1893) Chloroform. Später stellte Pfeiffer (1894) jedoch fest, daß nach einer Einwirkungszeit von 6—7 Std die Toxicität der Choleravibrionen nachließ. Die durch 5—10minütige Einwirkung von Chloroformdämpfen abgetöteten Agarkulturen waren nach Untersuchungen von Issaeff und Kolle (1894) außerordentlich toxisch. Eine Extraktion mit Kochsalzlösung und Chloroform ergab, daß kein Toxin in eine der beiden Phasen übergegangen war (Bürgers, 1911). Nicati und Rietsch (1886) dampften Peptonbouillonkulturen ein und extrahierten den Rückstand mit Äthylalkohol. Nach seiner Entfernung restierte eine ölige, nicht kristallisierbare Flüssigkeit, die toxische Eigenschaften besaß. Über Alkalibehandlung und andere früher angewandte Verfahren berichteten zusammenfassend Kolle und Prigge (1928). Säure- und Hitzebehandlung wurden von Freter (1955) angewendet; die in Peptonwasser zur Vermehrung gebrachten Choleravibrionen wurden abzentrifugiert, lyophilisiert und 95 mg Trockengewicht in 1 ml Aqua dest. aufgenommen; anschließend wurde die Suspension mit HCl auf pH 3,8 gebracht und 4 Std bei 37° C inkubiert. Nach Einstellung auf pH 7,0 mit NaOH wurde sie 30 min strömendem Dampf ausgesetzt.

Schafer und Lewis (1965) verwendeten die Flüssigkeit, welche sich nach Injektion von 5—10 ml einer 18 Std bebrüteten Choleravibrionen-Bouillonkultur im abgebundenen Darmsegment des saugenden Kaninchens gebildet hatte, als Ausgangsmaterial zur Toxingewinnung. Sie wurde teils zentrifugiert und der Überstand durch Milliporefilter (0,22 mµ) steril filtriert, ein Teil mit Ammoniumsulfat in der Kälte gesättigt, der Überstand verworfen und das Präcipitat in Aqua dest. gelöst. Die derart gewonnenen Präparate waren hitzelabil und verloren ihre Giftigkeit nach 30minütiger Einwirkung einer Temperatur von 55—62° C. Sie büßten bei Raumtemperatur sehr rasch ihre Toxicität ein, die im Kühlschrank über längere Zeit voll erhalten blieb. Die beiden Präparate waren dialysierbar und empfindlich gegenüber Säureeinfluß. Als weitere Verfahren wurden die Ätherextraktion, kombiniert mit Fällung in Äthylalkohol (Ribi et al., 1959; Finkelstein, 1965; Read, 1965), die Extraktion mit Trichloressigsäure und die tryptische Verdauung der Zellwände (Lavrovskaya und Blant, 1964; Burrows, 1965) angewendet, häufig in Verbindung mit physikalischen Verfahrensweisen.

g) Physikalische Verfahren

Die Ultraschallbehandlung der Vibrionen steht an erster Stelle. Als Beispiel für einen Präparationsgang sei der von Ghosh und Mukerjee (1959) mitgeteilte angeführt: Die in Roux-Flaschen auf Papain-Agar 24 Std bebrüteten Bakterien werden mit physiologischer Kochsalzlösung abgeschwemmt, zentrifugiert, in der gleichen Lösung resuspendiert und auf einen Gehalt von $1,7 \times 10^{10}$ Zellen eingestellt; 10 ml dieser Lösung werden $^1/_2$ Std beschallt (1 megacycle/sec) und während dieser Zeit durch einen Kühlmantel vor Überhitzung geschützt. Anschließend wird die Lyse mikroskopisch und durch Kultur überprüft. Die Suspension wird 30 min bei 4000 U/min zentrifugiert und der Überstand durch Seitzfilter gepreßt. Das klare Filtrat ist im Kühlschrank aufzubewahren. Im Tierexperiment zeigten der Überstand und das Sediment toxische Eigenschaften.

Einer ähnlichen Technik bedienten sich DE et al. (1960) sowie OZA und DUTTA (1963, 1965). Zur Herstellung eines Zellhomogenisates benutzte auch BURROWS (1965) das Ultraschallverfahren; für die Gewinnung von Zellwand- und intracellulärer Substanz zertrümmerte er frisch geerntete Vibrionen durch Schütteln mit Glasperlen. Das Homogenisat wurde zur Abtrennung der Glasperlen über einen Filter gegeben, gewaschen und Waschwasser mit Filtrat vereinigt. Die Zellwandfragmente wurden dann durch Zentrifugieren bei 4000 U/min abgetrennt; der gefriergetrocknete Überstand enthielt die intracelluläre Substanz. Nach diesem Verfahren ging auch READ (1965) vor, der die beiden Präparate jedoch zusätzlich dialysierte und Dialysat und Dialysand lyophilisierte; diese Fraktionen wurden anschließend in flüssigem Kulturmedium gelöst, über Milliporefilter (0,45 mμ) steril filtriert und die Filtrate 30 min in ein Wasserbad von 60° C eingestellt. Das Gesamtzellhomogenisat war vor der Gefriertrocknung 1 Std gekocht worden (s. S. 132).

h) Toxingewinnung aus Untersuchungsmaterial

Aus Ultrafiltraten diarrhoischer Ausscheidungen von Cholerakranken wurden Toxine isoliert, die im Tierversuch zu ähnlichen Veränderungen führten wie Vibrionenkulturfiltrate oder auf andere Weise gewonnene Toxine. Ihre Wirkung wurde hauptsächlich an der isolierten Froschhaut (s. S. 130) oder durch intracutane Injektion am Kaninchen (s. S. 123) überprüft. Über die Darstellung des Inhibitors der Natriumpumpe aus Dejekten von Cholerapatienten, die sich mit klassischen Choleravibrionen und dem Biotyp El Tor infiziert hatten, berichtete PHILLIPS (1963). Er konnte ihn auch aus dem Plasma von 3 Patienten isolieren, die an Cholera erkrankt waren. Im Stuhl Gesunder war er nicht nachzuweisen. BASU MALLIK und GANGULI (1964), CRAIG (1965) und FINKELSTEIN (1965) entdeckten in Reiswasserstühlen von Cholerakranken einen hitzelabilen, nicht dialysierbaren Faktor, der die Capillarpermeabilität steigerte und nach dem Vorschlag von CRAIG (1966) als „Cholera-Haut-Toxin" bezeichnet wurde.

4. Toxinwirkung

a) Meerschweinchen

Experimente mit diesem Versuchstier wurden überwiegend in der älteren Literatur beschrieben. Die Ergebnisse sind unterschiedlich und teilweise widersprüchlich. Im allgemeinen traten Erkrankung und Tod der Tiere ein, wenn sie einer Vorbehandlung wie bei der Infektion mit lebenden Vibrionen unterworfen wurden (s. S. 73).

α) Magen-Darm-Kanal

Die orale Gabe von 10 ml einer 2—4 Tage bebrüteten und 1 Std bei 80° C erhitzten Peptonbouillonkultur bewirkte innerhalb von 33—50 Std nur den Tod solcher Tiere, deren Magen alkalisiert und denen Opiumtinktur intraperitoneal injiziert worden war. Durch orale Alkoholgabe oder Injektion von Opium allein war dieses Ergebnis nicht zu erzielen (TIZZONI und CATTANI, 1888); also sind nicht nur die Vibrionen selber, sondern auch die Toxine säureempfindlich. Ultrafiltrate von hitzeabgetöteten Vibrionen waren nach Untersuchungen von SOBERNHEIM (1893a) gleich wirksam wie vermehrungsfähige Vibrionen. Wurde dagegen Toxin zusammen mit Futter gegeben, so konnte das Wohlbefinden der Meerschweinchen nicht beeinträchtigt werden (RANSOM, 1895; BÜRGERS, 1911). Nach Untersuchungen von BÜRGERS (1911) war auch nach Neutralisation des Magensaftes die orale Verabfolgung großer Mengen abgetöteter Vibrionen ergebnislos. Erst nach gleichzeitiger intraperitonealer Injektion von Opiumtinktur starben einzelne Meerschweinchen. Ähnliche Ergebnisse erreichte auch Puntoni (1913), der ihnen zusätzlich Natriumcarbonatlösung gab und sie einer Temperatur von 30—32° C und einer Luftfeuchte von 90—95% aussetzte. Zu negativen Resultaten kamen Pham (1935) und auch Freter (1955), die 300—400 g schweren Meerschweinchen bis zu 1200 mg Endotoxin (s. S. 114) per os applizierten. Selbst nach dieser hohen Dosis zeigten die Tiere keine krankhafte Reaktion.

Bei der Autopsie der Meerschweinchen wurden teils die gleichen pathologisch-anatomischen Veränderungen gefunden, wie sie nach Infektion mit lebenden Choleravibrionen zu beobachten waren (Tizzoni und Cattani, 1888; Sobern-heim, 1893a), teils war der Sektionsbefund völlig unauffällig (Freter, 1955). Die Diskrepanz dieser Ergebnisse könnte in der unterschiedlichen Virulenz der zur Toxingewinnung verwendeten Bakterienstämme begründet sein.

β) Parenterale Injektion

βα) Für die *intravenöse Injektion* von Choleravibrionen, die zur Abtötung 5 bis 10 min Chloroformdämpfen ausgesetzt waren, genügten $^1/_4$—$^1/_2$ Öse, um 300 g schwere Meerschweinchen innerhalb weniger Stunden zu töten (Issaeff und Kolle, 1894). Die tödliche Minimaldosis der abgetöteten Vibrionen entsprach bei intravenöser Injektion der lebender (Sanarelli, 1920). Nach den Untersuchungen dieses Autors trat die toxische Wirkung sehr rasch ein; die Versuchstiere ver-endeten unter den Zeichen einer akuten „Gastroenteritis". Die Läsionen an der intestinalen Mucosa waren die gleichen wie die nach intraperitonealer Injektion hitzeabgetöteter Vibrionen.

ββ) *Intraperitoneal injizierte*, abgetötete Choleravibrionen töteten Meerschwein-chen nach 14 Std bis 4 Tagen (Tizzoni und Cattani, 1888). Nach Injektion von 5 ml eines aus Eikulturen gewonnenen Toxins starben die Tiere innerhalb von 1—3 min (Scholl, 1892). Dieses Ergebnis wurde von Gruber (1892) auf die Wirkung des in Eikulturen gebildeten Schwefelwasserstoffs zurück-geführt. Gleichwohl gestand auch er diesem Toxin hohe Giftwirkung zu. Eine tödliche Erkrankung beim Meerschweinchen in Abhängigkeit von der injizierten Dosis Kulturfiltrat ermittelte Sobernheim (1893a). 285—338 g schwere Meer-schweinchen, die 5 bzw. 7 ml Kulturfiltrate erhalten hatten, gingen innerhalb von 20 Std zugrunde; ein 315 g schweres Tier, dem 3 ml injiziert wurden, erkrankte nur vorübergehend. Durch 1—2stündiges Erhitzen auf 75—80° C wurde die Giftig-keit der Filtrate nicht eingeschränkt. Wassermann (1893) ermittelte als sicher tödliche Dosis/100 g Körpergewicht 1—1$^1/_2$ Ösen durch Chloroform abgetötete Bakterien. Diese Mengenangabe wurde von Pfeiffer (1894) präzisiert, der als Dosis letalis für die intraperitoneale Injektion 2,5—5 mg abgetötete Bakterien/ 100 g Körpergewicht angab. Mit dem von Schurupow (1909) gewonnenen Endo-toxin genügten 0,2—0,3 ml, um 200 g schwere Meerschweinchen innerhalb 11—14 Std zu töten; nach Gabe von 0,5—1 ml starben die Tiere in 5—6 Std. Für hitzeabgetötete Vibrionen ermittelte dagegen Sanarelli (1920) eine wesent-lich höhere Dosis letalis minima als für vermehrungsfähige. Die Ergebnisse von Hahn und Hirsch (1927, 1929) sowie Soeleiman und Niekerk (1930) stimmen mit den positiven Resultaten früherer Autoren überein. Die Dosis letalis des von Bernard und Gallut (1943a, b) beschriebenen Toxins (s. S. 111) betrug für ein 250 g schweres Meerschweinchen 0,25 ml. Freter (1955) konnte nach intra-peritonealer Injektion von 3,3 mg des von ihm dargestellten Endotoxins Meer-schweinchen töten. Eine unterschiedliche Wirkung gegenüber Meerschweinchen, Kaninchen und Mäusen zeigte das von Ghosh und Mukerjee (1959) isolierte Toxin. Die Dosis letalis für 250—350 g schwere Meerschweinchen betrug 0,25 ml des Filtrates einer beschallten Bakteriensuspension, die $5,1 \times 10^{10}$ Vibrionen/ml enthielt.

In Publikationen, in denen über die Bestimmung der Dosis letalis berichtet wird, fehlen Angaben über den Krankheitsverlauf, da nur der Tod der Tiere von Interesse war. Dagegen wird in Untersuchungen über die Toxinwirkung angegeben, daß die Versuchstiere unter ähnlichen Symptomen wie nach der Injektion lebender Choleravibrionen zugrunde gingen (GAMALEIA, 1888c; RANSOM, 1895). Nach Beobachtungen von SCHOLL (1892) fielen die Tiere nach der Injektion zur Seite und verendeten unter leichten krampfartigen Zuckungen. Bei der Autopsie war eine Hyperämie des Dünndarms und der Nieren sowie ein blutiges Peritonealexsudat auffällig. PFEIFFER (1894) berichtete, daß die Tiere matt wurden, das Fell sträubten und ihre Haut sich kalt und schlaff anfühlte. Nach Injektion einer die tödliche Minimaldosis übersteigenden Menge wurden ein außerordentlich rascher Abfall der Körpertemperatur, oberflächliche und beschleunigte Atmung und generalisierte Krämpfe beobachtet (SCHURUPOW, 1909). Auch traten bei einigen Meerschweinchen Diarrhoen auf, denen bisweilen Blut beigemengt war. Gelegentlich wurde nur ein Absinken der Körpertemperatur registriert (FUKUHARA und ANDO, 1913; KABESHIMA, 1918a). Eine ausführliche Schilderung der Intoxikation stammt von HAHN und HIRSCH (1929):

Die Körpertemperatur sinkt innerhalb 2—3 Std nach der intraperitonealen Injektion auf bis zu 30° C ab. Gleichzeitig liegt das Tier auf seiner hinteren Körperpartie, wobei es sich mit den vorderen Extremitäten aufrecht hält; während der Muskeltonus im allgemeinen abnimmt, tritt infolge reichlicher Exsudation in die Bauchhöhle eine lokale Spannung der Bauchdecken auf. Nicht selten sind auch Exsudate auf den Konjunktiven zu finden. Im allgemeinen läßt 3 Std nach der Intoxikation diese progressive Symptomatik ziemlich plötzlich nach; die Temperatur steigt dabei um 2—3° C an. Die Versuchstiere sitzen dann zusammengekauert mit gesträubtem Fell, ohne daß ein Fortschreiten der Vergiftungserscheinungen wahrzunehmen ist. Nach weiteren Stunden sterben die Tiere meist unter den Zeichen von Atemkrämpfen. Durchfälle treten nach intraperitonealer Applikation des Giftes selten auf.

Bei der Autopsie fand sich in der Bauchhöhle, manchmal auch im Brustraum ein hellgelbliches bis rotes Exsudat, fibrinös eitrige Beläge auf der Leber, sowie Hyperämie von Magen und Darm. Die Schleimhäute waren mit dicken, grauen, von Blut untermischten Belägen bedeckt; ferner wurden punktförmige Blutungen in die Schleimhäute angetroffen (TIZZONI und CATTANI, 1888; SCHURUPOW, 1909; HAHN und HIRSCH, 1929; SOELEIMAN und NIEKERK, 1930; FRETER, 1955).

$\beta\gamma$) Die *subcutane Injektion* von abgetöteten Choleravibrionen führte nach den Ergebnissen von TIZZONI und CATTANI (1888) zu einer leichten Temperatursenkung. Eine tödliche Erkrankung konnte nur nach Vorbehandlung der Meerschweinchen mit Alkohol oder Alkali-Opium hervorgerufen werden. Auch wurde angegeben, daß für die letale Wirkung eine große Toxindosis erforderlich sei. Von 9 Tieren, deren Magensaft neutralisiert worden war, und die intraperitoneal Opiumtinktur erhalten hatten, gingen 7 nach Injektion von 1—6 ml abgetöteter Vibrionen (gewonnen aus einer 2—4 Tage alten Peptonwasserkultur) innerhalb von 5—33 Std zugrunde. Die beiden überlebenden Tiere hatten 0,5 und 0,7 ml erhalten (TIZZONI und CATTANI, 1888). Als Dosis letalis für ein 250 g schweres Meerschweinchen ermittelte RANSOM (1895) 0,5 ml Filtrat einer Vibrionenkultur, die 1 Std auf 100° C erhitzt worden war. Während SANARELLI (1920) nach subcutaner Injektion keine Krankheitserscheinungen beobachtete, vermerkten ANDU und NIEKERK (1929) sowie HAHN und HIRSCH (1929), daß als Letaldosis bei subcutaner Injektion etwa eine 5—10mal größere Menge benötigt wurde, als bei intraperitonealer Injektion. Die Temperatur sank ab, daneben wurden bisweilen erst 20 Std nach der Injektion Diarrhoen beobachtet (HAHN und HIRSCH, 1929).

Die Obduktion ergab an der Injektionsstelle eine entzündliche Infiltration der Subcutis, Flüssigkeitsansammlung in der Bauchhöhle, Hyperämie des Dünndarmes und blutig-tingierte Nebennieren (Ransom, 1895; Andu und Niekerk, 1929).

Um die Ursache der Anurie der Cholerakranken zu klären, untersuchte Fujii (1924) nach subcutaner Injektion von abgetöteten Choleravibrionen (1 mg/kg Körpergewicht) während eines längeren Zeitraums histologisch ausschließlich die Nieren. Wenngleich die Pathophysiologie des Nierenversagens bei der Choleraerkrankung heute bekannt ist, sei auf diese biometrisch und experimentell interessante Arbeit hingewiesen, da hier detailliert die histologischen Veränderungen der Niere beschrieben sind.

βδ) Intracutane Injektion. Ein hitzelabiles, aus Kulturfiltraten und Filtraten menschlicher Choleradejekte gewonnenes Toxin injizierte Craig (1965) Meerschweinchen intradermal. Damit konnte er ein Erythem erzeugen. Er stellte außerdem fest, daß die Capillargefäße für Wasser und Plasmaproteine eine verzögerte und verlängerte Permeabilität aufwiesen. Dieses Toxin wird durch Rekonvaleszentenserum neutralisiert. Die Prüfung zahlreicher Toxinpräparate von Choleravibrionen durch Bhatia et al. (1969) auf den Gehalt an „Cholera-Haut-Toxin" erbrachte, daß einzelne Fraktionen, auch das Endotoxinpräparat nach Gallut (1954), keine Reaktion verursachten, während bei anderen die Wirkung durch Erhitzen ($^1/_2$ Std 60° C) verlorenging. Die Wirkung des „Cholera-Haut-Toxins" ist auch vom Alter der Versuchstiere abhängig. Ghosh et al. (1972) untersuchten 10 Tage bis 6 Monate alte Albino-Meerschweinchen, denen in steigenden Dosen 0,01—0,1 mg „Cholera-Haut-Toxin" intradermal injiziert wurde. Die 10 Tage alten Tiere zeigten keine oder eine nur sehr schwache Hautreaktion ($\varnothing$ 2,5 mm). Bei den älteren bildete sich ein hämorrhagisches Ödem und Endothelzellproliferation aus. Der Durchmesser der Induration betrug annähernd 20 mm. Bei den jungen Tieren wurde eine leichte Reaktion erst nach Injektion von mehr als 0,1 mg sichtbar, während für ältere Meerschweinchen die entsprechende Dosis um den Faktor 10 geringer war.

γ) Intranervale Injektion

Einem 460 g schweren Meerschweinchen injizierte Pham (1935) 0,1 ml Endotoxin in den linken Nervus splanchnicus; eine Stunde später war das Tier im Schockzustand, mit Hypothermie, abdominaler Blähung und Anurie, 3 Std später ging es zugrunde. Bei der Obduktion war eine hämorrhagische Infiltration des unteren Dünndarmabschnittes, eine Desquamation der Dünndarmschleimhaut und eine Stauung der Peyerschen Plaques auffällig. Einer Toxindosis von 0,05 ml erlag 1 Versuchstier gleichen Gewichts nach 24 Std, einer von 0,02 ml nach 3—4 Tagen. Bei diesem Tier wurden Abmagerungen, Diarrhoen sowie Oligurie mit ausgeprägter Albuminurie beschrieben.

b) Kaninchen

α) Magen-Darm-Kanal

αα) Orale Applikation. Das junge, saugende Kaninchen ist für die Untersuchung der Wirkung des oral verabfolgten Choleratoxins ein besonders geeignetes Versuchstier. Zunächst gelang es auch mit sehr großen Toxinmengen nicht, Krankheitszeichen auszulösen (Schoffer, 1895; Bürgers, 1911; Hahn und Hirsch, 1928). Da keine näheren Angaben über das Alter der Kaninchen gemacht wurden, darf angenommen werden, daß ältere Tiere verwendet wurden. Für tierexperimentelle Untersuchungen sind saugende, bis zu 12 Tage alte Kaninchen geeignet. Dutta et al. (1959) gingen wie folgt vor: bei 8—12 Tage alten Kanin-

Tabelle 4. Die choleragene Wirkung von Toxin, das mit gereinigten Enzymen behandelt wurde, auf erwachsene Kaninchen. (Nach DUTTA und OZA, 1963)

Toxinbehandlung	Orale Dosis (in ml)	Diarrhoe	Letalität
Toxin + Trypsin	6—8	4	4/6
Toxin + Pepsin	6—8	4	4/5
Toxin + Pankreatin	6—8	0	0/5
Toxin + Phosphorylase	6—8	0	0/7
Toxin + Lipase	6—8	0	0/7
Toxin	6—8	12	12/12

chen wurde 12 Std vor Toxingabe eine Magenspülung vorgenommen. Im Anschluß daran stand ihnen nur Wasser zur Verfügung. Nach erneuter Magenspülung wurden in 2stündigem Abstand 5 ml „Gallut-Toxin" in 4 Portionen per os gegeben. Von 20 Tieren erlagen 16 der Intoxikation. In gleicher Weise wurde auch ein durch Ultraschallbehandlung gewonnenes Endotoxin (5 ml/100 g Körpergewicht) verfüttert (OZA und DUTTA, 1963). In diesem Zusammenhang ist eine weitere Arbeit dieser Autoren (DUTTA und OZA, 1963) bedeutungsvoll. Sie führten jungen Kaninchen 6—8 ml des mit einem gastrointestinalen Enzymgemisch vorbehandelten „Gallut-Toxin" oral zu. War das Toxin mit Fermentgemischen inkubiert worden, die aus jungen Kaninchen gewonnen waren, resultierte keine Abnahme der Toxinwirkung. Seine Giftigkeit ging dagegen verloren, wenn es mit reinen Enzymen behandelt wurde (Tabelle 4). Die choleragenen Eigenschaften gingen nach Abbau des Lipid- oder Polysaccharidkomplexes verloren; eine enzymatische Hydrolyse des Proteinanteils war ohne Einfluß auf die Giftigkeit des Toxinpräparates. Der Lipopolysaccharidkomplex ist nach diesen Untersuchungen ein bedeutungsvoller pathogenetischer Faktor.

Stuhlfiltrate von Cholerapatienten (1 ml/100 g Körpergewicht) verfütterte FINKELSTEIN (1965) nach Magenspülung an saugende Kaninchen. Das von ihm beschriebene Syncase-Choleragen wurde den Kaninchen teils bei intaktem Magen-Darm-Kanal, teils nach Unterbindung und nachfolgender Durchtrennung des Duodenums appliziert. Die Wirkung verschiedener Toxinpräparationen an 8 bis 10 Tage alten Kaninchen überprüften BHATIA et al. (1969), indem die Tiere jeweils 6 ml Probeflüssigkeit erhielten.

Die verschiedenen Toxinpräparate von BHATIA et al. (1969) lösten unterschiedliche Krankheitssymptome aus; einige bewirkten den Tod der Versuchstiere, andere Diarrhoe. Diese beiden Ereignisse korrelierten auch mitunter.

Nach Gabe eines durch Autolyse gewonnenen Toxins (DUTTA et al., 1959) wurden die Kaninchen teilnahmslos. Diarrhoe trat bisweilen 9 Std, in der Regel jedoch 12 Std nach der ersten Toxinverfütterung auf. Die zunächst milden Durchfälle wurden nach einiger Zeit reiswasserähnlich. Auf dem Höhepunkt der Intoxikation wirkten die Tiere total erschöpft, die Haut war kalt und das Fell gesträubt. Ab und zu traten Krämpfe der Skeletmuskulatur auf; außerdem bestand Anurie. Frühestens nach 12 und spätestens nach 24 Std trat der Tod bei 80% der Kaninchen ein. Der Gewichtsverlust schwankte zwischen 10 und 15%.

Der autoptische Befund war dem nach intraintestinaler Injektion vermehrungsfähiger Vibrionen und dem nach menschlicher Choleraerkrankung sehr ähnlich (DUTTA et al., 1959; OZA und DUTTA, 1963). Der Magen war leer, der Dünndarm im allgemeinen gestaut, die Gefäße erweitert und die Schleimhaut gallig verfärbt, das Colon gebläht und mit einer Flüssigkeit gefüllt, die Schleimhautfetzen und Fäkalien enthielt. Leber und Milz waren gestaut, die Nieren vergrößert und blaß. Histologisch fanden sich am Dünndarm eine teilweise abgehobene Mucosa und

Submucosa. Eine hydropische Degeneration wurde in der Markregion der Niere gesehen. In den Hili der Leber waren Eosinophileninfiltrate auffällig.

Bei Verwendung eines durch Ultraschall gewonnenen Toxins traten Diarrhoen schon nach 5 Std, der Tod nach 8—10 Std ein. Die Letalität betrug 100% (Oza und Dutta, 1963). Finkelstein (1965) konnte mit seinen Experimenten zeigen, daß Syncase-Choleragen am unterbundenen Magen keinerlei Wirkung zeigt, während es bei intaktem Magen-Darm-Kanal zu heftigen Diarrhoen führte. Herzblutuntersuchungen von Tieren im Kollapszustand ergaben, daß die Hämatokritkonzentration und des Reststickstoff signifikant erhöht waren.

αβ) Injektion in den Dünndarm. Hahn und Hirsch (1928), welche die Wirkung von Choleratoxin nach parenteraler Gabe als „enterotrop" bezeichneten, konnten nach Injektion in den Dünndarm des Kaninchens keine Intoxikation beobachten. Auch auf die intravesiculäre Instillierung von hitzeabgetöteten Choleravibrionen reagierten die Versuchstiere nicht (Violle, 1912).

αγ) Injektion in das abgebundene Dünndarmsegment. Um individuelle Faktoren auszuschließen und zu Kontrollzwecken, banden Ghosh und Mukerjee (1959) jeweils bei ein und demselben Kaninchen 3 Darmstücke ab. In das erste injizierten sie 0,5 ml durch Ultraschall gewonnenes Toxin, in das zweite 0,5 ml einer Suspension vermehrungsfähiger Choleravibrionen (10^9/ml) und in das dritte 0,5 ml sterile Nährbouillon. Bei der Autopsie der 18 Std später getöteten Tiere waren die mit Toxin behandelten und die Kontrollschlingen pathologisch-anatomisch unauffällig und enthielten lediglich Fäkalien. Die mit vermehrungsfähigen Mikroorganismen infizierten Segmente wiesen charakteristische Veränderungen auf. Durch die Untersuchungen von De et al. (1960) konnte dieser Befund nicht bestätigt werden. Das Filtrat einer mit 10 ml physiologischer Kochsalzlösung abgeschwemmten und mit Ultraschall behandelten Bakterienkultur erbrachte eine positive, das Ultrafiltrat von gewaschenen und mit Ultraschall behandelten Vibrionen dagegen keine Reaktion. Das Ultrafiltrat des Überstandes einer abgeschwemmten und zentrifugierten Choleravibrionenkultur führte mitunter zu typischen Veränderungen. Zahlreiche Kontrollversuche, die mit Filtraten des Kulturmediums durchgeführt wurden, bewirkten in keinem Fall eine Reaktion an der Dünndarmschlinge. Weiterhin konnte ermittelt werden, daß Kulturfiltrate von Choleravibrionen, die in 1%igem Peptonwasser zur Vermehrung gebracht worden waren, keine Wirkung zeigten, während Kulturfiltrate aus 5%igem Peptonwasser eine Flüssigkeitsansammlung verursachten.

Leitch (1965) band bei 2—3 kg schweren Kaninchen ein 30 cm langes Darmstück ab und sprach dann von einer Reaktion, wenn 24 Std nach Toxingabe 50—100 ml einer leicht gelblichen Flüssigkeit in dem betreffenden Darmsegment vorgefunden wurden. Durch Kochen gewonnene Lysate von E. coli- und El-Tor-Vibrionen bewirkten, im Gegensatz zu einigen NAG-Vibrionen, keine Reaktion. Die Injektion von V.-cholerae-Toxinen hatte stets dann eine Flüssigkeitsansammlung in dem Darmsegment zur Folge, wenn 2 mg in 5 ml physiologischer Kochsalzlösung suspendiertes gekochtes Gesamtzellysat verwendet wurde. Von unbehandeltem Gesamtzellysat waren 3 mg erforderlich. Nach Trennung des Gesamtzelllysates in Zellwand- und intracelluläre Substanz wurde das toxische Substrat in der intracellulären Substanz angetroffen. 0,5 mg bewirkten bei 1 von 5 Tieren, 2 mg bei allen Tieren die typischen Veränderungen. Durch 30minütiges Erhitzen auf 60° C ging die Toxinwirkung der intracellulären Substanz verloren. Ihre Auftrennung durch Dialyse in Dialysanden und Dialysat und die Untersuchungen beider Fraktionen zeigte, daß die toxische Substanz im Dialysanden enthalten war, von dem 1 mg in 4 von 7 Experimenten ein positives Resultat erbrachte, während die Injektion der gleichen Menge Dialysat ergebnislos blieb.

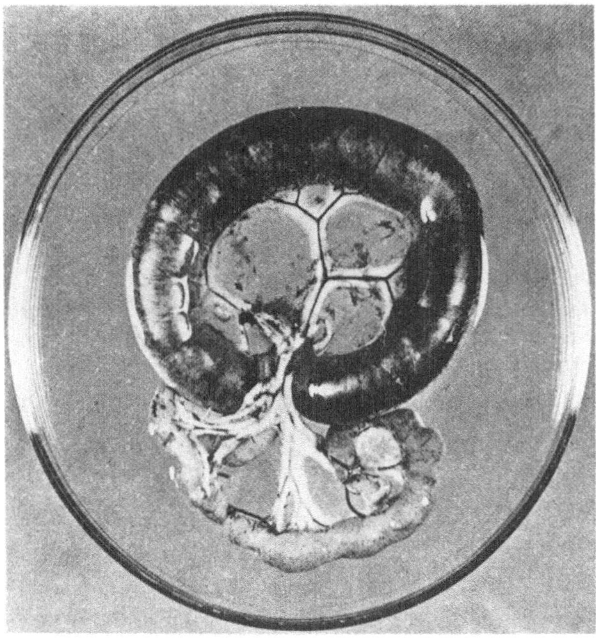

Abb. 5. Oben: Abgebundenes Dünndarmsegment eines jungen Kaninchens 18 Std nach Injektion von 1 ml Syncase-Choleragen. Unten: Kontrollsegment, in das Syncase-Medium
injiziert wurde. (FINKELSTEIN, 1965)

Auch die Injektion von 1 ml Syncase-Choleragen führte gegenüber der Kontrolle mit Syncase-Medium zu typischen Veränderungen (Abb. 5) des Dünndarm-
segments (FINKELSTEIN, 1965), ebenso wie fast alle von BHATIA et al. (1969) untersuchten Toxinpräparationen.

Das von DE et al. (1960) entworfene Modell des abgebundenen Dünndarm-
segments des saugenden Kaninchens zur Untersuchung des Choleratoxins unterzogen SCHAFER und LEWIS (1965) einer kritischen Betrachtung. Sie schreiben,
nach Inoculation der Testflüssigkeit in das Segment „wird das Abdomen verschlossen, der Untersucher geht nach Hause und zu Bett. Wenn er am nächsten
Morgen zurückkommt und seine Ergebnisse überprüft, findet er eine ‚positive‘
Dünndarmschlinge vor“. Um genauen Aufschluß über die Exsudation in das
Darmlumen zu erhalten, injizierten sie jedem Tier in 6 jeweils 2—4 cm lange
Darmstücke 2 ml Toxinflüssigkeit. Die Versuchstiere wurden dann nach 1—24, in
der Regel nach 6 Std getötet und das Flüssigkeitsvolumen in dem Darmsegment
bis auf 0,1 ml genau gemessen. Aus diesen Untersuchungen ergab sich, daß die
Flüssigkeitsansammlung im Darmsegment nach Injektion von nicht erhitztem
Toxin stets höher war als nach Applikation von erhitztem Toxin oder von physiologischer Kochsalzlösung. Jedoch wurde stets ein geringes Exsudat angetroffen,
wenn ein nach Ammoniumsulfatfällung wieder gelöstes und erhitztes Toxin verwendet wurde. Das Volumen der Exsudation steht nach diesen Untersuchungen
in direkter Beziehung zum Logarithmus der Injektionsdosis. Eine Menge von 2 ml
war gewöhnlich nach 1 Std vollständig resorbiert. Die Flüssigkeitsansammlung
setzte nach etwa 3—5 Std ein und erreichte ihr Maximum nach 6—8 Std. Das
Exsudationsvolumen war dosisabhängig und wurde durch die Kapazität des
Darmstücks limitiert.

β) Parenterale Injektion

βα) Die *intravenöse Injektion* wurde relativ selten angewandt. Sobernheim (1893a) berichtete, daß mehrere Milliliter einer erhitzten Choleravibrionenkultur vom Kaninchen ohne weiteres vertragen wurden. Zu ähnlichen Ergebnissen kamen auch Issaeff und Kolle (1894), die 350—2100 g schweren Kaninchen Choleratoxin verabfolgten. Lediglich eines von 10 Tieren starb 2 Tage nach der Injektion von 60 Ösen abgetöteter Bakterien. Auch Klemperer (1894a), Bürgers (1911) und Fukuhara und Ando (1913) berichteten, daß mit ihren Toxinzubereitungen unterschiedliche Ergebnisse erzielt wurden und meist große Toxindosen notwendig waren, um eine tödlich verlaufende Vergiftung beim Kaninchen zu erzeugen. Die teilweisen Mißerfolge sind mit großer Wahrscheinlichkeit auf den unterschiedlichen Virulenzgrad der verwendeten Bakterienstämme und die divergierenden Toxinpräparationen zurückzuführen.

Ghosh (1933) kam zu dem Ergebnis, daß die intravenöse Gabe von 0,5 ml des Filtrates ultraschallbehandelter Vibrionen ($5,1 \times 10^{10}$ V. cholerae/ml) 1—1,4 kg schwere Kaninchen innerhalb 3—24 Std tötete, nicht dagegen die Injektion von 0,1 ml.

Bemerkenswert war, daß auch bei den überlebenden Tieren kurze Zeit, mitunter 1 Std nach der Injektion, profuse Diarrhoen auftraten, während die Körpertemperatur teils nur gering (Issaeff und Kolle, 1894), teils erheblich absank (Hahn und Hirsch, 1928) oder leicht erhöht war (Ghosh, 1933). Den Darmentleerungen war zunächst Schleim beigemischt, wenig später wurden sie dünnflüssig und enthielten reisförmige Körner. Präfinal traten generalisierte Krämpfe, Kollaps und Paralyse der hinteren Extremitäten auf (Acton und Chopra, 1924; Ghosh und Mukerjee, 1959).

Bei der Autopsie der gestorbenen Tiere war der Dünndarm stark gerötet und mit einer Flüssigkeit prall gefüllt, in der nekrotische Epithelzellen schwammen. Leber und Milz waren gestaut, die Nieren anämisch.

ββ) Für die *intraperitoneale Injektion* bedienten sich De et al. (1951) eines Toxins, das durch 15minütiges Erhitzen auf 56° C aus einer Choleravibrionen-Abschwemmung hergestellt war, die 10^8 Mikroorganismen/ml enthielt. Die subletale Dosis betrug 0,75 ml/kg Körpergewicht, die sicher tödliche Dosis 5 ml/kg. Nach der Injektion kam es zur Ansammlung einer proteinreichen, zellarmen Flüssigkeit im Peritonealraum. Folge dieser Exsudation war eine Hämokonzentration und ein rascher Blutdruckabfall, der bei der Letaldosis innerhalb von 2 Std von 69 mm auf 15 mm Hg absank. Bei der histologischen Begutachtung der Niere zeigte sich, daß die corticalen Glomeruli ischämisch und meist kollabiert waren; am stärksten verändert war das Nephron in der Markregion; die Zellen im Bereich der Henleschen Schleifen waren geschwollen und granuliert, und die dem Lumen zugewandten Zellen abgelöst. Ödeme wurden im Myokard, in der Mucosa und Submucosa des Dünndarms gefunden. Die Capillarpermeabilität war erhöht und ermöglichte den Austritt einer plasmaähnlichen Flüssigkeit in das Gewebe. Im Peritonealraum wurden 5—6 ml einer klaren oder leicht getrübten Flüssigkeit angetroffen. Die Abdominalorgane waren gestaut, der Dünndarm enthielt nur wenig gelbliche Flüssigkeit.

βγ) Subcutane Injektion. Wie bei Meerschweinchen konnte Ransom (1895) auch bei 1500 g schweren Kaninchen durch subcutane Injektion von 4 ml abgetöteter Vibrionensuspension den Tod innerhalb 24 Std hervorrufen. Einen Schwund der chromaffinen Schicht der Nebenniere beobachtete Demetrescu (1915) nach Injektion von 10—25 ml einer Aufschwemmung hitzeabgetöteter Vibrionen bei fast allen Tieren. Ihr Kapselextrakt enthielt kaum noch Adrenalin, denn weder konnte nach Injektion des Extraktes in die V. jugularis eine Erhöhung des arteriellen Blutdrucks festgestellt werden, noch kam es an der Pupille des Frosches zur Mydriasis, und schließlich gab der Extrakt mit Phosphormolybdänsäure nicht die charakteristische Farbreaktion.

βδ) Nach *intracutaner Injektion* rufen vermehrungsfähige Vibrionen und Kulturfiltrate beim Kaninchen eine entzündliche Reaktion hervor. Diese wurde nach Injektion hitzebehandelter Toxinpräparate vermißt (GHOSH und MUKERJEE, 1959). Die intracutane Injektion des Filtrates ultraschallbehandelter Vibrionen $(1,7 \times 10^9/ml)$ bewirkte nach 2 Std eine unscharf begrenzte Rötung der Haut mit einem Durchmesser von 13—20 mm, die nach Verdünnung des Filtrates auf 1:10000 ausblieb.

Bei der Suche nach dem Toxin, das für die massive Flüssigkeitseinschwemmung in den Darm verantwortlich ist, injizierten BASU MALLIK und GANGULI (1964) 0,1 ml Choleravibrionen- und Cholerastuhlfiltrat Kaninchen intracutan in die rasierte Bauchhaut, nachdem 5 min zuvor intravenös 1%ige Evansblau-Lösung appliziert worden war. Sie beobachteten, daß der Farbstoff in den entzündeten Hautbereich übertrat und vermuteten daher in ihren Filtraten eine aktive, die Capillarpermeabilität steigernde Substanz. Diese Untersuchungen wurden von CRAIG (1965b), der den Permeabilitätsfaktor aus Stuhlfiltraten isolierte, weitergeführt und präzisiert. 6—8 Std nach Injektion von 0,1 ml Filtrat trat ein Erythem auf, das seinen Höhepunkt nach 18—24 Std hatte, innerhalb 48 Std an Intensität abnahm und noch 2—4 Tage andauerte. Bei einem Durchmesser zwischen 6 und 15 mm bestand eine lineare Beziehung zum Logarithmus der injizierten Filtratdosis. Ein Kontrollversuch zeigte, daß nach intracutaner Injektion von physiologischer Kochsalzlösung die gesteigerte Gefäßpermeabilität 30 min nach der Injektion verschwunden war. Zum Nachweis der Zunahme der Capillarpermeabilität wurde den Versuchstieren nach intracutaner Injektion des Toxins intravenös Pontamine Sky Blue 6 XB (0,12 ml einer 5%igen Lösung/100 g Körpergewicht) in unterschiedlichen Zeitabständen intravenös injiziert. Durch den Farbstoffübertritt in das entzündliche Infiltrat konnte gezeigt werden, daß ein Anstieg der Gefäßpermeabilität bereits nach 1 Std auftrat. Die Blaufärbung nahm in den nächsten 5—8 Std zu. Ihre Ausdehnung erreichte ein Maximum nach 8 Std. Die größte Farbintensität zeigte sich 18—24 Std später. Nach 24—48 Std ging die Blaufärbung wieder zurück. Mit dieser Untersuchungstechnik konnte CRAIG (1965) demonstrieren, daß das 30 min auf 56° C erhitzte Filtrat keine derartige Reaktion gab. Der wirksame, als „Cholera-Haut-Toxin" bezeichnete Faktor kann auch aus Kulturfiltraten von V. cholerae dargestellt werden, wenn diese in 5% Bacto-Pepton zur Vermehrung gebracht werden.

Für eine intradermale Reaktion genügten nach den Untersuchungen von BURROWS (1965) 0,01 mcg Gesamtzellysat, 0,0025 mcg intracelluläre Substanz oder 1,4 mcg der Zellwandfraktion. Somit ist die intracelluläre Substanz mit einer „ca. 600fach" höheren Aktivität als die Zellwandfraktion und einer „etwa 20fach" größeren Toxicität als das Gesamtzellysat Träger des „Cholera-Haut-Toxins". Von dem steril filtrierten Überstand eines Gesamtbakterienlysates wurden für eine Hautreaktion 150 mcg benötigt. Versuche, diese durch Zusatz von Adrenalin zu steigern, erbrachten zweifelhafte Ergebnisse (BURROWS, 1965).

Auf die unterschiedliche Reaktion verschieden alter Kaninchen, die wie Meerschweinchen bis zu einem Alter von 10 Tagen gegenüber dem Faktor resistent waren, wiesen GHOSH et al. (1972) hin. Die Hautreaktion konnte bei älteren Tieren nicht durch Histamin- oder 5-Hydroxytryptaminblocker unterbunden werden.

Auch Betamethason, ein Prednisolonderivat (1 mg über 5 Tage bzw. 1 mg für 1 Tag oral), verminderte die Hautreaktionen nicht, vielmehr war eine Verstärkung zu beobachten (Ghosh et al., 1972).

γ) Intranervale Injektion

Wie Meerschweinchen injizierte Pham (1935) auch Kaninchen 0,2 ml Endotoxin in den N. splanchnicus. Die Tiere gingen nach 24 Std zugrunde. Bei der Sektion wurden im wesentlichen Läsionen des Dünndarms, in geringem Umfang auch des Dickdarms beobachtet. Histologisch war eine Epitheldesquamation im Bereich des Dünndarms auffällig, die Capillaren der Submucosa waren erweitert und teilweise rupturiert. Die Glomeruli der Niere wiesen hyaline Degeneration, mitunter Ödem und Hämorrhagien auf. Bisweilen wurden eine parenchymatöse Hepatitis und gestaute Nebennieren beobachtet. Die anderen Organe waren unauffällig.

c) Maus

Für Untersuchungen mit Choleratoxinen fanden Mäuse früher kaum Anwendung. Heute werden sie für die quantitative Bestimmung des Choleratoxins und für die Überprüfung der Wirksamkeit von Impfstoffen im „Mäuse-Schutztest" herangezogen. Dabei werden Mäusen je 0,5 ml einzelner Verdünnungsstufen von verschiedenen Vaccinen intraperitoneal injiziert. 14 Tage später erfolgt die intraperitoneale Infektion mit einer definierten Zahl von vermehrungsfähigen Choleravibrionen, die unter standardisierten Bedingungen gezüchtet wurden. Die Mäuse werden dann 48 Std beobachtet und die Zahl der toten bzw. überlebenden Tiere festgestellt. Auf diese Weise kann die mittlere effektive immunisierende Dosis (ED_{50}) für jede Vaccine berechnet werden (Shrivastav et al., 1965).

α) Orale und subcutane Applikation

Die orale Verabfolgung hitzeabgetöteter Choleravibrionen beeinträchtigte das Wohlbefinden weißer Mäuse in keiner Weise (Loewenthal, 1889; Freter, 1955). Auch gegenüber subcutan injizierten waren sie nicht empfänglich (Ransom, 1895).

β) Intraperitoneale Injektion

Nach Injektion von 1,0 ml El-Tor-Vibrionentoxin (Kraus und Russ, 1908) starben die Tiere 3 Std und nach Gabe von 0,2 ml 24 Std später. Durch Toxinaufbereitungen von verschiedenen Cholerastämmen wurden weiße Mäuse nicht oder nach unterschiedlich langen Zeiträumen getötet (Baumgarten, 1921). Der Autor führte diese unterschiedlichen Ergebnisse auf Virulenzunterschiede der verwendeten Cholerastämme zurück. 0,05 ml eines aus Glucosebouillon gewonnenen Toxins waren nach den Untersuchungen von Bernard und Gallut (1943a, b) die tödliche Dosis für 15 g schwere weiße Mäuse.

In weiteren Experimenten wurde der Wandel der Toxicität von V. cholerae in verschiedenen Stadien der Cholera durch intraperitoneale Toxingabe studiert (Gallut, 1953). Aus 10 Cholerapatienten wurden in 24stündigen Abständen 40 Vibrionenstämme isoliert, die vor der tierexperimentellen Untersuchung einmal über Nährmedium geführt worden waren. Anschließend wurde das Toxin durch Autolyse in kohlenhydrathaltigen Nährmedien gewonnen, wobei 1 ml Toxin 8×10^{11} Vibrionen/ml entsprach. Für die Versuche wurden 24 Mäuse in 4 Gruppen unterteilt, die jeweils 0,2, 0,1, 0,05 und 0,025 ml Toxinlösung erhielten. Durch die ermittelte DL 50 hat sich gezeigt, daß die Toxicität der aus verschiedenen Patienten isolierten Vibrionenstämme unterschiedlich ist. 24 Std nach Ausbruch der Infektionskrankheit waren die isolierten Vibrionen im allgemeinen wenig

Tabelle 5. Einfluß der Bebrütungstemperatur auf die Toxinbildung von V. cholerae.
(Nach GALLUT und JUDE, 1955)

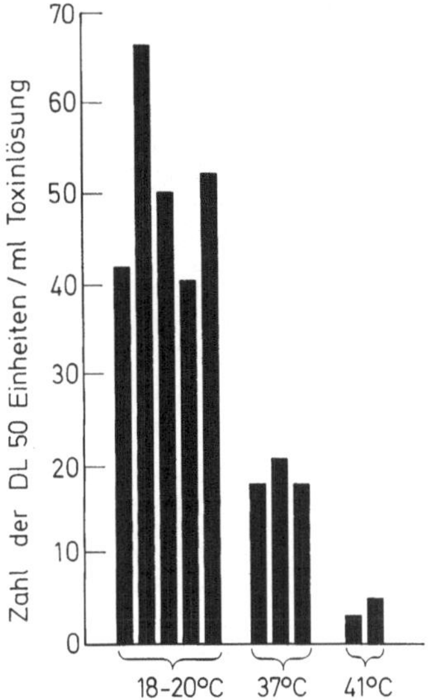

toxisch. Ihre Toxicität stieg erst im Verlauf des 2. Tages an, erreichte ein
Maximum um die 60. Std und fiel beim Abklingen der Krankheit im Verlauf des
4. und 5. Tages ab. Diese Untersuchungen bestätigen die schwache toxische
Wirkung, die allgemein bei Stämmen angetroffen wird, welche zu Beginn einer
Choleraerkrankung isoliert werden.

Die intraperitoneale Injektion von Toxinen aus Choleravibrionen, die bei verschiedenen Temperaturen gehalten worden waren, ergab, daß bei 18° C bebrütete
Stämme die größte Giftigkeit besaßen. Die geringste Giftwirkung hatten Toxine
aus Kulturen, die bei 41,5° C inkubiert worden waren. Eine Mittelstellung nahmen
Toxinisolate aus Kulturen ein, die bei 37° C gehalten wurden (GALLUT und JUDE,
1955). Diese Ergebnisse sind statistisch signifikant und in Tabelle 5 einander
gegenübergestellt.

Als DL 50 für 25—30 g schwere weiße Mäuse ermittelte FRETER (1955)
0,0625 ml, entsprechend 5,94 mg Vibrionentrockengewicht, DUTTA et al. (1959)
benötigten dazu 0,25 ml Gallut-Toxin für 16—18 g schwere weiße Mäuse. Die
Überprüfung der Toxicität der von GHOSH und MUKERJEE (1959) hergestellten
Toxinfraktionen erbrachte, daß die DL 50 für 25—35 g schwere männliche weiße
Mäuse bei hitzebehandelten Vibrionen 1,81 mg und für das Filtrat ultraschallbehandelter Vibrionen 2,12 mg betrug. In den Untersuchungen von BURROWS
(1965) war die DL 50 des Gesamtzellextraktes für 10—12 g schwere weiße Mäuse
2—5 mg, die der Zellwandsuspension 0,5—2 mg und die der intracellulären Substanz 5—10 mg. Da jedoch die Zellwand etwa 15—20% des Trockengewichtes der
intakten Vibrionenzellen ausmacht, ist die Toxinwirkung von Zellwand und intracellulärer Substanz gleichwertig. Das Toxin war hitzestabil und nicht dialysierbar.

Um den Einfluß von Nebennierenrindenhormon auf die Toxinwirkung bei
weißen Mäusen zu prüfen, applizierte GALLUT (1955) 15—18 g schweren Tieren
das von ihm präparierte Toxin und ermittelte die DL 50 unter folgenden Bedingungen: 1. 75 Tiere erhielten das Toxin; 2. bei 80 Mäusen wurden die Nebennieren entfernt, 8 Tage später wurden sie in 2 Gruppen eingeteilt, a) 52 Mäusen

Tabelle 6. Einfluß von Nebennierenrindenhormonen auf die Toxinwirkung von V. cholerae.
(Nach Gallut, 1955)

Versuch-Nr.	Behandlung	DL 50
1	Kontrolltiere	0,020
2a	Adrenektomie	0,002
2b	id. + 2 mg Cortison	0,140
3a	2 mg Cortison	0,520
3b	5 mg Cortison	0,086
4a	2 mg ACTH	0,018
4b	5 mg ACTH	0,1

wurde das Toxin verabfolgt, b) 28 Tiere erhielten subcutan 2 mg Cortison 1 Std
vor der Toxininjektion; 3. 125 Mäuse wurden mit Cortison behandelt. a) Von
diesen erhielten 75 2 mg Cortison 1 Std vor der Toxingabe und 50 Tiere 5 mg
während vier der Injektion vorausgegangenen Tagen; 4. 50 Mäuse erhielten ACTH,
25 von diesen 2 mg 1 Std vor der Toxingabe und 25 5 mg während vier der
Injektion vorausgegangenen Tagen. Über die Ergebnisse gibt Tabelle 6 Aufschluß.
Eine protektive Wirkung von Cortison und ACTH ist demnach erwiesen. Ein
geringer Effekt wurde bei der Gabe von 5 mg Cortison in Versuch 3 registriert,
während die Gabe von ACTH in der Versuchsanordnung 4 keine Wirkung bei der
Intoxikation zeigte.

d) Andere kleine Laboratoriumstiere

Ultraschallbehandelte Choleravibrionen wurden von Oza und Dutta (1967)
durch Dialyse in 2 Komponenten getrennt, von denen das hauptsächlich die Zellwandfraktion repräsentierende Dialysat keine antidiuretische Aktivität, der Dialysand — überwiegend Proteine — einen antidiuretischen Effekt aufwies. Dies
wurde an 2 Tiergruppen von 4 männlichen 140—240 g schweren Albinoratten
festgestellt, denen vor subcutaner Injektion der Toxinfraktionen 5 ml sterilisiertes
Aqua dest./100 g Körpergewicht durch die Schlundsonde gegeben worden war.
Die in 30minütigem Abstand während mindestens 3 Std vorgenommene Messung
der Ausscheidungen zeigte gegenüber einer Kontrollgruppe eine Verminderung
der Exkretion um 60%. Dieser Effekt wurde nach Injektion von 12 mg der Dia-
lysand-Fraktion pro 100 g Körpergewicht erreicht. Eine antidiuretische Wirkung
konnte auch durch subcutane Injektion von 40 mg Gallut-Toxin pro 100 g Körpergewicht erzielt werden.

Die Flüssigkeitsmenge in abgebundenen Darmsegmenten kleiner Laboratoriumstiere bestimmten Basu und Pickett (1969) 16 Std nach Injektion einer Cholera-
toxin-Rohfraktion (Coleman et al., 1968). Die Tiere wurden 24 Std vor und nach
der Injektion ohne Futter gehalten. Mit Ausnahme der weißen Maus reagierten

Tabelle 7. Reaktion des abgebundenen Ileumsegments auf die Injektion von Cholera-Rohtoxin.
(Nach Basu und Pickett, 1969)

Tier	Dosis (Öseneinheiten)	Flüssigkeitsmenge (ml/cm)	
		Toxin	Kontrolle
Wüstenmaus	0,25	0,2	<0,05
Ratte	0,5	0,3	<0,05
Hamster	0,5	0,3	<0,05
Meerschweinchen	0,5	0,45	<0,05
Chinchilla	0,5	0,8	<0,05
Katze	5	1,5	0,05
Weiße Maus	5	0,1	<0,05

sämtliche mit einer Exsudation in das Darmlumen (Tabelle 7). Die Injektion von hitzeabgetöteten Choleravibrionen (10^{10} Mikroorganismen, 10 min 100° C) war dagegen erfolglos.

e) Affe

POTTEVIN und VIOLLE (1913 b), die mit Affen der Arten Cynomolgus und Rhesus experimentierten, erhielten nach oraler Gabe von mit Äther abgetöteten Vibrionen die gleichen Ergebnisse einer tödlich verlaufenden Erkrankung wie nach Verfütterung von vermehrungsfähigen Choleravibrionen (s. S. 99).

f) Hund

α) Intravenöse Injektion

Hunde, denen NICATI und RIETSCH (1884 b) intravenös die Filtrate mindestens 8 Tage alter Bouillon- und Gelatinekulturen von V. cholerae injizierten, zeigten vorübergehend allgemeine Schwäche, erschwerte Atmung, Erbrechen und Diarrhoe. In extremen Fällen traten motorische Störungen auf. Ein Hund verendete bereits 12 Std nach der Injektion unter Anstieg der Körpertemperatur. Als Obduktionsbefunde waren hämorrhagische Bezirke im Duodenum und starke Hämorrhagien in der Rindensubstanz der Niere auffällig. Filtrate junger Kulturen blieben bei Hunden wirkungslos.

β) Intraperitoneale und subcutane Injektion

CANTANI (1886) injizierte zwei 3 kg schweren Hunden 60—70 ml einer erhitzten Vibrionenbouillonkultur. Bereits 15 min später kam es zu den Symptomen einer schweren Vergiftung. Sie zeigten allgemeine Schwäche, fibrilläres Muskelzittern und krampfartige Kontraktionen der hinteren Extremitäten. Wenige Minuten später stellte sich heftiges, in kurzen Intervallen auftretendes spastisches Erbrechen, jedoch keine Diarrhoe ein; die Extremitäten fühlten sich kühl an. Nach 24 Std waren die Tiere wieder wohlauf. Auf die Injektion von 60 ml Peptonbouillonkultur reagierte ein Kontrolltier nur mit einem einmaligen Erbrechen. KRAUS und RUSS (1908) beschrieben den Tod eines 7,5 kg schweren Hundes 2 Std nach intravenöser Injektion von 10 ml eines Filtrates, das aus einer 10 Tage alten El-Tor-Vibrionenkultur hergestellt war. 5 ml Filtrat töteten einen 6,8 kg schweren Hund nach 10 Std. Die subcutane Injektion von bakterienfreien Filtraten führte nach Untersuchungen von NICATI und RIETSCH (1884 b) bei Hunden zu keinerlei Krankheitszeichen.

g) Schwein

HECKLY et al. (1969) banden bei 2 Zwergschweinen mehrere Dünndarmstücke ab, in die sie einmal eine nach der Methode von CRAIG (1966) gewonnene Toxinrohfraktion und zum anderen den Dialysanden dieser Fraktion injizierten. Die Dosis für das erstgenannte Toxin, bezogen auf das Trockengewicht, betrug 0,1—100 mg, für das zweite 0,01—10 mg. Die nach 8 Std gemessenen Flüssigkeitsvolumina waren bei beiden Toxinpräparaten im Mittel gleich. Die Exsudation stellte sich erst nach hohen Toxindosen ein. In den einzelnen Darmsegmenten wurde kein signifikanter Unterschied der Flüssigkeitsmenge registriert.

h) Pferd

Bei seinen Untersuchungen „Zur Frage der Gewinnung eines Heilserums gegen die Cholera" injizierte SCHURUPOW (1909) insgesamt 15 Pferden 5—10 ml Choleratoxin in die V. jugularis. Es war aus Kulturabschwemmungen durch nachfolgende

Alkalibehandlung und anschließende Sterilfiltration gewonnen worden. Eine halbe Stunde nach der Injektion erkrankten die Pferde schwer; sie standen mit gesenktem Kopf da und verhielten sich gegenüber der Umgebung gleichgültig. Die Hautdecken, besonders der hinteren Extremitäten, fühlten sich kalt an, der Puls war kaum zu tasten; alle sichtbaren Schleimhäute waren livide verfärbt, die Augen leblos. Dann setzte 2—3 Std andauernder Durchfall ein. Während dieser Zeit sank die Körpertemperatur auf 36—35° C ab. 6 Std nach der Injektion begannen die Tiere am ganzen Körper zu zittern, und die Temperatur stieg auf über 40° C an; das Fieber dauerte mitunter 24 Std. Die Urinausscheidung sistierte während dieser Zeit und setzte erst 1 Tag später in geringem Umfang wieder ein. Nach 1—2 Tagen waren die meisten Tiere wieder wohlauf, zwei gingen jedoch zugrunde. Bei der Obduktion enthielt die Peritonealhöhle reichlich zähe, hellgelbe oder rote Flüssigkeit; Magen und Dünndarm waren dunkelblau gefärbt und mit Blut gefüllt; Milz und Leber wurden blutleer und verkleinert angetroffen. Die Harnblase war leer und geschrumpft.

i) Bebrütetes Hühnerei

Die Experimente von Wilson (1946) ergaben, daß in den Allantoissack injizierte hitzeabgetötete Vibrionen ohne Wirkung waren, während zellfreie Extrakte eine leichte, jedoch nicht konstante toxische Wirkung entfalteten. Mit intracellulären und Zellwandpräparaten dagegen beobachtete Burrows (1965) bei 10 Tage alten, bebrüteten Hühnereiern eine toxische Reaktion. Er injizierte 0,1 ml der entsprechenden Suspension in die Chorio-Allantois-Membran. Die Giftwirkung stellte sich rasch ein und konnte durch ein in der Eischale angebrachtes Fenster beobachtet werden. 4—5 Std post injectionem trat das Blut aus den Gefäßen aus, 10—20 Std später war der Embryo tot. Die DL 50 der intracellulären Substanz betrug 130 mcg, die der Zellwandfraktion 70 mcg.

j) Isolierte Organe

Für bestimmte Fragestellungen wird die Choleratoxinwirkung an isolierten Tierorganen überprüft. Während früher hierfür vorwiegend Darmstücke und Herzen von Warmblütern verwendet wurden, bedient man sich in neuerer Zeit der isolierten Haut von Kaltblütern, insbesondere der Froschhaut.

α) Säugetierherz

Eine geringe depressive Wirkung der Choleratoxine auf die Aktion des isolierten Kaninchenherzens teilten Pezzi und Savini (1910) mit. Dieser Effekt war nur durch hohe Konzentrationen des durch Frier-Tau-Verfahren gewonnenen Toxins zu erzielen. In einer anderen Studie (Cicconardi, 1913) dagegen wurde festgestellt, daß nach Applikation des Choleratoxins plötzlich eine Verlangsamung und Unregelmäßigkeit des Herzschlages eintrat. Dabei soll das Toxin auf das Reizleitungssystem und nicht auf das Myokard einwirken. Als Perfusionsflüssigkeit für das isolierte Kaninchenherz verwendeten Manwaring et al. (1923) Locke-Lösung mit Zusatz von 1—2% filtriertem und defibriniertem Blut des zu untersuchenden Tieres. In ihr schlägt das isolierte Kaninchenherz etwa 3 Std regelmäßig. Die Choleravibrionen waren in einer Locke-Lösung mit 1% Pepton und 0,25% Hefeextrakt zur Vermehrung gebracht worden. Als Toxin diente das Ultrafiltrat von 2—7 Tage bebrüteten Kulturen. Es erwies sich, daß der Giftstoff auf die Herzaktion selbst keinen Einfluß hatte. Sie war nach Toxinzugabe 90 min regelmäßig. Dagegen waren bereits 10 min nach Toxinzugabe ein Myokardödem und 30 min später Hämorrhagien zu beobachten. Bei der histologischen

Untersuchung erwiesen sich die Muskelfasern als ödematös, in den Bindegewebsspalten fanden sich vereinzelt Erythrocyten, welche auch unmittelbar unter dem Peri- und Endokard anzutreffen waren.

ACTON und CHOPRA (1924), die aus 10 Tage alten Vibrionenkulturen „nichtflüchtige" und „flüchtige" Toxinpräparate herstellten, fanden, daß durch den „nicht flüchtigen" Anteil eine leichte Abnahme der Herzaktionen erzeugt wurde. Die Toxinwirkung von 7 verschiedenen Cholerastämmen überprüften SOELEIMAN und NIEKERK (1930). Nur ein Stamm bewirkte eine Minderung der Herzfrequenz und manchmal auch einen 2:1- oder 3:1-Block. Die Toxine anderer Stämme verursachten mitunter eine Abnahme der Herzfrequenz.

β) Darm

HAHN und HIRSCH (1927) setzten ein durch Eindampfen von abgeschwemmten Choleravibrionen hergestelltes Trockentoxin in einer Konzentration von 0,2% einer Tyrode-Lösung zu, in die der Darm eines gesunden Kaninchens eingelegt war. Er reagierte mit einer Verkürzung der Kontraktionsamplitude, aus der sich eine komplette spastische Lähmung entwickelte. Der zeitliche Eintritt dieser Reaktion war weitgehend von der Konzentration des Giftes abhängig, das noch in einer Verdünnung von 1:400000 auf den isolierten Darm wirksam war. SOELEIMAN und NIEKERK (1930) fanden bei 6 Choleratoxinen keinerlei Wirkung auf das isolierte Darmstück des Kaninchens. Das Toxin eines weiteren Choleravibrionenstammes bewirkte in verschiedenen Experimenten an nur einem Darmabschnitt eine Hemmung der rhythmischen Kontraktionen.

Aufgrund dieser Befunde kamen die Autoren zu der Überzeugung, daß der isolierte Darm für Untersuchungen mit Choleratoxinen wenig geeignet ist, zumal es sich erwies, daß Bouillonzusatz allein eine stimulierende Wirkung auf die Darmkontraktion ausübte.

Auch BURROWS et al. (1944) gaben an, daß Choleratoxin keinen Einfluß auf die Peristaltik der isolierten Darmstücke von Meerschweinchen oder Kaninchen besaß.

γ) Epithelzellmembran

Aufgrund physiologischer Untersuchungen steht fest, daß Natrium aus vielen Epithelzellmembranen aktiv in das Plasma transportiert wird. Bei dem Natriumfluß vom Lumen in das Plasma wird ein elektrochemisches Potential gemessen, das ein Maß für den Umfang des Natriumtransports ist. Der Natriumfluß in das Lumen und aus dem Lumen ist eine lineare Funktion der NaCl-Konzentration innerhalb des Lumens. Die Wasserrückresorption geht passiv vor sich und folgt dem Netto-Salzfluß. Dieser ist die Differenz zwischen dem Natriumgehalt innerhalb des Lumens und dem aktiv rücktransportierten Natrium (CURRAN, 1960; CURRAN und SCHWARTZ, 1960; CUMMINS und VAUGHAN, 1963, 1965; CHOWDHURRY und SNELL, 1965; USSING, 1965, Übers. b. SCHULTZ und CURRAN, 1968). Da eine etwa dem zweifachen Plasmavolumen entsprechende elektrolytreiche Flüssigkeit täglich in den Darm sezerniert und wieder resorbiert wird, wird verständlich, welche Auswirkung auf den Organismus ein Wegfall der Resorption besitzt, wie es bei Diarrhoen zum Teil der Fall ist (KEIDEL, 1970).

Diese Erkenntnisse wirkten befruchtend auf die Klärung der Pathogenese der Cholera. Die isolierten Schleimhäute von Versuchstieren sind geeignete Versuchsmodelle, um die Wirkung von Choleratoxinen und Toxinfraktionen auf den Natriumtransport zu studieren. Auf diese Weise können Faktoren gefunden werden, welche für den enormen Wasser- und Salzverlust bei der Cholera verantwortlich sind.

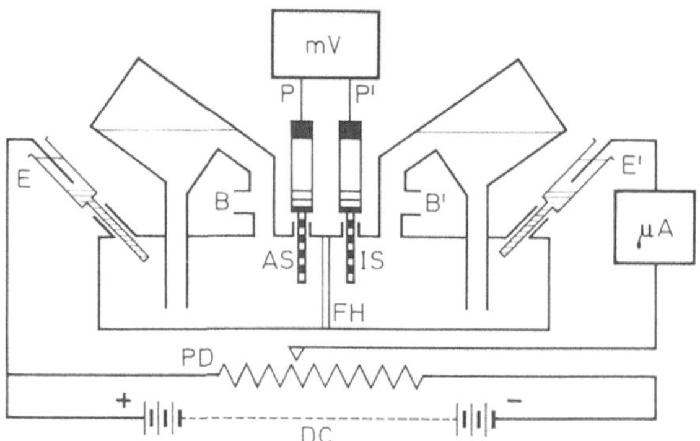

Abb. 6. Versuchsanordnung zur Messung des aktiven Na⁺-Transport (nach Phillips, 1965).
mV Millivoltmeter; *P, P'* Kalomel-Elektroden zur Ableitung des Haut-Potentials; *E, E'*
Silber-Silberchlorid-Elektroden zum Anlegen des äußeren Stroms; *B, B'* Belüftungsstutzen;
μA Mikroamperemeter; *FH* Froschhaut; *AS* u. *IS* Kammern, welche an die Außen- bzw.
Innenseite der Froschhaut grenzen; *PD* Potentiometer; *DC* Stromquelle

γα) Froschhaut. Wohl als erste teilten Burrows et al. (1944) mit, daß Choleratoxin die Permeabilität der isolierten abdominalen Froschhaut und des Dünndarms
von Meerschweinchen und Kaninchen steigerte. Eine detaillierte Beschreibung der
Versuchsanordnungen wurde von Fuhrman und Fuhrman (1960) gegeben: Entweder wurde die Magenschleimhaut des braunen europäischen Frosches (Rana
temporaria) oder ein Hautstück des amerikanischen Grasfrosches (Rana pipiens)
zwischen zwei konischen Zellen fixiert, die mit Ringer-Lösung gefüllt waren. Diese
wurde mit Luft durchperlt und die Potentialdifferenz zwischen den beiden Ge-
webeseiten abgeleitet (Abb. 6). In einer zusätzlichen Versuchsanordnung kann mit
Hilfe von Agarelektroden ein äußeres Potential angelegt werden, um die Potentialdifferenz bei Null zu halten.

Der dann von der unbehandelten Froschhaut bei Nullpotential („Kurzschlußstrom") produzierte Strom ist ein Maß für den „Netto-Natriumfluß" (Ussing und
Zehran, 1951) und zeigt Veränderungen im aktiven Natriumtransport auf. Fuhr-
man und Fuhrman (1960) maßen bei Kurzschlußstrom mit ²²Na den Natrium-
influx und -efflux an der Froschhaut. Dabei konnte der Natriumfluß in einer
Richtung aus folgender Gleichung berechnet werden: Nettofluß = Na-Influx — Na-
Efflux. Als Toxin verwendeten sie das lyophilisierte Ultrafiltrat von Cholera-
bouillonkulturen, das in einer Menge von 725 mcg pro ml Ringer-Lösung in die
Kammern gegeben wurde, welche an die Innen- und Außenseite der isolierten
Froschhaut grenzten. Als charakteristisches Zeichen für die Blockade des aktiven
Natriumtransports sanken Kurzschluß- und Potentialstrom rasch ab. Wurde das
Ultrafiltrat in gleicher Konzentration für die isolierte Magenschleimhaut des
Frosches benutzt, so war kurze Zeit später ein leichter Anstieg des Kurzschluß-
und Potentialstromes festzustellen, der sich nach wenigen Minuten wieder
normalisierte. Dieses Experiment zeigt, daß durch die Magenschleimhaut des
Frosches kein aktiver Natriumtransport stattfindet und daß das Toxin spezifisch
wirkt. Minimale noch effektive Konzentration für die Froschhaut waren
60 mcg/ml. Ferner konnte beobachtet werden, daß das Toxin nur an der Außenseite der Froschhaut wirksam war. Die Gabe in die an die Innenseite der Froschhaut grenzende Lösung führte zu keiner Abnahme des Natriumflusses. Durch die
Untersuchungen mit radioaktiv markiertem Natrium wurde verifiziert, daß das
Cholerafiltrat zur Abnahme des Natrium-Nettoflusses und des Natriumeinstromes

in die Zelle führt. Nach Dialyse des Toxins stellte sich heraus, daß die aktive Substanz im Dialysat enthalten war. Die Toxicität wurde durch Erhitzen auf 80° C 1 Std nicht beeinflußt.

Diese Untersuchungen wurden von LYNG (1964) weitergeführt, der dem dialysierbaren Inhibitor des Natriumtransports ein Molekulargewicht von einigen Hundert zuschrieb. Bei neutralem pH-Wert war er negativ geladen und stabil gegenüber Erhitzen, Säure und Alkali. Für die bioelektrischen Messungen verwendete er eine modifizierte Ringer-Lösung folgender Zusammensetzung: $NaHCO_3$ 0,2 g, KCl 0,2 g, NaCl 6,5 g, $CaCl_2$ 0,41 ml, mit doppelt destilliertem Wasser auf 1 000 ml aufgefüllt. Als Kupfersulfatlösung diente $CuSO^4 + 5 H_2$ 0,624 mg/l. 0,1 ml dieser Lösung wurde in 25 ml Ringer-Lösung gegeben. Auch bei diesen Experimenten wurde festgestellt, daß das Cholerafiltrat nur bei Zugabe in die Lösung, welche die Außenseite der Froschhaut begrenzte, wirksam war. Der Abfall des Potentials war irreversibel und deshalb eine Wiederholung an dem gleichen Froschhautstück unmöglich. Wurde jedoch Vasopressin, ein Hormon der Neurohypophyse, in die Kammerlösung gegeben, welche an die Innenseite grenzte, so stieg der Kurzschlußstrom nachträglich an. Durch 0,2 IU Vasopressin allein zur Froschhautinnenseite, stieg der Kurzschlußstrom um etwa 150 mA an. Zwischen der Blockade des Vasopressineffektes durch unterschiedliche Dosierungen des Cholerafiltrats und dem Abfall des Potentials bestand eine enge Beziehung. Durch Zugabe von Cu^{++} zur Ringer-Lösung wurde eine Stabilisierung des relativ unregelmäßigen Kurzschlußstromes erreicht, ohne daß die Empfindlichkeit der Froschhaut für das Choleratoxin beeinträchtigt wurde. Wurde jetzt 1 IU Vasopressin in die Kammerinnenseite und 0,5 ml Cholerafiltrat in die Kammeraußenseite gegeben, so war der ursprünglich im Leerversuch gefundene Vasopressineffekt aufgehoben, d.h., das Cholerafiltrat besaß gegenüber Vasopressin einen antagonistischen Effekt. Aufgrund dieses Antagonismus ist es möglich, den Inhibitor der Natriumpumpe quantitativ zu bestimmen.

Die Untersuchung der Stuhlfiltrate von Patienten, die an klassischer Cholera und El-Tor-Cholera erkrankt waren, erbrachte in beiden Fällen den Inhibitornachweis. Diese Experimente und histologische Untersuchungen widerlegten die Theorie, der Cholerastuhl des Menschen sei ein Transsudat, das nach Ablösung der Intestinalmucosa entstehe. Die Schleimhaut bleibt unversehrt. *Der enorme Elektrolyt- und Wasserverlust hat seine Ursache in der Blockade des aktiven Natriumrücktransports.*

Die Experimente von LEITCH (1965) erwiesen, daß die Verminderung des Membranpotentials der Froschhaut reversibel war, wenn intracelluläre Substanz von V. cholerae in die Kammerlösung gegeben wurde, welche an die Innenseite der Froschhaut grenzte. Der Effekt trat bei einer Konzentration von 1 mg/ml ein und war unabhängig von einer Sauerstoffdurchperlung der Lösung. Das Membranpotential war um 50% vermindert bei Zugabe von 3 mg/ml zur Kammerinnenseite und von 2 mg/ml zur Kammerinnen- und Außenseite. Die 1 Std gekochte Intracellulärfraktion verlor diesen toxischen Effekt nicht. Der Inhibitor wurde als dialysierbar beschrieben. Diese Befunde konnten von BURROWS (1965) bestätigt werden, welcher die Untersuchungen an der isolierten Abdominalhaut von Rana pipiens, Buffo americanus und Buffo marinus vornahm. Eine 50%ige Reduktion des Membranpotentials wurde bei Zugabe von 6—8 mg/ml Gesamtzellysat gemessen. An intracellulärer Substanz wurden dafür 1,5—2,5 mg/ml und an Zellwandfraktion 5—6 mg/ml benötigt. Aufgrund morphologischer und quantitativer Überlegungen kam er zu dem Schluß, daß die toxische Aktivität zu 95 oder mehr Prozent in der intracellulären Substanz vorliegt. Es zeigte sich ferner, daß nach Zugabe von 6 mg intracellulärer Substanz pro Milliliter Ringer-Lösung das

Membranpotential nach einem kurzen uncharakteristischen Anstieg 60—80 min später den niedrigsten Wert von etwa 8 mV erreichte, gegenüber einem Ausgangspotential von 60 mV. Bei Gabe geringerer Dosen verminderte sich das Membranpotential weniger stark. Wird die Abnahme des Potential- oder Kurzschlußstromes in Prozent angegeben, so besteht eine lineare Beziehung zum Logarithmus der Toxinkonzentration. Die Blockade der Natriumpumpe war nach den Untersuchungen von Burrows et al. (1965) reversibel, denn nach Ersetzen der toxinhaltigen Lösung durch frische Ringer-Lösung stieg das Membranpotential innerhalb weniger Minuten wieder an.

Da der aktive Natriumtransport im Darm des Menschen durch verschiedene Abführmittel gehemmt wird, untersuchten Phillips et al. (1965) deren Wirkung an der isolierten Froschhaut. Eine Blockade bis zu 80% gegenüber der Kontrolle wurde 30 min nach der Gabe von Cascara 12,5 mg/ml, Podophyllum 1 mg/ml, Phenolphthalein 10 mg/ml und Ricinusöl 0,05 mg/ml beobachtet.

γβ) Intestinalschleimhaut. Woolley und Gommi (1964) hatten am isolierten Rattenmagen festgestellt, daß in calciumfreien Lösungen Neuraminidase selektiv den Serotoninreceptor zerstörte. Dies führte zu einer Abnahme der durch Serotonin stimulierten contractilen Empfindlichkeit. Da Choleravibrionen in großem Umfang Neuraminidase bilden, könnten diese Befunde für die Pathogenese der Erkrankung von Bedeutung sein.

Al-Awqati et al. (1970) übertrugen die Experimente an der Froschhaut auf den isolierten Kaninchendarm und verwendeten 10—15 cm lange, distale Ileumstücke von etwa 2 kg schweren Tieren. Den Kurzschlußstrom leiteten sie folgendermaßen ab: 1. von der unverletzten Ileumschleimhaut, 2. von der unverletzten Schleimhaut plus 1 g Choleratoxin pro 30 ml Pufferlösung und 3. von der artifiziell geschädigten Schleimhaut. Aus den Ergebnissen zogen sie den Schluß, daß der Natriumfluß bei der destruierten Ileumschleimhaut ebenso vermindert ist wie nach Zugabe von Choleratoxin; der Ionenfluß im normalen Gewebe betrug 2,3 µÄqu/cm²/Std, in verletzten und mit Choleratoxinen behandelten Proben dagegen 1,6 µÄqu/cm²/Std. Noch nicht geklärt ist der interessante Befund, daß bei der Toxinvergiftung nach Zugabe von Glucose in die Kammer der Mucosaseite der Natriumtransport wieder in Gang kommt, während die Blockade bei dem verletzten Gewebe bestehen bleibt.

Die Behinderung des Natriumflusses beeinträchtigt nicht den aktiven Transport von Substanzen, welche vom oxydativen Stoffwechsel abhängig sind, wie Keusch et al. (1970) im Warburg-Gerät feststellten. Auch die mitochondriale und intestinale ATPase wird nach diesen Untersuchungen durch Choleratoxin nicht beeinflußt.

k) Zellkultur

Gelegentlich wurden Zellkulturen zur Überprüfung der Toxinwirkung von Choleravibrionen verwendet (Read, 1965). Als geeignet erwies sich der Clon 1 B von Earles L-Zellen. Auch Hep$_2$ (Human epidermoid carcinoma) und Affennierenzellen fanden Verwendung. Als Färbemittel ist eine 1:10 verdünnte Giemsa-Lösung geeignet. Read (1965) dialysierte die intracelluläre Substanz von Choleravibrionen und setzte Dialysand und Dialysat den Zellkulturen zu. 1 mg/ml intracellulärer Substanz oder Dialysand riefen eine rasche Vacuolisierung der Zellen hervor und lösten sie innerhalb von 5 Tagen vom Boden der Flasche; das Dialysat hatte diese Wirkung nicht.

Richardson und Evans (1965) präparierten für die Untersuchung der intestinalen ATPase-Aktivität die Villi saugender Kaninchen. Hierzu wurde der Dünndarm entnommen, der Länge nach aufgeschnitten und mit kaltem 0,01 M

Trispuffer, der 0,001 M EDTA enthielt (pH 7,5), gewaschen. Danach wurden die Villi in diesem Puffer abgeschabt, die gewonnene Mucosa homogenisiert und in der Kälte durch Zentrifugieren so lange gewaschen, bis der überstehende Puffer klar blieb. Der weißliche, flockige Niederschlag wurde anschließend in 0,25 M Saccharose, die 0,05 M Trispuffer enthielt, suspendiert und mit Ultraschall behandelt. Mit der so entstandenen gelblichen Suspension, die 0,5—2 mg Protein/ml enthielt, wurde experimentiert. Die Choleratoxine wurden für diese Untersuchungen nach DE et al. (1962) und FINKELSTEIN et al. (1964) präpariert.

Der Natriumtransport von der Mucosa zur Serosa ist ein energieabhängiger Vorgang. Dabei kommt der intestinalen ATPase eine entscheidende Bedeutung zu, da bei ihrer Blockierung der Transport abnimmt oder vollkommen sistiert. Aus diesem Grund wurde von RICHARDSON und EVANS (1965) nach Zugabe der einzelnen Toxine zur Suspension die ATPase-Aktivität gemessen. Das Toxin von DE et al. (1962) hemmte, die Toxinfraktion von FINKELSTEIN et al. (1964) stimulierte sie. Dieser Widerspruch kann durch die Verwendung verschiedener Kulturmedien für die Toxinpräparation erklärt werden, zumal festgestellt wurde, daß in den benutzten Medien Substanzen enthalten waren, die die Kaninchen-ATPase-Aktivität hemmten. In einer späteren Untersuchung wurde von RICHARDSON (1968) festgestellt, daß die ATPase-Aktivität der isolierten Kaninchenmucosa durch Cholerakulturfiltrate gehemmt wird. Verbindet man diesen Befund mit physiologischen Erkenntnissen (KEIDEL, 1970), so wäre es möglich, die Blockierung der Natriumpumpe zu erklären, da in Zellmembranen, durch die Na-Ionen aktiv transportiert werden, eine durch Na- und K-Ionen aktivierbare ATPase gefunden wird. Die Hemmung des Enzyms würde bedeuten, daß es die für den Natriumtransport erforderliche Stoffwechselenergie nicht mehr bereitstellen kann.

C. Infektion mit anderen vermehrungsfähigen Vibrionen

1. Allgemeines

Auch bei Versuchen mit anderen Vibrionenarten wurden besondere Methoden angewandt, um die Tiere empfänglich zu machen (s. S. 67). Mit tierpathogenen Mikroorganismen wie V. metschnikovii, V. anguillarum und V. piscium können Erkrankung und Tod der Versuchstiere ohne zusätzliche Maßnahmen hervorgerufen werden. Mit V. fetus werden dem natürlichen Krankheitsverlauf entsprechende Experimente an trächtigen Groß- und Laboratoriumstieren durchgeführt, um Aborte auszulösen. Zum Studium des Übertragungsmodus sind Genitalinfektionen bei weiblichen und männlichen Versuchstieren geeignet. Da in dem als Modell dienenden Tierexperiment möglichst die gleichen Symptome erzeugt werden sollen, wie bei natürlich infizierten Tieren, werden einige Angaben über die Krankheitsbilder der per vias naturales erkrankten Tiere einer Besprechung tierexperimenteller Untersuchungsergebnisse vorangestellt.

Allgemein ist festzuhalten, daß die bei verschiedenen Tierarten durch Vibrionen verursachten klinischen Bilder auch durch andere Bakterien hervorgerufen werden können. So stellte GAMALEIA (1888a) fest, daß das durch V. metschnikovii hervorgerufene Krankheitsbild bei Hühnern einer Infektion mit Past. multocida sehr ähnlich ist. Wie aus Untersuchungen von CANESTRINI (1892) und INGHILLERI (1903) hervorgeht, können die Symptome der durch Vibrionen hervorgerufenen Rotseuche der Fische auch durch grampositive oder gramnegative Stäbchenbakterien verursacht werden. Ähnliches ist von mikroaerophilen Vibrionen bekannt; Aborte beim Rind werden außer durch V. fetus auch durch Brucella abortus und andere Bakterienarten hervorgerufen. Für die Dysenterie des

Schweines wird neben V. coli auch Salmonella choleraesuis oder der gleichzeitige Befall mit Vibrionen und Salmonellen verantwortlich gemacht (Doyle, 1948; Boley et al., 1951).

Für das Ergebnis der Tierversuche ist die Virulenz der Bakterienstämme von wesentlicher Bedeutung. Die Virulenz verschiedener NAG-Vibrionenstämme, welche aus Stühlen von Cholerapatienten isoliert wurden, variierte beträchtlich, wie die intravenöse Injektion von Kochsalzabschwemmungen 24 Std bebrüteter Agarkulturen bei Kaninchen zeigte. Ein Teil der Bakterienstämme führte zum Tode der Tiere, während die Injektion anderer NAG-Vibrionen ohne weiteres vertragen wurde (Greig, 1917). Es liegen auch Berichte vor, daß Vibrionen durch Kulturpassagen eine Abschwächung ihrer Virulenz erleiden. Die gegenüber der Erstisolierung geringere Virulenz von V. piscium var. japonicus und V. ichthyodermis ist nach Smith (1961) eine Folge der wiederholten Kulturpassage. Bei V. fetus beobachtete Smith (1919a), daß durch fortlaufende Überimpfung zwar eine Adaptation an den Nährboden stattfand und sich dadurch die Bakterienmasse erhöhte, aber eine Minderung der Virulenz eintrat. Peckham (1958) stellte bei den vom Huhn isolierten mikroaerophilen Vibrionen eine Abschwächung der Virulenz bereits nach 4 Blutagar-Passagen fest.

Eine Virulenzsteigerung wird durch Tierpassagen angestrebt. Gamaleia (1888a) gelang es, die Virulenz von V. metschnikovii durch Taubenpassagen beträchtlich zu erhöhen. Er verwendete deshalb das vibrionenhaltige Blut von Tauben, die an der Infektion zugrunde gegangen waren. Ferner gab er den Hinweis, daß primär von Hühnern isolierte Vibrionen keine so hohe Virulenz aufwiesen, wie sie nach wiederholter Passage über Tauben erreicht wurde. Untersuchungen mit tierpathogenen Vibrionen werden aus diesem Grund häufig mit infektiösem Tiermaterial vorgenommen. Zur Infektion mit V. coli und V. jejuni werden Faeces der erkrankten oder der Infektion erlegenen Tiere für Versuchstiere verwendet. Bei Arbeiten mit V. fetus kommen Fetal- und Placentagewebe von Rind oder Schaf in Frage. Als Material mit mikroaerophilen hühnerpathogenen Vibrionen eignen sich Leberproben und Gallenflüssigkeit von infizierten Tieren. Der Infektionsmodus ist meist oral, jedoch werden auch parenterale und andere Techniken mitgeteilt. Auf mögliche Fehlerquellen wurde bereits hingewiesen (s. S. 72).

Zum Nachweis der NAG-Vibrionen werden für quantitative Untersuchungen feste Nährmedien bevorzugt, zur Anreicherung oder bei mischinfizierten Materialien sind flüssige, peptonhaltige Nährsubstrate erforderlich. Bei der Züchtung von fischpathogenen und anderen aus Wasser isolierten Vibrionen ist auf deren niedrigeres Temperaturoptimum und deren Halophilie zu achten (s. S. 61). Ist mit einer Begleitflora zu rechnen, so empfiehlt sich die Verwendung von Selektivnährböden (s. S. 62).

2. Aus Menschen isolierte aerobe Vibrionen

Tierversuche wurden besonders mit NAG-Vibrionen durchgeführt. Diese Bezeichnung ist ein Sammelbegriff für zahlreiche serologisch und biochemisch differente Stämme, die das gemeinsame Merkmal haben, durch Choleraseren (Typen Inaba und Ogawa) nicht agglutiniert zu werden. Versuchstiere sind Meerschweinchen und Kaninchen, die mit den üblichen Techniken infiziert werden (s. S. 72). Für die Untersuchungen wurden Stämme, die aus Menschen isoliert worden waren, und solche, deren Herkunft nicht mitgeteilt wurde, verwendet. Aus diesem Grunde wird auf eine Gliederung der Tierversuche nach Herkunft der NAG-Vibrionen verzichtet.

a) Meerschweinchen

α) Magen-Darm-Kanal

Eine orale Infektion der Versuchstiere mit V. proteus führte zu einer teilweise tödlich verlaufenden Erkrankung, wenn die Tiere vorbehandelt wurden (s. S. 73). Von 15 infizierten Tieren gingen nach den Untersuchungen von KOCH (1885) 5 Meerschweinchen zugrunde. Bei der Obduktion war der blaßgraue Darm mit einer wäßrigen Flüssigkeit gefüllt; die Gefäße waren bei weitem nicht so stark erweitert wie bei Choleratieren. Vom Darminhalt ging ein „penetranter Fäulnisgeruch" aus. ISSAEFF und IVANOFF (1894) registrierten nach der Gabe von V. proteus bei ihren Versuchstieren lediglich einen Temperaturabfall bis 35° C; sämtliche Versuchstiere überlebten.

Die intraduodenale Injektion von 1 ml einer 8 Tage bebrüteten und anschließend verflüssigten V. proteus-Gelatinekultur löste nach den Untersuchungen von DENEKE (1885) nur eine leichte, vorübergehende Temperaturerhöhung aus.

β) Parenterale Infektion

βα) Die *intraperitoneale Injektion* wurde früher hauptsächlich zur Abgrenzung der NAG-Vibrionen von Choleravibrionen herangezogen (s. S. 79). Aus den Untersuchungen von PFEIFFER (1892) ergibt sich, daß V. proteus sehr ähnliche Krankheitserscheinungen auszulösen vermag wie V. massauah (s. S. 170). Die Applikation von 0,5, 1,0 und 1,5 ml der Bouillonabschwemmung einer 24 Std bebrüteten Kultur bewirkte lediglich bei einer Dosis von 1,5 ml den Tod eines Tieres innerhalb 18 Std (SOBERNHEIM, 1893 b). Der Krankheitsverlauf und die pathologisch-anatomischen Veränderungen glichen denen nach intraperitonealer Infektion mit V. cholerae. V. proteus konnte aus Peritonealexsudat und Blut isoliert werden. BAERTHLEIN (1913) erreichte mit 5 von 6 NAG-Vibrionen-Stämmen in Mengen von $^1/_{10}$—$^1/_2$ Öse Kulturmaterial eine Erkrankung der Meerschweinchen. Der 6. Stamm führte auch nach Gabe von 2 Ösen nicht zum Tod des Versuchstieres.

Andere Vibrionen erwiesen sich als apathogen für Meerschweinchen. Die intraperitoneale Injektion von 1 ml einer 24 Std bebrüteten Agarkulturabschwemmung von V. sputigenus rief bei Meerschweinchen vorübergehend leichte Mattigkeit und Temperaturerhöhung hervor (BRIX, 1894). STEPHENS und SMITH (1896) berichteten, daß der aus der Mundhöhle isolierte V. tonsillaris, „in großen Mengen" intraperitoneal injiziert, keine Krankheitszeichen verursachte. Dies traf nach den Untersuchungen von CHALMERS und WATERFIELD (1916) auch für V. gindha zu.

ββ) Die *subcutane Injektion* erwies sich beim Meerschweinchen als unwirksam für V. tonsillaris und V. gindha (STEPHENS und SMITH, 1896; CHALMERS und WATERFIELD, 1916). Unter 22 NAG-Vibrionenstämmen fanden KOLLE und GOTSCHLICH (1903) 6, die für Meerschweinchen pathogen waren, wenn 1 Öse Kulturmasse in eine Hauttasche instilliert wurde.

b) Kaninchen

α) Injektion in das abgebundene Dünndarmsegment

GUPTA et al. (1956) untersuchten 7 von 36 NAG-Vibrionen (Gruppe V nach HEIBERG, 1934), die bei einer epidemisch aufgetretenen Gastroenteritis isoliert worden waren. Die abgebundenen Darmsegmente waren 4—6 cm lang. Injiziert wurde 1 ml Peptonwasser, in welches 1 Öse einer 24 Std bebrüteten flüssigen Bakterienkultur suspendiert war. Die Sektion ergab 24 Std später eine geringe Menge Peritonealexsudat; das infizierte Darmstück war gestaut und erheblich erweitert. Im Darmlumen fand sich reichlich blutige Flüssigkeit. Die Veränderungen

entsprachen denen nach Injektion von V. cholerae. Mikroskopisch war in allen
Darmsegmenten eine Degeneration der Epithelzellen auffällig; Leukocyten wurden
nicht gesehen. Auch im histologischen Präparat konnten keine entzündlichen
Reaktionen festgestellt werden. Der Albumingehalt des Exsudates schwankte
zwischen 0,5 und 1,5%. Die Isolierung der injizierten Mikroorganismen gelang
regelmäßig. Kontrolluntersuchungen mit V. metschnikovii, Prot. vulgaris, Staph.
aureus, Alcaligenes faecalis und E. coli verliefen ergebnislos. Ebenfalls zu keinem
Resultat führte die Injektion von Vibrionen mit den O-Antigenen 3 und 6 nach
GARDNER und VENKATRAMAN (1935). Vibrionen mit dem O-Antigen 2 riefen
eine geringe Erweiterung des isolierten Darmstücks ohne Stauungszeichen hervor. Vibrionen mit dem O-Antigen 5 dagegen bewirkten deutliche Kongestion
und Distension der Darmwand. Von SAKAZAKI (1965) wird ohne nähere Angaben
mitgeteilt, daß die Injektion von Bouillonkulturen von V. parahaemolyticus und
V. alginolyticus eine „Enteritis" in dem abgebundenen Darmsegment erzeugt.

β) Intravenöse Infektion

6 min nach Injektion von 0,75 ml einer konzentrierten Aufschwemmung von
V. proteus wurden in Blutkulturen massenhaft Vibrionen nachgewiesen, nach
30 min nur noch einzelne Exemplare. Spätere Kulturen blieben steril. Eine pathogene Wirkung dieser Vibrionen für das Kaninchen war demnach zu verneinen
(WYSSOKOWITSCH, 1886). Auch V. gindha rief nach intravenöser Injektion keine
Krankheitszeichen hervor (CHALMERS und WATERFIELD, 1916). Umfangreiche
Untersuchungen mit NAG-Vibrionen, die zum Teil aus Stuhl von Cholerapatienten
isoliert waren, wurden von GREIG (1914, 1915, 1916) vorgenommen. Den 1,1 bis
1,9 kg schweren Kaninchen injizierte er unterschiedliche Mengen einer 24 Std
bebrüteten Agarkulturabschwemmung. Die Versuchstiere starben in der Regel
24 Std, mitunter auch 48 Std später. Da die Erreger aus Herzblut, Gallenblase,
Dünndarminhalt, Leber, Milz, Lunge, Niere und Urin isoliert werden konnten,
wurde eine Generalisation der Infektion angenommen.

Bei Immunisierungsversuchen (GREIG, 1915) ging 1 Tier etwa 4 Wochen nach
der letzten Injektion zugrunde. Die Sektion zeigte eine stark erweiterte Gallenblase mit grauer Flüssigkeit und kleinen Kalksteinen; 1 Stein blockierte den
D. cysticus. Bereits mikroskopisch waren in der Galle Vibrionen zu sehen, die in
Reinkultur zur Vermehrung gebracht werden konnten und sich mit den zuvor
intravenös injizierten NAG-Vibrionen als identisch erwiesen. Nach Zertrümmerung
wurde im Zentrum der Steine mikroskopisch eine Aggregation von Vibrionen
angetroffen, so daß der Eindruck entstand, die Steine hätten sich um die Vibrionen
als Kristallisationspunkte gebildet. Die Sektion von Kaninchen, die mit 19 verschiedenen NAG-Vibrionen immunisiert wurden (GREIG, 1916), erfolgte bei 2 Tieren am 12. und 14. Tag, bei den übrigen nach 3—9 Monaten. Eine Cholecystitis
wurde bei 16 Tieren, Gallensteine bei 8 nachgewiesen. Der homologe Stamm konnte
nach der Sektion aus der Gallenblase von 17 Kaninchen isoliert werden. Diese
Befunde veranlaßten GREIG (1916) zu der Ansicht, die Gallenblase der Kaninchen
sei ein bevorzugter Ansiedlungsort für diese Vibrionen. Die intravenöse Injektion
von Kulturabschwemmungen erbrachte weiter, daß die Virulenz der NAG-
Stämme sehr verschieden ist. Die Injektion gleicher Erregermengen des einen
Stammes bewirkte den Tod der Versuchstiere, die des anderen Stammes keine
Krankheitserscheinungen (GREIG, 1917).

c) Maus, Affe, Hund, Katze

Mäuse, die 0,5 ml einer 18 Std bebrüteten Bouillonkultur von V. parahaemolyticus intraperitoneal erhielten, gingen innerhalb 24—48 Std zugrunde. Dagegen

überlebte die Mehrzahl der Tiere die Injektion von 0,05 ml. Die gleichen Ergebnisse wurden nach Injektion von V. alginolyticus erzielt (SAKAZAKI, 1965). Die subcutane Gabe einer Öse Kulturmaterial von V. sputigenus in eine Hauttasche der Schwanzwurzel der Maus wurde ohne weiteres vertragen (BRIX, 1894).

Nach Laparotomie injizierten CHALMERS und WATERFIELD (1916) 2 Affen V. gindha entweder in den oberen Teil des Dünndarmes oder in den unteren Teil des Colons. Krankheitserscheinungen traten nicht auf. Bei der Sektion waren die Vibrionen nicht mehr nachzuweisen. SAKAZAKI (1965) injizierte Affen, Hunden und Katzen V. parahaemolyticus. Eine Erkrankung wurde nicht beobachtet.

d) Taube

Unter 22 NAG-Vibrionen fanden KOLLE und GOTSCHLICH (1903) nur 6 Stämme, die nach Injektion in den Brustmuskel der Taube eine tödliche Septicämie auslösten. Zu unterschiedlichen Ergebnissen gelangte auch GREIG (1917); von 24 Tauben, die mit verschiedenen Stämmen infiziert worden waren, gingen 8 zugrunde, während 16 keine Reaktion zeigten, obschon sehr hohe Erregerdosen appliziert worden waren. V. gindha war für Tauben nach intramuskulärer Injektion apathogen (CHALMERS und WATERFIELD, 1916).

e) Bebrütetes Hühnerei

Die Injektion von 1 bis 5×10^4 Vibrionen der 6 Gruppen von GARDNER und VENKATRAMAN (1935) in den Allantoissack ist als tödliche Dosis für Hühnerembryonen anzusehen, die auf die Vibrioneninfektion empfindlich reagieren (WILSON, 1946).

3. Aus Menschen isolierte mikroaerophile Vibrionen

Über Vibrionen, die aus Menschen isoliert wurden, insbesondere V. fetus, liegen nur wenige tierexperimentelle Untersuchungen vor, die sich zudem meist auf nur geringe Tierzahlen stützen. In veterinärmedizinische Untersuchungen mit Groß- und Laboratoriumstieren wurden auch einige mikroaerophile Vibrionen einbezogen, die bei Erkrankungen des Menschen gezüchtet worden waren (MORSE und RISTIC, 1954; RISTIC et al., 1955; WINKENWERDER, 1967).

a) Meerschweinchen

Die *intraperitoneale Injektion* von 4 ml einer 48 Std bebrüteten V.-fetus-Kultur beeinträchtigte das Wohlbefinden von Meerschweinchen nicht, obwohl der Erreger 3—4 Std später aus dem Blut gezüchtet werden konnte (LEVY, 1946). Die Injektion von 1 ml eines von VINZENT et al. (1947) isolierten Stammes löste bei 3 graviden Meerschweinchen einen Abort aus. Der Erreger konnte anschließend aus dem Peritonealexsudat isoliert werden. Männliche Meerschweinchen dagegen waren für die intraperitoneale Infektion nicht empfänglich. Der von VINZENT et al. (1947) aus einer 39jährigen Patientin nach septischem Abort isolierte Stamm wurde als V. fetus identifiziert, jedoch sprechen die mitgeteilten Stoffwechselleistungen gegen diese Speciesbezeichnung. Mit einem gleichfalls nicht eindeutig definierten Vibrionenstamm erzielten MORSE und RISTIC (1954) ebenfalls Aborte bei trächtigen Meerschweinchen. Ein von KING und BRONSKY (1961) mit V. fetus intraperitoneal infiziertes Meerschweinchen ging innerhalb 72 Std zugrunde. Der Erregernachweis post mortem war jedoch weder bakterioskopisch noch kulturell, noch in histologischen Schnitten verschiedener Organe möglich. Zu negativen Ergebnissen nach intraperitonealer Infektion nicht trächtiger Meerschweinchen mit V. fetus kamen Bader et al. (1966) und Blasius et al. (1970), die 380 g schwere Tiere mit 0,1 ml einer 4 Tage bebrüteten Leberbouillonkultur infizierten.

b) Kaninchen, Maus

Die intravenöse Gabe von 2 ml einer 36 Std bebrüteten V.-fetus-Bouillon-kultur wurde ebenso wie die intraperitoneale Injektion von *Kaninchen* ohne weiteres toleriert. *Mäuse* waren nach intraperitonealer und subcutaner Infektion ebenfalls nicht empfänglich (Vinzent et al., 1947). V. fetus bewirkte auch während längerer Beobachtungszeit keine pathologischen Veränderungen und konnte in Gewebsproben nicht mehr nachgewiesen werden (King und Bronsky, 1961). Die intracerebrale und intraperitoneale Injektion einer V.-fetus-Suspension wurde von Babymäusen ohne Krankheitszeichen überstanden (Bader et al., 1966). Mit 7 vom Menschen isolierten V.-fetus-Stämmen sowie einem „related vibrio" infizierte Winkenwerder (1966a) weiße Mäuse oral, intraperitoneal und subcutan. Erreger-dosis waren jeweils 0,3 ml einer Kulturabschwemmung. Der Sektionsbefund der nach 14 Tagen getöteten Tiere war unauffällig. Bakteriologische Untersuchungen von Leber, Milz, Niere und Herzblut verliefen negativ.

c) Hund, Katze, Taube, Küken

Der von Levy (1946) mit 5 ml V.-fetus-Bouillonkultur in die Femoralvene infizierte *Hund* entwickelte innerhalb 24 Std eine tödlich verlaufende Diarrhoe. Bei der Sektion enthielt der erweiterte Magen und der Peritonealraum eine leicht blutig tingierte Flüssigkeit. Leber, Milz und Nieren waren nicht verändert, die Schleimhäute von Magen und Darm unauffällig. Eine kleine Menge muköser, fäkaler Flüssigkeit haftete an einigen Bezirken des Dünndarmes; Ulcerationen wurden nicht registriert. In Präparaten von Leber- und Milzoberfläche, von Darm-inhalt und Mucosa waren Vibrionen zu sehen. Die Kulturverfahren verliefen jedoch ergebnislos.

Die Verfütterung von je 10 ml V.-fetus-Kultur in 30 ml Milch an 3 *Katzen* sowie die intramuskuläre Injektion von 2 ml an 3 *Tauben* führte während 2 Wochen nicht zur Erkrankung (Levy, 1946). Auch 14 Tage alte *Küken* reagierten auf die Gabe von 0,3 ml V.-fetus-Kulturabschwemmung nicht. Der Obduktions-befund war unauffällig (Winkenwerder, 1966a).

d) Trächtiges Schaf

Intravenöse und intraruminale Infektion

Infektionsversuche an Großtieren mit V.-fetus-Stämmen, die von Menschen isoliert waren, wurden selten durchgeführt. Winkenwerder (1967) experimen-tierte mit 4 derartigen Erregern an trächtigen Schafen. Die intravenöse Injektion von $4,7 \times 10^{13}$ Mikroorganismen löste nach 32—72 Std Abort aus. Die Feten zeig-ten über die ganze Körperoberfläche verteilt punktförmige bis flächenhafte Blu-tungen. Der pathologisch-anatomische Befund eines während des Abortes ver-endeten Schafes wurde wie folgt beschrieben:

„Lunge — mittel- bis hochgradiges Ödem, geringgradiges alveoläres Emphysem, mäßig perivasculäre Infiltrate aus leuko-lymphocytären Zellen (verstärkt um die Gefäße), mäßige eitrige interstitielle Pneumonie; Herz — geringgradige, herdförmige, lymphocytäre Infiltrate; Niere — herdförmig hochgradige Hyperämie und Blutungen, in einzelnen Tubuli Eiweiß-ablagerungen; Leber — herdförmige Blutungen, Aktivierung der Kupfferschen Sternzellen, geringgradige, eitrige Hepatitis; Darm — in den oberen Epithellagen Nekrosen und Nekro-biosen, in den tieferen Schichten mittel- bis hochgradige lymphoplasmacelluläre Infiltrate."

Der Erreger konnte bei dem einen Feten aus der Eihaut, bei dem anderen außerdem aus Fruchtwasser und bei einem Muttertier aus Galle und Niere isoliert werden. Die intraruminale Gabe von 3,6 bis 14,3 × 10¹³ Vibrionen erzeugte bei trächtigen Schafen keinen Abort. Es kam zur normalen Geburt.

4. Aus Menschen isolierte anaerobe Vibrionen

Meerschweinchen, Kaninchen, Maus

Anaerobe Vibrionen sind unter den üblichen tierexperimentellen Bedingungen überwiegend apathogen. In Verbindung mit anderen Mikroorganismen können die apathogenen jedoch an Abszeßbildungen beteiligt sein.

V. niger wurde von RIST (1901) als pathogen für das Meerschweinchen beschrieben. Die Versuchstiere starben 14 Tage nach der Infektion, ohne daß makroskopisch Organveränderungen zu sehen waren. Als apathogen für Laboratoriumstiere erwies sich V. tenuis (VEILLON und REPACI, 1912). Auch V. crassus war nicht meerschweinchenpathogen (BEERENS und ALADAME, 1948). Der von SMITH (1930) aus einem Abszeß isolierte anaerobe Stamm rief nach intratrachealer Injektion bei Kaninchen teilweise Pneumonie und Gangrän hervor. Ein Abszeß in der Leistenbeuge des Meerschweinchens wurde durch die Implantation von kleinen Stückchen der Pseudomembran einer Angina Plaut-Vincenti erzeugt. Die in ihm enthaltenen Bakterien waren mit den Borrelien, fusiformen Stäbchenbakterien, Vibrionen und Kugelbakterien des Ausgangsmaterials identisch. Die Injektion der Vibrionen allein führte nicht zur Abszeßbildung (SMITH, 1930). Die subcutane oder intravenöse Injektion von 2 × 10¹² anaeroben Vibrionen löste beim Kaninchen keine Krankheitszeichen aus (CURTIS, 1913). Ebenso erwiesen sich 4 von MOORE (1954) überprüfte anaerobe Vibrionenstämme nach intravenöser, intraperitonealer und intramuskulärer Injektion als apathogen für Meerschweinchen, Kaninchen und Mäuse.

5. Aus Großtieren isolierte aerobe Vibrionen

Schwein, Meerschweinchen, Taube

Aus Großtieren isolierten aeroben Vibrionen kommt keine wesentliche pathogene Bedeutung zu. Über tierexperimentelle Untersuchungen wurde selten berichtet. SMITH (1891) war es nicht möglich, mit vom Schwein isolierten aeroben Vibrionen bei einem hungernden Schwein, das mit 300 ml Bouillonkultur gefüttert wurde, bei einem Meerschweinchen, welches 1,5 ml einer 3 Tage bebrüteten Bouillonkultur intraperitoneal erhielt, sowie bei Tauben, denen er jeweils 0,5 ml in die Flügelvene injizierte, irgendwelche Krankheitszeichen hervorrufen.

6. Aus Kühen und Bullen isolierte mikroaerophile Vibrionen

a) Allgemeines

Wie bereits erwähnt (s. S. 63), wird V. fetus nach seinem Standort unterteilt in V. fetus var. venerealis und V. fetus var. intestinalis. Da V. fetus var. venerealis Abort und Sterilität des Rindes verursacht, sind besonders jene tierexperimentellen Arbeiten von Interesse, die mit diesem Mikroorganismus vorgenommen wurden. Eine Einteilung der Tierversuche aufgrund der beiden Varianten ist jedoch nicht möglich, da diese in der Regel nicht bestimmt wurden. Auch ist die Herkunft der Bakterien, ob aus Genitaltrakt, Feten, Placenta oder Darm des Rindes oder Schafes, nicht immer klar ersichtlich. Ferner darf nicht außer acht gelassen werden, daß Schafe mit von Rindern isolierten V.-fetus-Stämmen infiziert wurden und umgekehrt.

Nur wenige Tierversuche liegen über V. bubulus vor, der im Darmkanal des Rindes parasitiert und mit Kot auch auf die Genitalien gelangen kann. V. jejuni wird von den Genitalvibrionen des Rindes serologisch unterschieden und bewirkt katarrhalische Entzündungen des Dünndarms bei Rind und Kalb (Rolle, 1964).

b) Färse und Kuh

Charakteristische pathologisch-anatomische Veränderungen an den Feten sind nach Vibrionenabort nicht festzustellen. Die Läsionen unterscheiden sich nicht von Aborten, welche durch andere Bakterien hervorgerufen werden. Smith (1918) nimmt an, daß durch die Zwischenschaltung des Placentarkreislaufes die schädigende Wirkung der Vibrionen auf das Chorion beschränkt bleibt. In der Regel können sie in Reinkultur aus Feten und aus der Placenta isoliert werden. V. fetus läßt sich auch aus dem Respirationstrakt der Feten isolieren, wenn Amnionflüssigkeit aspiriert wurde, selten dagegen aus dem Blut (Smith, 1918; Smith und Taylor, 1919). Im Falle einer Mischinfektion ist sein Nachweis mitunter unmöglich. Heute ist erwiesen, daß V. fetus eine Genitalinfektion des Rindes verursacht, die teils Unfruchtbarkeit, teils während der Trächtigkeit einen Abort verursachen kann. Neuere Forschungen haben gezeigt, daß die Vibriosis genitalis durch den Deckakt verbreitet wird; wie durch Felduntersuchungen festgestellt werden konnte, parasitiert der Erreger auf der Präputialschleimhaut des Bullen (Bisping et al., 1964).

Die Unfruchtbarkeit des Rindes kann akut, subakut oder chronisch sein (Lawson und MacKinnon, 1952). Die akute Verlaufsform tritt im allgemeinen dann auf, wenn die Infektion erstmals durch einen infizierten Bullen in eine Herde eingeschleppt wird. Ein verheerendes Absinken der Empfängnisrate, zum Teil unter 10%, ist die Folge. Dieser Zustand kann einige Monate oder länger dauern. Später entwickeln die Tiere eine lokale Immunität und es kommt allmählich wieder zur normalen Befruchtungsrate und Trächtigkeit. In Herden, in welchen der infizierte Zuchtbulle sowohl Kühe als auch Färsen deckt, wird festgestellt, daß die Mehrzahl der Kühe trächtig wird, während Jungkühe und zugekaufte Tiere unfruchtbar sind. Werden dagegen Färsen von nicht infizierten Bullen gedeckt, so tritt eine normale Trächtigkeit ein.

α) Orale Infektion

Lawson und MacKinnon (1952) verfütterten an 6 Jungkühe 10 Tage lang jeweils die Abschwemmung der in einer Roux-Flasche innerhalb von 5 Tagen gewachsenen V.-fetus-Kolonien. Nach dieser Behandlung wurden 3 Färsen bei der ersten und 1 Tier bei der zweiten Insemination trächtig. Die wiederholte Besamung der beiden anderen Tiere führte zu keiner Befruchtung, obwohl V. fetus nicht aus dem Vaginalschleim zu isolieren war.

Die orale Infektion von 6 trächtigen Rindern mit V. fetus var. intestinalis bewirkte keinen Abort. Die Mikroorganismen konnten allerdings mehrere Wochen lang aus den Stuhlproben dieser Tiere isoliert werden (Florent, 1959). Dieses Ergebnis steht im Gegensatz zu Befunden, welche bei der Infektion von trächtigen Schafen erhalten werden, wo es ohne Schwierigkeit gelingt, unter den gleichen Versuchsbedingungen einen Abort hervorzurufen (s. S. 145).

β) Intravenöse Infektion

Die Injektion von 4 verschiedenen V.-fetus-Stämmen an 4 trächtige Rinder verursachte nach Untersuchungen von Smith (1919a) keinen Abort. Es kam jeweils zur Spontangeburt. An den Placenten von 2 Kälbern wurde der Verlust von

Chorionepithel und eine Zellinfiltration mit beginnender Nekrose festgestellt. Die Mikroorganismen konnten nur mikroskopisch in der Placenta nachgewiesen werden. Dieses Ergebnis wurde von SMITH (1919a) mit der geringen Virulenz des verwendeten Stammes erklärt. In späteren Untersuchungen (SMITH, 1923) gelang es nämlich, durch Injektion von Stämmen, die über Meerschweinchen geführt waren, bei trächtigen Rindern teilweise einen Abort hervorzurufen. Auch wenn gesunde Kälber geboren wurden, waren pathologisch-anatomische Veränderungen an der Placenta, Ödem der fetalen Membranen, Exsudation zwischen Uterus und Chorion und fibrinöse Degeneration der Capillarintima vorhanden. Im Exsudat zwischen Chorion und Uterus wurden polynucleäre Zellen, Blutzellen und Epithelzelltrümmer des Chorion angetroffen. Die Vibrionen konnten regelmäßig aus der Placenta isoliert werden.

Unterschiedliche Ergebnisse wurden nach der Injektion von V. fetus var. intestinalis beobachtet (FLORENT, 1959). Mitunter konnte ein Abort des Rindes erzeugt werden, in anderen Experimenten gelang dies nicht. Nach dem Verwerfen waren die Vibrionen aus Placenta, Fruchtwasser, Lochien und Meconium des neugeborenen Kalbes zu isolieren. OSBURN und HOSKINS (1970) beobachteten 12—14 Tage nach intravenöser Injektion von 1 ml V.-fetus-var.-intestinalis-Suspension in die Vena jugularis bei 3 Kühen im 5., 6. und 8. Trächtigkeitsmonat Abort. Aufgrund der bereits eingetretenen Autolyse der Feten wurde der intrauterine Tod der Frucht auf 24—48 Std vor der Austreibung veranschlagt. Als pathologische Befunde wurden Encephalitis, generalisierte Hyperplasie des reticulo-endothelialen Gewebes, Lymphadenitis, Pneumonie und entzündliche Veränderungen an der Placenta erhoben. Die Vibrionen konnten aus Lunge, Magen und Leber der Feten isoliert werden.

Um die Toxinwirkung von V.-fetus-Stämmen zu prüfen, injizierten OSBORNE und SMIBERT (1964) sechs 2—4 Monate alten Kälbern 1,3—10 ml V.-fetus-Suspensionen (10^8—10^9/ml). Daraufhin entwickelte sich bei einigen Tieren ein tödlicher anaphylaktischer Schock. Eine einzige oder auch wiederholte Injektion der Bakterien bei 24—30 Tage alten Kälbern dagegen bewirkte einen leichten reversiblen Schockzustand. Blutkulturen, die 4 Std nach der Injektion angelegt wurden, erwiesen sich als steril. Eine Sepsis kann demnach bei Kälbern nicht erzeugt werden.

γ) Genital- und Placentainfektion

Über die durch V. fetus verursachte enzootische Sterilität bei Rindern berichteten wohl erstmals SJOLLEMA et al. (1949). Von 62 Herden, in denen V. fetus als Ursache des seuchenhaften Verwerfens festgestellt worden war, fiel bei 54 ein Rückgang der Fertilität auf. Die mikroskopische Untersuchung des Cervicalschleims der unfruchtbaren Kühe erbrachte den Nachweis von „V. fetus", während bei trächtigen Kühen der Mikroorganismus nicht zu sehen war. Die überwiegende Zahl der infizierten Kühe konzipierte nach der ersten Besamung nicht; falls sie doch trächtig wurden, abortierten von diesen Tieren 5—10% nach etwa 6 Monaten. Diejenigen Kühe, welche nach der ersten Besamung nicht empfangen hatten, zeigten in der Folgezeit einen unregelmäßigen Oestrus von 23—26 oder mehr Tagen. Da sie 4—6 Monate später nach Besamung durch einen infizierten Bullen trächtig wurden, konnte belegt werden, daß die enzootische Sterilität eine temporäre Unfruchtbarkeit ist. Wie weitere Untersuchungen ergaben, kann Infertilität auch nach künstlicher Besamung auftreten. Von 49 Tieren, denen infizierter Samen appliziert wurde, wurden lediglich 3 trächtig. Zwei dieser Muttertiere abortierten später. V. fetus konnte aus den Feten isoliert werden. Die übrigen 46 Tiere wurden anschließend mit dem Samen eines gesunden Bullen befruchtet.

Nach insgesamt 67 Inseminationen wurden schließlich 10 Kühe trächtig, was einer Besamungsrate von 6,7 pro Trächtigkeit entspricht. Bei 253 gesunden Kühen dagegen waren 1,8 Inseminationen pro Trächtigkeit erforderlich. Zu einer ähnlich schlechten Befruchtungsrate kamen Terpstra und Eisma (1951), wenn der Samen mit V.-fetus-Kulturen infiziert worden war. Eine weitere experimentelle Studie zur Infertilität der Kühe führten Lawson und MacKinnon (1952, 1953) mit Jungkühen aus einer nicht infizierten Herde durch. Sie wurden in Gruppen eingeteilt und diese isoliert. Als Samenspender dienten 1 gesunder Jungbulle und 2 ausgewachsene Bullen, die aus einer infizierten Herde stammten. Vor der Exposition wurde der Cervicalschleim der Jungkühe während 4 Monaten mit dem Agglutinationstest auf Antikörper gegen V. fetus und Trichomonas foetus mit negativem Ergebnis überprüft. Die Konzentration des Spermas war normal. Es wurde 1:6 mit Eidotter-Citratpuffer verdünnt und bei 4° C aufbewahrt. Die Ergebnisse dieser Untersuchungen sind in Tabelle 8 zusammengefaßt. Als Kriterium der Infektion galt die Isolierung der Mikroorganismen aus Vaginalschleim mit dem Kulturverfahren sowie der Nachweis agglutinierender Antikörper im Vaginalschleim. Im Gegensatz zu der hohen Inseminationsrate infizierter Tiere betrug die durchschnittliche Besamung von 48 nicht infizierten Kühen 2,1/Trächtigkeit. In einer weiteren Untersuchung (Lawson und MacKinnon, 1958) wurde bakteriologisch steriler Samen mit V. fetus infiziert und dem verdünnten Sperma 500 mcg Streptomycin, 500 IU Penicillin sowie 0,3% Sulphanylamid/ml zugefügt. Von 6 damit besamten Kühen wurden 2 infiziert; das gleiche Ergebnis wurde auch nach Verdopplung der Antibioticakonzentration erzielt. 12 Jungkühe erhielten den nicht mit Chemotherapeutica vorbehandelten Samen mit dem Erfolg, daß 11 Tiere infiziert wurden.

Ein signifikanter Anstieg der durchschnittlichen Inseminationsrate in Herden mit infizierten Bullen wurde auch von Frank et al. (1956) in einer breitangelegten Felduntersuchung festgestellt.

Zur Untersuchung der Verteilung und Überlebensfähigkeit von V. fetus im Genitaltrakt der Färsen bildeten Newsam und Peterson (1964) aus 59 6 Monate alten Tieren 4 Kollektive. Die Tiere der 1. Gruppe erhielten 5 ml einer V.-fetus-Suspension ($1,5 \times 10^8$/ml) in den vorderen Vaginalabschnitt. Sie wurden nach 13 Wochen getötet. Auf die gleiche Weise wurden den Tieren der 2. Gruppe 5 ml eines Hühnerei-adaptierten Stammes ($4,6 \times 10^8$/ml) verabfolgt. Sie wurden nach 68 Tagen getötet. Bei den Tieren des 3. Kollektivs wurden $1,5 \times 10^8$ Vibrionen auf die Vulva und angrenzende Vaginalschleimhaut aufgebracht. Die Färsen wurden 23, 48, 55 und 69 Tage später getötet. In der 4. Tiergruppe waren Kontrolltiere, welche sich frei zwischen den infizierten Tieren bewegen konnten. Die Resultate zeigten, daß ein frisch isolierter V.-fetus-Stamm schnell in den Uterus der Färsen eindrang und dort wenigstens 13 Wochen überlebte. Der Ei-adaptierte, alte Laboratoriumsstamm war 5 Tage nach der Exposition nicht mehr im Genitaltrakt nachzuweisen. Eine Infektion des Uterus konnte in keiner Versuchstiergruppe festgestellt werden.

Die histologische Untersuchung des Genitaltraktes der Tiere der 1. Versuchstiergruppe (Peterson und Newsam, 1964) erbrachte eine leichte, meist herdförmige und selten das ganze Endometrium umfassende Endometritis. Im Endometrium wurden lymphocytäre und plasmacelluläre Infiltrate, ähnliche celluläre Reaktionen auch in Cervix und Eileiter beobachtet. In der Vagina fanden sich keine Läsionen. Mitunter wurden trotz Anwesenheit von V. fetus keine Veränderungen registriert.

Estes et al. (1966) beschrieben die pathologischen Veränderungen nach intrauteriner Infektion von fünf 2—3 Jahre alten Färsen als subakute, diffuse Endo-

Tabelle 8. Tierexperimentelle Untersuchungen zur Übertragung von V. fetus durch Inseminationen nach LAWSON und MacKINNON (1952, 1953 in Anonym (1958)

Gruppe	Zahl der Färsen	Art der Insemination — Beschaffenheit des Samens	Zahl der Inseminationen	Zahl der infizierten Tiere	Zahl der trächtigen Tiere	Bemerkungen
I (a)	12	natürlich — infizierter Bulle	68	12	11	1 Tier nicht trächtig nach 10 Inseminationen
I (b)	12	künstlich — mit Samen eines infizierten Bullen	69	10	12	
I (c)	6	künstlich — nicht infizierter Samen	10	0	6	
II	12	künstlich — nicht infizierter Samen + V.-fetus-Kultur	88	12	11	1 Tier nicht trächtig nach 12 Inseminationen
III (a)	6	V.-fetus-Kultur oral; künstlich — nicht infizierter Samen	13	0	6	1 Tier verwarf einen mit V. fetus infizierten Feten am 187. Tag
III (b)	6	V.-fetus-Kultur in Conjunctivalsack; künstlich — nicht infizierter Samen	13	0	6	
IV	12	künstlich — nicht infizierter Samen + Filtrat von infiziertem Samen	26	0	11	1 Tier hatte keinen regulären Oestrus und wurde zweimal erfolglos besamt
V (a)	6	künstlich — infizierter Samen + 1000 IU Penicillin/ml verdünntem Samen	23	4	5	eines der 5 Tiere verwarf einen mit V. fetus infizierten Feten am 163. Tag
V (b)	6	künstlich — infizierter Samen + 1000 mcg Streptomycin/ml verdünntem Samen	33	4	6	
VI (a)	6	natürlich — nicht infizierter Bulle	19	0	6	
VI (b)	6	künstlich — nicht infizierter Samen	9	0	6	

metritis. Nach den Untersuchungen von Winter (1966) dauerte diese 2—13 Monate, durchschnittlich 5 Monate. 20 Wochen nach subcutaner Immunisierung mit vermehrungsfähigen V.-fetus-Kulturen infizierten Plastridge et al. (1966) 9 Färsen sowie 9 Kontrolltiere mit 1 ml V.-fetus-Suspension intracervical. Bei den immunisierten Färsen wurden die Vibrionen durchschnittlich 2 und bei Kontrolltieren etwa 21 Wochen lang im Genitaltrakt nachgewiesen. Entsprechend war auch die Befruchtungsrate nach artifizieller Insemination; bei den Tieren der 1. Untersuchungsgruppe waren 1,6 Besamungen erforderlich, sie wurden im Mittel nach 36 Tagen trächtig; bei Kontrolltieren stellte sich nach durchschnittlich 2,7 Inseminationen innerhalb 128 Tagen Trächtigkeit ein. Diese für die Kontrolltiere getroffenen Feststellungen wurden später von Clark et al. (1969) bestätigt.

Nach Laparotomie injizierten Osburn und Hoskins (1970) 3 Kühen im 5., 6. und 7. Trächtigkeitsmonat 1,0 ml V.-fetus-Suspension in die Placenta. Die Frucht wurde darauf im Mittel nach 15,6 Tagen verworfen. Die pathologischen und bakteriologischen Befunde waren die gleichen wie nach intravenöser Infektion trächtiger Kühe (s. S. 141).

δ) Intraconjunctivale Infektion

Das Zentrifugat einer 3 Tage bebrüteten V.-fetus-Kultur wurde in 0,5 ml physiologischer Kochsalzlösung aufgenommen (Lawson und MacKinnon, 1952) und 2mal im Abstand von 7 Tagen in den Conjunctivalsack von 6 Färsen eingeträufelt. Die folgende Fertilitätsprüfung ergab, daß 4 Jungkühe nach der ersten Insemination, 1 nach der zweiten und 1 weitere nach der dritten trächtig wurden. Da diese Ergebnisse nicht an einem größeren Tierkollektiv reproduziert wurden, scheint ein Kausalzusammenhang zwischen der intraconjunctivalen Infektion und der bei 2 Tieren beobachteten verzögerten Trächtigkeit fragwürdig.

c) Bulle

V. fetus parasitiert beim Bullen auf der Präputialschleimhaut. Er dringt nicht in die Testes oder akzessorischen Drüsen ein, Entzündungserscheinungen in anderen Abschnitten des Genitaltraktes sind nicht nachzuweisen (Winter, 1966). Mit Hilfe fluorescierender Antikörper kann gezeigt werden, daß die Erreger auf der epithelialen Oberfläche von Penis und Praeputium lokalisiert sind. Ihr Nachweis aus Präputialspülproben, abgeschabtem Material von Penis und Praeputium ist jedoch mitunter so schwierig, daß er erst nach Infektion von Färsen durch den Deckakt geführt werden kann (Florent, 1956).

d) Tierexperimente mit V. bubulus und V. jejuni

Via vaginale infizierte Florent (1953) 2 *Rinder* nach artifizieller Insemination mit 5 ml Bouillonkultur. Bei einem Tier war V. bubulus noch 65 Tage nach der Infektion in der Vagina nachzuweisen. Die Rinder blieben gesund, eines wurde trächtig. Beide wurden 4 Monate post infectionem getötet. In Vagina, Cervix und Uterus war V. bubulus nicht nachzuweisen.

Für Meerschweinchen (Thouvenot und Florent, 1954), weiße *Mäuse* und 10—14 Tage alte *Küken* ist V. bubulus nach intraperitonealer und subcutaner Injektion apathogen (Winkenwerder und Bisping, 1964).

Aufgrund histologischer Untersuchungen wurde die Ansiedlungsdauer nach intrauteriner V.-bubulus-Gabe bei 6 Kühen (10 ml einer 1:4 verdünnten, 72 Std bebrüteten Bouillonkultur) auf etwa 2 Wochen veranschlagt (Dozsa, 1965). Die Mikroorganismen konnten während 24 Tagen aus dem Genitaltrakt isoliert werden. Als einzige histologische Veränderung an der Uterusschleimhaut wurde eine leichte Entzündung festgestellt. Die alkalische Phosphatase des Endometriums war erniedrigt; einen charakteristischen Aussagewert hat dieser Befund jedoch nicht.

Der von JONES und LITTLE (1931a) bei einer Rinderdiarrhoe isolierte V. jejuni wurde kaum zu tierexperimentellen Untersuchungen verwendet. JONES und LITTLE (1931a) verfütterten unter anderem Ileum- und Jejunuminhalt eines erkrankten Tieres einem 4 Monate alten Kalb; 3 Tage später trat eine Diarrhoe auf. Die Obduktion des nach 16 Tagen geschlachteten Kalbes erbrachte eine ödematöse und blutige Darmschleimhaut; der Darminhalt war flüssig, dunkelbraun und enthielt blutigen Schleim. Aus Mucosateilen des Jejunums konnten die Vibrionen isoliert werden.

7. Aus Schafen isolierte mikroaerophile Vibrionen

a) Schaf

Die V.-fetus-Infektion nimmt beim Schaf einen anderen Verlauf als beim Rind. Der Abort, der in späten Stadien der Trächtigkeit eintritt, kann nicht als Folge einer venerischen Infektion gedeutet werden. Abgesehen von einem einzigen auf einer indirekten Beweisführung fußenden Bericht wird der venerischen Infektion beim Schaf keine Bedeutung zugemessen (BRYANS und SHEPARD, 1961). Die Erkrankung verläuft beim Schaf akut septisch mit Abort. Dies kann zu großen wirtschaftlichen Einbußen führen. Die Verluste betragen mitunter bis zu 60% der Lämmer (LINDENSTRUTH et al., 1949) und etwa 5% der Muttertiere (JENSEN et al., 1957). Obwohl der Infektionsweg im einzelnen noch nicht genau bekannt ist, wird eine orale Infektion angenommen.

α) Orale Infektion

Die Verfütterung von infiziertem Lammgewebe oder V.-fetus-Kultur ruft beim trächtigen Schaf Abort hervor (McFADYEAN und STOCKMAN, 1913). Werden gesunde, trächtige Schafe in demselben Pferch gehalten wie infizierte Tiere, so kommt es nach den Beobachtungen von STOCKMAN (1919) auch bei diesen Tieren zum Abort. Zu anderen Untersuchungsergebnissen gelangten WELCH und MARSH (1924), die 2 trächtige Schafe mit Mageninhalt von verworfenen Feten fütterten und dadurch keine Fehlgeburt erzielen konnten. Allerdings waren die Proben 3 Tage im Kühlschrank aufbewahrt und die Mikroorganismen mit großer Wahrscheinlichkeit geschädigt worden. Zwei weitere trächtige Schafe allerdings, die jeweils 20 ml V.-fetus-Kultur erhalten hatten, lammten gleichfalls normal. LEE und SCRIVNER (1941) gelang es nur dann einen Abort auszulösen, wenn vor der Verfütterung von V.-fetus-Kultur, Fetalgewebe oder Vaginalgeschabsel Kupfersulfat gegeben wurde. Die Tiere hatten dann nach 6—20 Tagen eine Fehlgeburt.

Über die Untersuchungsergebnisse der folgenden Infektionsverfahren wird im Anschluß daran berichtet. LINDENSTRUTH et al. (1949) teilten 20 gravide Schafe in 5 Gruppen ein. Als Erregerdosis diente eine V.-fetus-Suspension, die $1,5 \times 10^9$ Bakterien/ml enthielt. Annähernd 70 ml dieser Aufschwemmung wurden in wöchentlichem Intervall den Heu- und Wasserportionen der Tiere zugefügt. Die 1. Tiergruppe wurde damit einen, die 2. zwei, die 3. drei, die 4. vier Monate und die 5. Gruppe über die ganze Dauer der Trächtigkeit gefüttert. Ähnlich experimentierten TUCKER und ROBERTSTAD (1956) mit 50 jungen Mutterschafen, denen ein gesunder, nicht mit V. fetus infizierter Bock zugeführt wurde. Eine Mischung aus 4 V.-fetus-Stämmen, von denen einer bovinen, die anderen ovinen Ursprungs waren, wurde über das Heu versprüht. Die 1. Tiergruppe wurde nicht infiziert, die 2. zwischen dem 75. und 78. Trächtigkeitstag, die 3. zwischen dem 92. und 97.

und die 4. zwischen dem 124. und 127. Tag. Als Infektionsmaterial wurden von
Frank et al. (1957) Placenta, Mageninhalt und Leber abortierter Lammfeten verwendet. Eingehende Tierexperimente zur Klärung der Vibrionenübertragung
durch Kohabitation nahmen Jensen et al. (1957) vor. Je eine Gruppe von 2 Jahre
alten Schafen wurden einem infizierten bzw. nicht infizierten Bock zugeführt,
während eine 3. Gruppe zu Beginn des 5. Trächtigkeitsmonats 40 g frisches, mit
V. fetus infiziertes Lammgewebe oral erhielt. In ähnlichen Untersuchungen
wurden 2 Jahre alte Tiere 6 Monate vor dem Deckakt isoliert und im 5. Trächtigkeitsmonat mit 10 ml V.-fetus-Bouillonkultur gefüttert (Miller et al., 1959;
Miller und Jensen, 1961). Zum Studium der Übertragung des Erregers infizierten Bryans und Shepard (1961) 6—8 Monate alte Lämmer mit V. fetus-
Kulturen. In anderen Experimenten wurden Schafen V.-fetus-Kulturen verabfolgt, welche aus den Faeces artifiziell infizierter Elstern isoliert worden waren
(Waldhalm et al., 1964).

Von besonderem Interesse ist die Beantwortung der Frage, in welchem Monat
der Trächtigkeit es beim Schaf nach experimenteller Infektion zum Abort kommt
und welche Inkubationszeit die Vibriose besitzt. Die erwähnten Untersuchungen
zeigten, daß die einmalige Infektion im ersten Trächtigkeitsmonat sowie die Verfütterung der Vibrionen während 2 Monaten zu Beginn der Trächtigkeit ohne
Folgen vertragen wurde. Erst eine länger dauernde Verfütterung der Erreger,
besonders über den gesamten Trächtigkeitszeitraum hinweg, führte bei einem
Großteil der Tiere zum Abort (Lindenstruth et al., 1949). V. fetus wurde dann
zum Teil aus Labmagen, Leber und Lunge isoliert.

Als Inkubationszeit ermittelten Tucker und Robertstad (1956) 2—3 Wochen,
Jensen et al. (1957) 7—25 Tage, im Mittel 13,2 ± 4,4 Tage. Jensen et al. konnten
zeigen, daß durch einen infizierten Bock auf genitalem Weg keine Schafvibriose
erzeugt wird. Lediglich bei den Mutterschafen der Gruppe, die ovines Fetalgewebe
erhalten hatte, kam es bei annähernd 74% zum Abort. Sie besaßen noch 1 Jahr
später eine Immunität gegenüber V. fetus, da es während der 2. Trächtigkeit nach
Verfütterung von infiziertem ovinem Gewebe im 5. Trächtigkeitsmonat zu keinem
Verwerfen kam. Als kritischen Zeitpunkt für einen V.-fetus-Abort bei Schafen
geben Frank et al. (1957) die letzte Hälfte des 3. Trächtigkeitsmonats an. Als
Inkubationszeit wurden 19 Tage ermittelt, in einer späteren Mitteilung 8—60 Tage
(Frank et al., 1965).

Bei annähernd der Hälfte der Tiere wurde nach Verfütterung von infiziertem
Lammgewebe eine Septicämie beobachtet, während es nach Verfütterung von
V.-fetus-Kulturen bei 65% dazu kam. Meist trat die Septicämie am 3. Tag nach
der Infektion auf (Miller et al., 1959). Eine V.-fetus-Sepsis wurde auch bei denjenigen Tieren festgestellt, welche mit oral infizierten Schafen Kontakt hatten.
Bryans und Shepard (1961) nahmen an, daß die Mikroorganismen von den
infizierten Tieren mit den Faeces ausgeschieden und oral von nicht infizierten
Schafen aufgenommen wurden. V. fetus konnte bei einem Teil der Tiere gleichzeitig aus Blut und Faeces isoliert werden, bei anderen Schafen war die Blutkultur
24 Std nach der Stuhlkultur erfolgreich. Die Infektion der Lämmer konnte nur
durch die bakteriologische Untersuchung nachgewiesen werden, da sie gesund
blieben. Waldhalm et al. (1964) konnten die Vibrionen aus allen abortierten
Feten isolieren. Das Kulturverfahren war dagegen bei allen Lämmern ergebnislos,
die innerhalb von 24 Std post partum verendeten.

Myers et al. (1970) immunisierten Schafe erfolgreich mit verschiedenen An-
tigenaufbereitungen. Nach anschließender intraruminaler Infektion mit $1,5 \times 10^{10}$
Mikroorganismen abortierten die Tiere nicht. 36% der nicht immunisierten Kontrolltiere verwarfen.

Pathologisch-anatomische Veränderungen sind bei Schafen wenig untersucht worden. Im allgemeinen wurden „Veränderungen der Leber" beobachtet (TUCKER und ROBERTSTAD, 1956; MILLER et al., 1959).

β) Parenterale Infektion

βα) Intravenöse Injektion. Da dem Schafabort eine Vibrionensepsis vorausgeht, überrascht es nicht, daß trächtige Schafe nach intravenöser Injektion der Erreger meist mit einem Abort reagieren. MCFADYEAN und STOCKMAN (1913) lösten nach intravenöser Injektion einer V.-fetus-Kultur oder von infiziertem Lammgewebe bei 5 Schafen Abort aus. Nach Injektion von 5 ml einer Mischung aus 4 Vibrionenstämmen wurde der Erreger nach dem Abort in Reinkultur aus den Cotyledonen, der Amnionflüssigkeit und dem Magen der Feten sowie bis zu einem Monat nach dem Abort aus Vaginalabstrichen der Muttertiere gezüchtet (WELCH und MARSH, 1924). Durch intravenöse Injektion von V.-fetus-Kulturen konnten LEE und SCRIVNER (1941) ebenfalls seuchenhaftes Verwerfen hervorrufen; MILLER et al. (1964) injizierten am 110. Trächtigkeitstag 10 ml V.-fetus-Kultur (1,07 bis 2,53 × 10^9/ml) und bewirkten dadurch bei 98% der Tiere Abort.

Um die Verteilung der Vibrionen im Schaforganismus zu untersuchen, infizierten BRYNER et al. (1971) 2 Gruppen nicht trächtiger Tiere intravenös mit jeweils 10^{10} Mikroorganismen von V. fetus O-Antigen 1 und V. fetus O-Antigen 2. Von 7 mit V. fetus O-Antigen 2 infizierten Schafen verendeten 3 Tiere nach 12, 19 und 24 Std. Die anderen wurden nach 1—41 Tagen getötet und die Erreger aus Gallenblase und Dünndarm von 5 Tieren isoliert. Bei den Tieren der anderen Gruppe konnte V. fetus O-Antigen 1 dagegen aus keinem Organ gezüchtet werden.

ββ) Intraperitoneale Infektion. Aus 20 trächtigen Schafen bildeten LINDENSTRUTH et al. (1949) 5 Gruppen, die während der ersten 5 Trächtigkeitsmonate infiziert wurden. Ihnen wurden 2mal je 10 ml (1,5 × 10^9/ml) einer V.-fetus-Kulturabschwemmung injiziert. Den Tieren der ersten Gruppe wurden die Erreger während des 1. Trächtigkeitsmonats injiziert, den der anderen im 2., 3., 4 und 5. Monat. Abort konnte zwischen dem 3. und 5. Monat verursacht werden.

b) Bock

Dem männlichen Tier kommt bei der Übertragung der Schafvibriose nach den bisherigen Untersuchungen keine Bedeutung zu. Eine experimentelle Infektion wurde über die Geschlechtswege versucht, indem V.-fetus-Kulturmaterial vor dem Deckakt intrapräputial gegeben wurde. Eine Infektion des Schafes erfolgte dadurch nicht (BU et al., 1955). Auch die artifizielle Befruchtung mit infiziertem Samen und das Einbringen von V. fetus in die Cervix des trächtigen Tieres führten nicht zur Fehlgeburt (FIREHAMMER et al., 1956; JENSEN et al., 1957).

c) Meerschweinchen

Für die Diagnose der V.-fetus-Infektion sind Untersuchungen mit Laboratoriumstieren, insbesondere mit Meerschweinchen wenig geeignet. Diese bereits von SMITH (1918) getroffene Feststellung wurde in neuerer Zeit von TERPSTRA (1956) bestätigt, der zum Studium der Genitalinfektion des Rindes das weniger kostspielige Meerschweinchen heranzog und damit zu keinem brauchbaren Ergebnis gelangte.

α) Nicht trächtiges Meerschweinchen

40 Tiere, denen SMITH (1918) mit V. fetus infiziertes Gewebe und Körperflüssigkeiten intraperitoneal injizierte, erkrankten nicht. In einem späteren Ex-

periment (SMITH und TAYLOR, 1919) wurde eine dichte Aufschwemmung von infiziertem Placentagewebe 5 Meerschweinchen intraperitoneal gegeben. Bei zwei nach 3 und 4 Tagen getöteten Tieren konnte V. fetus aus Milz, Leber und Niere in Reinkultur gezüchtet werden, nicht aber bei dem dritten, am 5. Tag getöteten Tier. Die beiden anderen Versuchstiere wurden nach 2 Monaten getötet; pathologisch-anatomische Veränderungen konnten nicht festgestellt werden und V. fetus war nicht nachweisbar. Diese Befunde wurden durch Untersuchungen von MUNDT (1956) gestützt. Erregerdosis war eine Aufschwemmung, deren optische Dichte ca. 9×10^8 Mikroorganismen/ml entsprach. Die Tiere wurden oral mit 1 ml, intravenös mit 0,3 ml, intraperitoneal mit 0,5 ml und subcutan mit 1 ml infiziert. Bei der 3—30 Tage später vorgenommenen Obduktion war kein krankhafter Befund zu erheben. Der Nachweis von Vibrionen gelang nur aus der Milz bis zum 5. Tag post infectionem.

β) Trächtiges Meerschweinchen

Um einen Abort bei diesen Tieren auszulösen, wurden verschiedene Infektionstechniken angewandt. Ein Abort gelang GMINDER (1922) und WITTE (1923) durch subcutane Injektion von V.-fetus-Kulturmaterial. Auf die intraperitoneale Injektion reagierten trächtige Meerschweinchen empfindlicher als auf die subcutane (GRAHAM und THORP, 1930; LERCHE, 1937). Im Abstand von 2 Tagen injizierten RISTIC und MORSE (1953) jeweils 1 ml V.-fetus-Aufschwemmung (photometrisch standardisiert) intraperitoneal oder subcutan Versuchstieren, die in der 4. bis 7. Woche trächtig waren. Die Vibrionen waren ovinen und bovinen Ursprungs. Nach intraperitonealer Injektion abortierten 4 von 7 Meerschweinchen innerhalb 1—12 Tagen. Die subcutane Injektion löste bei 2 von 7 Versuchstieren 4—7 Tage später einen Abort aus. In einer weiteren Untersuchung (MORSE und RISTIC, 1954) wurde die Pathogenität von 31 verschiedenen aus Kühen, Schafen und Menschen isolierten V.-fetus-Stämmen überprüft. Als Dosis diente 1 ml einer Suspension von $1,8 \times 10^8$ Vibrionen/ml. Die Versuchstiere waren in der 4. bis 8. Woche trächtig. Bei ihnen wurde eine Abortrate von maximal 78% registriert. Das Verwerfen trat frühestens am 1. und spätestens 13. Tag post infectionem auf (MORSE und RISTIC, 1954). Bei einer allerdings nur kleinen Tiergruppe protokollierte MUNDT (1956) nach intravenöser, intraperitonealer und subcutaner Infektion stets seuchenhaftes Verwerfen.

Bei der Sektion der Muttertiere wurden im Abdomen und im Thorax 80—90 ml eines blutig-serösen Exsudats angetroffen (RISTIC und MORSE, 1953; MUNDT, 1956). Die Oberfläche der Bauchorgane war mit Fibrin bedeckt. Hämorrhagien wurden auf der Leberoberfläche und dem Epikard beobachtet. Der Magen enthielt eine gelbliche bis bräunliche, trübe Flüssigkeit. Mitunter war die Gallenblase erheblich dilatiert und entzündlich verändert. Im Uterus bestand eine hämorrhagische Endometritis mit Ödem und Nekrosen, wobei verschiedene Stadien der Entzündungsreaktion nebeneinander angetroffen wurden. Die Placenta war ebenfalls ödematös und zum Teil nekrotisch, die Eihäute waren blutig tingiert und mitunter nekrotisch. Beim Feten bestand ein Ödem der Haut mit Hämorrhagien.

V. fetus wurde nach dem Abort aus Uterus, Placenta und Eihäuten, vereinzelt aus der Gallenblase des Muttertieres und bisweilen aus dem Mageninhalt des Feten gezüchtet (RISTIC und MORSE, 1953; MUNDT, 1956).

γ) Genitale Infektion trächtiger und nicht trächtiger Meerschweinchen

Nach intravaginaler Gabe von 1 ml V.-fetus-Aufschwemmung an trächtige und nicht trächtige Meerschweinchen an 5 aufeinanderfolgenden Tagen wurde lediglich bei einem Tier 8 Tage nach der letzten Infektion eine Fehlgeburt verzeichnet (RISTIC und MORSE, 1953). In weiteren Experimenten wurden 7 Monate alte weibliche Meerschweinchen paarweise gehalten und ihnen je 1 männliches Tier zugegeben. Je eines der beiden Tiere erhielt an 5 aufeinanderfolgenden Tagen 1 ml V.-fetus-Suspension intravaginal. Die Hälfte der Tiere verwarf nach 32 bis 48 Trächtigkeitstagen. Dabei zeigte es sich, daß das Männchen V. fetus durch die Kohabitation auch auf das nicht infizierte Weibchen übertrug (RISTIC et al., 1954).

Die männlichen Meerschweinchen erkrankten nach Kontakt mit V. fetus nicht und zeigten keine Erhöhung des Antikörpertiters. Ein Teil der intravaginal infizierten Tiere verwarf. 4—5 Tage vor dem Abort wurde ein Ausfluß aus der Vagina festgestellt. Die pathologisch-anatomischen Veränderungen am Uterus glichen denen nach parenteraler Infektion (RISTIC und MORSE, 1953; RISTIC et al., 1954).

Die Vibrionen wurden bei Tieren, die verworfen hatten, stets aus dem Uterus und teilweise aus dem Magen der Feten isoliert. Aufgrund der bakteriologisch gesicherten Infektion der nicht artifiziell infizierten Tiere ist die Übertragung von V. fetus durch den Coitus anzunehmen.

d) Trächtiges Kaninchen

Während in früheren Untersuchungen die intraperitoneale und intravenöse Injektion von V. fetus beim trächtigen Kaninchen keinen Abort auslöste (McFADYEAN und STOCKMAN, 1912; GRAHAM und THORP, 1930), gelang es später, durch die intraperitoneale Injektion von 1,5 ml Vibrionensuspension nach 5 Tagen ein seuchenhaftes Verwerfen hervorzurufen (MUNDT, 1956). V. fetus konnte aus den Eihäuten, dem Uterus und dem Magen der Feten gezüchtet werden. Eine Suspension von 10^8—10^9 Vibrionen/ml verwendeten OSBORNE und SMIBERT (1964). Die einmalige intravenöse Injektion von 0,3 bzw. 0,5 ml erwies sich als tödliche Dosis. Wurde die Menge auf 0,8 ml gesteigert, so starben auch nicht tragende Tiere unter den Zeichen eines anaphylaktischen Schocks.

e) Maus

Die weiße Maus ist für V. fetus im allgemeinen nicht empfänglich (SMITH, 1918; LERCHE, 1927; JANSEN und KUNST, 1951). Von Rindern isolierte Stämme von V. fetus O-Antigen 1 und V. bubulus O-Antigen 3 injizierten WINKENWERDER und BISPING (1964) weißen Mäusen intraperitoneal und subcutan. In deren Organen konnten sie nach 14—15tägiger Beobachtungszeit keine Vibrionen nachweisen. Auch die histologische Untersuchung der inneren Organe erbrachte, bis auf einen kleinen lympho-histiocytären Herd in der Leber einer Maus und eine mäßige bis hochgradige follikuläre Hyperplasie der Milz einer anderen Maus, keinen pathologischen Befund.

f) Ratte

Ratten sind nach den Experimenten von SMITH (1918) für V. fetus nicht empfänglich.

g) Hamster

RISTIC et al. (1954) infizierten 3mal im Abstand von 2 Tagen 3—4 Monate alte männliche Hamster mit 0,3 ml einer V.-fetus-Suspension intraperitoneal. Nach der letzten Injektion wurde jedes Tier in eine Box mit 2 nicht infizierten weiblichen Versuchstieren gesetzt. 4 Gruppen wurden nach 7 Tagen, 3 nach 12 und die übrigen 3 nach 21 Tagen getötet. In einem weiteren Experiment wurde die

Pathogenität von 18 V.-fetus-Stämmen verschiedener Herkunft an männlichen Hamstern nach intraperitonealer Injektion untersucht (Ristic et al., 1955).

Aus den Befunden ergab sich, daß nach intraperitonealer Infektion des männlichen Hamsters eine Übertragung auf weibliche Tiere möglich war. Bei den Männchen wurde V. fetus noch nach 21 Tagen in Reinkultur aus dem Hoden isoliert. Bei nicht graviden weiblichen Tieren konnten die Mikroorganismen bis zum 21. Tag aus dem Uterus gezüchtet werden, während bei trächtigen Tieren der Erregernachweis nicht gelang. Bei 11 von 18 männlichen Hamstern (Ristic et al., 1955) wurde V. fetus aus den Testes gezüchtet. Von den untersuchten Stämmen waren die bovinen weniger virulent als die humanen und ovinen. Die Affinität von V. fetus zum Hoden der Hamster zeigte sich auch in pathologisch-anatomischen Veränderungen. Die Testes waren verkleinert und hart. Nach der Sektion waren ausgedehnte Fibrosen, Stauungen der Gefäße, Hämorrhagien und Nekrosen in der Subcapsularregion festzustellen. Die histologische Untersuchung ergab eine Zerstörung des Gewebeaufbaus, eine ausgedehnte Fibrose und Thrombosierung der Gefäße. Ferner wurden kleine Herde mit käsigem Eiter beobachtet (Ristic et al., 1954).

h) Küken

Winkenwerder und Bisping (1964) infizierten insgesamt 57 Küken im Alter von 10—14 Tagen mit vom Rind isolierten Stämmen von V. fetus (O-Antigen 1 und 2) und V. bubulus (O-Antigen 3). Sie infizierten die Tiere oral, intraperitoneal, intramuskulär und subcutan. Nach 14—21 Tagen waren bei den getöteten Tieren makroskopisch und histologisch keine mit der Infektion zusammenhängenden pathologischen Veränderungen festzustellen. Die Mikroorganismen konnten aus den Organen der Küken nicht isoliert werden.

i) Bebrütetes Hühnerei

Nach Injektion von V. fetus in die Allantoisflüssigkeit 12 Tage alter Hühnerembryonen starben diese 5 Tage später ab (Plastridge und Williams, 1943). Zum gleichen Ergebnis kamen Jansen und Kunst (1951) mit 7—9 Tage alten bebrüteten Eiern.

Die Injektion von 0,1 ml V.-fetus-Suspension in den Allantoissack von 219 Hühnerembryonen zeigte, daß die höchste Letalität 2—3 Std später auftrat. Am empfänglichsten waren 8—9 Tage bebrütete Hühnereier. Zwar zeigten die 6—7 Tage alten eine höhere Letalität, doch bestand auch bei einer Kontrollgruppe in dieser Altersstufe eine größere Sterblichkeit (Webster und Thorp, 1953). Die Chorio-Allantois-Membran wies eine Makrophageninfiltration auf, die Mesenchymalzellen waren proliferiert und das Mesoderm hämorrhagisch. Die Makrophagen nahmen das gesamte Lumen einiger Arteriolen ein, so daß hier Parallelen zu den Gefäßveränderungen der fetalen bovinen Placenta gezogen werden können. Häufig wurde bei den Embryonen eine Splenomegalie beobachtet. Leber und Niere waren meist vergrößert und gestaut. An den Glomeruli war das Gefäßendothel proliferiert und pyknotisch. Die Capillarschleifen zeigten eine Makrophageninfiltration. Insbesondere in der Haut der Extremitäten, aber auch in der Magenwand und in der Lunge, im Gehirn und im Epikard waren petechiale Blutungen zu sehen.

j) Schwein

Junge und erwachsene Schweine (Osborne und Smibert, 1964) sowie trächtige Tiere (Graham und Thorp, 1930) reagierten auf eine intravenöse Injektion von V. fetus nicht.

8. Aus Schweinen isolierte mikroaerophile Vibrionen

Die durch V. coli verursachte Dysenterie der Schweine wurde von DOYLE (1944, 1948) als eine auf das Colon lokalisierte Erkrankung beschrieben. Sie ist durch den Abgang von halbflüssigen, gelblichen, mit großen Mengen Schleim oder Blut durchsetzten Faeces charakterisiert. Die Körpertemperatur schwankt zwischen 38 und 41° C (ROBERTS, 1956a), bisweilen ist sie normal. Die Tiere verlieren an Gewicht, die Letalität beträgt durchschnittlich 25%, unter besonders ungünstigen Verhältnissen bis zu 50%. Der Obduktionsbefund zeigt Veränderungen ausschließlich im Verdauungstrakt. Der Dünndarm ist normal. Distal der Ileo-Cöcal-Klappe ist die Schleimhaut gerötet und das Colon gestaut. Der Inhalt des Dickdarmes ist breiartig und blutig, die Mucosa gelblich verfärbt und stellenweise nekrotisch. An der Leber finden sich blasse, erhabene Zonen von annähernd 1 cm Durchmesser. Auffällig ist die Leukocyteninfiltration der Mucosa. Einzelne Abschnitte scheinen fast ausschließlich aus großen erweiterten Becherzellen zu bestehen. Die schleimige Ablagerung auf der Mucosa enthält Bakterien, Epithelzellen, Leukocyten und Erythrocyten. Die Vibrionen sind bisweilen fischzugartig angeordnet (DOYLE, 1944).

a) Schwein

α) Orale Infektion

Die Verfütterung von V.-coli-Kulturen an Schweine löste bei 6 von 8 Tieren Diarrhoen aus, die nach 3—5 Tagen einsetzten und meist ebensolange andauerten. Bei einem Schwein wiederholte sich der Durchfall nach einer Woche (DOYLE, 1944). Von 60 Ferkeln, die mit V.-coli-Kulturen gefüttert wurden, welche in Magenschleim inkubiert waren, entwickelten 50 eine Dysenterie. Die Zahl der Erkrankungen stand mit der nach oraler Gabe von infizierten Coecum- oder Colonstücken in Einklang (JAMES und DOYLE, 1947). Eine milde Form der Diarrhoe mit leichtem Fieberanstieg erzielte v. BALLMOOS (1950) bei 10 Wochen alten Schweinen, die jeden 2. Tag während eines Zeitraums von 7 Wochen infiziert wurden. Die Ergebnisse von DOYLE wurden durch ROBERTS (1956a) bestätigt, der teils eine Faeces-Mischung von 4 Schweinen, teils V.-coli-Mucin-Suspensionen zur Infektion seiner Tiere verwendete. Auch SCHIB (1956) konnte bei 2 Absatzferkeln nach einmaliger Gabe der Erreger schwere Diarrhoen hervorrufen. Es sei in diesem Zusammenhang jedoch darauf hingewiesen, daß auch eine plötzliche Futterumstellung bei Ferkeln zu Durchfällen führen kann.

Die klinischen und Obduktionsbefunde bei oral infizierten Tieren stimmen mit denen der natürlich erkrankten überein. In den Untersuchungen von JAMES und DOYLE (1947) wurden keine Angaben über die Isolierung von V. coli gemacht. Sein Nachweis aus Darmlymphknoten gelang v. BALLMOOS (1950), während ROBERTS (1956a) zu negativen Ergebnissen kam. Beide Untersucher jedoch konnten V. coli aus Coloninhalt, SCHIB (1956) aus Faeces isolieren. In Leber, Milz und Nieren war kein Vibrionennachweis möglich (v. BALLMOOS, 1950; ROBERTS, 1956a), ebensowenig im Herzblut (ROBERTS, 1956a).

β) Parenterale Infektion

Bei 2 Jungschweinen, die innerhalb 64 Tagen 3 Injektionen von jeweils 3, 6 und 8 ml Vibrionenaufschwemmung subcutan erhalten hatten, kam es nach jeder Injektion zu einer vorübergehenden, leichten Temperaturerhöhung. 3 Tage nach der letzten Injektion traten Durchfälle auf; am 9. Tag, auf dem Höhepunkt der Erkrankung, waren die Tiere apathisch und verweigerten die Futteraufnahme (MESSERLI, 1953). Eine einmalige Gabe von 4 ml Bakteriensuspension blieb nach SCHIB (1956) wirkungslos.

b) Großtiere

Die Verfütterung von V. coli an ein Kalb verursachte keine Krankheitserscheinungen (Doyle, 1948). Auch das Schaf war, abgesehen von einer leichten Temperaturerhöhung, nicht empfänglich, wie die intravenöse Injektion von 10 ml Kulturabschwemmung und eine 8 Tage später vorgenommene subcutane Injektion von 5 ml ergab (Messerli, 1953). Dagegen berichtete Schib (1956), daß 1 Schaf kurze Zeit nach intravenöser Injektion von 10 ml V.-coli-Aufschwemmung unruhig wurde, die Körpertemperatur auf 40° C stieg und 10 Std nach der Infektion das Tier zugrunde ging. Ein weiteres Schaf erhielt 5 ml subcutan; es reagierte mit vorübergehender Temperaturerhöhung. Nachdem 6 Tage später 5 ml intravenös injiziert worden waren, verendete das Tier innerhalb 24 Std im Schock. Andere Schafe, die 2 ml subcutan im Abstand von 2 Wochen erhalten hatten, wiesen nur Temperaturerhöhung, Neutrophilie und Lymphopenie auf. V. coli wurde weder aus dem Darm noch aus den inneren Organen isoliert.

c) Meerschweinchen, Maus, Ratte, Goldhamster, Huhn, Küken

Die Virulenz von V. coli für kleine Versuchstiere ist gering. Die parenterale Injektion bewirkte bei Meerschweinchen, weißen Mäusen, Ratten und Hühnern keine Erkrankung (Doyle, 1948). Zum gleichen Ergebnis kam bei diesen Tieren und bei Kaninchen nach oraler, intrakardialer, intraperitonealer und subcutaner Infektion auch v. Ballmoos (1950). Die Organe der nach 10 Wochen getöteten Tiere zeigten keine pathologisch-anatomischen Veränderungen. Vibrionen waren nicht nachzuweisen. Diese Ergebnisse wurden von Roberts (1956b) und Schib (1956) bestätigt. Morse und Ristic (1954) dagegen berichteten, daß es nach intraperitonealer Injektion von nicht näher definierten Schweinevibrionen bei trächtigen Meerschweinchen zum Abort kam. Die Pathogenität von 6 V.-coli-Stämmen unterschiedlicher Herkunft prüften Maciak und Winkenwerder (1964) an weißen Mäusen, Goldhamstern und Küken, die intraperitoneal, subcutan und per os infiziert wurden. Während der Versuchsdauer von 10—14 Tagen verendeten 4 von 12 Mäusen, 1 von 3 Goldhamstern und 19 von 24 zwei bis drei Tage alten Küken, jedoch keins der 4 Wochen alten. Die überlebenden Tiere wurden am Ende der Versuchszeit getötet und der Erregernachweis aus Leber, Gallenblase, Milz und Herzblut versucht. V. coli konnte aus den Organen der während des Versuchs verendeten 4 und bei 1 von 8 zu Versuchsende noch lebenden weißen Maus, aus einem verendeten und einem der beiden überlebenden Goldhamster isoliert werden. Auch war das Ergebnis bei 6 von 19 verendeten und bei einem der 5 überlebenden 3—5 Tage alten Küken positiv. Dagegen konnte V. coli in den Organen der 4 Wochen alten Tiere in keinem Fall gefunden werden. Pathologisch-anatomische Veränderungen wurden nie beobachtet.

9. Aus Vögeln isolierte aerobe Vibrionen

Gamalaia (1888a) beschrieb die Symptome und den Sektionsbefund des von ihm als „gastroentérite cholérique" bezeichneten, durch V. metschnikovii hervorgerufenen Krankheitsbildes bei natürlich infizierten Hühnern folgendermaßen:

Die kranken Tiere sitzen mit gesträubtem Gefieder unbeweglich da und wirken wie eingeschlafen. Während dieses Dämmerzustandes, der 48 Std und länger andauern kann, haben sie erniedrigte Körpertemperatur, ferner bestehen Diarrhoen. Bei der Sektion findet sich eine akute Entzündung des ganzen Darmtraktes, insbesondere in den dem Magen am nächsten liegenden Abschnitten; vornehmlich der Dünndarm enthält eine große Menge graugelber Flüssigkeit, die mit Epithelflocken und Blut durchsetzt ist. Auch der Kropf ist mit einer serösen Flüssigkeit gefüllt. Die inneren Organe sind ohne auffälligen Befund.

Während die Blutproben erwachsener Hühner in der Regel steril waren, ließ sich V. metschnikovii bei jungen Tieren isolieren. Demnach sind diese für die Infektion besonders empfänglich. Nach den Beobachtungen von GAMALAIA (1888a) können bis zu 10% eines Bestandes der Erkrankung erliegen. Über eine Infektion mit einem V. metschnikovii nahestehenden Erreger bei 500 Sonnenvögeln (Chinesische Nachtigall, Leiothrix luteus L.) berichteten KRAUSE und WINDRATH (1919). Die Tiere waren auf dem Transport oder während der ersten beiden Tage nach der Ankunft am Bestimmungsort verendet. Bei der Sektion war eine blutige Darmentzündung auffällig. Bereits mikroskopisch waren in Darminhalt und Blutausstrichen massenhaft Vibrionen zu sehen, die auch gezüchtet werden konnten.

a) Huhn

α) Orale, subcutane und intramuskuläre Infektion

Für die orale Infektion mit Kultur- oder infektiösem Tiermaterial sind nur junge Hühner empfänglich. Nach Trinken von vibrionenhaltigem Taubenblut verendeten sie innerhalb von 2 Tagen (GAMALAIA, 1888a). Bei der Obduktion war der Darm hyperämisch und enthielt reichlich mit grauen Flocken durchsetzte Flüssigkeit. Der Erreger konnte aus dem Blut isoliert werden. Erwachsene Hühner erkrankten auch nach Gabe großer Erregerdosen und bei Verwendung eines über Tauben geführten Stammes nicht. Durch Verfütterung vibrionenreicher Taubenorgane konnte PFEIFFER (1889) bei einem erwachsenen und einem jungen Huhn keine Erkrankung hervorrufen.

Für eine erfolgreiche subcutane und intramuskuläre Infektion wurden für junge Hühner mehr als 1 ml vibrionenhaltiges Taubenblut benötigt; erwachsene Hühner dagegen vertrugen bis zu 3 ml intramuskulär (GAMALAIA, 1888a). Die Injektion von je 1 ml Bouillonkultur in den Brustmuskel eines jungen und eines ausgewachsenen Huhnes führte nur bei ersterem zum Tod. An der Injektionsstelle wurde eine lokale entzündliche Reaktion angetroffen, der Darm war äußerlich blaß, die Schleimhaut zeigte eine fleckige Hyperämie; mikroskopisch waren zahlreich desquamierte Epithelzellen zu sehen. Vibrionen konnten mit dem Kulturverfahren nicht nachgewiesen werden.

β) Intratracheale Infektion

Obwohl unter natürlichen Bedingungen auch erwachsene Hühner an einer Infektion mit V. metschnikovii zugrunde gehen, war es GAMALAIA (1888a) zunächst nicht gelungen, bei ihnen eine tödliche Erkrankung auszulösen. Nach intratrachealer Applikation von 1 ml vibrionenhaltigem Taubenblut bei 2 Hühnern, einem Hahn und zwei 3—4 Monate alten Hühnern, starben die Tiere, mit Ausnahme eines nach 2 Tagen verendeten Huhnes, innerhalb von 20 Std. Auch hier zeigten sich bei der Obduktion die bereits geschilderten Veränderungen. GAMALAIA (1888b) glaubte aus diesen Befunden schließen zu können, daß die natürliche Infektion des Huhnes über die Atemwege erfolge.

b) Taube

α) Orale Infektion

Bei oraler Gabe sehr großer, mit dem Futter vermengter Erregerdosen erkrankten Tauben nicht (GAMALAIA, 1888a, b). Dieser Befund wurde auch von PFEIFFER (1889) erhoben, der den Tod von 2 Tauben aus einem oral infizierten Kollektiv aufgrund des Sektionsbefundes als Septicämie und Intoxikation deutete. Er war der Meinung, daß die Vibrionen durch Schlingbewegungen in die Trachea und über das Lungenparenchym in die Blutbahn gelangt seien.

β) Intramuskuläre Infektion

Für eine intramuskuläre Infektion sind Tauben empfänglich. Wenige Tropfen einer Kulturaufschwemmung genügten, um sie innerhalb 8—12 Std zu töten (Gamalaia, 1888a). Auch nach Injektion von vibrionenhaltigem Blut starben sie innerhalb 20 Std. Nach Pfeiffer (1889) war als Erregerdosis „etwa soviel, wie an der Spitze einer Platinnadel hängenbleibt", ausreichend, um den Tod herbeizuführen. Bei der Obduktion zeigte sich regelmäßig eine beträchtliche Schwellung des geimpften Brustmuskels. Er war gelblich verfärbt, nekrotisch und mit einer blutigen Ödemflüssigkeit durchsetzt, in der sich massenhaft Vibrionen nachweisen ließen. Der Darm war nach Untersuchungen von Gamalaia (1888a) blutig verfärbt und mit einer serösen, purulenten Flüssigkeit angefüllt. Pfeiffer (1889) dagegen beschrieb dieses Organ als meist blaß und den Inhalt als graugelb und mehlsuppenähnlich. V. metschnikovii konnte aus dem Darm (Gamalaia, 1888a; Pfeiffer, 1889) und auch aus Herzblut (Gamalaia, 1888a) gezüchtet werden.

γ) Intratracheale Infektion

Nach intratrachealer Gabe von 0,25 ml vibrionenhaltigem Taubenblut ging das infizierte Tier innerhalb 24 Std zugrunde (Gamalaia, 1888b). Bei der Obduktion fanden sich am Darm choleraähnliche Veränderungen; ferner waren eine anämische Milz, eine Hyperämie der Lunge und eine seröse Pleuritis auffällig. Die Erreger ließen sich aus Blut, Pleuraexsudat und Darminhalt züchten. Eine weitere, mit diesem Darminhalt intratracheal infizierte Taube verendete ebenfalls; jedoch waren bei ihr Lunge und Pleura pathologisch-anatomisch unauffällig.

c) Meerschweinchen

α) Orale Infektion

Durch orale Gabe weniger Milliliter einer 48 Std bebrüteten V.-metschnikovii-Kultur wurden Meerschweinchen innerhalb 24 Std getötet (Gamalaia, 1888a). Dieser Versuch gelang Pfeiffer (1889) erst nach Vorbehandlung der Versuchstiere mit Sodalösung und intraperitonealer Injektion von Opiumtinktur. Die Obduktion erbrachte einen entzündeten, purpurrot verfärbten Darmtrakt, dessen Flüssigkeit Epithelzellen enthielt. Vibrionen konnten aus Darminhalt und Herzblut isoliert werden (Gamalaia, 1888a; Pfeiffer, 1889).

β) Subcutane Infektion

Auf subcutane Infektion reagierten Meerschweinchen besonders empfindlich (Gamalaia, 1888a). Wurde 1 ml einer Bouillonaufschwemmung injiziert, so gingen alle Tiere zugrunde (Pfeiffer, 1889). Bei kleineren Dosen war der letale Ausgang nicht mehr sicher. Erhielten die Tiere die gleiche Dosis wie Tauben, so überlebten etwa 10% (Pfeiffer, 1889). Bereits 2 Std nach der Infektion traten die ersten Krankheitszeichen auf: die Tiere wurden zunehmend apathisch und saßen zusammengekauert da. Die hinteren Extremitäten schienen wie gelähmt. Es trat eine vorübergehende Temperaturerhöhung von 1—2° C auf; anschließend sank sie bis auf etwa 33° C ab. Nach 18 bis höchstens 24 Std trat unter Muskelzuckungen der Tod ein. Bei der Obduktion wurde ein von der Injektionsstelle ausgehendes, sanguinolentes Ödem festgestellt, das sich häufig auf den halben Tierkörper erstreckte. Die hyperämischen Lungen und das klare seröse Pleuraexsudat wurden als Zeichen einer Intoxikation gewertet; die Darmschleimhaut war blaß. Die Mikroorganismen konnten aus der Ödemflüssigkeit und dem Blut reichlich, aus dem Darminhalt dagegen nur sehr spärlich nachgewiesen werden.

d) Kaninchen, Maus

Bei Kaninchen konnte GAMALAIA (1888b) nur durch sehr hohe Erregerdosen nach intratrachealer Gabe und subcutaner Injektion von vibrionenhaltigem Taubenblut eine tödliche Erkrankung auslösen. Mäuse konnte er durch intraperitoneale Injektion von 1 ml vibrionenhaltigem Taubenblut innerhalb 24 Std töten. Die Mikroorganismen waren aus dem hyperämischen Darm und Blut zu isolieren. PFEIFFER (1889) dagegen stellte fest, daß Mäuse für eine Infektion mit V. metschnikovii nicht empfänglich waren. Die Tiere wurden nach der Injektion in die Schwanzwurzel zwar mehrere Tage „sichtlich" krank, erholten sich jedoch wieder.

e) Sonnenvögel

Der von KRAUSE und WINDRATH (1919) aus Sonnenvögeln isolierte aerobe Vibrio unterschied sich nach Ansicht der Autoren von V. metschnikovii durch eine geringere Pathogenität für Tauben und Meerschweinchen und eine erhöhte für Mäuse. Tauben wurden durch intramuskuläre Injektion von $^1/_{10}$ Öse Kulturmaterial innerhalb von 48 Std getötet; bei größeren Erregerdosen ($^1/_2$ Öse) starben sie nach 18—20 Std. Der infizierte Brustmuskel wurde als stark angeschwollen beschrieben. Aus ihm konnten die Vibrionen in Reinkultur isoliert werden. Für die Chinesische Nachtigall (Leiothrix luteus L.) genügten bei intramuskulärer Injektion „Spuren von Kultur", um den Tod in 18—20 Std herbeizuführen. Für weiße Mäuse betrug die Dosis letalis etwa $^1/_{33}$ Öse nach subcutaner Injektion. Ratten und Meerschweinchen verendeten spätestens 20 Std nach intraperitonealer Injektion von $^1/_5$ Öse. Als Krankheitszeichen wurden Lähmung der hinteren Extremitäten und Absinken der Körpertemperatur mitgeteilt. Hühner und Kaninchen waren nach subcutaner und intramuskulärer Infektion nicht empfänglich (KRAUSE und WINDRATH, 1919).

10. Aus Vögeln isolierte mikroaerophile Vibrionen

Klinische Manifestation und pathologisch-anatomische Veränderungen bei einer Vibrionenhepatitis der Hühner waren schon häufig beschrieben worden, bevor es HOFSTAD (1956) und wohl gleichzeitig — wie dem Versuchsprotokoll zu entnehmen ist — auch PECKHAM (1958) gelang, aus der Leber der infizierten Tiere mikroaerophile Vibrionen zu isolieren. Durch Übertragungsversuche konnte der Kausalzusammenhang zwischen Vibrioneninfektion und Hühnerhepatitis erhärtet werden (HOFSTAD et al., 1958). Der Mikroorganismus kann aus Leber- und Gallenproben gezüchtet werden (PECKHAM, 1958; WHENHAM et al., 1961).

Das klinische Bild ist bei erkrankten Hühnern wenig charakteristisch. Im Vordergrund steht ein Rückgang der Legeleistung, der zwischen 15 und 25% betragen kann (HOFSTAD et al., 1958; PECKHAM, 1958; VIELITZ et al., 1965). Gelegentlich werden auch Diarrhoen beobachtet (WHENHAM et al., 1961; BISPING et al., 1963). Die Letalität infizierter Bestände wird mit 2—5% angegeben (PECKHAM, 1958; VOUTE und GRIMBERGEN, 1959; KÖLBL, 1964; VIELITZ et al., 1965), kann jedoch, besonders zu Beginn der Infektion, auch 10—15% betragen (HOFSTAD et al., 1958; WHENHAM et al., 1961).

Pathologisch-anatomische Veränderungen bei natürlich infizierten Hühnern werden hauptsächlich an Leber und Darm festgestellt. Die Leber ist geschwollen, oft dunkelbraun verfärbt und besitzt durch unregelmäßig große, weißliche Nekroseherde ein gesprenkeltes Aussehen. Die Größe der Herde beträgt im Durchmesser einen oder mehrere Zentimeter. Gelegentlich werden auch subcapsuläre Blutungen beobachtet (HOFSTAD et al., 1958; PECKHAM, 1958; WHENHAM et al., 1961; VIELITZ et al., 1965). Am Dünndarm findet sich eine katarrhalische Entzündung

(Whenham et al., 1961; Vielitz et al., 1965), die Nieren sind anämisch und leicht vergrößert, die Eifollikel häufig degeneriert (Peckham, 1958; Vielitz et al., 1965). In der Portalregion werden die ersten histologischen Veränderungen beobachtet, die mit einer Proliferation des Bindegewebes und einer Lymphocyten- und Eosinophileninfiltration einhergehen. Häufig dehnt sich das Bindegewebe in das Parenchym aus; in diesem Gebiet ist dann eine Verfettung der Leberzellen zu sehen. Die Blutgefäße sind gewöhnlich außerordentlich gestaut (Whenham et al., 1961).

Zum Erregernachweis eignet sich Blutagar, auf den Gallenflüssigkeit aufgetropft wird. Er wird bei 37,5° C in einem Brutschrank gehalten, der 27% Luft, 10% CO_2 und 63% Methan enthält (Peckham, 1958; Whenham et al., 1961). Für den kulturellen Nachweis verwendeten Vielitz et al. (1965) Hammelblutagar ohne Traubenzuckerzusatz. In Galle-Nativpräparaten wurde der Erregernachweis durch Untersuchung mit dem Phasenkontrastmikroskop geführt.

a) Huhn

Die orale Infektion 6—7 Monate alter Hühner gelang nicht, wie die Sektion der 1—3 Wochen später getöteten Tiere ergab (Voute und Grimbergen, 1959). Diese Ergebnisse wurden von Winkenwerder und Bisping (1964) bestätigt, die je 2 Junghennen kurz vor der Legereife mit einem über Küken geführten Stamm oral, intraperitoneal und intravenös infizierten. Pathologisch-anatomische Veränderungen wurden bei den nach 29—35tägiger Versuchsdauer getöteten Tieren nicht gefunden. Ein Vibrionennachweis gelang in keinem Fall.

b) Küken

Von Peckham (1958) wurden 7 Tage alte Küken mit 0,2 ml Eigelb-Vibrionensuspension intramuskulär infiziert, andere mit einer Kulturabschwemmung. Voute und Grimbergen (1959) injizierten 2 Wochen alten Küken eine Kulturabschwemmung intramuskulär. 3 Tierkollektive bildeten Whenham et al. (1961) aus 20 Tage alten Küken. Die 1. Gruppe erhielt 2 ml gewaschene Vibrionensuspension intravenös, die 2. subcutan und die 3. die gleiche Dosis oral. In einem zweiten Experiment wurden 3 von verschiedenen Hühnern isolierte Kulturen verwendet, die im Dottersack von 6 Tage alten Hühnerembryonen zur Vermehrung gebracht worden waren. 0,25 ml infiziertes Eigelb wurden intraperitoneal injiziert. Zur Prüfung der Pathogenität der bei Hühnerhepatitis isolierten Vibrionen infizierten Winkenwerder und Bisping (1964) 84 2—14 Tage alte Küken in verschiedenen Versuchsreihen oral, intraperitoneal, subcutan und intramuskulär.

Übertragungsversuche führten Vielitz et al. (1965) durch, indem sie Leberstückchen und die Galle von infizierten Hühnern homogenisierten und im Verhältnis 1:10 mit physiologischer Kochsalzlösung aufschwemmten. Von dieser Suspension erhielten Eintagsküken 0,2 ml intraperitoneal. Die infizierten Küken ließen innerhalb der ersten Woche gegenüber Kontrolltieren ein unausgeglichenes Wachstum mit geringerer Gewichtszunahme erkennen (Kölbl, 1964). Sechs Tage post infectionem wurden sie nach der Beobachtung von Vielitz et al. (1965) teilnahmslos, am 7. Tag traten die ersten Todesfälle auf. Der Obduktionsbefund der nach 7—10 Tagen getöteten Küken ergab eine vergrößerte Leber mit fokalen Nekroseherden und eine vergrößerte Milz. Das Myokard war auch auffallend blaß und im Perikard wurde ein klarer Erguß angetroffen. Die Herzveränderungen wurden nur bei artifiziell infizierten Tieren beobachtet (Peckham, 1958; Hofstad et al., 1958; Whenham et al., 1961; Vielitz et al., 1965). Winkenwerder und Bisping (1964) fanden bei lediglich 4 Tieren, die während des Versuches gestorben waren, und einem Küken, das nach Versuchsabschluß getötet worden war, Zeichen einer geringgradigen Enteritis, bei je einem Tier eine gelbliche Verfärbung der Leber, eine blasse Entfärbung des Herzmuskels sowie geringgradige Petechien der Leber. Die histologischen Veränderungen glichen denen der natürlich infizierten Tiere (PECKHAM, 1958). Im Gegensatz dazu konnten WINKENWERDER und BISPING (1964) an der Leber keine oder nur unspezifische Veränderungen beobachten, wie sie sowohl bei infizierten als auch bei Kontrolltieren angetroffen wurden. An der Herzmuskulatur waren, abgesehen von einer Epikarditis (1 Küken) und geringgradigen herdförmigen Infiltraten mit mononucleären Zellen (2 Küken) oder heterophilen Granulocyten (1 Küken), keine Läsionen zu verzeichnen.

Die Isolierung der Vibrionen gelang in der Regel aus Leber und Galle (HOFSTADT et al., 1958; PECKHAM, 1958; VIELITZ et al., 1965). Besonders geeignet war die Übertragung von Leber, Milz, Perikard und Gallenflüssigkeit in den Dottersack von 5—7 Tage alten Hühnerembryonen (PECKHAM, 1958). Aus 27 von 48 infizierten Küken isolierten WINKENWERDER und MACIAK (1964) den Erreger. Dabei konnte er 17mal aus Herzblut und Galle, 15mal aus der Muskulatur, 14mal aus der Leber und 13mal aus der Milz gezüchtet werden. KÖLBL (1964) gelang nur in einem Fall der Nachweis von Vibrionen aus Leber und Galle, bei anderen Küken wurden sie dagegen im Blinddarm gefunden.

c) Bebrütetes Hühnerei

Die Injektion von infektiösem Tiermaterial oder Vibrionenkultur führt bei 6—7 Tage alten Hühnerembryonen innerhalb von 4—5 Tagen zum Tod. Bei älteren, bis zu 15 Tage alten, werden in Abhängigkeit von der Erregerdosis unterschiedliche Ergebnisse erzielt. Diese Infektionsmethode ist insbesondere geeignet, die Dosis letalis zu bestimmen (HOFSTAD et al., 1958). Bei den abgestorbenen Embryonen imponieren Leberläsionen und Milzschwellungen. PECKHAM (1958) injizierte 0,2 ml Lebersuspension in den Dottersack 6 Tage alter Embryonen. Sie starben am 2. Tag. Eidotter und Allantoisflüssigkeit wurden lyophilisiert und anschließend wieder auf Kulturmedium gebracht. Die Mikroorganismen aus dem Eigelb-Lyophilisat vermehrten sich in größerer Zahl und rascher als die aus der Allantoisflüssigkeit. Über eine Virulenzsteigerung durch wiederholte Hühnerembryopassagen berichteten HOFSTAD et al. (1958). KÖLBL (1964) führte Vibrionen unterschiedlich lang über künstliche Nährmedien und überprüfte durch Infektion verschieden alter Hühnerembryonen die Virulenzminderung und den Einfluß des Alters auf den Zeitpunkt des Todes. Nach 6 Passagen wurden Dottersack und Allantoishöhle von 7, 8, 9 und 12 Tage alten Embryonen infiziert. Von den 7, 8 und 9 Tage alten Embryonen starben alle am 1. und 2. Tag, von den 12 Tage alten 8 am 1.—5. Tag, 12 blieben am Leben. Nach 11 Passagen überlebten 11 Tage alte Embryonen und 7 Tage alte starben erst nach 2—4 Tagen. Das bebrütete Hühnerei verwendeten VIELITZ et al. (1965) als „Anreicherungsmethode", um wenige Vibrionen nachweisen zu können. Von fraglich infizierten Tieren wurde 0,1 ml Gallenflüssigkeit in den Dottersack von 5—7 Tage bebrüteten Hühnereiern instilliert. Waren Vibrionen vorhanden, so starben die Embryonen nach 3—5 Tagen. Sie konnten dann mit dem Phasenkontrastmikroskop in Massen in Dottersack und Gallenblase, in geringer Zahl in Allantois- und Amnionhöhle, und häufig auch in Organen gesehen werden.

d) Maus

Von PECKHAM (1958) wurde erwähnt, daß nach intracerebraler Injektion der bei Hühnerhepatitis isolierten Vibrionen weiße Mäuse nervöse Symptome zeigten, und daß sie aus dem Gehirn wieder isoliert werden können. Als Erregerdosis verwendeten Winkenwerder und Bisping (1964) jeweils 0,5—0,8 ml einer gut bewachsenen Petrischalenkultur, die 15 weißen Mäusen intraperitoneal und subcutan injiziert wurden. Vier Tiere starben während des Versuches, die übrigen wurden nach 7—12 Tagen getötet. Die histologische Untersuchung der Leber von 6 Mäusen erbrachte herdförmige, lympho-histiocytäre Infiltrate, multiple Nekroseherde mit leuko-histiocytärer Demarkation und eitrige Granulome. In der Milz war eine follikuläre Hyperplasie auffällig. Herz und Nieren waren ohne pathologischen Befund. Bei zwei während des Versuchs verendeten Tieren wurden Vibrionen isoliert, außerdem bei 8 der übrigen 11 Mäuse. Sie wurden 10mal aus der Leber, 5mal aus Herzblut, 4mal aus Niere und 3mal aus Milz gezüchtet.

11. Aus anderen Vögeln isolierte Vibrionen

a) Trappen

Bei verendeten Trappenküken stellten Grünberg und Otte (1963) als Todesursache eine durch Vibrionen hervorgerufene nekrotisierende Hepatitis fest. Die pathologisch-anatomische Untersuchung der Leber zeigte zahlreiche, gleichmäßig über das Organ verteilte graugelbe Nekroseherde, die von kleinen, subcapsulären Hämorrhagien umgeben waren, wodurch das Organ ein eigenartig marmoriertes Aussehen erhielt. Die Nekrosen waren unregelmäßig begrenzt und glichen denen bei der infektiösen Leberentzündung der Hühner. Bei 2 älteren Küken schien die Darmschleimhaut leicht gerötet. Das jüngere davon hatte eine akute katarrhalische Entzündung des Dünndarms. Die Milz war blaß und wie die Nieren stark vergrößert. Mit dem aus diesen Tieren isolierten Vibrionenstamm wurden ohne nähere Angabe der Erregerdosis Küken und Junghühner oral, intravenös und intraperitoneal infiziert. Von den Eintagsküken gingen 2 am 6. bzw. 8. Tag zugrunde, bei einigen stellte sich 5 Tage nach der Infektion Mattigkeit und Freßunlust ein. Die pathologisch-anatomischen Veränderungen entsprachen denen der natürlich infizierten Trappenküken. Lediglich im Interstitium des Myokards trat eine lymphocytäre Infiltration stärker hervor, als es bei den Spontanerkrankungen der Fall war. Bei infizierten Junghühnern wurde sie erst nach 12—15 Tagen manifest. Die getöteten Tiere hatten weniger stark ausgeprägte Veränderungen als die Küken. Doch gelang es auch bei diesen regelmäßig, die Mikroorganismen aus den veränderten Organen zu züchten.

Fünf bis sieben Tage alte Hühnerembryonen starben 2—3 Tage nach Injektion von 0,1 ml Kulturabschwemmung in den Dottersack ab. An ihrer Körperoberfläche bestand eine herdförmige Hyperämie, in der Rückenregion fanden sich kleinere Petechien. Aus den Dottersäcken konnten die Vibrionen in Reinkultur isoliert werden.

b) Haussperling

Mit aus Herzblut, Leber, Jejunum und Colon von Haussperlingen isolierten Vibrionen, die sich kulturell, biochemisch und serologisch von Hühnervibrionen unterschieden, wurden Hühnerküken oral, subcutan und intraperitoneal infiziert (Abdallah und Winkenwerder, 1966). Aus 7 von 18 Tieren konnten sie wieder isoliert werden. In der Leber wurden lympho-leukocytäre Infiltrate im Parenchym, periportal und perivasculär festgestellt, in der Milz eines Tieres ausgedehnte Nekrosen. Auf die gleiche Weise wurden je 3 erwachsene weiße Mäuse infiziert; bei einem Drittel der nach 15 Tagen getöteten Tiere waren Vibrionen nachzuweisen. Leber und Milz zeigten die gleichen histologischen Veränderungen wie die infizierter Hühnerküken.

c) Truthuhn

TRUSCOTT et al. (1964) ermittelten mikroaerophile Vibrionen als Ursache einer übertragbaren Enteritis bei Truthühnern. Befallen werden alle Altersstufen. Die Letalität bei jungen Tieren ist besonders groß. Mit den aus Duodenum und Gallenflüssigkeit isolierten Vibrionen sowie mit Intestinalsuspension natürlich infizierter Truthühner wurden tierexperimentelle Untersuchungen angestellt. Als Erregerdosis erhielten 100 Truthühner je 1 ml 20 %ige Intestinalsuspension in den Kropf. Mit ihnen wurden 100 nicht infizierte in Kontakt gebracht. Anschließend wurden über einen Zeitraum von 7 Tagen aus beiden Kollektiven täglich 5 Tiere getötet und Darminhalt, Herz, Leber und Gallenflüssigkeit untersucht. Bei der infizierten Tiergruppe konnten die Mikroorganismen bereits nach 24 Std aus Leber und Darminhalt und nach 48 Std auch aus Gallenflüssigkeit gezüchtet werden. Der Darminhalt von Kontakttieren zeigte nach 2 Tagen und die Gallenflüssigkeit nach 3 Tagen ein positives Kulturergebnis. Von den infizierten Tieren starben 52 innerhalb 15 Tagen, von den Kontakttieren 45 während des gleichen Zeitraumes. Die größte Sterblichkeit wurde bei dem ersten Kollektiv nach 2—5 Tagen, bei dem zweiten nach 5—7 Tagen beobachtet. Wenn anstelle von infektiösem Darmmaterial 0,6 ml Vibrionensuspension $(3,4 \times 10^{10}/ml)$ in 5 % Mucin gegeben wurde, konnten die gleichen Beobachtungen getroffen werden. In einem weiteren Experiment wurde gezeigt, daß bei 82 % der infizierten Truthühner noch bis zu 20 Wochen post infectionem die Vibrionen isoliert werden konnten.

12. Aus Wasser isolierte Vibrionen

Viele aus Wasser isolierte Vibrionen werden ohne Speciesbezeichnung als NAG-Vibrionen aufgeführt. Einige wurden sowohl vom Menschen als auch aus Wasser isoliert, oder aber als identisch angesehen mit Vibrionen, die aus Tieren gezüchtet wurden, so z.B. V. nordhafen mit V. metschnikovii (PFEIFFER, 1892). Aus Meerwasser, Fischen und Menschen können V. parahaemolyticus und V. alginolyticus isoliert werden. Ihr Biotop ist das Meerwasser (ZEN-YOJI et al., 1965; SAKAZAKI, 1968). Zu tierexperimentellen Untersuchungen mit NAG-Vibrionen finden im allgemeinen die bereits bei anderen Vibrionen geschilderten Methoden Anwendung.

a) Meerschweinchen

Für Meerschweinchen erwies sich V. aquatilis nach oraler und intraperitonealer Applikation als apathogen (GÜNTHER, 1892). Auch mit V. berolinensis konnte NEISSER (1893) nach oraler Gabe von 5 ml Bouillonkultur und Alkali-Opium-Vorbehandlung keine Erkrankung hervorrufen. Die intraperitoneale Injektion von 2,5 ml erbrachte ebenfalls ein negatives Ergebnis, jedoch führte die Injektion einer höheren Konzentration (1 Öse Kulturmaterial in 1 ml Bouillon aufgeschwemmt) zum Tod des Meerschweinchens. Der Erreger war aus Peritonealexsudat und Herzblut zu züchten. Als Dosis letalis minima für 300—400 g schwere Meerschweinchen ermittelte GÜNTHER (1893) bei intraperitonealer Injektion 1 Öse einer 24 Std bebrüteten Agarkultur. Bei großen Erregermengen gingen die Tiere unter raschem Temperaturabfall innerhalb von 24 Std zugrunde. Bei geringeren Dosen setzte die Temperatursenkung langsamer ein und die Tiere verendeten nach 2—3 Tagen. Wurden subletale Erregermengen gegeben, so erholten sie sich nach einem vorübergehenden Temperaturabfall.

Bei der Obduktion verendeter Meerschweinchen fand sich in der Bauchhöhle eine geringe Menge trübe, schmutzig-braune, leukocytenreiche Flüssigkeit. Ferner waren fibrinös-eitrige Beläge auf der Serosa der Bauchorgane, hauptsächlich der

Leber auffällig. In mikroskopischen Präparaten dieser Beläge waren neben Eiterzellen massenhaft Vibrionen zu sehen. Bei einigen Versuchstieren fiel eine blutigödematöse Durchtränkung des subcutanen Gewebes an der Injektionsstelle auf. Die Vibrionen konnten aus dieser, aus Peritonealexsudat und bisweilen aus Herzblut isoliert werden. Mit einem „dem Choleravibrio ähnlichen Vibrio", der aus Wasser isoliert worden war, verlief die orale und intraperitoneale Infektion ergebnislos (KIESSLING, 1893). PANJA und PAUL (1943) verwendeten aus dem Hoghly-River bei Kalkutta isolierte, nicht näher definierte Vibrionen. Sie infizierten Meerschweinchen oral und subcutan. Die Sterblichkeitsrate der Tiere betrug 75%. Vibrionen konnten aus Blut, Peritonealhöhle und Gallenblase gezüchtet werden. Der Sektionsbefund war ähnlich dem einer experimentellen Cholera. SAYAMOV (1963a), der 5 aus Wasser isolierte Vibrionenstämme in verschiedenen Dosen Meerschweinchen in ein abgebundenes Darmsegment injizierte, stellte bei 85% der Tiere keine Veränderungen fest. Bei den übrigen wurden mitunter leichte Hämorrhagien und vermehrte Gefäßzeichnung der Mucosa protokolliert. Der Darminhalt bestand in der Regel aus einer dicken braunen Masse. Bei einigen Tieren fand sich eine leicht gelbliche Flüssigkeit mit wenig Eiterzellen. Bei fast allen jedoch wurde der injizierte Vibrio aus dem abgebundenen Darmsegment gezüchtet. Wie Bakterienzählungen ergaben, vermehrten sich die Wasservibrionen in einigen Experimenten im Darmstück, in anderen starben sie ab, so daß beispielsweise von $2,5 \times 10^7$ injizierten Vibrionen/ml nur noch 300/ml zu zählen waren. Bei 2 Tieren konnten Vibrionen nicht mehr gefunden werden. Der histologische Befund zeigte mitunter kleine Hämorrhagien in Serosa und Muskelschicht. Das Darmepithel war stets intakt. Im Darmlumen wurden Schleim und gelegentlich Leukocyten angetroffen. Auf der Oberfläche der Mucosa waren vereinzelt Leukocytenanhäufungen zu erkennen. Eine Parallele zur experimentellen Cholera war nicht ersichtlich.

b) Kaninchen

Für Kaninchen war V. aquatilis nach intravenöser Injektion nicht pathogen (GÜNTHER, 1892). Auch V. berolinensis führte nach intraperitonealer Injektion zu keinen Krankheitszeichen (NEISSER, 1893). Der von KIESSLING (1893) isolierte NAG-Vibrio löste ebenfalls nach intravenöser und intraperitonealer Injektion keine Erkrankung aus. Die Injektion von drei aus Wasser isolierten NAG-Vibrionenstämmen in das abgebundene Darmsegment erbrachte keine pathologisch-anatomischen Veränderungen (GUPTA et al., 1956; SAYAMOV, 1963a).

c) Andere kleine Laboratoriumstiere

Weiße Mäuse und Feldmäuse waren für eine Infektion mit V. aquatilis (GÜNTHER, 1892) und V. berolinensis (NEISSER, 1893) nach subcutaner Injektion nicht empfänglich. Auch Tauben zeigten nach intramuskulärer Injektion dieser beiden Mikroorganismen keine Krankheitserscheinungen. Eine intravenöse und intraperitoneale Applikation wurde sowohl von diesen Tieren als auch von weißen Ratten ohne weiteres toleriert (KIESSLING, 1893).

13. Aus Fischen isolierte Vibrionen

Die bei Aalen durch V. anguillarum verursachte epizootische Erkrankung wird als „Rotseuche" bezeichnet. Es hat sich jedoch eingebürgert, als Rotseuche alle Erkrankungen von Fischen zu bezeichnen, die mit einer Rotfärbung des Bauches und der Flossen einhergehen und als deren Ursache verschiedene Bakterien in Frage kommen (SCHÄPERCLAUS, 1927). BERGMAN (1909) trennte die von ihm bei

Aalen beobachtete, durch V. anguillarum hervorgerufene Erkrankung von den anderen Rotseuchen ab und führte dafür den Begriff der „roten Beulenkrankheit" ein. Nach Schäperclaus (1927) handelt es sich lediglich um eine Verschiebung der Akzente bei der makroskopischen Beurteilung. Die Krankheitssymptome bei Aalen sind Hyperämie und Petechien, besonders an Flossen, Kiemen und After. Mitunter treten Ulcerationen, vornehmlich an Rückenflossen und Flanken auf. Der Tod tritt ein, wenn sich die Entzündung im subcutanen Bindegewebe über den größten Teil des Aalkörpers erstreckt. Nach Eröffnen des Abdomens wird in der Peritonealhöhle eine rötliche, seröse Flüssigkeit angetroffen; Leber, Nieren und Darm sind leicht gestaut (Bergman, 1909; Lagarde und Chakroun, 1965).

Bei allen untersuchten erkrankten Aalen konnte Bergman (1909) V. anguillarum aus „Beulen" in Reinkultur züchten; falls ein Ulcus vorhanden war, enthielt es neben Vibrionen in geringer Zahl auch andere Mikroorganismen. Bei verendeten Aalen gelang die Isolierung aus Peritonealexsudat, Leber, Herzbeutel und bisweilen aus Blut (Bergman, 1909; Lagarde und Chakroun, 1965).

Aus Hautulcerationen von Dorschen (Gadus callarias, L.) isolierten Bagge und Bagge (1956) ebenfalls V. anguillarum. Eine Variante dieses Bacteriums, V. anguillarum Typ C, war in Bachforellen zu finden, die im Spätsommer oder Frühherbst tot angespült wurden und weder äußerlich noch innerlich Veränderungen aufwiesen. Die Mikroorganismen wurden jedoch häufig in Reinkultur aus Milz, Leber, Niere, Herzblut und mitunter aus Muskelfleisch gezüchtet (Smith, 1961).

Die Infektion von Fischen mit V. piscium wurde erstmals von David (1927) bei Karpfen beobachtet und eingehend beschrieben. Nach einer Inkubationszeit von 1—3 Wochen wurden die Fische auffallend matt, die Atmung war angestrengt, sie atmeten mit dem Maul über dem Wasserspiegel, schwammen dem Ufer zu und ließen sich, ohne zu flüchten, mit der Hand ergreifen. Später legten sie sich auf die Seite und gingen nach einigen Tagen unter zunehmender Mattigkeit zugrunde. Bei einigen Karpfen waren punkt- oder flächenhafte Blutungen auf der Haut zu sehen, ohne Beulen- oder Abszeßbildung. Häufig entleerte sich aus dem After eine schleimig-blutige Flüssigkeit, die mit Epithelmassen durchsetzt war. Der pathologisch-anatomische Befund war nicht besonders typisch. Gewöhnlich bestand eine Hyperämie der Leber und des Darmes; Milz, Leber und Niere waren meist erheblich vergrößert. Mitunter wurden auch Blutungen an Kiemen, Herzmuskel und Peritoneum, ferner bei einzelnen Tieren eine Entzündung des Dickdarmes und eine Peritonitis festgestellt. Die Mikroorganismen konnten stets aus Galle isoliert werden, meist auch aus Herz, Niere und Milz.

Die gleiche „Vibrionenseuche" mit ähnlichen Symptomen und pathologisch-anatomischen Veränderungen wurde auch bei Hechten ermittelt (David, 1927). Bei jungen und erwachsenen Regenbogenforellen traten beulenartige, hämorrhagische Veränderungen im Muskelfleisch auf. Hoshina (1956, 1957) gab dem verantwortlichen Bacterium die Bezeichnung V. piscium var. japonicus. Sowohl aus dem Seewasser von Tanks als auch aus den jungen, darin befindlichen Lachsen wiesen Rucker et al. (1954) eine halophile Vibrionenart nach. Das Muskelfleisch und die inneren Organe der befallenen Fische zeigten ausgedehnte Blutungen. Die Letalität war außerordentlich hoch. Eine Krankheit mit ähnlichen Symptomen wurde auch bei Regenbogen- und Stahlkopfforellen beobachtet, die wahrscheinlich von wandernden Lachsen infiziert worden waren.

a) Infektion mit V. anguillarum

Zu den üblichen Infektionsmethoden kommen Experimente, bei denen die Vibrionen dem Wasser zugefügt werden, in welches die Fische eingesetzt sind

(Schäperclaus, 1927; David, 1927). Teils wird Süßwasser, teils Salzwasser verwendet, um den Einfluß dieses Milieus auf den Ausbruch der „Rotseuche" zu studieren.

α) Aal

Durch Verfütterung der Vibrionen an Aale wurden keine Erkrankungen verursacht, während die intraperitoneale Injektion bei 9 Aalen innerhalb 1—10 Tagen zu einer tödlich verlaufenden Erkrankung führte (Bergman, 1909). Nach subcutaner Injektion starben von 18 Aalen 11 innerhalb 4—28 Tagen, 1 Tier ging 24 Std nach der Infektion zugrunde, 6 überlebten. Die verendeten Aale boten die gleichen Krankheitszeichen und Sektionsbefunde wie natürlich infizierte. Bei den 6 überlebenden bildete sich am Ort der Injektion eine Beule aus, die nach einiger Zeit wieder verschwand.

In Abhängigkeit von der Größe der Aale injizierte Schäperclaus (1927) 0,1—0,3 ml Kulturabschwemmung intraperitoneal. Sie wurden in Süßwasser und in Salzwasser eingesetzt. Nach 3—6 Tagen gingen die in Süßwasser gehaltenen unter den Symptomen der Rotseuche zugrunde. In Salzwasser lebten sie 1—2 Tage länger. Bei diesen waren im Gegensatz zu den in Süßwasser gehaltenen Fischen nur wenige Vibrionen im Blut zu finden. Weitere Tiere wurden derart infiziert, daß in einen Einschnitt der Muskulatur in Höhe des Afters etwas Kulturmaterial eingestrichen wurde. Die so geimpften Aale starben im Süßwasser nach 5—6 Tagen. Die Infektionsstelle war nicht entzündet (Schäperclaus, 1927). In einer weiteren Versuchsanordnung waren dem Süßwasser Vibrionenkulturen zugegeben worden. Die darin gehaltenen Aale erkrankten nicht. Die Wiederholung des Experiments im Salzwasser verlief bis auf einen Aal, der nach 65 Tagen einging, ergebnislos. Die Infektion hatte sich zuerst am Maul manifestiert; später war es zu einer allgemeinen Erkrankung gekommen. Schäperclaus (1927) diskutierte eine Wundinfektion, deren Ulceration durch Salzwasser gefördert wird, was mit den Beobachtungen von Bergman (1909) in Einklang zu bringen ist, der bei den aus Salzwasser gefangenen Aalen meist Geschwüre beobachtete. Nach subcutaner Injektion (0,2 ml Bouillonkultur) von Vibrionen, die aus Dorschen isoliert worden waren, starben Aale ebenfalls. Zuvor hatte sich eine Beule gebildet, die nach kurzer Zeit ulcerierte (Bagge und Bagge, 1956). Die gleichen Mikroorganismen verwendete Smith (1961) für die intramuskuläre Infektion von 4 Aalen, die 2 bis 7 Tage später eingingen. An der Injektionsseite waren bei 2 Tieren Hämorrhagien zu sehen, Hautschwellung und Hyperämie bei dem dritten und keine Symptome bei dem vierten. Allerdings wurden die Mikroorganismen nach der Obduktion aus Milz, Leber und Muskelfleisch aller Tiere isoliert. Nach intraperitonealer Injektion von V. anguillarum starben Aale innerhalb 6—24 Std ohne Krankheitszeichen (Lagarde und Chakroun, 1965). Die Vibrionen wurden bei allen aus Herzblut isoliert. Auch nach intramuskulärer Gabe starben die Fische innerhalb 24 Std. Bei der Sektion waren hämorrhagische Flecken im Abdominalbereich auffällig. Nach subcutaner Injektion überlebten sie 36—48 Std. An der Impfstelle waren beulenartige Veränderungen. Die Infektion des Augapfels (1 Tier) verlief ergebnislos (Lagarde und Chakroun, 1965).

β) Andere Fische

Die subcutane Injektion von wenigen Tropfen V.-anguillarum-Kultur führte bei Plötzen innerhalb 36 Std zum Tod. Die Schuppen waren an der Impfstelle durch Flüssigkeitsansammlung in den Schuppentaschen aufgerichtet. Nach Abschaben der Schuppen erschienen die Kanten der Schuppentaschen rot angeschwollen. Das subcutane Bindegewebe der Infektionsseite war rot und ödematös;

Tabelle 9. Experimentelle Infektion von Fischen mit V. anguillarum-Typ C. (Nach Smith, 1961)

Fisch	Anzahl	Injektionsart	Todeszeitpunkt (Tage)	Äußere Symptome
Lachs	3	intraperitoneal	1—6	Zwei zeigten Hämorrhagien an der Bauchseite, einer keine Symptome
Lachs	1	intramuskulär	2	Entzündung der Muskulatur der Injektionsseite
Steinforelle	2	intraperitoneal	4—6	keine
Barsch	2	intraperitoneal	2	keine
Scholle	1	intramuskulär	22	„Penny-große" geschwollene, hämorrhagische Zone mit bläulich-schwarzem Zentrum; Hämorrhagien der umgebenden Muskulatur
Köhler	2	intraperitoneal	2—6	einer symptomlos, der andere wies eine gräulich verfärbte Zone am Rücken auf

die Entzündung erstreckte sich bis in die Muskulatur. Nach Eröffnen des Abdomens wurde eine katarrhalisch-entzündete Darmschleimhaut angetroffen. Der Erregernachweis gelang stets aus Blut (Bergman, 1909). Auf gleiche Weise infizierte *Seeskorpione* (Cottus scorpius L.) starben nach 4 Tagen. Die pathologisch-anatomischen Veränderungen ähnelten denen der infizierten Aale und Plötzen, In weiteren Experimenten infizierte Bergman (1909) 11—15 cm große *Karauschen* (Carassius vulgaris) subcutan und intramuskulär. Nach 24 Std verhielten sie sich außerordentlich ruhig und vermieden es, die Schwanzflosse zu bewegen. Von 5 Tieren starben 4 nach 3 Tagen; das 5. war einen Tag vor dem Tod hyperästhetisch: es führte außerordentlich schnelle Bewegungen durch, sobald das Aquarium nur berührt wurde. Die Obduktions- und bakteriologischen Befunde glichen den bereits bei Aalen beschriebenen. Intraperitoneal infizierte Karauschen starben nach $2^1/_2$—3 Tagen. Dagegen blieben in ein Wasserbad eingesetzte Tiere, dem zwei 3 Tage alte Gelatinekulturen zugefügt waren und das erst nach 3 Tagen gegen Frischwasser ausgewechselt wurde, ohne Krankheitszeichen (Bergman, 1909). Die von Schäperclaus (1927) mit 0,3 ml einer 72 Std bebrüteten Bouillonkultur infizierten Karauschen verendeten nach 8 Tagen an Rotseuche. Über die experimentellen Untersuchungen von Smith (1961) gibt die Tabelle 9 Aufschluß. Nach dem Tod wurden die Vibrionen stets aus dem Fischorganismus isoliert. Eine erfolgreiche Infektion gelang Lagarde und Chakroun (1965) auch bei Goldfischen nach subcutaner Injektion von V. anguillarum.

γ) Frosch

Wenige Tropfen V.-anguillarum-Bouillonkultur wurden von Bergman (1909) 4 jungen, 25—35 mm großen Fröschen (Rana temporaria L.) unter die Rückenhaut gespritzt. Alle 4 starben innerhalb 12 Std. Durch eine Flüssigkeitsansammlung in der Subcutis wirkten sie stark aufgetrieben. Das Exsudat enthielt neben wenigen weißen Blutkörperchen Vibrionen, die auch aus Blut gezüchtet wurden. Die Injektion von 0,5 ml bei 2 erwachsenen Fröschen und 2 Kröten (Buffo vulgaris Laur.), die sich im Winterschlaf befanden, wurde toleriert.

b) Infektion mit V. piscium

α) Fische

Für *Karpfen* verwendete David (1927) als Erregerdosis bei subcutaner und intraperitonealer Infektion 0,1—0,5 Ösen einer 3 Tage bei Zimmertemperatur gehaltenen Bouillonkultur bzw. $^1/_5$ Öse einer 48stündigen Agarkultur. Sie verendeten nach 8 Tagen. Der Sektionsbefund war identisch mit dem der natürlich erkrankten Fische (s. S. 161). *Schleien* erkrankten auch nach Injektion größerer Bakterienmengen nicht, jedoch konnten die Vibrionen noch nach 2 Monaten aus Galle isoliert werden. *Rotfedern, Plötzen, Barsche, Forellen* und *Bitterlinge* erkrankten unter natürlichen Bedingungen nicht, vermochten allerdings andere, empfängliche Fische zu infizieren. David (1927) fischte die anscheinend gesunden Tiere aus einem Teich ab, in dem sich infizierte Karpfen befunden hatten, und setzte sie in ein wasserdurchströmtes Aquarium ein. Innerhalb von 8 Monaten waren keine Krankheitszeichen festzustellen. Drei später zugesetzte gesunde *Zwergwelse* anderer Herkunft erkrankten. Bereits nach 5 Tagen zeigten sie Blutungen an den Flossen, später auch an den Seitenflächen. Sie lagen tagelang wie betäubt auf der Seite. Einer von drei verendete nach 10 Tagen, die beiden anderen, ebenfalls schwerkranken Welse wurden getötet. Durch den bakteriologischen Nachweis von V. piscium wurde dessen ätiologische Bedeutung gesichert. Die Untersuchung der als Überträger in Frage kommenden, anscheinend gesunden Fische zeigte, daß in allen Fällen V. piscium aus Galle gezüchtet werden konnte, während Herz, Milz und Niere steril waren. V. piscium var. japonicus war nach den Untersuchungen von Hoshina (1957) für *Aale* apathogen.

β) Frosch, Krebs

Auf die Empfänglichkeit von *Fröschen* für die Infektion mit V. piscium wurde David (1927) schon durch die Beobachtung hingewiesen, daß während eines Fischsterbens keine Frösche in dem den Weiher umgebenden Park zu finden waren, während sie zuvor dort massenhaft angetroffen worden waren. Nach experimenteller Infektion des dorsalen Lymphsacks waren die Frösche (Rana ridibunda und temporaria) nach 24 Std durch eine Gasansammlung immens aufgetrieben und starben innerhalb 4—10 Tagen. Der Sektionsbefund erbrachte eine Gastroenteritis mit Blutungen in den inneren Organen. Zu dem gleichen Ergebnis kamen bei der Gattung Rana temporaria auch Lagarde und Chakroun (1965) nach subcutaner Injektion des Erregers.

Mit V. anguillarum infizierte Bergman (1909) *Krebse* (Astacis fluviatilis Fabr.), indem er wenige Tropfen Kulturmaterial unter das Schildpatt in die Körperhöhle oder unter die Schale der Schwanzunterseite oder in eine Schere injizierte. Im ersten Experiment verendeten die Tiere nach 10—24 Std, im zweiten nach 36—44 und im dritten nach 42—48 Std. Die Muskulatur war an der Injektionsstelle meist gerötet und etwas ödematös. Die Vibrionen wurden im Muskelfleisch und Blut nachgewiesen.

c) Infektion mit V. ichthyodermis

Der von Hodgkiss und Shewan (1950) aus einer Scholle isolierte V. ichthyodermis war apathogen für Aale, während eine von vier intraperitoneal infizierten Forellen einging (Smith, 1961).

d) Andere Vibrionen

Bei einer Augenkrankheit der Dorsche (Gadus morrhua L.) konnte Bergman (1912) einen Vibrionenstamm isolieren, der sich von V. anguillarum durch fehlende Lactosespaltung unterschied. Bergman beschrieb das Krankheitsbild der natürlich infizierten Fische folgendermaßen:

„Das rechte Auge zeigte ein frühes Entwicklungsstadium der Krankheit. Das Auge hatte eine normale Größe und Form. Die nächste Umgebung war etwas ödematös und an einer Stelle hellrot. Die Cornea hatte eine milchweiße Farbe und war in ihrem peripheren Teil glatt und glänzend. Ein $1,5 \times 0,8$ cm großer Teil in der Mitte hatte eine unebene, fast wollige Oberfläche und ragte über den anderen Teil, von welchem er auch durch eine mehr oder weniger deutlich hervortretende Spalte getrennt war, hervor. Er hatte also den Charakter eines Sequesters."

Bei einem weiter fortgeschrittenen Krankheitszustand wurden die pathologisch-anatomischen Veränderungen wie folgt angegeben:

„Anstatt der Cornea fand sich ein großes rundes Loch mit einem dicken, grauen, zum Teil aus der Sclera, zum Teil aus Cornea-Resten gebildetem Rande. Aus dem Inneren des Auges ragte eine grau-schwarz-grün und blutrot marmorierte Gewebsmasse, deren Oberfläche in Zerfall begriffen war. Linse und Glaskörper fehlten. Von der Iris waren nur einige Reste vorhanden. Als der Bubulus enucleiert wurde, wurde Ödem in der Umgebung gefunden. Der Durchmesser des Bulbus hatte eine Länge, bedeutend unter der normalen, und zwar nur 8 mm."

Fisch

Infektionsmaterial waren wenige Tropfen einer mit physiologischer Kochsalzlösung abgeschwemmten, 2 Tage alten Vibrionen-Agar-Kultur (BERGMAN, 1912). Die Cornea derjenigen *Dorsche*, welche die Vibrionen in den Glaskörper injiziert erhielten, wurde schon am 2. Tag grau und undurchsichtig. Anschließend bildete sich ein Ödem, das mitunter zurückging, aber meist zum Zerfall der Cornea führte, bis schließlich die trübe Linse und der ganze zerstörte Glaskörper durch eine Perforation ausflossen. Das Hornhautepithel trübte sich 48 Std nach intracornealer Impfung. Dann wurde es durch Exsudat stark angespannt und von dem darunterliegenden, noch durchsichtigen Teil der Cornea abgehoben. Nach Resorption des Exsudates löste sich das Hornhautepithel. Meist setzte dann von außen nach innen fortschreitend ein Zerfall der Cornea ein, wodurch Linse und Glaskörper, die nicht getrübt waren, herausgedrängt wurden. Als unmittelbare Folge dieses Ereignisses trat eine Panophthalmie ein.

Subcutan infizierte *Aale* starben nach 4—16 Tagen. Bei den länger überlebenden Tieren entstanden an der Impfstelle, um den After und an den Flossen rotfleckige Efflorescenzen. Nach 8—10 Tagen war die Injektionsstelle geschwollen und fluktuierend; die Beule brach 12—16 Tage später auf. Die Muskulatur um das Ulcus war gerötet und ödematös. Bei der Obduktion wurden an dem parietalen Peritoneum rote Flecken beobachtet. Die Vibrionen konnten im Blut aller Tiere festgestellt werden.

Nach intraoculärer Injektion trat bei *Aalen* eine Schwellung und Trübung der Cornea mit Epitheldefekten auf, jedoch keine Perforation während 3wöchiger Beobachtungszeit.

Intraperitoneal infizierte *Plötzen* verendeten zwischen 2 und 10 Tagen. Der Sektionsbefund glich dem der mit V. anguillarum infizierten Aale. Intraoculär infizierte erkrankten innerhalb 8—24 Tagen meist an einer Panophthalmie, häufig mit Perforation der Cornea.

e) Infektion von Laboratoriumstieren

Für Kaltblüter pathogene Mikroorganismen verursachen beim Warmblüter meist keine Erkrankung. Ein wesentliches Kriterium für die Infektion, die Vermehrung, ist nicht erfüllt, da das Temperaturoptimum der Bakterien im Warmblüterorganismus erheblich überschritten wird. Falls dennoch Krankheitszeichen, wie Temperaturanstieg, festgestellt werden, oder die Tiere zugrunde gehen, ist eine Intoxikation in Erwägung zu ziehen. Die Infektion von *Meerschweinchen* mit V. anguillarum (BERGMAN, 1909) und V. piscium (DAVID, 1927) verlief nach subcutaner und intraperitonealer Injektion (auch bei Gabe „hoher Erregerdosen") ergebnislos. Die nach einem längeren Beobachtungszeitraum getöteten Tiere wiesen keine pathologisch-anatomischen Veränderungen auf. Auch ein auf die Bebrütungstemperatur von 30—34° C adaptierter V.-piscium-Stamm war für diese Versuchstiere nicht pathogen (David, 1927). Ergebnislos war auch die subcutane und intraperitoneale Infektion von *Kaninchen* mit V. anguillarum (Bergman, 1909). Nach Untersuchungen dieses Autors (1909, 1912) waren *weiße Mäuse* für eine orale Infektion mit V. anguillarum nicht empfänglich. Die intraperitoneale Injektion von 1 ml Kulturmaterial führte bei 2 Mäusen nach 14 bzw. 19 Std zum Tod. Auffällig waren ein rot verfärbtes Peritoneum und eine große, dunkelrote Milz. Bei der mikroskopischen Untersuchung wurden keine Bakterien im Blut oder in der Milz gesehen. Blutkulturen blieben steril. Aufgrund dieses Befundes vermutete Bergman (1912) zu Recht eine Intoxikation. Im Gegensatz dazu stehen die Befunde von Lagarde und Chakroun (1965), die weiße Mäuse intraperitoneal mit V. anguillarum infizierten und auf eine pathogene Wirkung schlossen, da die Tiere innerhalb 18—24 Std verendeten.

Die Verfütterung von infizierten, kurz zuvor verendeten Aalen an *weiße* und *graue Ratten* beeinträchtigte deren Wohlbefinden nicht (Schäperclaus, 1927). Ebensowenig reagierten *Hühner* auf eine subcutane oder intraperitoneale Infektion mit V. anguillarum (Bergman, 1909). *Tauben* zeigten nach intraperitonealer Injektion von V. anguillarum (Bergman, 1909) und nach intramuskulärer Injektion von V. piscium (David, 1927) bis auf einen vorübergehenden Schwächezustand keine Krankheitssymptome.

Klein (1905) injizierte den aus der Herzmuschel isolierten V. cardii (1 Öse Kulturmaterial einer 24—48 Std bebrüteten Vibrionenkultur) *Meerschweinchen* intraperitoneal. Sie starben innerhalb 20 Std; bei der Sektion waren Peritoneum und Darm stark gerötet und mit Ekchymosen besetzt. Die subcutane Injektion auch großer Erregermengen rief lediglich eine Schwellung an der Injektionsstelle hervor. Zu ähnlichen Ergebnissen kamen Remlinger und Nouri (1908 b), die aus Austern und Muscheln gezüchtete Vibrionen Meerschweinchen intraperitoneal injizierten. Bei diesem Experiment waren die Vibrionen aus dem Blut der Versuchstiere zu isolieren. Defressine und Cazeneuve (1914) konnten bei Meerschweinchen nach intraperitonealer Injektion aus Muscheln isolierter Vibrionen eine tödliche Erkrankung hervorrufen. Post mortem war der Erreger aus Gallenflüssigkeit nachzuweisen.

14. Aus anderen Tieren isolierte Vibrionen

a) Aerobe Vibrionen

Aus kranken und toten Raupen (Pyrausta nubialis Hübn.) wurde V. leonardi gezüchtet, der 1—2, mitunter auch 3 Geißeln aufweist (Métalnikov und Chorine, 1928) und folglich irrtümlich noch den Vibrionen zugerechnet wird (Bergey, 1957). Kleinste Erregerdosen, oral verabfolgt, genügten, um Raupen der Gattung Galleria tödlich zu infizieren; sie verendeten meist innerhalb 12—24 Std. Dieser Befund war Anlaß zu der Überlegung, diese Vibrionenart für die Bekämpfung von Raupenplagen einzusetzen. V. xenopus (Schrire und Greenfield, 1930) erwies sich für Meerschweinchen als nicht pathogen. Infizierte Frösche erlagen nur dann der Infektion, wenn zusammen mit den Vibrionen „Bacillus fulminans" intraperitoneal injiziert wurde. Zwei Meerschweinchen applizierte Deneke (1885) intraduodenal V. tyrogenus; sie erkrankten vorübergehend leicht, erholten sich jedoch sehr rasch wieder. Die von Koch (1885) oral infizierten Meerschweinchen zeigten Krankheitszeichen erst nach Alkali-Opium-Behandlung und Gabe großer Erregerdosen. Von 15 infizierten Tieren verendeten 3.

b) Mikroaerophile Vibrionen

Aufgrund des Rückganges der Geburtenrate in einer Antilopenherde auf 48 Kälber pro 100 Muttertiere (normal: 80—100 Kälber pro 100 Muttertiere) untersuchten TRUEBLOOD und POST (1959) bei Antilopen im 3. und 4. Trächtigkeitsmonat Blut, Uterusgeschabsel, Amnionflüssigkeit und Mageninhalt der Feten. Bei einem Großteil konnte V. fetus nachgewiesen werden. Bei trächtigen Tieren konnte allerdings nach oraler Gabe von 100 ml einer Aufschwemmung dieser Bakterien kein Abort ausgelöst werden.

Unter semiaeroben Bedingungen züchteten WINKENWERDER und BÖTTCHER (1965) aus dem Genitaltrakt von Stuten und Hengsten in 1,95% und aus dem Verdauungskanal in 4% Vibrionen. Die „Pferdevibrionen" waren serologisch von V. fetus, V. bubulus und V. coli abzugrenzen. Ein Zusammenhang zwischen dem Auftreten von Aborten bei Stuten und der Infektion mit diesem Mikroorganismus wurde nicht beobachtet. Die experimentelle Infektion von weißen Mäusen und 3 Wochen alten Küken war ergebnislos.

15. Die Wirkung von abgetöteten Vibrionen, bakterienfreien Filtraten und Zellextrakten auf Versuchstiere

Die Toxinpräparationen wurden meist in der gleichen Weise vorgenommen, wie für Choleravibrionen beschrieben (s. S. 110). Auch hier werden Antigenpräparationen verwirrend häufig als Toxine bezeichnet. Treffender sollte von der toxischen Wirkung eines Antigens gesprochen werden. Für NAG-Vibrionen liegen sehr wenige Untersuchungen vor. Sie beziehen sich auf die Wirkung des Endotoxins von V. metschnikovii und die des Hämolysins von V. parahaemolyticus. Im Vordergrund experimenteller Versuche steht bei den Mikroaerophilen V. fetus. Nur wenige Autoren beschäftigen sich mit der Fragestellung, ob V.-fetus-Toxine für Abort oder Infertilität verantwortlich sind, meist werden Antigenpräparationen auf ihre Tauglichkeit für die aktive Immunisierung von Rindern und Schafen untersucht (MILLER und JENSEN, 1961, 1963; MILLER et al., 1964; OSBORNE, 1965; CLARK et al., 1968; CLARK et al., 1970; MYERS et al., 1970; MEINERSHAGEN et al., 1971).

a) Aerobe Vibrionen

Die zuerst von FUJINO et al. (1951) beschriebene hämolytische Aktivität von V. parahaemolyticus wurde von KATO et al. (1966), SAKAZAKI et al. (1968) und ZEN-YOJI et al. (1971) weiter untersucht. Das Hämolysin ist ein thermostabiler Eiweißkörper, ohne Kohlenhydrat- und Lipidkomponenten, der keinen organischen Phosphor gebunden hat (KATO et al., 1966; ZEN-YOJI et al., 1971). Es ist offenbar an den Standort der Bakterienstämme gebunden, da 96,5% der aus dem Menschen isolierten Stämme Hämolyse zeigen, während dies bei 99% der aus Seewasser oder Seefischen isolierten nicht der Fall ist (SAKAZAKI et al., 1968). Das Protein besitzt eine starke hämolytische Wirkung für Erythrocyten von Ratte, Hund, Maus und Affe, eine mäßige für die von Mensch, Kaninchen, Meerschweinchen und Huhn, eine geringe für die von Schafen und keine für die von Pferden (ZEN-YOJI et al., 1971).

Die DLM für die 20 g schweren Mäuse wurde als Stickstoffgehalt des Proteins angegeben und betrug 0,62 mg (ZEN-YOJI et al., 1971).

Die Kulturabschwemmung von V. metschnikovii wurde von FUKUHARA und ANDO (1913) in unterschiedlicher Weise behandelt. Erstens wurde die Suspension 1 Std auf 60° C oder 10 min auf 100° C erhitzt; zweitens wurde sie zentrifugiert und der Überstand sowie das mit physiologischer Kochsalzlösung gewaschene und anschließend zerriebene Sediment nach Erhitzen untersucht. Die Dosis letalis der auf 60° C erhitzten Bakterien betrug nach intravenöser Injektion für *Kaninchen* $^1/_{10}$ Kulturabschwemmung/kg Körpergewicht. Die gleiche DL wurde für den auf 60° C und 100° C erhitzten Überstand der Suspension ermittelt, während vom Bakterienrückstand $^1/_5$ Kulturabschwemmung (60° C) bzw. $^2/_5$ (100° C) erforderlich waren. Bei der Obduktion wurden die inneren Organe hyperämisch angetroffen, die Milz war vergrößert; Leber und Milz zeigten eine parenchymatöse Degeneration. Die DL für *Meerschweinchen* betrug nach intraperitonealer Injektion der abgetöteten Bakterien $^1/_2$, für das Sediment (60° C) 4 und für den Überstand (60° C) 2 Kulturabschwemmungen. Der Obduktionsbefund war ähnlich dem der Kaninchen, hinzu kamen Blutungen in der Lunge. Von Leitch (1965) wurde mitgeteilt, daß nach Injektion von 2 mg des Zellwandlysates von NAG X_{45}-Vibrio in ein abgebundenes Dünndarmsegment des Kaninchens eine Flüssigkeitsansammlung und Hyperämie zu beobachten war.

b) Mikroaerophile Vibrionen

α) Rind und Schaf

Durch Inseminationsversuche konnten Lawson und MacKinnon (1952) zeigen, daß das die Unfruchtbarkeit auslösende Agens von V. fetus nicht filtrierbar ist. Infizierter Bullensamen wurde über Seitz-E.-K.-Filter gegeben und das Filtrat mit 1 ml bakteriologisch einwandfreiem Samen vermischt. Die Trächtigkeitsrate der artifiziell befruchteten Färsen war normal. Den Überstand einer flüssigen V.-fetus-Bouillonkultur injizierten Osborne und Smibert (1962) 1—6 Monate alten Kälbern und 3—12 Jahre alten Kühen intravenös. Bei allen Tieren wurden die klinischen Symptome eines anaphylaktischen Schocks festgestellt, dessen Verlauf dosisabhängig war. 1 ml/22,6 kg Körpergewicht war die Dosis letalis für 136,6 kg schwere Kälber. Nach intracutaner Injektion in die Haut des Halses entwickelte sich nach 1—2 Std ein Erythem. In einer späteren Untersuchung (Osborne und Smibert, 1964) wurden die Vibrionen bei 18000 × g niedergeschlagen und der Überstand über Milliporefilter (0,22 μm) gegeben. Die Injektion von 4 ml Ultrafiltrat rief bei 2—4 Monate alten Kälbern einen schweren, zum Teil irreversiblen Schock, eine 2. Injektion, die 3—7 Tage später vorgenommen wurde, einen leichten Schock hervor. Die ersten Symptome traten 11 min nach der Injektion auf; die Kälber röchelten intermittierend oder kontinuierlich. Anschließend setzte eine Hyperventilation ein. Beim reversiblen Schock waren 2 Fiebergipfel, $^1/_2$ Std und 3 Std nach der Toxingabe, festzustellen. Die Kälber mit schwerem oder irreversiblem Schock röchelten dauernd mit offenem Maul, die Ohren hingen herunter, der Nacken war nach vorne gestreckt. Von den Lippen tropfte Speichel, der bisweilen mit Blut tingiert war; Harn und Stuhl gingen ab. Im irreversiblen Schockzustand wurden eine extreme Anoxie, Atemschwäche und Sichaufbäumen beobachtet.

Histopathologisch schienen besonders die kleinen Blutgefäße betroffen, in denen Stase, Thrombosen und Embolien zu beobachten waren. Als Folge einer erhöhten Capillarpermeabilität traten Ödeme auf (Osborne, 1965). Estes et al. (1966) fanden nach intrauteriner Gabe von V.-fetus-Endotoxin, Zellwandfraktion und intracellulärer Substanz bei jeweils 5 Färsen keine pathologisch-anatomischen Veränderungen des Organs.

An trächtige *Schafe* verfütterten erstmals MacFadyean und Stockman (1913) das Ultrafiltrat von infiziertem Lammgewebe. Sie konnten dadurch keinen Abort auslösen. Im Gegensatz dazu stehen die Ergebnisse von Jensen et al. (1957): Nach Gabe von 50 ml Ultrafiltrat von infiziertem Gewebe trat bei 3 Schafen Abort auf.

Die intravenöse Injektion von 1 und 1,5 ml zellfreiem Überstand einer V.-fetus-Kultur verursachte bei 2 trächtigen Schafen nach 15—18 min einen schweren anaphylaktischen Schock (Osborne und Smibert, 1964). Das Mutterschaf, welches 1,5 ml erhalten hatte, verwarf 3 Tage später. Das andere Tier abortierte nicht und wurde nach 21 Tagen getötet. In dem normalen graviden Uterus wurde ein regelrecht entwickelter lebender Fetus vorgefunden.

β) Kleine Laboratoriumstiere

Die Toxicität und Pyrogenität des durch Phenol-Wasser-Extraktion gewonnenen Lipopolysaccharids von V. fetus wurde durch 5minütiges Erhitzen auf 80° C gesteigert (Dennis, 1959). Die DL des nicht erhitzten Toxins betrug für *Kaninchen* nach intravenöser Injektion 400 mcg/kg und verminderte sich für das erhitzte auf 40 mcg/kg. Mit Fieberanstieg um 1,5—4° C reagierten sie nach intravenöser Injektion von 4 mcg unbehandelten Toxins/kg, während für das erhitzte nur 0,005 mcg/kg erforderlich waren. Die Temperatur stieg während der ersten Stunde rasch an, erreichte das Maximum nach 3 und die Norm wieder nach 24 Std. Winter (1966) dagegen beschrieb den Temperaturverlauf nach intravenöser Injektion von 10 mcg Lipopolysaccharid bei zwei 3,3 bzw. 3,5 kg schweren Kaninchen als biphasisch; das erste Maximum wurde nach 1,5, das zweite nach 3,5 Std erreicht. Ein anaphylaktischer Schock wurde nach Injektion von 100 mcg Endotoxin nicht beobachtet, während ein Kaninchen nach 2maliger Injektion von je 1 mg 24 Std nach der letzten Toxingabe verendete. Bei der Obduktion wirkte die Cortex der Nieren durch abwechselnd rote und blasse Areale gesprenkelt. Die histologische Untersuchung zeigte fibrinoide Thromben in den meisten Glomeruli und in anderen inneren Organen.

In einigen anderen Experimenten wurde die hypersensitive Wirkung des Toxins durch intracutane Injektion untersucht. Ristic et al. (1955) injizierten *Hamstern*, die mit V. fetus infiziert waren, teils durch Formalin, teils durch Hitze abgetötete Vibrionen. Mit beiden Präparaten wurde eine Hautreaktion ausgelöst, die nach 10 Std sichtbar wurde und ein Maximum zwischen 24 und 48 Std erreichte. Das Erythem hatte einen Durchmesser von 5—8 mm und eine zentrale Nekrose. Bei 4 von 24 nicht infizierten Kontrolltieren wurde gleichfalls eine Hautreaktion festgestellt.

Nach der Injektion von 0,1 ml der wäßrigen Phase einer Phenol-Wasser-Extraktion von V.-fetus-Kultur in die Haut von *Kaninchen* entwickelte sich ebenfalls nach 48 Std ein Erythem (Winter und Dunne, 1962). In einer späteren Untersuchung injizierte Winter (1966) 10 mcg Lipopolysaccharid. 4 Std später war die Injektionsstelle erythematös. Nach 24 Std war das Erythem bei einem Tier verschwunden, bei einem anderen hatte es noch einen Durchmesser von 10 mm.

Mäuse reagierten nach den Untersuchungen von Dennis (1959) auf das Lipopolysaccharid weniger empfindlich als Kaninchen. Die DL betrug annähernd 2 mg. Winter und Dunne (1962) gaben als DL 50 für 23—28 g schwere Mäuse 0,04—0,05 ml der wäßrigen Phase einer Phenol-Wasser-Extraktion an. Nach intraperitonealer Injektion wurden die Mäuse dyspnoisch und teilnahmslos. 4—6 Std später stellte sich eine Paralyse ein. Im allgemeinen verendeten sie innerhalb 24 Std. Für 13—15 g schwere weiße Mäuse war die DL 50 0,38 mg Lipopolysaccharid (Winter, 1966).

16. Tierexperimente mit V. massauah

Auch nachdem der Erreger der Cholera bekannt und seine Züchtung auf festen Nährböden möglich war, wurden Tierexperimente mit Bakterien durchgeführt, die beim Menschen ein der Cholera ähnliches Krankheitsbild verursacht hatten. Sie wurden wiederholt für Choleraerreger gehalten.

Als Beispiel sei V. massauah angeführt. Dieser Stamm wurde wegen seiner Virulenz für Versuchstiere in verschiedenen Laboratorien verwendet. Die Untersuchungen wurden in dem Glauben durchgeführt, daß er mit V. cholerae identisch sei, obwohl nach Pfeiffer (1892) bereits Koch geäußert habe, daß es sich bei V. massauah nicht um den Erreger der Cholera handle. Die nach Infektion von Versuchstieren beobachteten klinischen Symptome und der Sektionsbefund wurden als typisch für eine experimentelle Cholera erachtet. Auffallend war jedoch, daß Massauah-Vibrionen früher als Cholera-Vibrionen zur Bakteriämie führten. Einer oralen Gabe erlagen *Meerschweinchen* nach Vorbehandlung gewöhnlich innerhalb 1—3 Tagen (Brieger et al., 1892; Vincenzi, 1892; Metschnikoff, 1894). Nach intraperitonealer Injektion starben sie meist innerhalb 20 Std (Neisser, 1893). Das Krankheitsbild wurde als dem Stadium algidum der menschlichen Cholera sehr ähnlich beschrieben (Pfeiffer, 1892). Die ersten Symptome traten $1^1/_2$—2 Std nach der Infektion auf: Die Tiere wurden teilnahmslos, frühzeitig war eine Muskelschwäche bemerkbar. Die Körpertemperatur sank bisweilen unter 30° C ab. Die hinteren Extremitäten zeigten Lähmungen; das Abdomen war stark aufgetrieben. Die Meerschweinchen verendeten innerhalb 24 Std im Kreislaufkollaps. Bei der Obduktion wurde ein für „Cholera" charakteristischer Befund erhoben (Brieger et al., 1892; Pfeiffer, 1892; Neisser, 1893).

Die subcutane Injektion von V. massauah rief bei Meerschweinchen ein „kolossales" Ödem hervor; die Tiere verendeten nach 20—30 Std. Aus Blut und Darmproben konnten die Erreger gezüchtet werden (Vincenzi, 1892). Metschnikoff (1894) konnte bei *Kaninchen* nach oraler Gabe von V. massauah ein der Cholera ähnliches Krankheitsbild erzeugen.

Auch andere Tiere wurden in die experimentellen Untersuchungen mit V. massauah einbezogen, so *Mäuse* (Vincenzi, 1892; Metchnikoff, 1894), *Katzen* (Metchnikoff, 1894; Karlinski, 1896), *Hunde* (Emmerich und Tsuboi, 1893) sowie *Tauben* (Vincenzi, 1892). Hervorgehoben seien schließlich die Befunde von Emmerich und Tsuboi (1893), die bei oraler Gabe von Nitraten und Vibrionen sowie in Nitratbouillonkulturen eine außerordentlich rasche Reduktion zu Nitriten feststellten. Dadurch kam es bei Hunden zu hochgradiger Cyanose, Beschleunigung der Respiration und, wie spektroskopisch nachgewiesen werden konnte, zur Bildung von Methämoglobin.

Literatur

Abdallah, I. S., Winkenwerder, W.: Haussperlinge (Passer domesticus L.) als Überträger von Vibrionen. Zbl. Vet.-Med. B **13**, 338 (1966).

Abraham, K. C.: The viability of Vibrio cholerae in the clam (Meretrix casta). Indian J. med. Res. **42**, 491 (1954).

Acton, M. W., Chopra, R. N.: The nature and pharmacological action of cholera toxin. Indian J. med. Res. **12**, 235 (1924).

Al-Awqati, Q., Garcia-Bunuel, R., Field, M., Greenough, W. B. III.: The influence of structural abnormality on ion transport in rabbit ileum. Proc. Soc. exp. Biol. (N.Y.) **135**, 598 (1970).

Aldova, E., Zakhariev, Z. A., Dinev, T. S., Zlatanov, Z. T.: Vibrio parahaemolyticus im Schwarzen Meer. Zbl. Bakt., I. Abt. Orig. **218**, 176 (1971).

Andu, A. B., Niekerk, J. van: Choleratoxine I. Zbl. Bakt., I. Abt. Orig. **112**, 519 (1929).

Anonym: The pathogenicity of Vibrio fetus. Vet. Rec. **70**, 393 (1958).

Arnold, L., Shapiro: An experimental study of host susceptibility to cholera. Indian med. Gaz. **65**, 496 (1930).

Aziz, K. M. S., Mohsin, A. K. M., Hare, W. K., Phillips, R. A.: Using the rat as a cholera "model". Nature (Lond.) **220**, 814 (1968).

BADER, R.-E.: Bakterien als Krankheitserreger. In: Handbuch der allgemeinen Pathologie, Bd. XI, Teil 2, S. 172, hrsg. von F. BÜCHNER, E. LETTERER, F. ROULET. Berlin-Heidelberg-New York: Springer 1965.

BADER, R.-E.: Isolierung von Vibrionen der Heiberg-Gruppe II bei einer Durchfallerkrankung. Münch. med. Wschr. 114, 914 (1972).

BADER, R.-E., WINKLER, H., MARGET, W.: Vibrio fetus als Erreger einer Säuglingsmeningitis. Zbl. Bakt., I. Abt. Orig. 199, 202 (1966).

BAERTHLEIN: Ueber choleraähnliche Vibrionen. Zbl. Bakt., I. Abt. Orig. 67, 321 (1913).

BAGGE, J., BAGGE, O.: Vibrio anguillarum som årsag til ulcussygdom hos torsk (Gadus callarias, Linné). Nord. Vet.-Med. 8, 481 (1956).

BALLMOOS, P. v.: Über die Vibrionen-Dysenterie des Schweines. Inaug.-Diss. (Bern 1950).

BARONI, V., CEAPARU, V.: Elimination des vibrions cholériques introduits dans le sang des lapins adultes. C. R. Soc. Biol. (Paris) 72, 894 (1912).

BAROSS, J., LISTON, J.: Occurrence of Vibrio parahaemolyticus and related hemolytic vibrios in marine environments of Washington State. Appl. Microbiol. 20, 179 (1970).

BARTLEY, C. H., SLANETZ, L. W.: Occurrence of Vibrio parahaemolyticus in estuarine waters and oysters of New Hampshire. Appl. Microbiol. 21, 965 (1971).

BASU, S., PICKETT, M. J.: Reaction of Vibrio cholerae and choleragenic toxin in ileal loop of laboratory animals. J. Bact. 100, 1142 (1969).

BASU MALLIK, K. C., GANGULI, N. C.: Some observations on the pathogenesis of cholera. Indian J. med. Res. 52, 894 (1964).

BAUMGARTEN, W.: Die intraperitoneale Cholerainfektion und der Pfeiffersche Versuch bei der Maus. Z. Hyg. Infekt.-Kr. 93, 87 (1921).

BEAUDETTE, F. R., HUDSON, C. B.: Zit. nach TUDOR, D. C. (1954).

BEERENS, H., ALADAME, N.: Recherches sur Vibrio crassus (Veillon et Repaci) Prévot 1940. Ann. Inst. Pasteur 75, 391 (1948).

BERG, R. L., JUTILA, J. W., FIREHAMMER, B. D.: A revised classification of Vibrio fetus. Amer. J. vet. Res. 32, 11 (1971).

BERGEY's manual of determinative bacteriology, ed. by R. S. BREED, E. G. D. MURRAY, and N. R. SMITH. Baltimore: Williams & Wilkins Co. 1957.

BERGMAN, A. M.: Die rote Beulenkrankheit des Aals. Ber. a. d. Kgl. Bayer. Biol. Versuchsstat. München 2, 10 (1909).

BERGMAN, A. M.: Eine ansteckende Augenkrankheit, Keratomalacie, bei Dorschen an der Südküste Schwedens. Zbl. Bakt., I. Abt. Orig. 62, 200 (1912).

BERNARD, P. N., GALLUT, J.: Sur un mode de préparation de la toxine cholérique. C. R. Soc. Biol. (Paris) 137, 10 (1943a).

BERNARD, P. N., GALLUT, J.: Conditions favorables à la production de la toxine cholérique. C. R. Soc. Biol. (Paris) 137, 11 (1943b).

BEZZOLA, C.: Contribution à la connaissance des modifications de la résistance des animaux vis-à-vis des microorganismes pathogènes. II. Choléra. Zbl. Bakt., I. Abt. Orig. 61, 133 (1912).

BHAT, J. V., BARKER, H. A.: Studies on a new oxalate-decomposing bacterium, Vibrio oxaliticus. J. Bact. 55, 359 (1948).

BHATIA, R. Y. P., BHATIA, A. L., THOMAS, A. K.: Isolation and concentration of V. cholerae toxin and study of its effect on skin permeability in guinea-pigs. Indian. J. med. Res. 57, 2018 (1969).

BISPING, W., FREITAG, U., KRAUSS, H.: Feststellung der Vibrionenhepatitis der Hühner in Nordwestdeutschland. Berl. Münch. tierärztl. Wschr. 76, 456 (1963).

BISPING, W., LANGENEGGER, J., WINKENWERDER, W.: Nachweis und Vorkommen der Vibrio-fetus-Infektion beim Bullen in Nordwestdeutschland und Vorschläge zu deren Bekämpfung. Dtsch. tierärztl. Wschr. 71, 285 (1964).

BLASIUS, C., ULLMANN, U., ACHINGER, R.: Vibrio-fetus-Sepsis bei Thrombophlebitis. Zbl. Bakt., I. Abt. Orig. 214, 17 (1970).

BOCKEMÜHL, J.: Isolierung und Identifizierung von Cholera-Vibrionen. Zbl. Bakt., I. Abt. Orig. 218, 251 (1971).

BOIVIN, A., MESROBEANU, I., MESROBEANU, L., NESTORESCU, B.: Extraction d'un complexe polysaccharidique toxique et antigénique, a partir de diverses bactéries autres, que le bacille d'Aertrycke. C. R. Soc. Biol. (Paris) 115, 306 (1934).

BOLEY, L. E., WOODS, G. T., HATCH, R. D., GRAHAM, R.: Studies on porcine enteritis. II. Experimental therapy with sulfathalidine, sulfamethazine, sodium arsanilate, and bacitracin in a natural outbreak of swine dysentry. Cornell Vet. 41, 231 (1951).

BRIEGER, L., KITASATO, S., WASSERMANN, A.: Über Immunität und Giftfestigung. Z. Hyg. Infekt.-Kr. 12, 137 (1892).

BRIX: Über einen neuen Vibrio aus Sputum. Hyg. Rundschau 4, 913 (1894).

BRYANS, J. T., SHEPHARD, B. P.: Isolation of Vibrio fetus from the feces of lambs and pen-contact transmission of the infection. Cornell Vet. 51, 376 (1961).

Bryner, J. H., Estes, P. C., Foley, J. W., O'Berry, P. A.: Infectivity of three Vibrio fetus biotypes for gallbladder and intestines of cattle, sheep, rabbits, guinea pigs, and mice. Amer. J. vet. Res. **32**, 465 (1971).

Bryner, J. H., Frank, A. H.: A preliminary report on the identification of Vibrio fetus. Amer. J. vet. Res. **16**, 76 (1955).

Bu, A. I., Garm, O., Lindqvist, K., Skjerven, O.: Podningsforsøk på sau med bovine Vibrio fetus-stammer. Nord. Vet.-Med. **7**, 948 (1955).

Buchanan, R. E., Holt, J. G., Lessel, E. F.: Index Bergeyana. An annotated alphabetic listing of names of the taxa of the bacteria. Baltimore: Williams & Wilkins Co. 1966.

Bürgers, T.: Über das Choleragift. Verhandlungen der Gesellschaft deutscher Naturforscher und Ärzte 82. Versammlung zu Königsberg 20.—26. 9. 1910, zweiter Teil, 2. Hälfte Mediz. Abt. (1911).

Bujwid, O.: Neue Methode zum Diagnosticiren und Isoliren der Cholerabakterien. Cbl. Bakt. **4**, 494 (1888).

Bundesseuchengesetz: Gesetz zur Verhütung und Bekämpfung übertragbarer Krankheiten beim Menschen v. 18. 7. 1961 (BGBl. I S. 1012 bzw. Berichtigung des BSG v. 18. 7. 1961).

Burrows, W.: Cholera vibrio toxicities. In: Proc. Cholera Res. Symp., Honolulu (1965), p. 120. Publ. Hlth. Serv. (Wash.) Publ. No. 1328.

Burrows, W., Deupree, N. G., Moore, D. E.: The effect of X-irradiation on fecal and urinary antibody response. J. infect. Dis. **87**, 169 (1950).

Burrows, W., Elliott, M. E., Havens, I.: Studies on immunity to Asiatic cholera. IV. The excretion of coproantibody in experimental enteric cholera in the guinea pig. J. infect. Dis. **81**, 261 (1947).

Burrows, W., Musteikis, G. M., Oza, N. B., Dutta, N. K.: Cholera toxins: Quantitation of the frog skin reaction and its relation to experimental enteric toxicity. J. infect. Dis. **115**, 1 (1965).

Burrows, W., Wagner, S. M., Mather, A. N.: The endotoxin of the cholera vibrio: action on living semipermeable membranes. Proc. Soc. exp. Biol. (N.Y.) **57**, 311 (1944).

Calvano, U.: Il colera sperimentale nel coniglio. G. Batt. Immun. **11**, 264 (1933). Zit. nach Pollitzer (1959).

Canestrini, G.: La malattia dominante delle anguille. Atti del R. Inst. Veneto di Scienze **4**, Ser. 7 (1892). Zit. nach Bergmann (1909).

Cano, U.: Ueber die Wanderung des Choleravibrios im Körper des befallenen Tieres. Zbl. Bakt., I. Abt. Orig. **72**, 124 (1914).

Cano, U., Martinez, G.: Einfluß der Wasserfauna auf Choleravibrionen. Zbl. Bakt., I. Abt. Orig. **67**, 431 (1913).

Cantacuzene, J., Marie, A.: Choléra gastro-intestinal expérimental chez le cobaye. C. R. Soc. Biol. (Paris) **76**, 307 (1914).

Cantani, A.: I. Giftigkeit der Cholerabacillen. Dtsch. med. Wschr. **12**, 789 (1886).

Cao, G.: Über den Durchtritt von Mikroorganismen durch den Darm einiger Insekten. L'Ufficiale Sanitario Anno **11** (1898), ref. Zbl. Bakt., I. Abt. **26**, 456 (1899).

Caselitz, F. H.: Laboratoriumsdiagnose der Cholera. Z. Tropenmed. Parasit. **11**, 109 (1960).

Chalmers, A. J., Waterfield, N. E.: Paracholera caused by Vibrio gindha Pfeiffer 1896. J. trop. Med. Hyg. **19**, 165 (1916).

Chowdhury, T. K., Snell, F. M.: A microelectrode study of electrical potentials in frog skin and toad bladder. Biochim. biophys. Acta (Amst.) **94**, 461 (1965).

Cicconardi: Zit. nach Galeotti, G. (1913).

Clark, B. L., Dufty, J. H., Monsbourgh, M. J.: Experimental Vibrio fetus (venerealis) infection in heifers. The immunising properties of killed organisms injected subcutaneously. Aust. vet. J. **44**, 110 (1968).

Clark, B. L., Dufty, J. H., Monsbourgh, M. J.: Observations on the isolation of Vibrio fetus (venerealis) from the vaginal mucus of experimentally infected heifers. Aust. vet. J. **45**, 209 (1969).

Clark, B. L., Dufty, J. H., Monsbourgh, M. J.: Vaccination of heifers with Vibrio fetus (intestinal type) against infection with Vibrio fetus (genital type). J. comp. Path. **80**, 47 (1970).

Cohendy, Wollman, E.: Quelques résultats acquis par la méthode des élevages aseptiques. I. Scorbut expérimental. II. Infection cholérique du cobaye aseptique. C. R. Acad. Sci. (Paris) **174**, 1082 (1922).

Coleman, W. H., Kaur, J., Iwert, M. E., Kasai, G. J., Burrows, W.: Cholera toxins: Purification and preliminary characterization of ileal loop reactive type 2 toxin. J. Bact. **96**, 1137 (1968).

Craig, J. O.: The effect of cholera stool and culture filtrates on the skin of guinea pigs and rabbits. In: Proc. Cholera Res. Symp., Honolulu (1965a), p. 153. Publ. Hlth. Serv. (Wash.) Publ. No 1328.

CRAIG, J. P.: A permeability factor (toxin) found in cholera stools and culture filtrates and its neutralization by convalescent cholera sera. Nature (Lond.) **207**, 614 (1965 b).

CRAIG, J. P.: Preparation of the vascular permeability factor of Vibrio cholerae. J. Bact. **92**, 793 (1966).

CRAIG, TH. C.: The transmission of the cholera spirillum by the alimentary contents and intestinal dejecta of the common house-fly. Med. Rec. (N.Y.) **46**, 38 (1894).

CRENDIROPOULO, M.: Assainissement général, prophylaxie. Rapport concernant des expériences sur les porteurs de vibrions cholériques. Bull. off. int. Hyg. publ. **13**, 247 (1921).

CUMMINS, J. T., VAUGHAN, B. E.: Relation of sodium to the bioelectric parameters of rat stomach. Nature (Lond.) **198**, 1197 (1963).

CUMMINS, J. T., VAUGHAN, B. E.: Ionic relationships of the bioelectrogenic mechanism in isolated rat stomach. Biochim. biophys. Acta (Amst.) **94**, 280 (1965).

CUNNINGHAM, D. D.: On the effects sometimes following injection of choleraic comma-bacilli into the subcutaneous tissues in guinea-pigs. In: Sci. memoirs of the med. officers of India, Calcutta **2**, 1 (1886).

CURRAN, P. F.: Na, Cl, and water transport by rat ileum in vitro. J. gen. Physiol. **43**, 1137 (1960).

CURRAN, P. F., SCHWARTZ, G. F.: Na, Cl, and water transport by rat colon. J. gen. Physiol. **43**, 555 (1960).

CURTIS, A. H.: A motile curved anaerobic bacillus in uterine discharges. J. infect. Dis. **12**, 165 (1913).

DAVID, H.: Über eine durch choleraähnliche Vibrionen hervorgerufene Fischseuche. Zbl. Bakt., I. Abt. Orig. **102**, 46 (1927).

DE, S. N.: Enterotoxicity of bacteria-free culture-filtrate of Vibrio cholerae. Nature (Lond.) **183**, 1533 (1959).

DE, S. N., BHATTACHARYA, K., ROYCHANDHURY, P. K.: The haemolytic activities of Vibrio cholerae and related vibrios. J. Bact. **67**, 117 (1954).

DE, S. N., CHATTERJE, D. N.: An experimental study of the mechanism of action of Vibrio cholerae on the intestinal mucous membrane. J. Path. Bact. **66**, 559 (1953).

DE, S. N., GHOSE, M. L., CHANDRA, J.: Further observations on cholera enterotoxin. Trans. roy. Soc. trop. Med. Hyg. **56**, 241 (1962).

DE, S. N., GHOSE, M. L., SEN, A.: Activities of bacteria-free preparations from Vibrio cholerae. J. Path. Bact. **79**, 373 (1960).

DE, S. N., SARKAR, J. K., TRIBEDI, B. P.: An experimental study of the action of cholera toxin. J. Path. Bact. **63**, 707 (1951).

DEFRESSINE, C., CAZENEUVE, H.: Vibrions cholériques et paracholériques. Vibrions des moules des pares de Brégaillon. Arch. Méd. Pharm. nav. **101**, 46, 103 (1914). Zit. nach CHALMERS und WATERFIELD (1916).

DEMETRESCU, C. A.: Action des endotoxines typhique et cholérique sur les capsules surrénales. C. R. Soc. Biol. (Paris) **77**, 591 (1915).

DENEKE, TH.: Über eine neue den Choleraspirillen ähnliche Spaltpilzart. Dtsch. med. Wschr. **11**, 33 (1885).

DENNIS, S. M.: Isolation of a lipopolysaccharide from Vibrio fetus. Nature (Lond.) **183**, 186 (1959).

DENYS, SLUYTS: La cellule vol. 10. Zit. nach KLEMPERER (1894 a, b).

DIATROPTOFF, P.: Zur Frage über die Bacteriologie der Cholera. Dtsch. med. Wschr. **20**, 691 (1894).

DIEUDONNE, A.: Blutalkaliagar, ein Elektivnährboden für Choleravibrionen. Zbl. Bakt., I. Abt. Orig. **50**, 107 (1909).

DOYEN, E.: Recherches anatomiques et expérimentales sur le choléra epidémique. Arch. Phys. Path., troisième série **6**, 179 (1885).

DOYLE, L. P.: A vibrio associated with swine dysentery. Amer. J. vet. Res. **5**, 3 (1944).

DOYLE, L. P.: The etiology of swine dysentery. Amer. J. vet. Res. **9**, 50 (1948).

DOZSA, L.: The effect of Vibrio bubulus on the bovine endometrium. J. Amer. vet. med. Ass. **147**, 620 (1965).

DUFTY, J. H.: Diagnosis of vibriosis in the bull. Aust. vet. J. **43**, 433 (1967).

DUNBAR: Zur Differentialdiagnose zwischen den Choleravibrionen und anderen denselben nahestehenden Vibrionen. Z. Hyg. Infekt.-Kr. **21**, 295 (1896).

DUTTA, N. K., HABBU, M. K.: Experimental cholera in infant rabbits: A method for chemotherapeutic investigation. Brit. J. Pharmacol. **10**, 153 (1955).

DUTTA, N. K., OZA, N. B.: The effect of gastrointestinal enzymes on cholera toxin. Bull. Wld Hlth Org. **28**, 307 (1963).

DUTTA, N. K., PANSE, M. V.: An experimental study usefulness on the of bacteriophage in the prophylaxis and treatment of cholera. Bull. Wld Hlth Org. **28**, 357 (1963).

DUTTA, N. K., PANSE, M. V., KULKARNI, D. R.: Role of cholera toxin in experimental cholera. J. Bact. **78**, 594 (1959).

Emmerich, R., Tsuboi, J.: Ist die Nitritbildung der Cholerabacillen von wesentlicher Bedeutung für das Zustandekommen der Cholera? Eine Widerlegung der Einwendungen G. Klemperer's in der Berliner klinischen Wochenschrift No. 31. Münch. med. Wschr. 40, 602 (1893).

Ermengem, C. van: IV. Recherches sur le bacille-virgule du choléra asiatique. Conclusions principales du travail présenté à la Société Belge de Microscopie dans sa séance de 26 octobre 1884. Dtsch. med. Wschr. 10, 749 (1884). Ref. von Gaffky.

Ermengem, C. van: Recherches sur le microbe du choléra asiatique. (Bruxelles 1885.) Zit. nach Scholl, H. (1892).

Estes, P. C., Bryner, J. H., O'Berry, P. A.: Histopathology of bovine vibriosis and the effects of Vibrio fetus extracts on the female genital tract. Cornell Vet. 56, 610 (1966).

Feeley, J. C.: Passive protective activity of antisera in infant rabbits infected orally with Vibrio cholerae. In: Proc. Cholera Res. Symp., Honolulu (1965), p. 231. Publ. Hlth. Serv. (Wash.) Publ. No 1328.

Felsenfeld, O.: A review of recent trends in cholera research and control. Bull. Wld Hlth Org. 34, 161 (1966).

Finkelstein, R. A.: Observations on the nature and mode of action of the choleragenic product(s) of cholera vibrios. In: Proc. Cholera Res. Symp., Honolulu (1965), p. 264. Publ. Hlth. Serv. (Wash.) Publ. No 1328.

Finkelstein, R. A.: Preselection of hemolytic variants of El Tor Vibrios. J. Bact. 92, 513 (1966).

Finkelstein, R. A., Norris, H. Th., Dutta, N. K.: Pathogenesis of experimental cholera in infant rabbits. I. Observations on the intraintestinal infection and experimental cholera produced with cell-free products. J. infect. Dis. 114, 203 (1964).

Finkelstein, R. A., Ransom, J. P.: Non-specific resistance to experimental cholera in embryonated eggs. J. exp. Med. 112, 315 (1960).

Finkler: Ueber den Bacillus der Cholera nostras und seine Cultur. Dtsch. med. Wschr. 10, 632 (1884).

Finkler, Prior: Forschungen über Cholerabacterien. Cbl. f. allg. Gesundheitspflege, Bd. I, H. 5 u. 6 (1885). Zit. nach Tizzoni und Cattani (1888).

Firehammer, B. D., Marsh, H., Tunnicliff, E. A.: The role of the ram in vibriosis of sheep. Amer. J. vet. Res. 17, 573 (1956).

Florent, A.: Isolement d'un vibrion saprophyte du sperme du taureau et du vagin de la vache (Vibrio bubulus). C. R. Soc. Biol. (Paris) 147, 2066 (1953).

Florent, A.: Méthode d'isolement de Vibrio foetus à partir d'échantillons polymicrobiens, spécialement du liquide préputial. Milieu sélectif „coeur-sang-gélose au vert brillant" en microaérobiose. C. R. Soc. Biol. (Paris) 150, 1059 (1956).

Florent, A.: Analogies entre certaines souches de Vibrio coli et certaines souches de Vibrio foetus. Adaption des premières à l'intestin de la bête bovine. C. R. Soc. Biol. (Paris) 151, 1055 (1957).

Florent, A.: Les deux vibrioses genitales de la bête bovine: La vibriose vénérienne, due à V. foetus venerialis, et la vibriose d'origine intestinale due à V. foetus intestinalis. Proc. XVIth Int. Vet. Congr. (Madrid) 2, 489 (1959).

Formal, S. B., Kundel, D., Schneider, H., Kunev, N., Sprinz, H.: Studies with Vibrio cholerae in the ligated loop of the rabbit intestine. Brit. J. exp. Path. 42, 504 (1961).

Frank, F. W., Bailey, J. W., Heithecker, D.: Experimental oral transmission of vibrionic abortion of sheep. J. Amer. vet. med. Ass. 131, 472 (1957).

Frank, A. H., Bryner, J. H., Caruthers, B.: Proc. III. Int. Cong. Anim. Reprod. Cambridge Sect. 2, 18 (1956).

Frank, F. W., Waldhalm, D. G., Meinershagen, W. A., Scrivner, L. H.: Newer knowledge of ovine vibriosis. J. Amer. vet. med. Ass. 147, 1313 (1965).

Fraser, G.: Isolation of an anaerobic vibrio from a king penguin (Aptenodytes longirostris). Avian Dis. 5, 243 (1961).

Freter, R.: The fatal enteric cholera infection in the guinea pig, achieved by inhibition of normal enteric flora. J. infect. Dis. 97, 57 (1955).

Freter, R.: Experimental enteric shigella and vibrio infections in mice and guinea pigs. J. exp. Med. 104, 411 (1956).

Friedrich, P.: Vergleichende Untersuchungen über den Vibrio cholerae asiaticae (Kommabacillus Koch), mit besonderer Berücksichtigung der diagnostischen Merkmale desselben. Arb. Gesundh.-Amte (Berl.) 8, 87 (1893).

Fuhrman, G. J., Fuhrman, F. A.: Inhibition of active sodium transport by cholera toxin. Nature (Lond.) 188, 71 (1960).

Fujii, S.: Findings of an experimental study of the kidney affected by cholera toxin. J. Orient. med. 2, 209 (1924).

Fujino, T. et al.: On the bacteriological examination of shrasu food poisoning. J. Japan Ass. infect. Dis. 25, 11 (1951). Zit. nach Sakazaki (1965).

Fukuhara, Y., Ando, J.: Über die Bakteriengifte, insbesondere die Bakterienleibesgifte. Z. Immun.-Forsch. 18, 350 (1913).

Galeotti, G.: Über das Nukleoproteid der Cholerabacillen. Zbl. Bakt., I. Abt. Orig. 67, 225 (1913).

Gallut, J.: Variation du pouvoir toxique de Vibrio cholerae au cours de la maladie. C. R. Acad. Sci. (Paris) 237, 1038 (1953).

Gallut, J.: Contribution à l'étude de la toxine cholérique: Variation du pouvoir toxique de Vibrio cholerae (Ogawa) au cours de la maladie. Ann. Inst. Pasteur 86, 561 (1954).

Gallut, J.: Du rôle de la glande surrénale dans l'intoxication cholérique expérimentale de la souris. C. R. Soc. Biol. (Paris) 149, 1414 (1955).

Gallut, J.: Antigenic structure of vibrios. In: Proc. Cholera Res. Symp., Honolulu (1965), p. 235. Publ. Hlth. Serv. (Wash.) Publ. No. 1328.

Gallut, J., Grabar, P.: Recherches immunochimiques sur le vibrion cholérique. III. Mise en évidence de deux constituants toxiques de nature différente dans la toxine cholérique. Ann. Inst. Pasteur 71, 83, 321 (1945).

Gallut, J., A. Jude: Contribution à l'étude de la virulence et du pouvoir toxigène du vibrion cholérique: II. Influence de la température d'incubation sur le pouvoir toxigène in vitro de Vibrio cholerae (Ogawa). Ann. Inst. Pasteur 88, 282 (1955).

Gamaleia, N.: Vibrio Metschnikovi (n. sp.) et ses rapports avec le microbe du choléra asiatique. Ann. Inst. Pasteur 2, 482 (1888a).

Gamaleia, N.: Vibrio Metschnikovi. Son mode naturel d'infection. Ann. Inst. Pasteur 2, 552 (1888b).

Gamaleia, N. (1888c): Zit. nach Pfeiffer, R., u. Nocht (1889).

Gamaleia: Verh. des internat. med. Congr. (1890). Zit. nach Issaeff u. W. Kolle (1894).

Gamaleia, N.: Sur la vaccination cholérique. C. R. Soc. Biol. (Paris) 41, 694 (1889).

Gamaleia, N.: Du choléra chez les chiens. C. R. Soc. Biol. (Paris) 44, 739 (1892).

Gardner, A. D., Venkatraman, K. V.: The antigens of the cholera group of vibrios. J. Hyg. (Lond.) 35, 262 (1935).

Gardner, E. W., Lyles, S. T., Lankford, C. E.: A comparison of virulence of Vibrio cholerae strains for the embryonated egg. J. Infect. Dis. 114, 412 (1964).

Gauld, L., Schlingman, A. S., Jackson, E. B., Manning, M. C., Batson, H. C., Campbell, Ch. C.: Chloramphenicol (Chloromycetin) in experimental cholera infections. J. Bact. 57, 349 (1949).

Ghosh, A. K., Bhattacharya, S., Sircar, B. K., Mazumder, R. N., Mondal, A.: Observations on the cutaneous reactions to cholera toxin in suckling and adult animals. Ann. Inst. Pasteur 122, 43 (1972).

Ghosh, H.: Préparation de la toxine cholérique. Action pathogène expérimentale. C. R. Soc. Biol. (Paris) 112, 1176 (1933).

Ghosh, S. N., Mukerjee, S.: Studies on the nature of ultrasonic extract of cholera vibrio. Part I: Studies on toxicity and pathogenicity. Ann. Biochem. 19, 173 (1959).

Gill, C. A., Lal, R. B.: The epidemiology of cholera, with special reference to transmission. A preliminary report. Indian J. med. Res. 18, 1255 (1931).

Gillmore, J.: Zit. nach Phillips, R. A. (1965).

Gminder, A.: Nachweis von Spirillen als Ursache des ansteckenden Verkalbens auch in Deutschland. Berl. Münch. tierärztl. Wschr. 38, 184 (1922).

Goere, J.: Le choléra et la fièvre typhoïde peuvent-ils être propagés par les lézards? C. R. Soc. Biol. (Paris) 74, 91 (1913).

Gohar, M. A., Makkawi, M.: Experimental infection of animals with the cholera vibrio. J. Egypt. med. Ass. 31, 599 (1948).

Golovanoff, M.: De l'action de la bile prise par la bouche sur la réceptivité vis-à-vis des vibrions cholériques injectés dans les veines. C. R. Soc. Biol. (Paris) 89, 1263 (1923).

Gotschlich, E., Weigand, J.: Über die Beziehungen zwischen Virulenz und Individuenzahl einer Cholerakultur. Z. Hyg. Infekt.-Kr. 20, 376 (1895).

Graham, R., Thorp, F., Jr.: Vibrionic abortion in sheep. J. Amer. vet. med. Ass. 76, 568 (1930).

Greer, W. E., Jiricka, Z., Felsenfeld, O.: Gallbladder damage and prolonged excretion of cholera vibrios in Erythrocebus patas. Proc. Soc. exp. Biol. (N.Y.) 127, 551 (1968).

Greig, E. D. W.: Lesions of the gall-bladder and biliary passages in cholera: A bacteriological, histological and experimental study. Indian J. med. Res. 2, 28 (1914).

Greig, E. D. W.: On the production of gall-stones in rabbits following intravenous inoculations of cholera-like vibrios. Indian J. med. Res. 3, 259 (1915).

Greig, E. D. W.: Further observations on lesions of the biliary passages of rabbits dying after repeated intravenous injections of living vibrios: A contribution to the study of experimental cholera infection. Indian J. med. Res. 3, 397 (1916).

Greig, E. D. W.: Bacteriological studies of cholera-like vibrios isolated from the stools of cholera cases in Calcutta. IV. Virulence experiments. Indian J. med. Res. 5, 340 (1917).

Griffitts, J. J.: The use of mucin in experimental infections of mice with Vibrio cholerae. Publ. Hlth Rep. (Wash.) **57**, 707 (1942a).

Griffitts, J. J.: Laboratory studies of the effect of sulfonamide drugs on V. cholerae. Publ. Hlth Rep. (Wash.) **57**, 814 (1942b).

Gruber, M.: Weitere Mittheilungen über vermeintliche und wirkliche Choleragifte. Wien. klin. Wschr. **5**, 685, 706 (1892).

Gruber, M.: Theorie der activen und passiven Immunität gegen Cholera, Typhus und verwandte Krankheitsprozesse. Münch. med. Wschr. **43**, 206 (1896).

Gruber, M., Wiener, E.: Ueber die intraperitoneale Cholerainfection der Meerschweine. Wien. klin. Wschr. **5**, 543 (1892a).

Gruber, M., Wiener, E.: Cholerastudien. I. Über die intraperitoneale Cholerainfection der Meerschweine. Arch. Hyg. (Berl.) **15**, 241 (1892b).

Grünberg, W., Otte, E.: Vibrionen-Hepatitis bei Trappenkücken (Otis tarda L.). Wien. tierärztl. Mschr. **50**, 862 (1963).

Günther, C.: Über eine neue, im Wasser gefundene Kommabacillenart. Dtsch. med. Wschr. **18**, 1124 (1892).

Günther, C.: Weitere Studien über den Vibrio Berolinensis. Arch. Hyg. (Berl.) **19**, 214 (1893).

Günther, O.: Die Cholera. In: Die Infektionskrankheiten des Menschen und ihre Erreger. Bd. I, S. 808, hrsg. von A. Grumbach, O. Bonin. Stuttgart: Thieme 1969.

Gupta, N. P., Gupta, S. P., Mangalik, V. S., Prasad, B. G., Yajnik, B. S.: Investigations into the nature of the vibrio strains isolated from the epidemic of gastro-enteritis in Kumbh Fair at Allahabad in 1954. Indian J. med. Sci. **10**, 781 (1956).

Hahn, M.: Ueber einige Beobachtungen während der diesjährigen Choleraepidemie in Südrußland und russisch Mittelasien. Berl. klin. Wschr. **42**, 25 (1905).

Hahn, M.: Über den Übergang der Choleravibrionen vom Blut in den Darm bei Meerschweinchen (nach Versuchen von Dr. Olsen und Dr. Ray). Zbl. Bakt., I. Abt. Ref. **81**, 91 (1926).

Hahn, M., Hirsch, J.: Gewinnung von Choleragift. Klin. Wschr. **5**, 1569 (1926).

Hahn, M., Hirsch, J.: Gewinnung und Prüfung von Choleragift (II. Mitteilung). Klin. Wschr. **6**, 312 (1927).

Hahn, M., Hirsch, J.: Die Enterotropie und die parenterale Wirkung des Choleragiftes (III. Mitteilung). Klin. Wschr. **7**, 2483 (1928).

Hahn, M., Hirsch, J.: Studien über das Choleragift. Z. Hyg. Infekt.-Kr. **110**, 355 (1929).

Hasan, S. I., Greenough III, W. B., Gordon, R. S., Jr., Benenson, A. S.: The resus monkey as an experimental cholera model. In: Proc. Cholera Res. Symp., Honolulu (1965), p. 276. Publ. Hlth. Serv. (Wash.) Publ. No 1328.

Heckly, R. J., Wolochow, H., Christiansen, C.: Vibrio enterotoxin in miniature pigs. J. Bact. **100**, 1140 (1969).

Heiberg, B.: Des réactions de fermentation chez les vibrions. C. R. Soc. Biol. (Paris) **115**, 984 (1934).

Hendrie, M. S., Hodkiss, W., Shewan, J. M.: Proposal that the species Vibrio anguillarum Bergman 1909, Vibrio piscium David 1927, and Vibrio ichthyodermis (Wells and ZoBell) Shewan, Hobbs, and Hodgkiss 1960 be combined as a single species. Int. J. Syst. Bact. **21**, 64 (1971).

Heyningen, W. E. van, Mellanby, J.: Exotoxine. In: Die Infektionskrankheiten des Menschen und ihre Erreger, Bd. I, S. 249, hrsg. von A. Grumbach, O. Bonin. Stuttgart: Thieme 1969.

Hodgkiss, W., Shewan, J. M.: Pseudomonas infection in a plaice. J. Path. Bact. **62**, 655 (1950).

Hofstad, M. S. (1956): Zit. nach Hofstad, M. S., et al. (1958).

Hofstad, M. S., McGehee, E. H., Bennett, P. C.: Avian infectious hepatitis. Avian Dis. **2**, 358 (1958).

Horowitz, L.: Zur Frage über Cholera-Toxine und -Antitoxine. Z. Immun.-Forsch. **19**, 44 (1913).

Horowitz-Wlassowa, L.-M., Pirojnikowa, E. A.: De la vaccination contre le choléra par la voie buccale. C. R. Soc. Biol. (Paris) **94**, 1067 (1926).

Hoshina, T.: An epidemic disease affecting rainbow trout in Japan. J. Tokyo Univ. Fish. **42**, 15 (1956). Zit. nach Smith, I. W. (1961).

Hoshina, T.: Further observations on the causative bacteria of the epidemic disease like furunculosis of rainbow trout. J. Tokyo Univ. Fish. **43**, 59 (1957). Zit. nach Smith, I. W. (1961).

Hueppe, F.: Cholerabacillen und Cholera nostras. Dtsch. med. Wschr. **10**, 643 (1884).

Hueppe, F.: III. Ueber Fortschritte in der Kenntniss der Ursachen der Cholera asiatica. Berl. klin. Wschr. **24**, 164 (1887a).

Hueppe, F.: IV. Ueber Fortschritte in der Kenntniss der Ursachen der Cholera asiatica. Berl. klin. Wschr. **24**, 185 (1887b).

Hueppe, F.: Ueber Giftbildung durch Bacterien und über giftige Bacterien. Berl. klin. Wschr. **29**, 409 (1892).

Index Bergeyana s. Buchanan et al. (1966).

Inghilleri: Sulla eziologia e patogenesi della peste rossa delle anguille. Atti della R. accademia dei Lincei, Serie 5, Vol. 12 (1903). Zit. nach Bergman (1909).

Issaeff, Kolle, W.: Experimentelle Untersuchungen mit Choleravibrionen an Kaninchen. Z. Hyg. Infekt.-Kr. **18**, 17 (1894).

Issaeff, Ivanoff: Untersuchungen über die Immunisierung der Meerschweinchen gegen den Vibrio Ivanoff. Z. Hyg. **17**, 117 (1894).

James, H. D., Doyle, L. P.: Further studies with a vibrio as the etiologic agent of swine dysentery. J. Amer. vet. med. Ass. **111**, 47 (1947).

Jansen, J., Kunst, H.: On the egg as a culture medium for Vibrio fetus. T. Diergeneesk. **76**, 778 (1951).

Jenkin, C. R., Rowley, D.: Possible factors in the pathogenesis of cholera. Brit. J. exp. Path. **40**, 474 (1959).

Jenkin, C. R., Rowley, D.: The importance of antibody in the prevention of experimental cholera in rabbits. Brit. J. exp. Path. **41**, 24 (1960).

Jensen, R., Miller, V. A., Hammarlund, M. A., Graham, W. R.: Vibrionic abortion in sheep. I. Transmission and immunity. Amer. J. vet. Res. **18**, 326 (1957).

Jones, F. S., Little, R. B.: The etiology of infectious diarrhea (winter scours) in cattle. J. exp. Med. **53**, 835 (1931a).

Jones, F. S., Little, R. B.: Vibrionic enteritis in calves. J. exp. Med. **53**, 845 (1931b).

Jude, A., Gallut, J.: Contribution à l'étude de la virulence et du pouvoir toxigène du vibrion cholérique: I. Influence de la température d'incubation sur la virulence expérimentale de Vibrio cholerae (Ogawa). Ann. Inst. Pasteur 88, 145 (1955).

Kabeshima, T.: Notes sur la nature biologique des vibrions d',,El Tor''. C. R. Soc. Biol. (Paris) **81**, 616 (1918a).

Kabeshima, T.: Le poisson de mer considéré dans ses rapports avec les vibrions cholériques qui peuvent exister dans l'eau. Bull. Off. int. Hyg. publ. **10**, 908 (1918b).

Kamel, M. M.: Isolierung und Differenzierung der beim Rinde vorkommenden Vibrionen. Inaug.-Diss. (Hannover 1960).

Kamen, L.: Bakteriologisches aus der Cholerazeit. Zbl. Bakt., I. Abt. **18**, 417 (1895).

Karlinski, J.: Die Vibrioneninfektion per os bei jungen Tieren. Zbl. Bakt., I. Abt. **20**, 150 (1896).

Kato, T., Obara, Y., Ichinoe, H., Yamai, S., Nagashima, K., Sakazaki, R.: Hemolytic activity and toxicity of V. parahaemolyticus. Jap. J. Bact. **21**, 442 (1966).

Keidel, W. D.: Kurzgefaßtes Lehrbuch der Physiologie, S. 189. Stuttgart: Thieme 1970.

Keusch, G. T., Rahal, J. J., Jr., Weinstein, L., Grady, G. F.: Biochemical effects of cholera enterotoxin: oxidative metabolism in the infant rabbit. Amer. J. Physiol. **218**, 703 (1970).

Kiessling, F.: Ein dem Choleravibrio ähnlicher Kommabacillus. Arb. Gesundh.-Amte (Berl.) **8**, 430 (1893).

King, E. O.: Human infections with Vibrio fetus and a closely related vibrio. J. infect. Dis. **101**, 119 (1957).

King, S., Bronsky, D.: Vibrio fetus isolated from a patient with localized septic arthritis. J. Amer. med. Ass. **175**, 1045 (1961).

Kitasato, S.: Die Widerstandsfähigkeit der Cholerabacterien gegen das Eintrocknen und gegen Hitze. Z. Hyg. Infekt.-Kr. **5**, 134 (1889).

Klein, E.: Ueber einen neuen tierpathogenen Vibrio — Vibrio cardii. Zbl. Bakt., I. Abt. Orig. **38**, 173 (1905).

Klemperer, G.: Untersuchungen über Infection und Immunität bei der asiatischen Cholera. Z. klin. Med. **25**, 449 (1894a).

Klemperer, G.: Zur Kenntniss der natürlichen Immunität gegen asiatische Cholera. Dtsch. med. Wschr. **20**, 435 (1894b).

Koch, R.: In: I. Die Conferenz zur Erörterung der Cholerafrage. Dtsch. med. Wschr. **10**, 499, 519 (1884).

Koch, R.: In: Conferenz zur Erörterung der Cholerafrage (zweites Jahr). Dtsch. med. Wschr. **11**, No. 37A, 1 (1885).

Koch, R., Gaffky, G.: Bericht über die Tätigkeit der zur Erforschung der Cholera im Jahre 1883 nach Ägypten und Indien entsandten Kommission. Arb. Gesundh.-Amte (Berl.) **3**, 1 (1887).

Koch, W., Kaplan, D.: Enumerating variable bacteria. Nature (Lond.) **203**, 896 (1964).

Kölbl, O.: Nachweis der Vibrionenhepatitis bei Hühnern in Österreich. Wien. tierärztl. Mschr. **51**, 165 (1964).

Kolle, W.: Beiträge zu den experimentellen Cholerastudien an Meerschweinchen. Z. Hyg. Infekt.-Kr. **16**, 329 (1894).

Kolle, W., Gotschlich, E.: Untersuchungen über die bakteriologische Choleradiagnostik und Specifität des Koch'schen Choleravibrio. Z. Hyg. Infekt.-Kr. 44, 1 (1903).

Kolle, W., Prigge, R.: In: Handbuch der pathog. Mikroorganismen, 3. Aufl., Bd. 4, hrsg. von W. Kolle, R. Kraus u. P. Uhlenhuth. Jena: Fischer 1928.

Kolle, W., Schürmann, W.: Cholera asiatica. In: Handbuch der pathog. Mikroorganismen, 2. Aufl., Bd. 4, hrsg. von W. Kolle u. A. v. Wassermann. Jena: Fischer 1912.

Kotlyarova, R. I., Ledovskaya, A. P.: Increasing the virulence of Vibrio cholerae by its passage on animals with reduced protective reactions. Zh. Mikrobiol. (Mosk.) 32, 80 (1961).

Krantz, G., Colwell, R. R., Lovalace, T. E.: Vibrio parahaemolyticus from the blue crab Callinectes sapidus in Chesapeake Bay. Science 164, 1286 (1969).

Kraus, R., Russ, V. K.: Ueber Toxine und Antitoxine des Choleravibrio. Zbl. Bakt., I. Abt. Orig. 45, 258, 332 (1908).

Krause, W., Windrath, H.: Über eine durch einen Vibrio veranlaßte Seuche der Sonnenvögel (Leiothrix luteus L., chinesische Nachtigall). Berl. tierärztl. Wschr. 35, 468 (1919).

Kubitschek, H. E.: Electronic counting and sizing of bacteria. Nature (Lond.) 182, 234 (1958).

Kujumgiev, I.: Von Vibrio metschnikovi verursachte Paracholera (Vibrionencholera) beim Geflügel in Bulgarien. Bull. Inst. Microbiol. Bulg. Acad. Sci. 8, 103 (1957).

Labrec, E. H., Sprinz, H., Schneider, H., Formal, S. B.: Localization of vibrios in experimental cholera: A fluorescent antibody study in guinea pigs. In: Proc. Cholera Res. Symp., Honolulu Publ. Hlth. Serv. (Wash.), p. 272 (1965).

Lagarde, E., Chakroun, F.: Une épizootie à Vibrio anguillarum chez les anguilles de l'étang du canet (Pyrénées orientales). Ann. Inst. Pasteur 108, 135 (1965).

Laing, J. A. (Ed.): Vibrio fetus infection of cattle. Food and Agriculture Organization, Rome 1960.

Lavrovskaya, V. M., Blant, M. E.: The effect of the initial culture of cholera vibrio on the quantity and specific activity of antigenic complexes. Z. Mikrobiol. (Mosk.) 41, 108 (1964).

Lawson, J. R., MacKinnon, D. J.: Vibrio foetus infection in cattle. Vet. Rec. 64, 763 (1952).

Lawson, J. R., MacKinnon, D. J.: Rep. 15th Int. Vet. Cong. Stockholm Pt. I. Vol. II, 821 (1953). Zit. nach Vet. Rec. 70, 393 (1958) (Anonym).

Lawson, J. R., MacKinnon, D. J.: Zit. nach Vet. Rec. 70, 393 (1958) (Anonym).

Lee, A. M., Scrivner, L. H.: Experimental work upon recent outbreaks of abortion in ewes. Amer. J. vet. Res. 2, 50 (1941).

Leitch, G. J.: Effect of cholera toxin on epithelial cell permeability and transport. In: Proc. Cholera Res. Symp., Honolulu (1965), p. 148. Publ. Hlth. Serv. (Wash.) Publ. No. 1328.

Lerche, P.: Beitrag zum Spirillenabortus beim Rinde. Dtsch. tierärztl. Wschr. 35, 484 (1927).

Lerche, P.: Beitrag zum Spirillenabortus beim Rinde. Dtsch. med. Wschr. 33, 118 (1937).

Levy, A. J.: A gastro-enteritis outbreak probably due to a bovine strain of Vibrio. Yale J. Biol. Med. 18, 243 (1946).

Lewis, T.: "Comma-shaped Bacillus", alleged to be the cause of cholera. Lancet 1884 II, 513.

Lindenstruth, R. W., Ashcraft, J. B., Ward, B. Q.: Studies on vibrionic abortion of sheep. J. Amer. vet. med. Ass. 114, 204 (1949).

Loeffler, F.: Eine neue Methode zum Färben der Mikroorganismen im besonderen ihrer Wimperhaare und Geisseln. Zbl. Bakt. Orig. 6, 209 (1889).

Loesche, W. J., Gibbons, R. J., Socransky, S. S.: Biochemical characteristics of Vibrio sputorum and relationship to Vibrio bubulus and Vibrio fetus. J. Bact. 89, 1109 (1965).

Loewenthal, W.: IV. Experimentelle Cholerastudien. Dtsch. med. Wschr. 15, 496, 520 (1889).

Loghem, J. J. van: Ueber den Unterschied zwischen El Tor- und Choleravibrionen. Zbl. Bakt. Orig. 57, 289 (1911).

Loghem, J. J. van: Ueber den Unterschied zwischen Cholera- und El Tor-Vibrionen. II. Mitteilung. Zbl. Bakt. Orig. 67, 410 (1913).

Lyng, J.: Cholera filtrate and vasopressin. Acta path. microbiol. scand. 62, 349 (1964).

Maciak, T., Petzold, K., Winkenwerder, W.: Vergleichende kulturell-biochemische und elektronenoptische Untersuchungen an von Rindern, Pferden, Schweinen und Hühnern isolierten Vibrionen. Arch. exp. Vet.-Med. 20, 797 (1966).

Maciak, T., Winkenwerder, W.: Kulturelle, tierexperimentelle und vergleichende serologische Untersuchungen an Schweinevibrionen. Zbl. Vet.-Med. 11, 693 (1964).

Maddox, R. L.: XII. Experiments on feeding some insects with the curved or "comma" bacillus, and also with another bacillus (B. subtilis?). J. roy. micr. Soc., 2nd ser. 5, 602 (1885).

Manwaring, W. H., Boyd, W. H., Okami, S.: Study of bacterial products by means of excised mammalian heart. I. Endotheliotoxin of S. cholerae. J. infect. Dis. 32, 307 (1923).

Masaki, S.: Du mécanisme de l'infection cholérique et de la vaccination contre le choléra par la voie buccale. Ann. Inst. Pasteur 36, 399 (1922).

MASHIMO, S.: Cholera bacteriemia and appearance of its bacteria by bile. Jap. med. Wld. **3**, 10 (1923).

MATSUMOTO, K., ANDO, K., SHIRAIWA, T.: Zur Frage der Durchlässigkeit der intakten Haut für Typhus-, Paratyphus- und Cholerabazillen. Sci. Rep. Inst. infect. Dis. Tokyo Univ. **6**, 35 (1927). Zit. nach POLLITZER, R. (1959).

McFADYEAN, J., STOCKMAN, S.: A report of the departmental committee appointed by the board of agriculture and fisheries to inquire into epozootic abortion. Part. III and appendix to part. III, abortion in sheep. London: Wyman and Sons, Ltd. 1912. Zit. nach LEE und SCRIVNER (1941).

McFADYEAN, J., STOCKMAN, St.: Abortion in sheep. In "Report of the departmental committee appointed to inquire into epizootic abortion". Part 3. Great Britain board of agriculture and fisheries, his Majesty's stationery office. London 1913. Zit. nach JENSEN et al. (1957).

McINTYRE, O. R., FEELEY, J. C.: Passive serum protection of the infant rabbit against experimental cholera. J. infect. Dis. **114**, 468 (1964).

MEINERSHAGEN, W. A., WALDHALM, D. G., FRANK, F. W., THOMAS, L. A., PHILIP, R. N.: Efficacy of combined bacterins for experimental immunization of sheep against ovine vibriosis and chlamydial abortion of ewes. Amer. J. vet. Res. **32**, 51 (1971).

MENDOZA, A.: Nota acerca del cólera experimental en el mono. Bol. del. Inst. nat. de Hyg. (Madrid) **9**, 117 (1913). Zit. nach KOLLE, W., u. R. PRIGGE (1928).

MESSERLI, W.: Bakteriologische und serologische Untersuchung über den Vibrio coli des Schweines. Inaug.-Diss. Bern (1953).

METALNIKOV, S., CHORINE, V.: Maladies microbiennes chez les Pyrales de mais. Ann. Inst. Pasteur **42**, 1635 (1928).

METALNIKOW, S., GASCHEN, H.: Sur la rapidité d'immunisation chez la chenille de Galleria. C. R. Soc. Biol. (Paris) **85**, 224 (1921).

METCHNIKOFF, E.: Recherches sur le choléra et les vibrions. Quatrième mémoire sur l'immunité et la réceptivité vis-à-vis du choléra intestinal. Ann. Inst. Pasteur 8, 529 (1894).

METCHNIKOFF, E., ROUX, E., TAURELLI-SALIMBENI: Toxine et antitoxine cholérique. Ann. Inst. Pasteur 10, 257 (1896).

MILLER, V. A., JENSEN, R.: Experimental immunization against ovine vibriosis. I. The use of live and formalin-killed Vibrio fetus vaccines. Amer. J. vet. Res. **22**, 43 (1961).

MILLER, A. V., JENSEN, R.: Experimental immunization against ovine vibriosis. II. Formalin-killed Vibrio fetus adjuvant vaccines. Amer. J. vet. Res. **24**, 65 (1963).

MILLER, V. A., JENSEN, R., GILROY, J. J.: Bacteremia in pregnant sheep following oral administration of Vibrio fetus. Amer. J. vet. Res. **20**, 677 (1959).

MILLER, V. A., JENSEN, R., OGG, J. E.: Immunization of sheep against ovine vibriosis with bacterins containing serotype I and serotype V in mineral oil. Amer. J. vet. Res. **25**, 664 (1964).

MITSCHERLICH, E., LIESS, B.: Die serologische Differenzierung von Vibrio fetus-Stämmen. Dtsch. tierärztl. Wschr. **65**, 2 (1958a).

MITSCHERLICH, E., LIESS, B.: Die serologische Differenzierung von Vibrio fetus-Stämmen. II. Vergleich der serologischen Differenzierung von Vibrionenstämmen mit der Komplementbindungsmethode und dem Agglutinationstest. Dtsch. tierärztl. Wschr. **65**, 36 (1958b).

MITSCHERLICH, E., LIESS, B.: Der serologische Nachweis der Vibrio-fetus-Infektion des Rindes und Schafes. Mh. Tierheilk. **10**, 303 (1958c).

MONOD, J.: The growth of bacterial cultures. Ann. Rev. Microbiol. **3**, 371 (1949).

MOORE, B.: Observations on a group of anaerobic vaginal vibrios. J. Path. Bact. **67**, 461 (1954).

MORSE, E. V., RISTIC, M.: Experimental Vibrio fetus infection in guinea pigs. III. Pathogenicity studies and the effect of guinea pigs passage upon agglutinogens. Amer. J. vet. Res. **15**, 599 (1954).

MUDD, St., WARREN, S.: A readily cultivable vibrio, filtrable through Berkefeld "V" candles, Vibrio percolans (new species). J. Bact. **8**, 447 (1923).

MUNDT, W.: Untersuchungen der Tierpathogenität von Vibrio foetus und Spirillum suis aus dem Schweinedarm an Meerschweinchen und Kaninchen. Prakt. Tierarzt **7**, 89 (1956).

MYERS, L. L., BERG, R. L., FIREHAMMER, B. D.: Immunoserologic properties of antigens from Vibrio fetus of ovine origin. Amer. J. vet. Res. **31**, 1773 (1970).

NAKANISHI, H., LEISTNER, L., HECHELMANN, H., BAUMGART, J.: Weitere Untersuchungen über das Vorkommen von Vibrio parahaemolyticus und Vibrio alginolyticus bei Seefischen in Deutschland. Arch. Lebensmitt.-Hyg. **19**, 49 (1968).

NASAROFF, JURGELUNAS: Zit. nach SEWASTIANOFF, E. P. (1910).

NEISSER, M.: Über einen neuen Wasser-Vibrio, der die Nitrosoindol-Reaction liefert. Arch. Hyg. (Berl.) **19**, 194 (1893).

NEWSAM, I. D. B., PETERSON, J. E.: Persistence of Vibrio fetus in the genital tract of experimentally infected heifers. Brit. vet. J. **120**, 223 (1964).

Nicati, Rietsch: Sur l'inoculation du bacille virgule du choléra. Sem. méd. (Paris) 2nd series 4, 370 (1884a), identisch mit: Dtsch. med. Wschr. 10, 634 (1884a).

Nicati, W., Rietsch, M.: Odeur et effets toxiques des produits de la fermentation produite par les bacilles en virgule. C. R. Acad. Sci. (Paris) 99, 928 (1884b).

Nicati, W., Rietsch, M.: Recherches sur le choléra. Expériences d'inoculation. Rev. Méd. (Paris) 5, 449 (1885a).

Nicati, W., Rietsch, M.: Recherches sur le choléra. Le bacille en virgule dans l'organisme, sa culture, ses produits de fermentation, et leur action sur les animaux. Arch. Physiol. norm. path. 6, 72 (1885b).

Nicati, W., Rietsch, M.: Recherches sur le choléra (Paris 1886). Zit. nach Scholl, H. (1892).

Nichols, H. J.: Experimental observations on the pathogenesis of gall-bladder infections in typhoid, cholera and dysentery. J. exp. Med. 24, 497 (1916).

Osborne, J. C.: Pathologic responses in animals after Vibrio fetus toxin shock. Amer. J. vet. Res. 26, 1056 (1965).

Osborne, J. C., Smibert, R. M.: Vibrio fetus endotoxin. Nature (Lond.) 195, 1106 (1962).

Osborne, J. C., Smibert, R. M.: Vibrio fetus toxin. I. Hypersensitivity and abortifacient action. Cornell Vet. 54, 561 (1964).

Osburn, B. I., Hoskins, R. K.: Experimentally induced Vibrio fetus var. intestinalis infection in pregnant cows. Amer. J. vet. Res. 31, 1733 (1970).

Oza, N. B., Dutta, N. K.: Experimental cholera produced by toxin prepared by ultrasonic disintegration of Vibrio comma. J. Bact. 85, 497 (1963).

Oza, N. B., Dutta, N. K.: Choleragenic activity in infant rabbits of El Tor vibrios from Southeast Asia. In: Proc. Cholera Res. Symp., Honolulu (1965), p. 271. Publ. Hlth. Serv. (Wash.) Publ. No. 1328.

Oza, N. B., Dutta, N. K.: Characterization of the antidiuretic factor in the lysate of V. cholerae. Indian. J. Physiol. Pharmacol. 11, 101 (1967).

Panja, G., Paul, B. M.: A study of the invasiveness and toxicity of cholera, paracholera and saprophytic vibrios in animals. Indian med. Gaz. 78, 190 (1943). Zit. n. Pollitzer, R. (1959).

Park, R. W. A.: A study of certain heterotrophic polarly flagellate water bacteria: Aeromonas, Pseudomonas and Comamonas. J. gen. Microbiol. 27, 121 (1962).

Park, R. W. A., Munro, J. B., Melrose, D. R., Stewart, D. L.: Observations on the ability of two biochemical types of Vibrio fetus to proliferate in the genital tract of cattle and their importance with respect to infertility. Brit. vet. J. 118, 411 (1962).

Passek: Veränderung der Virulenz der Choleravibrionen im Darme der Fliege (Russisches militär-medizinisches Journal, März 1911). Arch. Schiffs- u. Tropenhyg. 15, 531 (1911) (Ref.).

Peckham, M. C.: Avian vibrionic hepatitis. Avian Dis. 2, 348 (1958).

Peterson, J. E., Newsam, I. D. B.: The histopathology of genital vibriosis in virgin heifers. Brit. vet. J. 120, 229 (1964).

Pezzi, C., Savini, E.: Sur l'action des endotoxines typhique et cholérique, chauffées et non chauffées, sur le coeur de mammifère. C. R. Soc. Biol. (Paris) 69, 270 (1910).

Pfeiffer, R.: Ueber den Vibrio Metschnikoff und sein Verhältniss zur Cholera asiatica. Z. Hyg. Infekt.-Kr. 7, 347 (1889).

Pfeiffer, R.: Untersuchungen über das Choleragift. Z. Hyg. Infekt.-Kr. 11, 393 (1892).

Pfeiffer, R.: Studien zur Choleraätiologie. Z. Hyg. Infekt.-Kr. 16, 268 (1894a).

Pfeiffer, R.: Weitere Untersuchungen über das Wesen der Choleraimmunität und über specifisch bactericide Processe. Z. Hyg. Infekt.-Kr. 18, 1 (1894b).

Pfeiffer, R., Issaeff: Ueber die specifische Bedeutung der Choleraimmunität. Z. Hyg. Infekt.-Kr. 17, 355 (1894).

Pfeiffer, R., Nocht: Ueber das Verhalten der Choleravibrionen im Taubenkörper. Z. Hyg. Infekt.-Kr. 7, 259 (1889).

Pfeiffer, R., Wassermann, A.: Untersuchungen über das Wesen der Choleraimmunität. Z. Hyg. Infekt.-Kr. 14, 46 (1893).

Pham, H. C.: L'action de l'endotoxine cholérique sur le système neuro-végétatif abdominal. C. R. Soc. Biol. (Paris) 119, 78 (1935).

Phillips, R. A.: The patho-physiology of cholera. Bull. Wld Hlth Org. 28, 297 (1963).

Phillips, R. A.: Pathophysiology of cholera. In: Proc. Cholera Res. Symp., Honolulu (1965), p. 82. Publ. Hlth. Serv. (Wash.) Publ. No. 1328.

Phillips, R. A., Love, A. H. G., Mitchell, T. G., Neptune, E. M., Jr.: Cathartics and the sodium pump. In: Proc. Cholera Res. Symp., Honolulu (1965), p. 85. Publ. Hlth. Serv. (Wash.) Publ. No. 1328.

Plastridge, W. N., Kersting, E. J., Williams, L. F.: Resistance of vaccinated heifers to vibriosis. Amer. J. vet. Res. 27, 186 (1966).

Plastridge, W. N., Williams, L. F.: Observations on Vibrio fetus infection in cattle. J. Amer. vet. med. Ass. 102, 89 (1943).

Pollitzer, R.: Cholera. Wld Hlth Org. Monogr. Ser. No. 43 (1959).

POTTEVIN, H., VIOLLE, H.: Transmission du choléra aux singes par la voie gastro-intestinale. Soc. Path. exot. **6**, 482 (1913a).

POTTEVIN, H., VIOLLE, H.: Choléra expérimental des singes inférieurs. C. R. Acad. Sci. (Paris) **157**, 343 (1913b).

PREVOT, A. R.: Etudes de systématique bactérienne. V. Essai de classification des Vibrions anaérobies. Ann. Inst. Pasteur **64**, 117 (1940).

PREVOT, A. R.: Vibrioses anaérobies (1955). In: Biologie des maladies dues aux anaérobies, chapitre 3, p. 451. Paris: Edit. méd. flammarion 1955.

Proceedings of the Cholera Research Symposium, January 24—29, 1965, Honolulu, Hawaii (Publ. Hlth. Serv. Wash.). Publ. No. 1328.

PUNTONI, V.: Azione della tossina colerica sull'intestino degli animali sotto l'influenza del caldo umido. Gazz. Osp. Clin. **140**, 1466 (1913). Zit. nach POLLITZER (1959).

RANSOM: Choleragift und Choleraantitoxin. Dtsch. med. Wschr. **21**, 457 (1895).

READ, J. K.: The effects of cholera toxin on mammalian cells in culture. In: Proc. Cholera Res. Symp., Honolulu (1965), p. 151. Publ. Hlth. Serv. (Wash.) Publ. No. 1328.

REMLINGER, P., NOURI, O.: Les poissons peuvent-ils transmettre la fièvre typhoide ou le choléra? C. R. Soc. Biol. (Paris) **64**, 361 (1908a).

REMLINGER, P., NOURI, O.: Vibrions cholériques où pseudo-cholériques dans les huîtres et les moules à Constantinople. C. R. Soc. Biol. (Paris) **64**, 550 (1908b).

Report Scientific Advisory Board (1946): New Delhi: Indian Research Fund Association Secretariat. Zit. nach DUTTA, N. K., u. M. K. HABBU (1955).

RIBI, E., MILNER, K. C., PERRINE, TH. D.: Endotoxic and antigenic fractions from the cell wall of Salmonella enteritidis. Methods for separation and some biologic activities. J. Immunol. **82**, 75 (1959).

RICHARDS: Zit. nach Lancet I, 859 (1884).

RICHARDSON, ST. H.: An ion translocase system from rabbit intestinal mucosa. Preparation and properties of the (Na$^+$—K+)-activated ATPase. Biochim. biophys. Acta (Amst.) **150**, 572 (1968).

RICHARDSON, ST. H., EVANS, D. J., JR.: The effects of Vibrio cholerae extracts on membrane transport mechanisms. In: Proc. Cholera Res. Symp., Honolulu (1965), p. 139. Publ. Hlth. Serv. (Wash.) Publ. No. 1328.

RINDFLEISCH, W.: Die Pathogenität der Choleravibrionen für Tauben. Z. Hyg. Infekt.-Kr. **21**, 247 (1896).

RIST, E.: Neue Methoden und neue Ergebnisse im Gebiete der bakteriologischen Untersuchung gangränöser und fötider Eiterungen. Zbl. Bakt. I. Abt. **30**, 287 (1901).

RISTIC, M., MORSE, E. V.: Experimental Vibrio fetus infection in guinea pigs. I. Bacteriological aspects. Amer. J. vet. Res. **14**, 399 (1953).

RISTIC, M., MORSE, E. V., WIPF, L., McNUTT, S. H.: Transmission of experimental Vibrio fetus infection among guinea pigs and hamsters. Amer. J. vet. Res. **15**, 309 (1954).

RISTIC, M., SANDERS, D. A., YOUNG, F.: Experimental Vibrio fetus infection in male hamsters. Amer. J. vet. Res. **16**, 189 (1955).

ROBERTS, D. S.: Vibrionic dysentery in swine. Aust. vet. J. **32**, 27 (1956a).

ROBERTS, D. S.: Studies on vibrionic dysentery of swine. Aust. vet. J. **32**, 114 (1956b).

ROLLE, M.: Vergleichende Untersuchungen der Eigenschaften von Genital- und Darmvibrionen des Rindes. Wien. tierärztl. Mschr. **51**, 61 (1964).

ROTKY, K.: Immunisierungsversuche gegen El Tor. Prag. med. Wschr. **38**, 391 (1913).

RUCKER, R. R.: Vibrio infections among marine and fresh-water fish. Progressive Fish-Culturist **21**, 22 (1959).

RUCKER, R. R., EARP, B. J., ORDAL, E. J.: Infectious diseases of pacific salmon. Trans. Amer. Fish. Soc. **83**, 297 (1954).

SABOLOTNY, D.: Infektions- und Immunisierungsversuche am Ziesel (Spermophilus guttatus) gegen den Choleravibrio. Zbl. Bakt. **15**, 150 (1894).

SAKAZAKI, R.: Vibrio parahaemolyticus, a non-choleragenic, enteropathogenic Vibrio. In: Proc. Cholera Res. Symp., Honolulu (1965), p. 30. Publ. Hlth. Serv. (Wash.) Publ. No. 1328.

SAKAZAKI, R.: Proposal of Vibrio alginolyticus for the biotype 2 of Vibrio parahaemolyticus. Jap. J. med. Sci. Biol. **21**, 359 (1968).

SAKAZAKI, R., IWANAMI, S., FUKUMI, H.: Studies on the enteropathogenic, facultatively halophilic bacteria. Vibrio parahaemolyticus. I. Morphological, cultural, and biochemical properties and its taxonomical position. Jap. J. Med. Sci. Biol. **16**, 161 (1963). Zit. nach ZEN-YOJI et al. (1965).

SAKAZAKI, R., TAMURA, K., KATO, T., OBARA, Y., YAMAI, S., HOBO, K.: Studies on the enteropathogenic, facultatively halophilic bacteria, Vibrio parahaemolyticus. III. Enteropathogenicity. Jap. J. med. Sci. Biol. **21**, 325 (1968).

SALUS, H.: Ueber das Verhalten der Choleravibrionen im Taubenkörper und ihre Beziehungen zum Vibrio Metschnikovi. Arch. Hyg. (Berl.) **19**, 333 (1893).

Sanarelli, G.: Pathogénie du choléra. Reproduction expérimentale de la maladie. C. R. Acad. Sci. (Paris) **163**, 538 (1916).

Sanarelli, G.: De la pathogénie du choléra. (Deuxième mémoire.) La „peritonite cholérique" du cobaye. Ann. Inst. Pasteur **34**, 271 (1920a).

Sanarelli, G.: De la pathogénie du choléra. (Troisième mémoire.) Le protéide du vibrion cholérique. Ann. Inst. Pasteur **34**, 370 (1920b).

Sanarelli, G.: De la pathogénie du choléra. (Cinquième mémoire.) Le „choléra intestinal" des jeunes animaux. Ann. Inst. Pasteur **35**, 745 (1921).

Sanarelli, G.: De la pathogénie du choléra. (Sixième mémoire.) Le „choléra intestinal" des jeunes chiens. Ann. Inst. Pasteur **36**, 386 (1922).

Sanarelli, G.: De la pathogénie du choléra. (Septième mémoire.) Voies de pénétration et de sortie des vibrions cholériques dans l'organisme animal. Ann. Inst. Pasteur **37**, 364 (1923a).

Sanarelli, G.: De la pathogénie du choléra. (Huitième mémoire.) L'algidité cholérique. Ann. Inst. Pasteur **37**, 806 (1923b).

Sawtschenko, J.: Die Beziehung der Fliegen zur Verbreitung der Cholera. Zbl. Bakt. **12**, 893 (1892).

Sayamov, R. M.: Laboratory studies on the El Tor vibrio. Bull. Wld Hlth Org. **28**, 311 (1963a).

Sayamov, R. M.: Treatment and prophylaxis of cholera with bacteriophage. Bull. Wld Hlth Org. **28**, 361 (1963b).

Schäperclaus, W.: IV. Die Rotseuche des Aales im Bezirk von Rügen und Stralsund. Z. Fischerei **25**, 99 (1927).

Schafer, D. E., Lewis, G. W.: Studies on the properties of V. cholerae enterotoxin and the time- and dose-dependence of its effects on the ligated intestinal loop. In: Proc. Cholera Res. Symp., Honolulu (1965), p. 160. Publ. Hlth. Serv. (Wash.) Publ. No. 1328.

Schib, W.: Über die experimentelle Infektion von Schweinen, Schafen und Kaninchen mit Vibrio coli. Inaug.-Diss. (Bern 1956).

Schöbl, O.: Experimental cholera-carriers. J. infect. Dis. **18**, 307 (1916a).

Schöbl, O.: Further study on experimental cholera-carriers. J. infect. Dis. **19**, 145 (1916b).

Schöbl, O., Nukada, M.: Versuche über Fische als Choleraträger. Kitasato Arch. exp. Med. **12**, 313 (1935).

Schoffer: Versuche über die Empfänglichkeit junger Kaninchen für die Infektion mit Choleravibrionen. Ein Beitrag zur Aetiologie der Cholera. Arb. Gesundh.-Amte (Berl.) **11**, 460 (1895).

Scholl, H.: Untersuchungen über giftige Eiweißkörper bei Cholera asiatica und einigen Fäulnisprocessen. Arch. Hyg. (Berl.) **15**, 172 (1892).

Schottelius, M.: Zum mikroskopischen Nachweis von Cholerabacillen in Dejectionen. Dtsch. med. Wschr. **11**, 213 (1885).

Schrire, Th., Greenfield, E. C.: On bacillus fulminans and certain other new organisms isolated from Xenopus laevis. Trans. roy. Soc. S. Afr. **17**, 309 (1930).

Schuckmann, W. von: Über Fliegen, besonders ihre Rolle als Krankheitsüberträger und Krankheitserreger und über ihre Bekämpfung. Zbl. Bakt., I. Abt. Ref. **81**, 529 (1926).

Schultz, S. G., Curran, P. F.: Intestinal absorption of sodium chloride and water. Handbook of physiology, vol. 3, p. 1245. Washington 1968.

Schurupow, J. S.: Zur Frage der Gewinnung eines Heilserums gegen die Cholera. Zbl. Bakt., I. Abt. Orig. **49**, 623 (1909).

Sdrodowski, P., Brenn, E.: Zur Pathogenese der Cholera. Zbl. Bakt., I. Abt. Orig. **94**, 155 (1925).

Sewastianoff, E. P.: Zur Frage des Durchdringungsvermögens der R. Kochschen Choleravibrionen durch die Darmwand in die Gewebe und Organe. Z. Hyg. Infekt.-Kr. **65**, 127 (1910).

Shewan, J. M., Hobbs, G., Hodgkiss, W.: A determinative scheme for the identification of certain genera of gramnegative bacteria, with special reference to the Pseudomonadaceae. J. appl. Bact. **23**, 379 (1960).

Shrivastav, J. B., Bhatia, A. L., Nath, M. L.: Large-scale manufacture and standardization of Kasauli agar-grown cholera vaccine. In: Proc. Cholera Res. Symp., Honolulu (1965), p. 176. Publ. Hlth. Serv. (Wash.) Publ. No. 1328.

Sjollema, P., Stegenga, Th.. Terpstra, J.: Infectious sterility in cattle, caused by Vibrio foetus. Proc. 14th Int. Vet. Congr. London **3**, 123 (1949).

Sluyts, Ch.: Etude sur les propriétés du poison du chol. as. (Louv. 1893). Zit. nach Issaeff u. W. Kolle (1894).

Smibert, R. M.: Vibrio fetus var. intestinalis isolated from fecal and intestinal contents of clinically normal sheep: Isolation of microaerophilic vibrios. Amer. J. vet. Res. **26**, 315 (1965).

Smith, D. T.: Fusospirochetal disease of the lungs produced with cultures from Vincent's angina. J. infect. Dis. **46**, 303 (1930).

SMITH, I. W.: A disease of finnock due to Vibrio anguillarum. J. gen. Microbiol. **24**, 247 (1961).
SMITH, TH.: Kleine bakteriologische Mitteilungen. 3. Ueber einen neuen Kommabacillus. Zbl. Bakt. **10**, 177 (1891).
SMITH, TH.: Spirilla associated with disease of the fetal membranes in cattle (infectious abortion). J. exp. Med. **28**, 701 (1918).
SMITH, TH.: The etiological relation of spirilla (Vibrio fetus) to bovine abortion. J. exp. Med. **30**, 313 (1919a).
SMITH, TH.: The bacteriology of bovine abortion, with special reference to acquired immunity. J. exp. Med. **30**, 325 (1919b).
SMITH, TH.: Further studies on the etiological significance of Vibrio fetus. J. exp. Med. **37**, 341 (1923).
SMITH, TH., TAYLOR, M. S.: Some morphological and biological characters of the spirilla (Vibrio fetus, N. sp.) associated with disease of the fetal membranes in cattle. J. exp. Med. **30**, 299 (1919).
SOBERNHEIM, G.: Experimentelle Untersuchungen über Choleragift und Choleraschutz. Z. Hyg. Infekt.-Kr. **14**, 485 (1893a).
SOBERNHEIM, G.: Zur intraperitonealen Cholerainfection der Meerschweinchen. Hyg. Rdsch. **3**, 997 (1893b).
SÖDERLIND, O.: The isolation of Vibrio coli from pigs. Vet. Rec. **77**, 193 (1965).
SOLARINO, G.: Sulla patogenesi del cholera. Contributo alla conoscenza dell'evoluzione del colera sperimentale nel coniglio. G. Batt. Immun. **23**, 1 (1939).
SOELEIMAN, M. M., NIEKERK, J. VAN: Choleratoxine. Zbl. Bakt., I. Abt. Orig. **117**, 19 (1930).
STEPHENS, J. W. W., SMITH, R. F. W.: Vibrio tonsillaris (Klein), Beschreibung eines aus der Mundhöhle isolierten Vibrios. Zbl. Bakt., I. Abt. **19**, 929 (1896).
STEINER, M.: Über eine neue Bakterienzählkammer. Ein Beitrag zur Methodik der direkten Keimzahlermittlung. Zbl. Bakt., I. Abt. Orig. **113**, 306 (1929).
STICKER, G.: Abhandlungen aus der Seuchengeschichte und Seuchenlehre. II. Band: Die Cholera. Gießen 1912.
STILLE, W., HELM, E. B.: Sepsis und Meningitis durch Vibrio fetus. Dtsch. med. Wschr. **94**, 2484 (1969).
STOCKMAN, S.: Vibrionic abortion. J. Amer. vet. med. Ass. **55**, 499 (1919).
TAYLOR, J., WILKINS, M. P., PAYNE, J. M.: Relation of rabbit gut reaction to enteropathogenic Escherichia coli. Brit. J. Exp. Path. **42**, 43 (1961).
TERPSTRA, J. I.: Some aspects of genital infections in cattle. Proc. Third Int. Congr. Anim. Reprod. (Cambridge) Plenary papers, p. 34 (1956).
TERPSTRA, J. I., EISMA, W. A.: Vibrio foetus infection in cattle and enzootic infertility. T. Diergeneesk. **76**, 433 (1951).
THIERSCH, C.: Infektionsversuche an Thieren mit dem Inhalte des Choleradarmes. München 1856. Zit. nach NICATI und RIETSCH (1885a).
THOMAS: Ueber die Erzeugung der Cholera von der Blutbahn aus und die prädisponierende Rolle des Alkohols. Naunyn-Schmiedebergs Arch. exp. Path. Pharmak. **32**, 38 (1893).
THOUVENOT, H., FLORENT, A.: Etude d'un anaerobie du sperme du taureau et du vagin de la vache Vibrio bubulus Florent 1953. Ann. Inst. Pasteur **86**, 237 (1954).
TIZZONI, G., CATTANI, J.: Untersuchungen über Cholera. Zbl. med. Wiss. **43**, 769 (1886).
TIZZONI, G., CATTANI, G.: Recherches sur le choléra asiatique. Beitr. path. Anat. **3**, 189 (1888).
TRUEBLOOD, M. S., POST, G.: Vibriosis as a factor in the reproduction of antelope (Antilocapra americana). J. Amer. vet. med. Ass. **134**, 562 (1959).
TRUSCOTT, R. B., MORIN, E. W.: A bacterial agent causing bluecomb disease in Turkeys. II. Transmission and studies of the etiological agent. Avian Dis. 8, 27 (1964).
TUCKER, J. O., ROBERTSTAD, G. W.: Experimental vibriosis in sheep. J. Amer. vet. med. Ass. **129**, 511 (1956).
TUDOR, D. C.: A liver degeneration of unknown origin in chickens. J. Amer. vet. med. Ass. **125**, 219 (1954).
TUNNICLIFF, R.: An anaerobic vibrio isolated from a case of acute bronchitis. J. infect. Dis. **15**, 350 (1914).
ULLMANN, U.: Vibrio fetus als Krankheitserreger des Menschen. Dtsch. med. Wschr. **94**, 2399 (1969).
ULLMANN, U.: Ein Verfahren zur kontinuierlichen Registrierung der optischen Dichte sich vermehrender Bakterienkulturen und seine Anwendungsmöglichkeiten. Zbl. Bakt., I. Abt. Orig. **218**, 356 (1971).
URBAIN, A.: Infection cholérique expérimentale par la voie intra-rachidienne. Essai de vaccination locale de la cavité meningée contre le vibrion cholérique. C. R. Soc. Biol. (Paris) **100**, 991 (1929).
USSING, H. H.: Active sodium transport through epithelia. In: Proc. Cholera Res. Symp., Honolulu (1965), p. 99. Publ. Hlth. Serv. (Wash.) Publ. No. 1328.

Ussing, H. H., Zehran, K.: Active transport of sodium as the source of electric current in the short-circuited isolated frog skin. Acta physiol. scand. **23**, 110 (1951).

Vallee, A., LeCain, A., Thibault, P., Second, L.: Isolement chez la chatte d'un vibrion voisin de Vibrio foetus. Bull. Acad. vét. Fr. **34**, 151 (1961).

Veillon, A., Repaci, G.: Des infections secondaires dans la tuberculose ulcéreuse du poumon. Ann. Inst. Pasteur **26**, 300 (1912).

Vielitz, E., Landgraf, H., Kirsch, R.: Zur Diagnostik und Therapie der Vibrionenhepatitis. Tierärztl. Umsch. **20**, 216 (1965).

Vincenzi, L.: Ueber intraperitoneale Einspritzungen von Kochschen Kommabacillen bei Meerschweinchen. Dtsch. med. Wschr. **13**, 351, 573 (1887).

Vincenzi, L.: III. Ueber Cholera (Vorläufige Mittheilung). Dtsch. med. Wschr. **18**, 394 (1892).

Vinzent, R., Dumas, J., Picard, N.: Septicémie grave au cours de la grossesse, due à un vibrion. Avortement consécutif. Bull. Acad. nat. Méd. (Paris) **131**, 90 (1947).

Violle, H.: De la vésicule biliaire envisagée comme lieu d'inoculation. Contribution à l'étude de l'immunité et à la physiologie générale. Ann. Inst. Pasteur **26**, 381, 467 (1912).

Violle, H.: Sur la pathogénie du choléra. C. R. Acad. Sci. (Paris) **158**, 1710 (1914a).

Violle, H.: Essais sur la pathogénie du choléra. Ann. Inst. Pasteur **28**, 759 (1914b).

Violle, H., Crendiropoulo: Note sur le choléra expérimental. C. R. Soc. Biol. (Paris) **78**, 331 (1915).

Voute, E. J., Grimbergen, A. H. M.: Vibrio hepatitis bij kippen. T. Diergeneesk. **84**, 1380 (1959).

Waldhalm, D. G., Mason, D. R., Meinershagen, W. A., Scrivner, L. H.: Magpies as carriers of ovine Vibrio fetus. J. Amer. vet. med. Ass. **144**, 497 (1964).

Wassermann, A.: Untersuchungen über Immunität gegen Cholera asiatica. Zschr. Hyg. Infekt.-Kr. **14**, 35 (1893).

Webster, H. D., Thorp, F., Jr.: A study of the pathology of embryonating chicken eggs inoculated with Vibrio fetus. Amer. J. vet. Res. **14**, 118 (1953).

Welch, H., Marsh, H.: Vibrionic abortion in sheep. J. Amer. vet. med. Ass. **65**, 203 (1924).

Wells, N. A., ZoBell, C. E.: Achromobacter ichthyodermis, n. sp., the etiological agent of an infectious dermatitis of certain marine fishes. Proc. nat. Acad. Sci. (Wash.) **20**, 123 (1934).

Whenham, G. R., Carlson, H. C., Aksel, A.: Avian vibrionic hepatitis in Alberta. Canad. vet. J. **2**, 3 (1961).

Wiener, E.: Die Vibrioneninfektion per os bei jungen Katzen. Zbl. Bakt., I. Abt. **19**, 205 (1896a).

Wiener, E.: Zur Vibrioneninfektion per os bei jungen Kaninchen. Zbl. Bakt., I. Abt. **19**, 595 (1896b).

Wilson, A. T.: Experimental vibrio infections of developing chick embryos. J. exp. Med. **84**, 293 (1946).

Winkenwerder, W.: Untersuchungen an von Menschen isolierten Stämmen des Vibrio fetus. Z. med. Mikrobiol. Immunol. **152**, 273 (1966a).

Winkenwerder, W.: Vibrionen und Spirillen bei Hund und Katze. Zbl. Bakt., I. Abt. Orig. **199**, 391 (1966b).

Winkenwerder, W.: Infektionsversuche an Schafen mit Vibrio fetus-Stämmen humaner und aviärer Herkunft. Zbl. Vet.-Med. **14**, 737 (1967).

Winkenwerder, W., Bisping, W.: Kulturelle, serologische und tierexperimentelle Untersuchungen mit von Hühnern und Rindern isolierten Vibrionen. Zbl. Vet.-Med. B **11**, 603 (1964).

Winkenwerder, W., Böttcher, R.: Vibrionen bei Pferden. Berl. Münch. tierärztl. Wschr. **78**, 361 (1965).

Winkenwerder, W., Maciak, T.: Vibrionenfunde bei Hühnern aus erkrankten Beständen und bei Schlachthühnern. Dtsch. tierärztl. Wschr. **71**, 625 (1964).

Winter, A. J.: Characterization of the antibody for Vibrio fetus endotoxin in sera of normal and V. fetus infected cattle. J. Immunol. **95**, 1002 (1966).

Winter, A. J., Dunne, H. W.: An antigenic analysis of Vibrio fetus. I. Properties of soluble extracts of the organism. Amer. J. vet. Res. **23**, 150 (1962).

Witte, J.: Spirillen als Ursache des Abortus beim Rinde. Berl. tierärztl. Wschr. **39**, 553 (1923).

Woolley, D. W., Gommi, B. W.: Serotonin receptors: V. Selective destruction by neuraminidase plus EDTA and reactivation with tissue lipids. Nature (Lond.) **202**, 1074 (1964).

Wyssokowitsch, W.: Ueber die Schicksale der in's Blut injicirten Mikroorganismen im Körper der Warmblüter. Z. Hyg. Infekt.-Kr. **1**, 3 (1886).

Zen-Yoji, H., Hitokoto, H., Morozumi, S., Le Clair, R. A.: Purification and characterization of a hemolysin produced by Vibrio parahaemolyticus. J. infect. Dis. **123**, 665 (1971).

Zen-Yoji, H., Sakai, S., Terayama, T., Kudo, Y., Ito, T., Benoki, M., Nagasaki, M.: Epidemiology, enteropathogenicity, and classification of Vibrio parahaemolyticus. J. infect. Dis. **115**, 436 (1965).

Experimentelle Infektionen durch Bakteroidazeen

HERBERT WERNER

Mit 10 Abbildungen

I. Einleitung

Anaerobe gramnegative sporenlose Stäbchen (Bakteroidazeen) leben auf der Mund-, Rachen- und Darmschleimhaut des Menschen sowie in den weiblichen Genitalien. Sie bilden einen Teil der jeweiligen Standortflora. Während sie auf der Schleimhaut des Oropharynx sowie in den weiblichen Genitalien normalerweise zahlenmäßig hinter den Leitkeimen dieser Regionen — Streptokokken einerseits und *Lactobacillus*-Arten (Döderleinsche Stäbchen) andererseits — zurückstehen, stellen sie im Coloninhalt und in den Faeces den vorherrschenden Keimanteil dar:

Tabelle 1. Obligate Darmbakterien im Stuhl des gesunden mischkosternährten Menschen[a]

Anzahl der züchtbaren Bakterien	$\approx 10^{10}$/g Stuhl
Davon:	
anaerobe Bakterien	80—99%
aerobe Bakterien	1—10—20%
Anaerobier	
Sporenlose gramnegative Stäbchen (*Bacteroides*-Arten)	40—80%
Sporenlose grampositive Stäbchen (Bifidobakterien)	30—70% $\Big\}$ 80—99%
Clostridien (vorwiegend *C. perfringens*)	$0{,}01^0/_{00}$
Aerobier	
Escherichia coli	$<$1—5%
Enterokokken	$<$1—5%
Lactobacillus acidophilus und *L. fermenti*	$0{,}1$—$1^0/_{00}$

[a] Abweichungen von diesen Verhältnissen stellen sich bei Enteritis und Colitis, gelegentlich bei extrem einseitiger Ernährung und stets beim rein mit Muttermilch ernährten Säugling ein.

Innerhalb der intestinalen *Bacteroides*-Gruppe sind mit kulturell-biochemischen Methoden mehrere Arten abgrenzbar, unter denen *Bacteroides vulgatus* und *B. thetaiotaomicron* vorherrschen (Tabelle 2).

Tabelle 2. Zusammensetzung des *Bacteroides*-Keimanteils der menschlichen Darmflora[a]

Bacteroides-Art	Anzahl der Isolierungen	Anteil %
B. vulgatus	278	43
B. thetaiotaomicron	185	29
B. fragilis	86	13
B. variabilis	18	3
B. distasonis	15	2
B. uniformis	15	2
Sonstige Arten[b]	41	8
	638	

[a] Nach größtenteils bisher unveröffentlichten Untersuchungen.
[b] B. tumidus, B. incommunis u.a.

Darmbewohnende *Bacteroides*-Arten gehören zu den Eiter- und Sepsis-
erregern. Besonders häufig findet man sie, zu einem beachtlichen Teil in Reinkultur, bei postappendicitischen Abscessen, infizierten Hämatomen und Pyo-
salpinx. Mehr als 80% der aus pathologischem Material isolierten *Bacteroides*-
Keime sind Angehörige der Species *B. fragilis* (Tabelle 3).

Tabelle 3. Vorkommen von intestinalen *Bacteroides*-Arten in pathologischem Material[a]

Bacteroides-Art	Anzahl der Isolierungen, in Klammern: davon in Reinkultur	Vorkommen %
B. fragilis	133 (54)	82,6
B. thetaiotaomicron	28 (11)	17,4

[a] Nach z.T. bereits veröffentlichten Ergebnissen (vgl. Werner, 1967; Werner et al., 1970 b; Werner u. Pulverer, 1971).

Daneben kommt *B. thetaiotaomicron* vor. Die Species *B. vulgatus* wurde bisher
in darmfernen Eiterungen und bei Sepsis nicht nachgewiesen. Unter den intestinalen *Bacteroides*-Arten besitzt demnach *B. fragilis* die größte Virulenz (Werner,
1967; Werner et al., 1970 b).

Sphaerophorus- und *Fusobacterium*-Arten, deren normaler Standort die
Schleimhaut des Oropharynx ist, wurden bei Sepsis, Angina, Peritonitis, Pleuritis,
Pleuraempyem, Lungenabsceß, nekrotisierender Hepatitis, Meningitis und Aktino-
mykose gefunden. In aktinomykotischen Eiterungen kommt fast regelmäßig
B. melaninogenicus vor.

Die pathogene Bedeutung anaerober gramnegativer sporenloser Stäbchen ist
bei Nachweis in normalerweise sterilen Körperflüssigkeiten (Liquor, Blut) und bei
Vorliegen der entsprechenden Krankheitsbilder (Meningitis, Sepsis) evident.
Dagegen wird man in mischinfizierten Eiterungen vielfach lediglich Schrittmacherdienste von seiten der Bakteroidazeen annehmen dürfen. In anderen Fällen (z.B.
bei schleimhautnahen Prozessen) kann es sich um akzidentelle, ätiologisch weitgehend bedeutungslose Keimbeimengungen handeln.

Bacteroides-, *Fusobacterium*- und *Sphaerophorus*-Infektionen kommen, wie
leicht ersichtlich, endogen zustande. Über die Bedingungen für die Entstehung
einer endogenen Infektion weiß man kaum etwas Sicheres. Als Voraussetzung
von seiten des Makroorganismus wird lokale oder allgemeine Resistenzminderung,
u.a. auf dem Boden von Traumen, Mangelernährung, konsumierenden Krankheiten und Erkältungen, angenommen. Die für den Wechsel vom unschädlichen
Epiphyt zum Krankheitserreger verantwortlichen Veränderungen des Bacteriums
werden unter dem Begriff Virulenzsteigerung subsumiert. Zur Virulenzsteigerung
können neben unbekannten Größen die Adaptation an die Verhältnisse in bestimmten Geweben, eventuell auch Schrittmacherdienste von seiten anderer
Mikroorganismen beitragen.

Trotz der beachtlichen Schwierigkeiten, die dem Tierversuch bei der Erforschung von endogenen Infektionen entgegenstehen, wurden immer wieder Versuche unternommen, die Pathogenität bzw. Virulenz von *Bacteroides*-, *Fusobacterium*- und *Sphaerophorus*-Arten tierexperimentell nachzuweisen. Der experimentellen Mis infektion wurde dabei große Bedeutung beigemessen. In neuerer

Zeit hat die Charakterisierung von Virulenzfaktoren zunehmendes Interesse gefunden. Darüber hinaus wurde die Wirkung von Chemotherapeutica, der Einfluß resistenzmindernder Faktoren und Gast-Wirt-Beziehungen untersucht.

II. Methoden der Züchtung, Isolierung und Identifizierung anaerober gramnegativer sporenloser Stäbchen

Für Tierversuche können entweder frische Isolate oder Sammlungsstämme anaerober gramnegativer sporenloser Stäbchen benutzt werden.

Sammlungsstämme sind bei der *American Type Culture Collection*, 12301 Parklawn Drive, Rockville, Maryland 20852, U.S.A., bei der *National Collection of Type Cultures*, Central Public Health Laboratory, Colindale Avenue, London, N.W. 9, und im *Institut Pasteur de Paris* (Rue du Docteur Roux, Paris 15^e) erhältlich. Über die verfügbaren Species informieren die Kataloge der genannten Kulturensammlungen.

In kaum einem anderen Bereich der Bakteriologie ist jedoch gegenüber der Benennung der Stämme und damit ihrer Specieszugehörigkeit so viel Skepsis am Platz wie bei anaeroben gramnegativen sporenlosen Stäbchen. Sammlungsstämme sollten daher vor der Benutzung für Tierversuche und dergleichen stets kulturell-biochemisch unter Berücksichtigung der unten geschilderten Methoden überprüft werden. Möglichst eingehende Kenntnisse über Differenzierung, Taxonomie und Nomenklatur dieser Keimgruppe erleichtern dem Benutzer von Sammlungskulturen die Deutung der eigenen Befunde.

Da auch die genannten, international renommierten Kulturensammlungen bisher nur über wenige Species anaerober gramnegativer sporenloser Stäbchen verfügen, muß sich der Interessierte meist noch andere Quellen eröffnen. Hinzu kommt, daß Sammlungsstämme ihre ursprünglich nachweisbare Virulenz vielfach verlieren. Frische Isolate aus pathologischem Material werden daher den Bedürfnissen des an Tierversuchen interessierten Untersuchers häufig eher entsprechen. Daneben dürften gelegentlich auch Isolate aus Schleimhautabstrichen und Stuhlproben zu berücksichtigen sein. Auch diese Kulturen müssen nach Züchtung und Isolierung zur Identifizierung kulturell-biochemisch überprüft werden.

1. Züchtung

Die strikt anaeroben gramnegativen sporenlosen Stäbchen der Gattungen *Bacteroides*, *Fusobacterium* und *Sphaerophorus* sind nur mit Hilfe leistungsfähiger Anaerobierkulturverfahren züchtbar. Zwar können strikte Anaerobier in Mischkulturen mit gewissen Aerobiern auch „aerob" wachsen — die Grundlage dieses Phänomens ist das durch die Aerobier geschaffene anaerobe Mikroklima —, doch gilt für die Isolierung und die Weiterzüchtung von Reinkulturen uneingeschränkt die obige Bedingung. Die Stoffwechselmechanismen, die das strikt anaerobe Kulturverhalten dieser Keime bedingen, sind im einzelnen nicht bekannt. Die Energiegewinnung beruht wahrscheinlich so gut wie ausschließlich auf der Wirkung von Dehydrogenasen, wobei infolge Fehlens oxydierender Fermente Pyruvat, Acetaldehyd u.a. als Wasserstoffacceptoren dienen.

Kennzeichen eines leistungsfähigen Anaerobierkulturverfahrens ist die Erniedrigung des Oxydoreduktionspotentials auf ein rH unter 7, besser unterhalb von 5. Häufig reicht bereits ein etwas höherer rH-Wert (um 7) für das Ingangsetzen der anaeroben Stoffwechselvorgänge aus.

Zur Erniedrigung des Redoxpotentials sind drei verschiedene Methoden bekannt:

a) Physikalische Verfahren: Hierbei wird der Luftsauerstoff durch Evakuieren aus Anaerostaten, z. B. Zeissler-Töpfen, Brewer Anaerobic Jars der Baltimore Biological Laboratories u. a., oder durch 20 min Auskochen aus einem agarhaltigen Medium, z. B. Hochschichtagar, und aus Nährlösungen usw. entfernt.

b) Chemische Verfahren: Zum Beispiel Pyrogallol-Pottasche-Verfahren, das auf der sauerstoffbindenden Wirkung des Pyrogallols in alkalischem Milieu beruht, oder Zusatz reduzierender Substanzen (Natriumthioglykolat, Ascorbinsäure, Leberstückchen) zum Nährboden.

c) Mikrobiologische Verfahren: Hierbei werden sauerstoffverbrauchende und CO_2- und wasserstoffbildende Bakterien in einem geschlossenen System gemeinsam mit Anaerobiern bebrütet (Fortner-Verfahren).

Bei der Züchtung und Isolierung anaerober gramnegativer sporenloser Stäbchen werden besonders günstige Resultate durch die kombinierte Verwendung von zwei verschiedenen Verfahren, z. B. einer physikalischen und einer mikrobiologischen Methode, erzielt. Hierzu werden beispielsweise zwei mit *Escherichia coli* beimpfte Platten zu Anaerobierkulturen in den Anaerostaten gestellt. Die Wirkung von Anaerostaten wird ähnlich vorteilhaft verstärkt, wenn mit Pyrogallol, Pottasche und Kieselgur im Verhältnis 1:2:4 gefüllte Filterpapierbriefchen in die Deckel der Petrischalen eingelegt werden. Nährböden für die anaerobe Oberflächenkultur sollten bereits vor der Beimpfung in Anaerostaten aufbewahrt werden.

Die zur Züchtung von Bakteroidazeen brauchbaren Nährböden enthalten über die sonst üblichen Bestandteile hinaus bestimmte Zusätze, wie Blut, Serum, Ascites, Hefeextrakt, Glucose und Cysteinchlorhydrat. Entsprechende Medien sind sowohl für die Oberflächenkultur als auch für feste, halbfeste und flüssige Tiefenkulturen angegeben worden.

Nachfolgend werden einige empfehlenswerte Nährböden aufgeführt.

a) Für Oberflächenkulturen:

5—7%iger *Schaf-* oder *Menschenblutagar* zur Züchtung aller Arten anaerober gramnegativer sporenloser Stäbchen: Peptonagar (Pepton e carne 25 g, NaCl 5 g, Agar 17,5—20 g auf 1 000 ml Aqua dest.; pH 7,4—7,5 einstellen, 1—2 Std im Dampftopf kochen; filtrieren, autoklavieren) verflüssigen, auf 48° C abkühlen und defibriniertes Hammel- oder Menschenblut zugeben.

Dextrose-Blutagar zur Züchtung aller Arten anaerober gramnegativer sporenloser Stäbchen: Zusatz von 1% Glucose zum obengenannten Medium.

Hämolysierter Blutagar nach Schäfer (1948) zur Züchtung aller Arten, insbesondere von *B. melaninogenicus*:

Teil A	3%iger Fleischwasser-Agar (im Autoklav sterilisiert)	70 ml
	20%ige Nährgelatine (im Dampftopf sterilisiert)	20 ml
Teil B	steriles, hämolysiertes Hammelblut (1 Teil Blut + 2 Teile Aqua dest.)	21 ml

Teil A und B werden getrennt unter ständigem Schwenken $^1/_2$ Std auf 48° C erwärmt, miteinander vermengt und in Petrischalen gegossen. Das End-pH des Nährbodens soll 7,5 betragen.

Hefeextrakt-Cystein-Blutagar nach Beerens (1962):

Pepton tryptisch	10 g
NaCl	5 g
Fleischextrakt (Liebig oder Difco)	2 g
Hefeextrakt (Liebig oder Difco)	5 g
Cysteinchlorhydrat	0,3 g
Glucose	2 g
Bacto-Agar (Difco)	20 g
Aqua dest. ad	1 000 ml

Aufkochen, filtrieren, 20 min bei 115° C autoklavieren. Vor Gebrauch 10% defibriniertes Schaf- oder Pferdeblut hinzufügen. In Petrischalen gießen.

b) Für Tiefenkulturen:

Rosenow-Medium in der Modifikation von BEERENS (1962):

Pepton tryptisch	10 g
Rindfleischextrakt	3 g
Glucose	2 g
NaCl	2 g
Cysteinchlorhydrat	0,3 g
Aqua dest. ad	1 000 ml

Zur Lösung kurz aufkochen; pH auf 7,2 einstellen; filtrieren; erst dann 10 ml des Indicators nach ANDRADE (0,5 g saures Fuchsin auf 100 ml Aqua dest.) hinzufügen. Bei richtig eingestelltem pH nimmt das Medium eine rosa Farbe an. In Röhrchen abfüllen, in die zuvor ein etwa haselnußgroßes Stück Rinder- oder Schafshirn und ein kleines Stückchen Calciumcarbonat eingelegt wurde. Bei 115° C autoklavieren.

Zur Erzielung optimalen Bakterienwachstums sind Oberflächen- und Tiefenkulturen bei 37° C zu bebrüten. Bei 30° C oder 42° C wird nur noch schwaches Wachstum beobachtet.

Die Bebrütungszeit ist je nach Untersuchungsmaterial verschieden. Während Reinkulturen bestimmter *Bacteroides*-Arten auf geeigneten Nährböden bereits nach 18—24 Std makroskopisch erkennbare Kolonien ausbilden, ist zur möglichst umfassenden Anzüchtung aus Mischkulturen eine längere Bebrütungszeit (5 bis 8 Tage) erforderlich.

Sammlungsstämme werden heutzutage im allgemeinen als Lyophilisat zur Verfügung gestellt. Anaerobe gramnegative sporenlose Stäbchen vertragen jedoch die Lyophilisation häufig nicht sehr gut, so daß meist nur mit wenigen lebensfähigen Zellen pro Lyophilisat gerechnet werden kann. Der Inhalt der Ampulle sollte daher nur auf ein Röhrchen mit Rosenowbouillon verimpft werden. Die Rosenowbouillon ist vor der Beschickung mit dem Lyophilisat 20 min im kochenden Wasserbad zu halten, anschließend abzukühlen und nach dem Beimpfen mit erhitztem Paraffinum durum zu verschließen.

Nachdem Wachstum aufgetreten ist, wird das Paraffinsiegel mit einem erhitzten Eisenstab von etwa 3 mm Durchmesser durchbohrt und so für die ausgezogene Spitze einer Pasteur-Pipette durchgängig gemacht. Mit Hilfe einer Pasteur-Pipette wird Kulturmaterial entnommen und auf die Oberfläche von Blut- und Dextroseblutagar (s. oben) gebracht. Nach Bebrütung werden die anaeroben Oberflächenkulturen makroskopisch und mikroskopisch auf Reinheit kontrolliert. Reinkulturen werden biochemisch geprüft und identifiziert (s. unten).

2. Isolierung

Da für Tierversuche frische Isolate häufig besser geeignet sind als Sammlungskulturen, sind die Methoden der Isolierung anaerober gramnegativer sporenloser Stäbchen ebenfalls kurz abzuhandeln.

In pathologischem Material (Eiter, Liquor, Punktate, Blut) können diese Keime entweder allein oder in Mischkultur mit anderen Bakterien vorkommen. In Stuhlproben und an Schleimhautabstrichen liegen *Bacteroides*-Arten und verwandte Keime zunächst stets in Mischkultur vor.

Zur Isolierung und Reinzüchtung sind Oberflächenkulturen vergleichsweise am besten geeignet. An Medien können entweder die oben bei der Züchtung beschriebenen Optimalnährböden oder aber Selektivnährböden verwendet werden. Jedoch gilt bei den anspruchsvollen und empfindlichen anaeroben gramnegativen sporenlosen Stäbchen noch mehr als sonst in der Bakteriologie, daß die Keime, deren selektive Züchtung angestrebt wird, durch hemmende Zusätze zum Nährboden ebenfalls geschädigt werden. Daher sind auch zur Isolierung aus Keimgemischen Nährböden ohne hemmende Zusätze, d.h. also Optimalmedien, vorzuziehen.

Dabei können Reinkulturen nur über Subkulturen gewonnen werden. In der
einschlägigen Literatur wird immer wieder auf die Schwierigkeit hingewiesen,
daß Subkulturen von Primärkulturen häufig nicht angehen. Als Ursache für dieses
„Abreißen" der Kultur wird der Verlust symbiontischer Einflüsse von seiten der
Begleitkeime vermutet. Nach eigenen Erfahrungen (Werner, 1966, 1967) ist
diese Schwierigkeit ohne weiteres zu umgehen, *wenn die Abimpfungen aus dem
Keimgemisch der Primärkulturen unmittelbar nach dem Öffnen des Anaerostaten
angelegt werden*, die mikroskopische Kontrolle der abgeimpften Kolonien somit
erst später erfolgt. Auf diese Weise werden aus sehr artenreichen Keimgemischen,
wie sie z.B. in Stuhlproben vorliegen, zwar gelegentlich Subkulturen auch von
Aerobiern oder von grampositiven Stäbchen angelegt, die Abimpfungen gramnegativer anaerober sporenloser Stäbchen gehen dabei aber praktisch ausnahmslos
an (Werner, 1967). Daraus folgt, daß die in der Literatur vielfach beschriebenen
Mißerfolge beim Versuch der Reinzüchtung auf den für empfindliche Anaerobier
zu langen Zeitraum zwischen Herstellung und Beurteilung eines Grampräparates
und dem Anlegen der Subkultur zurückzuführen sind. Diese Exposition gegen
Luftsauerstoff entfällt, wenn verdächtige Kolonien zuerst abgeimpft und erst
danach mikroskopisch kontrolliert werden.

Manche Untersucher werden es dennoch vorziehen, mit Selektivnährböden zu
arbeiten, oder sie werden Selektivmedien neben den Optimalmedien verwenden.
Daher werden nachfolgend die Formeln einiger bewährter Selektivmedien angegeben:

Brillantgrün-Natriumazid-Agar nach Beerens (1957) zur selektiven Züchtung von *Fusobacterium*- und *Sphaerophorus*-Arten:

Pepton tryptisch	10 g
NaCl	5 g
Fleischextrakt (Liebig oder Difco)	2 g
Hefeextrakt (Liebig oder Difco)	5 g
Cysteinchlorhydrat	0,3 g
Glucose	2 g
Bacto-Agar (Difco)	20 g
Aqua dest. ad	1 000 ml

Aufkochen, filtrieren, 20 min bei 115° C autoklavieren. Zum verflüssigten und auf 50° C
abgekühlten Nährboden 10% defibriniertes Schaf- oder Pferdeblut sowie 10 Vol.-% der folgenden Brillantgrün-Natriumazid-Lösung zufügen:

Natriumazid	0,4	g
Brillantgrün	0,032	g
Aqua dest.	100	ml

Rindergalle-Natriumazid-Agar nach Beerens (1957) zur selektiven Züchtung der durch
Rindergalle im Wachstum geförderten *Bacteroides*-Arten:
Zum obigen Medium an Stelle der Brillantgrün-Natriumazid-Lösung 10 Vol.-% der folgenden Lösung zufügen:

Sterile Rindergalle	100 ml
Natriumazid	0,1 g

Neomycin-Brillantgrün-Natriumtaurocholat-Eggerth-Gagnon-Agar von MITSUOKA et al.
(1964) zur selektiven Züchtung von *Bacteroides*-Arten aus Faeces:

Pferdefleischwasser	930	ml
Proteose Peptone Nr. 3 (Difco)	10	g
Hefeextrakt (Difco)	5	g
Na$_2$HPO$_4$	4	g
Lösliche Stärke	0,5	g
Glucose	1,5	g
Cystin (in HCl-Lösung)	0,2	g
Antifoam B (Dow Corning; in 10%iger Lösung)	10	ml
Bacto-Agar (Difco)	15	g
Pferdeblut	50	ml
Cysteinhydrochlorid (in 5%iger Lösung)	10	ml
Neomycinsulfatlösung 1%ig	20	ml
Brillantgrünlösung 0,01%ig	10	ml
Natriumtaurocholat (10%ige Lösung)	10	ml

Die Bestandteile des Nährbodens außer Pferdeblut, Cysteinhydrochlorid und den drei letztgenannten Lösungen in Wasser lösen, auf pH 7,6—7,8 einstellen und 10 min bei 120° C sterilisieren. Nach Abkühlung auf 50° C die 5 fehlenden Bestandteile gleichzeitig zugeben. Sterilisation der Lösungen durch Seitz-Filtration (Neomycinsulfatlösung) bzw. im kochenden Wasserbad (Natriumtaurocholatlösung).

Erwähnenswert ist weiter der Glucose-Cystein-Agar mit Hefeextrakt und Tomatensaft,
den LEWIS et al. (1940) zur Züchtung von intestinalen *Bacteroides*-Arten empfahlen. SMITH u.
CRABB (1961) entwickelten einen Neomycin-Blutagar zur Züchtung von *Bacteroides*-Keimen
aus menschlichen Stuhlproben. Zur selektiven Züchtung von *B. fragilis* ist nach FINEGOLD
et al. (1965) ein Blutagar mit Zusatz von 100 µg Kanamycin und 7,5µg Vancomycin pro ml
geeignet.

Zur Reinzüchtung von Fusobakterien aus Keimgemischen empfahlen BØE (1941) und BER-
GER (1956) einen 20%igen Ascitesagar mit Zusatz von Gentianaviolett 1:15000. Schon nach
1—2 Subkulturen auf diesem Medium sollen sonstige Keimbeimengungen eliminiert sein.
Nach FINEGOLD et al. (1965) eignet sich Blutagar mit Zusatz von 100 µg Paromomycin oder
Neomycin zusammen mit 7,5 µg Vancomycin pro ml Nährboden zur selektiven Anzüchtung
von Fusobakterien. McCARTHY u. SNYDER (1963) sahen auf 5%igen Kochblutplatten mit
Zusatz von 7,5 µg Vancomycin und 20 µg Streptomycin pro ml nur Wachstum von *Fusobacterium*- und *Leptotrichia*-Arten. Nach ARAUJO u. GIBBONS (1962) wirkt bei den Kristallviolett (= Gentianaviolett) und Streptomycin enthaltenden Selektivmedien z.B. von OMATA
u. DISRAELY (1956) sowie BAIRD-PARKER (1957) nur Kristallviolett (in der Verdünnung
1:100000) selektierend, während Streptomycin unter anaeroben Bedingungen praktisch
wirkungslos ist. SUTTER et al. (1971) empfahlen einen 50 µg Rifampicin/ml enthaltenden
Blutagar zur selektiven Züchtung von *Sphaerophorus varius* aus mischinfiziertem Material.
Da die intestinalen *Bacteroides*-Arten durch die angegebene Rifampicin-Konzentration gehemmt werden (WERNER, 1972b), eignet sich das Selektivmedium auch zum Nachweis von
Sph. varius aus Stuhl (SUTTER et al., 1971).

3. Identifizierung

Zur Identifizierung von *Bacteroides*-, *Fusobacterium*- und *Sphaerophorus*-Arten
können folgende Merkmale dienen:

a) mikroskopische und makroskopische Morphologie,
b) biochemisches Verhalten,
c) serologisches Verhalten,
d) Chemotherapeutica-Empfindlichkeit,
e) Phagensensibilität.

Für eine verläßliche Differenzierung anaerober gramnegativer sporenloser
Stäbchen müssen mindestens das morphologische und biochemische Verhalten
sowie die Chemotherapeutica-Empfindlichkeit geprüft werden.

a) Morphologie

Die Prüfung der mikroskopischen und makroskopischen Morphologie hat eine gewisse Bedeutung für die Differenzierung der drei Gattungen anaerober gram-negativer sporenloser Stäbchen (*Bacteroides, Fusobacterium, Sphaerophorus*), ist für eine Speciesdifferenzierung jedoch nur in Verbindung mit anderen Methoden brauchbar.

Durch wiederholte mikroskopische Kontrolle von gramgefärbten Ausstrichen und Nativpräparaten junger Kulturen auf Optimalmedien ist die Abgrenzung stäbchenförmiger Zellen (Angehörige der Gattungen *Bacteroides* oder *Sphaerophorus*) von fusiformen Bakterien (in der Hauptsache *F. fusiforme*) ohne weiteres möglich. Die Unterschiede zwischen „isomorphen" *Bacteroides*-Zellen und fusiformen Bakterien sind auch elektronenoptisch deutlich darstellbar.

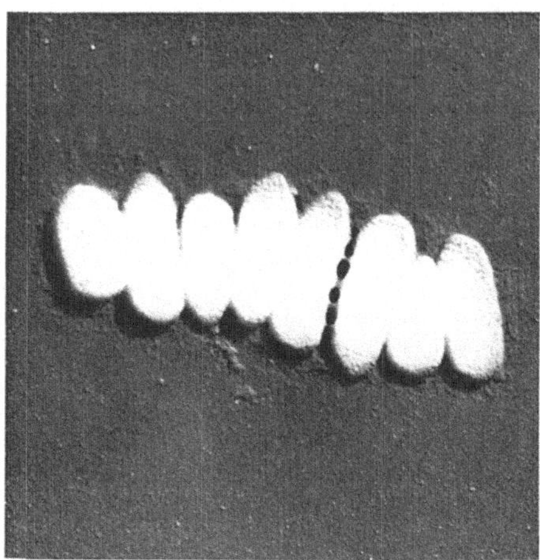

Abb. 1. Elektronenoptische Darstellung eines 24 Std bei 37° C in Thioglykolatbouillon ge-züchteten Stammes von *B. fragilis*. Kurze Stäbchen und kokkoide Zellen. Palladium-bedampfung. Vergr. 9000:1

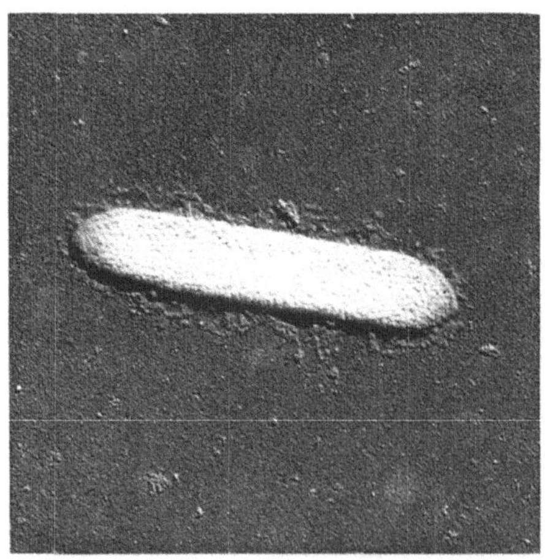

Abb. 2. Stäbchenförmige Zelle eines weiteren *B. fragilis*-Stammes. Kulturbedingungen wie in Abb. 1. Vergr. 12000:1

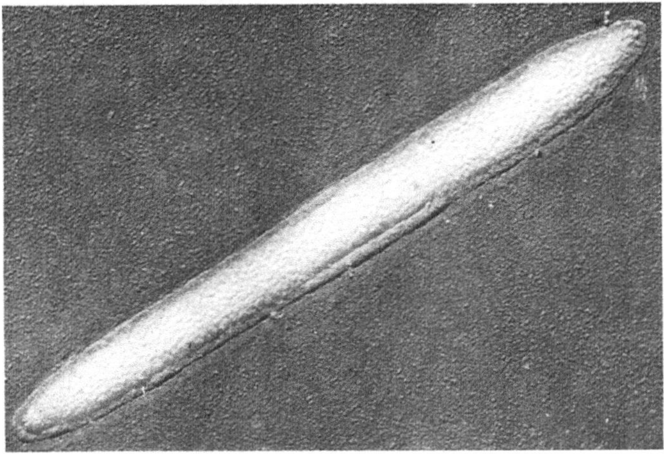

Abb. 3. *F. fusiforme.* Langgestreckt-spindelförmige Zelle mit zugespitzten Enden. 20 Std Bebrütung bei 37° C in Thioglykolatbouillon. Palladiumbedampfung. Vergr. 18000:1

Dagegen ist die mikroskopische Differenzierung der beiden stäbchenförmigen Gattungen *Bacteroides* und *Sphaerophorus* meist sehr schwierig. Der in Abb. 4 wiedergegebene *Sph. necrophorus*-Stamm zeigt nur wenig Sphäroplasten und keine Fadenformen; es überwiegen kokkoide und schlanke Stäbchen:

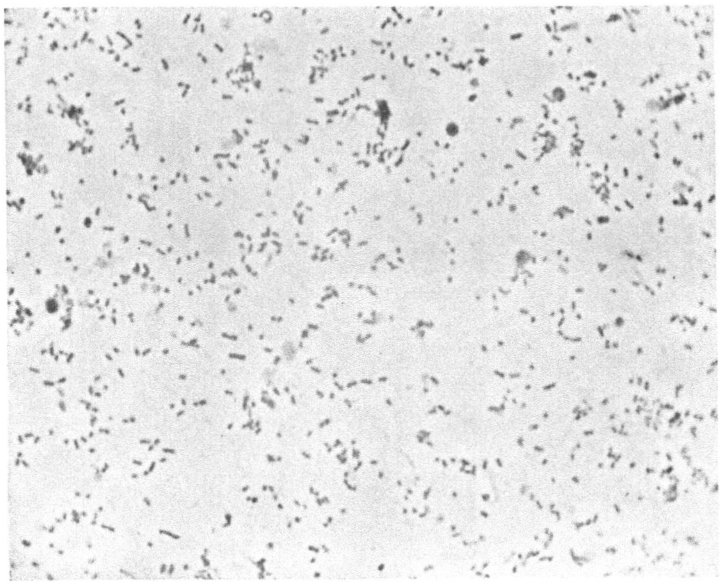

Abb. 4. Mikroskopische Morphologie eines aus Empyemeiter gezüchteten Stammes von *Sph. necrophorus.* Schafblutagarkultur nach 6tägiger Bebrütung bei 37° C im Brewer-Anaerostaten. Vergr. 1400:1. Gramfärbung. Phasenkontrast. Außer kokkoiden und schlanken Stäbchen sind einzelne Sphäroplasten sichtbar. In älteren Kulturen wird ausgeprägtere Pleomorphie beobachtet. (Nach WERNER et al., 1971a)

Kokkoide Stäbchen sind auch die typische Zellform von *B. fragilis*-Stämmen:

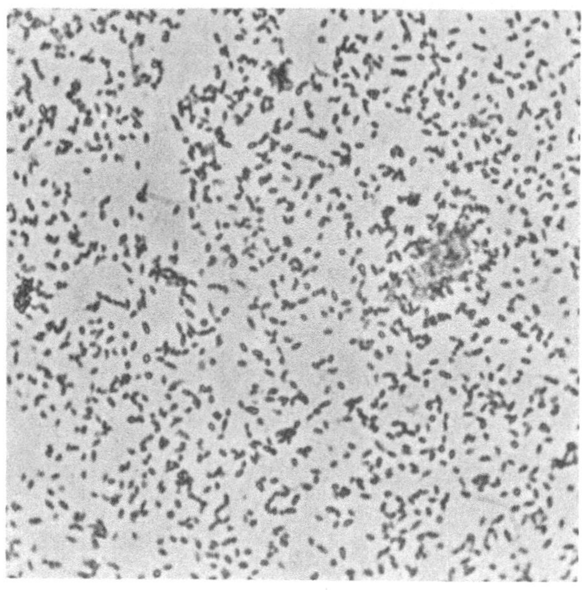

Abb. 5a

Viel eindrucksvollere mikroskopisch-morphologische Unterschiede als bei Angehörigen verschiedener Species werden häufig bei ein und demselben Stamm nach Züchtung in unterschiedlichen Medien beobachtet. So treten z.B. nach Züchtung in glucosehaltigem Medium bei *Bacteroides-* und *Sphaerophorus*-Kulturen regelmäßig deutliche Formveränderungen (große pleomorphe Zellen) auf:

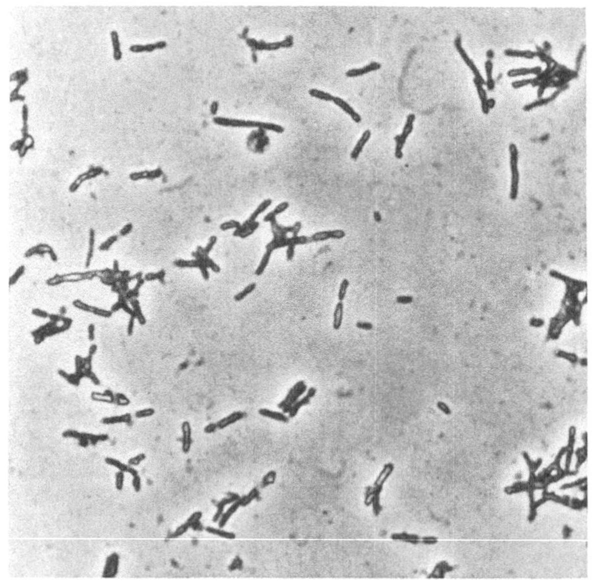

Abb. 5b

Abb. 5. a Mikroskopische Morphologie eines *B. fragilis*-Stammes nach 3wöchiger Bebrütung bei 37° C in halbfestem Pepton-Hefeextrakt-Medium. Überwiegend kokkoide Stäbchen. Vergr. 1400:1. Gramfärbung. Phasenkontrast. (Nach Müller u. Werner, 1970b). b Vergleichsweise große Zellen und beginnende Pleomorphie bei dem gleichen *B. fragilis*-Stamm nach Züchtung in glucosehaltigem Pepton-Hefeextrakt-Medium. Bebrütungszeit, Vergrößerung usw. wie in Abb. 5a

Unterschiede in der Kolonieform dürfen nur bei Verwendung desselben Mediums differentialdiagnostisch verwertet werden. Auf Medien unterschiedlicher Zusammensetzung bildet auch ein und derselbe Stamm differente Kolonieformen aus.

Die saccharolytischen intestinalen *Bacteroides*-Arten (*B. fragilis*, *B. thetaiotaomicron* u.a.) wachsen im Brewer-Anaerostaten auf Schafblutagar in flachgewölbten, grauweiß-transparenten, glattrandigen, weichen Kolonien, die nach 3—4 Tagen Bebrütung bei 37° C einen Durchmesser von 1—2 mm aufweisen. Im Gegensatz zu *B. melaninogenicus*- sowie den *Fusobacterium*- und *Sphaerophorus*-Arten zeigen *B. fragilis* und verwandte Arten auf Hefeextrakt-Cystein-Blutagar mit Glucosezusatz (s. S. 188) keine wesentliche Wachstumsförderung. Das diagnostisch wichtige beige-bräunliche bis schwarze Pigment — nach Tracy (1969) handelt es sich um Eisensulfid — wird von *B. melaninogenicus* auf Schafblutagar meist früher gebildet als auf Hefeextrakt-Cystein-Blutagar mit Glucosezusatz. Die Kolonien von *B. melaninogenicus* auf Schafblutagar sind flach oder flachgewölbt und glattrandig; auf Hefeextrakt-Cystein-Blutagar tritt vergleichsweise reichliches Wachstum in glattrandigen, deutlich gewölbten Kolonien auf.

F. fusiforme und *Sph. necrophorus* zeigen auf Hefeextrakt-Cystein-Blutagar mit Glucosezusatz im Vergleich mit der anaeroben Schafblutagarkultur eine deutliche Wachstumsförderung. *F. fusiforme* bildet auf Hefeextrakt-Cystein-Blutagar nach 4—6 Tagen Bebrütung bei 37° C gelbgrüne, relativ große (3—6 mm Durchmesser) Kolonien mit unregelmäßigem Rand und erhöhtem Zentrum. Dagegen wachsen auf einfachem Schafblutagar manche *F. fusiforme*-Kulturen nicht an; andere Stämme bilden lediglich kleine, flache Kolonien. Bei *Sph. necrophorus*-Stämmen wird auf Hefeextrakt-Cystein-Blutagar mit Glucosezusatz gutes Wachstum in Form von gelbgrünen Kolonien mit gewölbtem Zentrum und flach auslaufender radiär gestreifter Peripherie beobachtet. Die Kolonien sind meistens von einem Hämolysehof umgeben. Auf Schafblutagar werden kleine, flache Kolonien mit unregelmäßigem Rand gebildet. Charakteristisch sowohl für *Sph. necrophorus* als auch für die medizinisch weniger wichtigen Arten *Sph. varius* und *Sph. freundii* ist das gleichzeitige Vorkommen von relativ großen und vielen sehr kleinen Kolonien auf der gleichen Hefeextrakt-Cystein-Blutagar-Kultur.

Die medizinisch wichtigen Bakteroidazeen-Arten sind unbeweglich.

b) Biochemisches Verhalten

Die Prüfung des kulturell-biochemischen Verhaltens ist die praktisch und theoretisch wichtigste Methode zur Differenzierung anaerober gramnegativer sporenloser Stäbchen. Besondere Bedeutung hat dabei der Nachweis der in komplexen Kulturmedien gebildeten bzw. angehäuften niederen Fettsäuren. Bakteroidazeen zeichnen sich nämlich biochemisch u.a. dadurch aus, daß sie außer Acetat noch weitere niedere Fettsäuren bilden bzw. anhäufen. Als Quelle für die in Bakteroidazeen-Kulturen angereicherten niederen Fettsäuren kommen in erster Linie Aminosäuren in Betracht:

Tabelle 4. Metabolische Herkunft der in Bakteroidazeen-Kulturen angereicherten niederen Fettsäuren

Fettsäure	Substrat
Propionsäure	Aminosäuren (Alanin, Serin, Threonin)
Isobuttersäure	Valin
Buttersäure	Glucose Aminosäuren (Threonin, Glutaminsäure, Lysin)
Isovaleriansäure	Leucin

Alle Angehörigen der Gattung *Bacteroides* sind durch Isobutter- und Iso-valeriansäurebildung charakterisiert, d.h. *Bacteroides*-Arten bauen die Amino-säuren Valin und Leucin nur bis zu den korrespondierenden verzweigten Fett-säuren ab (Werner u. Reichertz, 1971; Werner, 1972a). *Sph. necrophorus* und *F. fusiforme* bilden stets reichlich Buttersäure, häufen dagegen Isobutyrat und Isovalerianat nicht an:

Tabelle 5. Differenzierung medizinisch wichtiger Bakteroidazeen auf Grund der Fettsäurebildung

Bakteroidazeen-Species	Fettsäurebildung			
B. fragilis	C_2	C_3	$isoC_4$	$isoC_5$
B. thetaiotaomicron	C_2	C_3	$isoC_4$	$isoC_5$
B. melaninogenicus	C_2	C_3	$isoC_4$	C_4 $isoC_5$
Sph. necrophorus	C_2	C_3	C_4	
F. fusiforme	C_2	$[C_3]$	C_4	

C_2, C_3, C_4 = Essig-, Propion-, Buttersäure.
$isoC_4$, $isoC_5$ = Isobutter-, Isovaleriansäure.

Die im Kulturmedium angereicherten Fettsäuren werden gaschromato-graphisch nachgewiesen (Methode nach Werner, 1969c).

Die zu prüfenden Stämme werden (in 10 cm hoher Schicht) in einem Medium der folgenden Zusammensetzung gezüchtet:

Pepton tryptisch	15	g
NaCl	5	g
Fleischextrakt	2	g
Hefeextrakt	10	g
Cysteinchlorhydrat	0,3	g
Glucose	10	g
Bacto-Agar	0,5	g
Aqua dest. ad	1000	ml
pH 7,4		

Jeder Stamm wird außerdem in einem glucosefreien Medium sonst gleicher Zusammen-setzung gezüchtet. Nach 1—3—7 Tagen Bebrütung bei 37° C werden die Kulturen mit 50%iger H_2SO_4 auf pH 2 angesäuert und mit 3 ml Äthyläther pro Röhrchen ausgeschüttelt. Diese schwefelsauren Ätherextrakte werden gaschromatographisch analysiert (z.B. in dem Gas-chromatograph Modell 900 der Firma Bodenseewerk Perkin-Elmer & Co. mit Flammen-ionisations-Detektor auf einer 120° C heißen kieselgurgepackten Stahlsäule mit Diäthylhexyl-sebacinat und Sebacinsäure als stationärer Phase und Stickstoff als Trägergas).

Für jede Bakteroidazeen-Species werden mit dieser Methode qualitativ und quantitativ charakteristische, reproduzierbare Kurven gewonnen (Abb. 6, 7, 8 u. 9). Die saccharolytischen *Bacteroides*-Arten (*B. fragilis*, *B. thetaiotaomicron* u.a.) bilden bei Gegenwart von Glucose vergleichsweise reichlich Acetat; in glucose-freiem Medium werden dagegen Propion-, Isobutter- und Isovaleriansäure ver-stärkt angehäuft (Abb. 6). *B. melaninogenicus* ist durch Bildung aller verzweigten und unverzweigten Fettsäuren bis $IsoC_5$ gekennzeichnet (Abb. 7). Die Species ist an Hand dieses Fettsäurespektrums sicherer zu identifizieren als durch die Pig-mentbildung (Werner et al., 1971c). *Sph. necrophorus* und *F. fusiforme* weisen sehr ähnliche Pikrogramme auf (Abb. 8 und 9). *Sph. necrophorus* wird von den (selteneren) Species *Sph. varius* und *Sph. freundii* u.a. durch den Buttersäure-Quotienten (= Butyrat in Pepton-Hefeextrakt-Glucose-Medium : Butyrat in Pepton-Hefeextrakt-Medium) abgegrenzt (Werner, 1972c).

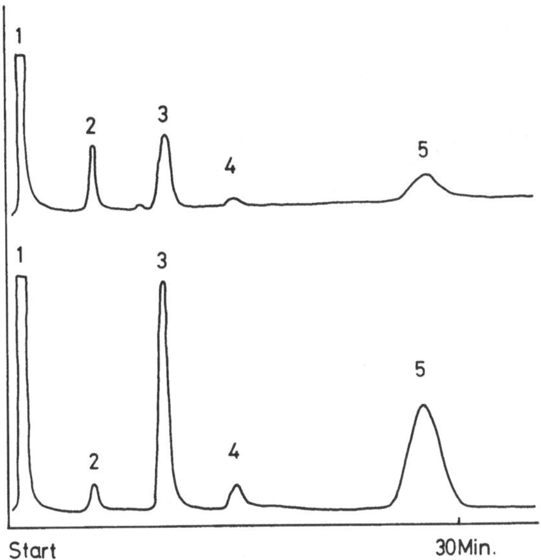

Abb. 6. Gaschromatographische Analyse der von *B. fragilis* in glucosehaltigem (obere Kurve)
bzw. in glucosefreiem Medium (untere Kurve) gebildeten niederen Fettsäuren. *1* Äther (Lösungsmittel), *2* Essigsäure, *3* Propionsäure, *4* Isobuttersäure, *5* Isovaleriansäure. So gut wie
identische Kurven („Pikrogramme") werden mit *B. thetaiotaomicron* und den anderen saccharolytischen intestinalen *Bacteroides*-Arten (*B. vulgatus, B. variabilis, B. distasonis* usw.)
gewonnen. Die Ergebnisse sind von der Bebrütungszeit weitgehend unabhängig

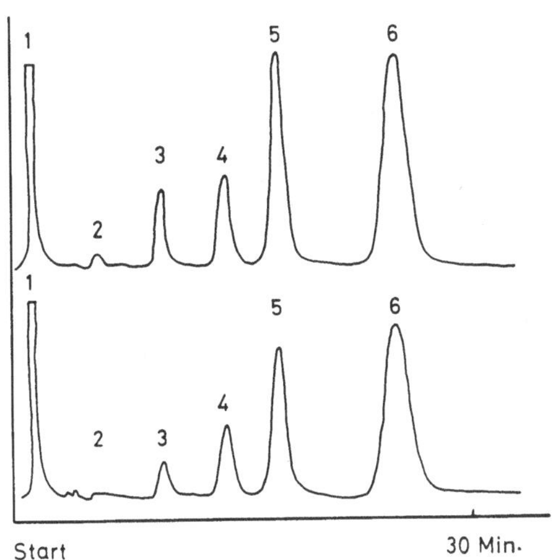

Abb. 7. Pikrogramme eines *B. melaninogenicus*-Stammes. Kulturbedingungen wie in Abb. 6,
1 Äther (Lösungsmittel), *2* Essigsäure, *3* Propionsäure, *4* Isobuttersäure, *5* Buttersäure.
6 Isovaleriansäure

Bedeutung für die biochemische Identifizierung von *Sphaerophorus*- und *Fuso-*
bacterium-Arten besitzt darüber hinaus der Nachweis der Threoninspaltung (BEE-
RENS et al., 1959), der neuerdings ebenfalls gaschromatographisch geführt wird
(Methode modifiziert nach WERNER, 1972a):

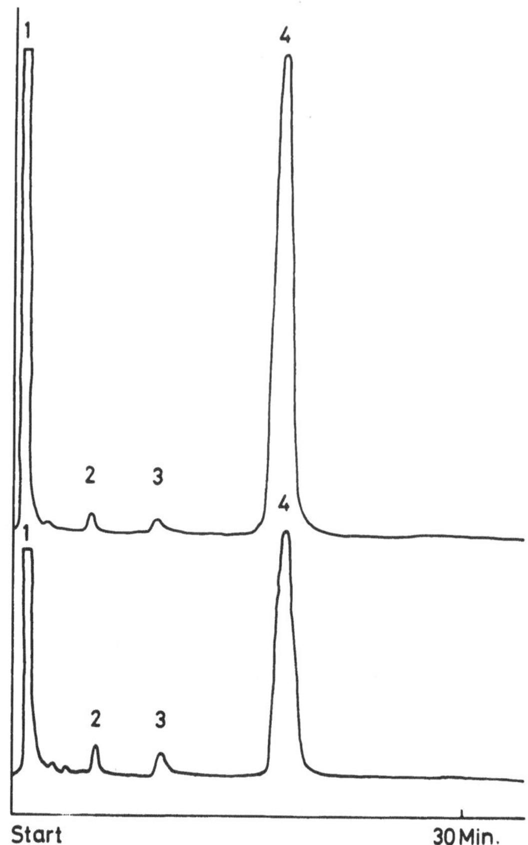

Abb. 8. Pikrogramme eines *F. fusiforme*-Stammes. *1* Äther (Lösungsmittel), *2* Essigsäure,
3 Propionsäure, *4* Buttersäure

Die zu prüfenden Stämme werden 18—24 Std in einem Pepton-Hefeextrakt-Medium
(s. S. 196) gezüchtet und in kurz zuvor autoklaviertem Sørensen-Phosphat-Puffer pH 7,4
zweimal gewaschen. Anschließend werden die Kulturen mit 2 ml einer sterilfiltrierten 1%igen
Threoninlösung versetzt und 48 Std bei 37° C im Brewer-Anaerostaten bebrütet. Danach
werden die Suspensionen mit 1 Tr. 50%iger H_2SO_4 angesäuert und mit 1,5 ml Äther ausgeschüttelt. Die Extrakte werden in Mengen von 3 µl gaschromatographisch auf Carbonsäuren
analysiert (vgl. S. 196).

Bacteroides-Arten bauen Threonin nicht zu Propionat ab. Dagegen spaltet
Sph. necrophorus Threonin unter Bildung von Propion- und Buttersäure (Werner,
1972c). *Sph. varius* und *Sph. freundii* bilden aus Threonin lediglich Propionat.
Das gleiche gilt für *F. fusiforme*; manche Stämme dieser Species bleiben allerdings
negativ (Werner et al., 1971b).

Die einleitende Reaktion beim Abbau des Threonins zu Propionsäure besteht
in der Desaminierung des Substrats und in Bildung von α-Ketobuttersäure.
Suzuki et al. (1966) schlugen daher vor, die Threoninspaltung bei anaeroben
gramnegativen sporenlosen Stäbchen nicht erst durch das Endprodukt Propionsäure, sondern durch das erste Abbauprodukt, nämlich Ammoniak, nachzuweisen.

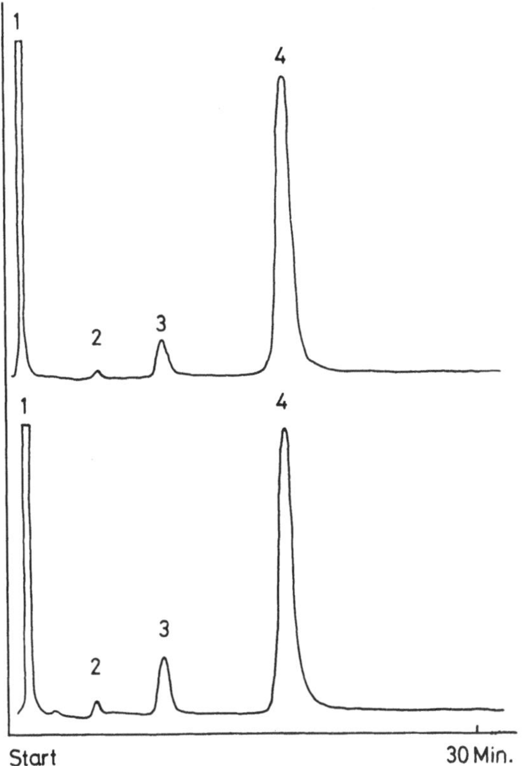

Abb. 9. Fettsäurebildung durch *Sph. necrophorus*. Kulturbedingungen wie in Abb. 6. *1* Äther (Lösungsmittel), *2* Essigsäure, *3* Propionsäure, *4* Buttersäure

Die zu prüfenden Keime werden in einem Medium folgender Zusammensetzung gezüchtet:

Trypticase BBL	1	g
Yeast Extract Difco	0,5	g
Glucose	0,5	g
Fleischextrakt	0,5	g
Phytone BBL	0,2	g
Stärke (löslich)	0,5	g
$Na_2HPO_4 \cdot 12H_2O$	0,5	g
L-Cystein · HCl	0,03	g
Hämin	0,001	g
Aqua dest.	100	ml

pH auf 7,3—7,5 einstellen. Zu 20 ml in Röhrchen abfüllen und 20 min autoklavieren. 15—20 Std bei 37° C bewachsene Kulturen zweimal in 1/15 mol Phosphatpuffer (pH 7,5) waschen und in 1 ml Puffer resuspendieren (Dichte mindestens McFarland-Röhrchen Nr. 10). 0,5 ml der Suspension und 0,5 ml Threoninlösung (200 mg DL-Threonin in 10 ml Phosphatpuffer pH 7,5) in einem Röhrchen mischen. 0,5 ml Suspension + 0,5 ml Phosphatpuffer werden als Kontrolle verwendet. Nach 3 Std Bebrütung bei 37° C 0,05 ml einer 20%igen NaOH-Lösung und 0,1 ml Neßlers Reagenz hinzufügen und mischen. Rotfärbung der Suspension bzw. Bildung eines braunen Sediments bedeuten positiven Ausfall der Reaktion.

Wertvolle Dienste bei der Differenzierung von *Bacteroides*-Arten leistet der Glutaminsäuredecarboxylase-Test (WERNER, 1969c, 1970a).

Bacteroides-Kulturen werden 24—48 Std in Pepton-Hefeextrakt-Medium (s. S. 196) gezüchtet, in Sørensen-Phosphat-Puffer pH 7,4 gewaschen und in 2 ml gepufferter Natriumglutaminatlösung aufgeschwemmt.

Natriumglutaminatlösung:

l-Na-Glutaminat	1 g
Acetatpuffer	50 ml
Aqua dest.	50 ml
pH 4,4—4,5	

Acetatpuffer: 19,5 Teile der Lösung I + 30,5 Teile der Lösung II.
Lösung I: 16,4 g Natriumacetat (wasserfrei) in 1000 ml Aqua dest.
Lösung II: 12 g Essigsäure (96%) in 1000 ml Aqua dest.

Nach 17, 20 und 24 Std *aerober* Bebrütung bei 37° C werden die Suspensionen zentrifugiert. Vom Überstand werden 0,02 ml punktförmig auf Schleicher & Schüll-Papier 2043 b aufgetragen und absteigend in dem Solvens Äthanol 180 : Ammoniakwasser (28%) 10 : Aqua dest. 10 chromatographiert. Als Eichsubstanzen werden l-Glutaminsäure und γ-Aminobuttersäure, zu je 5 mg/ml in Acetatpuffer gelöst, verwendet. Unbeimpfte gepufferte Natriumglutaminatlösung dient als 0-Wert. Das getrocknete Chromatogramm wird mit einer 0,2%igen Lösung von Ninhydrin in Äthanol besprüht und bei 100° C im Trockenschrank 10 min entwickelt. Die l-Glutaminsäure erscheint in R_f 0,0425, die γ-Aminobuttersäure in R_f 0,2 als rotvioletter Fleck.

Eine positive Reaktion geben die saccharolytischen intestinalen *Bacteroides*-Arten (*B. fragilis, B. thetaiotaomicron* usw.). Dagegen setzt *B. melaninogenicus* aus Natrium-Glutaminat keine γ-Aminobuttersäure frei und unterscheidet sich insbesondere hierdurch von der ebenfalls asaccharolytischen Species *B. putredinis* (WERNER, 1970 b). Für die biochemische Identifizierung von *Sphaerophorus*- und *Fusobacterium*-Stämmen hat der Glutaminatdecarboxylase-Test nur geringe Bedeutung (WERNER et al., 1971 a, b).

An Hand der Glucosespaltung werden saccharolytische von asaccharolytischen Arten differenziert. Starke Säurebildung in Pepton-Hefeextrakt-Medium mit Zusatz von 1% Glucose zeigen *B. fragilis, B. thetaiotaomicron, B. vulgatus* und verwandte Arten, schwache Säure- und starke Gasbildung die *Sphaerophorus*-Arten (*Sph. necrophorus, Sph. varius, Sph. freundii*); schwache Säurebildung ohne Gasentwicklung ist kennzeichnend für *Fusobacterium fusiforme*. Der Nachweis der Spaltung weiterer Kohlenhydrate ist wichtig für die Differenzierung der intestinalen *Bacteroides*-Species und der *Sphaerophorus*-Arten:

Tabelle 6. Differenzierung der vier wichtigsten saccharolytischen intestinalen *Bacteroides*-Arten auf Grund der Kohlenhydratfermentation. (Nach WERNER et al., 1970 b)

Differential-diagnostisch wichtige Kohlenhydrate[a]	B. fragilis	B. thetaiotaomicron	B. vulgatus	B. distasonis
Arabinose	−	+	+	−
Xylose	+	+	+	+
Rhamnose	−	+	+	+
Trehalose	−	+	−	+
Cellobiose	+	+	−	+
Glykogen	+	+	+	−

\+ = Säuerung um pH 5 oder darunter (bis pH 4,7). — = Keine Säuerung (pH 7,2—6,0) oder Säuerung nicht unterhalb von pH 5,5.

[a] Die genannten sowie die übrigen saccharolytischen *Bacteroides*-Arten (*B. variabilis, B. uniformis, B. incommunis* u.a.) spalten Glucose, Fructose, Galaktose, Lactose, Saccharose, Mannose, Raffinose, Dextrin und Stärke. Mannit und Inosit werden nicht gespalten.

Tabelle 7. Differenzierung der *Sphaerophorus*-Arten an Hand der Spaltung von
Di- und Trisacchariden. (Nach WERNER, 1972c)

Schwache Säure- und starke Gasbildung in Pepton-Hefeextrakt-Medium mit Zusatz von 1%	Sph. necrophorus	Sph. varius	Sph. freundii
Maltose	+	−	− oder +
Saccharose	−	−	+
Trehalose	−	−	+ oder −
Cellobiose	−	−	+
Lactose	−	−	+ oder −
Raffinose	−	−	+

Die verschiedenen Mono-, Di-, Oligo- und Polysaccharide werden in 1%iger Konzentration
in einem Basismedium (Pepton tryptisch 10 g, NaCl 5 g, Fleischextrakt 2 g, Hefeextrakt 5 g,
Cysteinchlorhydrat 0,3 g, Aqua dest. ad 1000 ml; Bromkresolpurpur als Indicator) geprüft.
Die Röhrchen werden vor der Beimpfung 20 min bei 100° C gehalten, anschließend auf etwa
30° C abgekühlt und mittels Pasteurpipetten mit einer Vorkultur in Rosenowbouillon beimpft.
Die Röhrchen werden nach der Beimpfung mit sterilem, erhitztem Paraffinum durum über-
schichtet und bei 37° C im Wärmeschrank bebrütet. In täglichen oder mehrtägigen Abständen
werden Wachstum der Keime und der Indicatorumschlag kontrolliert. Nach 12—14 Tagen
Bebrütung erfolgt die endgültige Ablesung der pH-Werte mit der Glaselektrode.

Der Nachweis von Indol-, Acetoin- und Schwefelwasserstoffbildung, Gelatine-
spaltung, Harnstoffhydrolyse und Nitratreduktion hat für die Identifizierung
anaerober gramnegativer sporenloser Stäbchen nur untergeordnete Bedeutung.
Auf die Wiedergabe der Methoden kann daher hier verzichtet werden. Geeignete
Testmedien hat WERNER (1965) zusammengestellt.

c) Serologisches Verhalten

Die heutige Vorstellung von der Existenz verschiedener Bakteroidazeen-
Species und -Gattungen beruht zu einem wesentlichen Teil auf der Erforschung
serologischer Merkmale (Antigene). So zeigen etwa *Bacteroides*-Arten keine Kreuz-
reaktionen mit *Sphaerophorus*-Species (WERNER u. SEBALD, 1968), wodurch die
Eigenständigkeit der beiden Gattungen stäbchenförmiger, nichtfusiformer Bakteroidazeen unterstrichen wird. *B. melaninogenicus* weist keine Antigengemein-
schaften mit den saccharolytischen *Bacteroides*-Arten auf (WERNER, 1966). Auch
die biochemisch nur wenig differenten saccharolytischen *Bacteroides*-Species
(*B. fragilis*, *B. thetaiotaomicron*, *B. vulgatus* usw.) können serologisch differenziert
werden (WERNER, 1969a; BEERENS et al., 1971); das gleiche gilt für die drei
Species der Gattung *Sphaerophorus* (*Sph. necrophorus*, *Sph. varius* und *Sph. freundii*; vgl. WERNER, 1972d). Dagegen sind vom Menschen isolierte Fusobakterien
untereinander serologisch nahe verwandt und wohl zu Recht als Angehörige einer
Species: *F. fusiforme*, zu betrachten (WERNER et al., 1971b).

Methodisch bewährt haben sich bei der Antigenanalyse von Bakteroidazeen
insbesondere die Agargelpräcipitation und die Agglutinationsreaktion. Da innerhalb einzelner Species zahlreiche antigenetisch differente „Serotypen" vorkommen
(die wiederum nur zum Teil bisher untersucht sind), konnten Antiseren zur Er-
fassung aller Angehörigen einer Species oder Gattung noch nicht hergestellt
werden. Die Antigenanalyse stellt daher bei Bakteroidazeen noch keine routine-
mäßig verfügbare Differenzierungsmethode dar.

d) Chemotherapeutica-Empfindlichkeit

Die Antibiotica-Empfindlichkeit medizinisch wichtiger Bakterien hat nicht nur therapeutische, sondern auch diagnostische Implikationen. Für die Identifizierung von Bakteroidazeen stellt die Prüfung der Chemotherapeutica-Empfindlichkeit eine wesentliche, ja unentbehrliche Methode dar (s. auch S. 203).

Sph. necrophorus, F. fusiforme und *B. melaninogenicus* sind gegen die meisten therapeutisch wichtigen Antibiotica, insbesondere gegen Penicilline, Cephalosporine und Tetracycline, empfindlich:

Tabelle 8. Minimale Hemmungskonzentrationen (µg/ml) von 11 Antibiotica gegenüber den medizinisch wichtigen Arten der Gattung *Bacteroides*, *Sphaerophorus* und *Fusobacterium*. (*Nach* Werner u. Boll, 1968; Werner et al., 1971a, c)

Antibioticum	B. fragilis[a]	B. melanino-genicus	Sph. necro-phorus	F. fusi-forme
Penicillin G	10—50	0,01—0,02	0,005—0,01	0,1
Ampicillin	10—50	0,01—0,02	0,02	0,1
Carbenicillin	50—125	0,01—0,05	0,02—0,05	0,2
Cephalothin	50—500	0,02—0,05	0,02—0,05	0,05
Cephaloridin	50—500	0,01—0,02	0,05	0,05
Chlortetracyclin	0,2—1	0,02—0,1	0,005	0,005
Chloramphenicol	2,5—10	0,1 —1	1	3
Erythromycin	2—10	0,01—0,05	3	6
Streptomycin		20 —100	10	15
Neomycin	200— > 500	10 —50	15	15
Colistin		20 —100	0,5—1	1,5

[a] Ein sehr ähnliches Verhalten weisen die übrigen saccharolytischen intestinalen *Bacteroides*-Arten (*B. thetaiotaomicron* usw.) auf; einzelne *B. fragilis*-Stämme können tetracyclinresistent sein (MHK 10—50 µg/ml).

Eine geringere Wirkung entfalten lediglich die Aminoglykosid-Antibiotica (Streptomycin, Neomycin); gegen Polymyxin B/Colistin sind nur *Sph. necrophorus* und *F. fusiforme* empfindlich.

Demgegenüber weisen die Angehörigen der Species *B. fragilis* (und *B. thetaiotaomicron*) eine insgesamt stark herabgesetzte Antibiotica-Empfindlichkeit, in vielen Fällen (vgl. die minimalen Hemmungskonzentrationen der Aminoglykoside und Cephalosporine sowie des Colistins in Tabelle 8) sogar deutliche Resistenz auf. Außer Tetracyclin, Chloramphenicol und Erythromycin sind noch Lincomycin und Fusidinsäure als (schwach) wirksam einzustufen.

Bei der Resistenzbestimmung von Bakteroidazeen werden wie bei aeroben Keimen Reihenverdünnungs- und Agardiffusionsteste angewendet. Damit Oberflächen- und Bouillonkulturen von *Bacteroides-*, *Fusobacterium-* und *Sphaerophorus*-Arten anwachsen, ist allerdings eine vergleichsweise reichliche Einsaat nötig. Bei Resistenzbestimmungen sollte jedoch das zum Anwachsen gerade notwendige Inokulum (das in antibioticumfreien Kontrollröhrchen bestimmt wird) nicht wesentlich überschritten werden. In den für Resistenzbestimmungen üblicherweise verwendeten antagonistenfreien Medien wachsen Bakteroidazeen häufig nicht an, so daß für Reihenverdünnungsversuche auf Thioglykolatbouillon mit Zusatz von 10% sterilem Rinderserum und für Agardiffusionsteste auf Hefeextrakt-Cystein-Blutagar zurückgegriffen werden muß. Reihenverdünnungsversuche werden bei 37° C so lange bebrütet, bis die antibioticumfreien Kontrollröhrchen gutes bis reichliches Wachstum zeigen. Für Agardiffusionsteste werden die üblichen Antibioticaträger (Testblättchen, Teststerne) verwendet; die Inkubationszeit beträgt 3—4 Tage bei 37° C in Brewer-Anaerostaten.

e) Phagensensibilität

Nacescu et al. (1972) isolierten aus Abwasser zwei Bakteriophagen, die sich als streng spezifisch für *B. fragilis*-Stämme erwiesen; Angehörige der Species *B. vulgatus, B. thetaiotaomicron, B. distasonis* u. a. waren resistent:

Tabelle 9. Lytische Aktivität des Phagen φA_1. (Nach Nacescu et al., 1972)

Bacteroides-Art	Anzahl der geprüften Stämme	Lysis-Reaktion bei
B. fragilis	68	23
B. thetaiotaomicron	31	—
B. vulgatus	24	—
B. distasonis	10	—
B. tumidus	1	—
B. variabilis	1	—

Mit Hilfe des Phagen φA_1 wiesen Nagescu et al. (1972) das Vorhandensein von *B. fragilis* in einer zuvor als *B. thetaiotaomicron* identifizierten (Misch-) Kultur nach. Zur praktischen Nutzbarmachung dieser offenbar hochempfindlichen Identifizierungsmethode bedarf es jedoch der Auffindung weiterer spezifischer *Bacteroides*-Phagen.

Besondere Bedeutung besitzen unter den aufgeführten Differenzierungsmethoden neben gewissen morphologischen Kennzeichen die kulturell-biochemische Prüfung und die Testung der Penicillin-, Cephalosporin- und Polymyxin-Empfindlichkeit. Die wissenschaftlich exakte Differenzierung der medizinisch wichtigen Bakteroidazeen, das sind *B. fragilis* und verwandte Arten, *B. melaninogenicus*, *Sph. necrophorus* und *F. fusiforme*, beruht dabei auf den in Tabelle 10 angegebenen Merkmalen.

Tabelle 10. Differenzierung der medizinisch wichtigen Bakteroidazeen

Differentialdiagnostisch bedeutsame Merkmale	B. fragilis[a]	B. melaninogenicus	Sph. necrophorus	F. fusiforme
Bildung von				
Buttersäure	—	+	+	+
Isobuttersäure	+	+	—	—
Isovaleriansäure	+	+	—	—
Säurebildung in Pepton-Hefeextrakt-Glucose-Medium	+	—	(+)	(+)
Glutaminatdecarboxylase	+	—	—	—
Threonindesaminierung	—	—	+	+ oder —
Bildung von Propionsäure aus Threonin	—	—	+	+ oder —
Gasbildung aus Rosenowbouillon	(+)	(+)	+++	—
Minimale Hemmungskonzentrationen (in µg/ml) von				
Penicillin G	10—50	0,01	0,01	0,1
Cephalothin	50—500	0,02	0,05	0,05
Colistin	200—500	20—100	1	1,5

[a] Identisches Verhalten in den hier angegebenen Merkmalen zeigen die übrigen saccharolytischen intestinalen *Bacteroides*-Arten (*B. thetaiotamicron, B. vulgatus* usw.).

III. Tierversuche mit Bacteroides-, Fusobacterium- und Sphaerophorus-Arten

Wie in den beiden vorangegangenen Abschnitten dargelegt wurde, beschränkt sich nach neuerer Konzeption die Liste der medizinisch wichtigen Bakteroidazeen auf wenige Arten, nämlich *B. fragilis*, *B. thetaiotaomicron*, *B. melaninogenicus*[1], *F. fusiforme* und *Sph. necrophorus*. Die wissenschaftliche Literatur als Ganzes zeichnet jedoch unter Verwendung zahlreicher weiterer Artnamen ein ungleich mannigfaltigeres Bild. Dies bezeugen auch die Lehrbücher der Bakteriensystematik, z.B. die 7. Auflage von Bergeys Manual of Determinative Bacteriology (Breed et al., 1957), das Manuel de Classification et de Détermination des Bactéries An-aérobies von Prévot (1957), der Traité de Systématique Bactérienne des gleichen Autors (Prévot, 1961) und die umfangreiche Monographie „Les Bactéries An-aérobies" von Prévot et al. (1967). Daß die Anzahl der Species sowie die Ab-grenzung von Gattungen und Familien anaerober gramnegativer sporenloser Stäbchen vielfach von Auflage zu Auflage wechselten, war lange Zeit nicht so sehr Beweis für eine zunehmende Kenntnis dieser Keimgruppe, als vielmehr Ausdruck uneinheitlicher Befunde und widersprüchlicher Deutungen. Isolierte Kulturen konnten an Hand der meist unvollständigen älteren Speciesbeschreibungen häufig nicht sicher identifiziert werden. Daher wurden nicht wenige altbekannte Arten, manchmal sogar mehrfach, „neu" beschrieben. Einige dieser Doppel- und Mehr-fachbeschreibungen wurden in neuerer Zeit wissenschaftlich widerlegt (z.B. sind *B. convexus*, *Ristella pseudoinsolita* und *Sph. intermedius* spätere und daher un-gültige Synonyme von *B. fragilis*; vgl. Werner, 1969b—d). Von anderen, wahr-scheinlich ebenfalls nicht eigenständigen Arten blieben keine Typ- oder Referenz-stämme erhalten, so daß Vergleichsuntersuchungen nicht mehr möglich sind und die Frage der taxonomischen Stellung letztlich offenbleiben muß.

Obwohl daher die Interpretation mancher Untersuchungsbefunde unsicher bleibt, wird nachfolgend der Versuch unternommen, auch die ältere Literatur über Tierexperimente mit menschenpathogenen Bakteroidazeen in die moderne Kon-zeption von der Existenz nur weniger Arten einzuordnen.

1. Bacteroides fragilis

a) Definition und Synonyme

B. fragilis wurde von Veillon u. Zuber (1898) als *Bacillus fragilis* erstmals beschrieben und von Castellani u. Chalmers (1919) zur Typspecies der Gattung *Bacteroides* erhoben. Die an Merkmalen arme Erstbeschreibung des *Bacillus fragilis* (Veillon u. Zuber, 1898) wurde von Cohen (1932) sowie von Weinberg et al. (1937) geringfügig erweitert und letztmalig von Werner (1969c) emendiert.

Von Veillon u. Zuber (1898) wurde *Bacillus fragilis* folgendermaßen charakterisiert: Im Originalmaterial (appendicitischer Eiter!) finden sich schlanke regelmäßige Stäbchen, die etwas kleiner als Diphtheriebakterien sind. Manchmal sind die Stäbchen etwas gebogen; sie liegen isoliert oder zu zweien an einem Pol verbunden. In der Kultur gleicher mikroskopischer Befund; allerdings sind die Stäbchen ein wenig größer und manche Zellen länger. Keine Eigen-bewegung. Schwache Anfärbung mit Gentianaviolett und Löfflers Methylenblau; stärkere An-färbung mit Ziehlscher Lösung; in der Gramfärbung negativ. Schwer züchtbar. Deutliche Koloniebildung erst nach 3—4 Tagen anaerober Bebrütung bei 37° C. Die Kolonien sind punktförmig, rund oder etwas unregelmäßig, ovoid, gelbbräunlich, opak, glattrandig. Isoliert stehende Kolonien können 1 mm Durchmesser erreichen. Sobald Kolonien sichtbar sind, müssen Subkulturen angelegt werden. Nach 7—8 Tagen Aufenthalt im Brutschrank ist die Kultur nicht mehr lebensfähig.

---

1 *B. putredinis* wird nur sehr selten aus pathologischem Material isoliert (Werner, 1970b); Angehörige des sog. *B. corrodens* sind meist nicht strikt anaerob, so daß diese Species nicht zur Gattung *Bacteroides* gerechnet werden kann.

Cohen (1932) sowie Weinberg et al. (1937) stellten fest, daß als *Bacillus* (*Bacteroides*) *fragilis* angesprochene Stämme keine proteolytische Aktivität zeigten, jedoch Glucose und einige andere Kohlenhydrate spalteten. Die Untersuchungen dieser Autoren stellen noch die Grundlage für die Speciesbeschreibung in der 7. Auflage von Bergeys Manual of Determinative Bacteriology (Breed et al., 1957) dar. Danach soll *B. fragilis* aus Glucose, Fructose, Galaktose, Arabinose, Maltose und Saccharose Säure bilden. Einige Stämme fermentieren angeblich auch Lactose. „Sonstige Kohlenhydrate" (Weinberg et al., 1937) werden nicht gespalten.

Eine solche nur wenige Merkmale enthaltende Speciesbeschreibung hat vor allem den Nachteil, daß sie auf viele Kulturen, die möglicherweise differente Arten repräsentieren, zutrifft. So werden von amerikanischen Bakteriologen (vgl. z.B. Finegold et al., 1965) alle aus pathologischem Material und aus Stuhlproben züchtbaren, nicht sero- oder hämophilen anaeroben gramnegativen sporenlosen Stäbchen, die in 1%iger Glucosebouillon ein pH unter 5 erzeugen, summarisch als *B. fragilis* bezeichnet.

Die Speciesbeschreibung des *B. fragilis* wurde von Werner (1969c) folgendermaßen erweitert: Es handelt sich um strikt anaerob wachsende kokkoide gramnegative sporenlose unbewegliche Stäbchen mit geringer Neigung zur Pleomorphie, die durch Zusatz von 10—20% Rindergalle zum Medium im Wachstum gefördert werden, Nitrat nicht reduzieren, Glutaminsäuredecarboxylase-Aktivität zeigen und Essig-, Propion-, Isobutter- und Isovaleriansäure bilden, und zwar mit Ausnahme der Essigsäure in glucosefreien Medien reichlicher als bei Anwesenheit von Glucose. pH 5 wird in Medien erreicht, die folgende Kohlenhydrate in 1%iger Konzentration enthalten: Glucose, Fructose, Galaktose, Mannose, Lactose, Maltose, Saccharose, Xylose, Raffinose, Dextrin und Stärke. Zur Abgrenzung gegen andere saccharolytische intestinale *Bacteroides*-Arten (s. S. 200) ist wichtig, daß bei Anwesenheit von Arabinose, Rhamnose, Trehalose und Melecitose der pH-Wert nicht unter 5,5 sinkt.

Dieser Speciesbeschreibung entsprechen u.a. die *B. fragilis*-Stämme 8560, 9343 und 9344 der National Collection of Type Cultures in London. Das Subkomitee für gramnegative anaerobe Stäbchen des Internationalen Komitees für bakteriologische Nomenklatur hat vorgeschlagen (Report 1970), den Stamm NCTC 9343 als Neotyp der Species *B. fragilis* anzuerkennen.

Die Speciesbeschreibung des *B. fragilis* wurde u.a. deswegen jahrzehntelang nicht mehr weiterentwickelt, weil mehrere Synonyme geprägt worden waren, die an Stelle von *B. fragilis* benutzt wurden.

In diesem Zusammenhang fällt zunächst auf, daß Eggerth u. Gagnon (1933) bei der Beschreibung von intestinalen *Bacteroides*-Arten den *B. fragilis* nicht berücksichtigten. Dafür dürfte die Tatsache verantwortlich sein, daß *B. fragilis* in der 1. Auflage von Bergeys Manual of Determinative Bacteriology (Bergey et al., 1923) sowohl im Identifizierungsschlüssel der damals noch grampositive und gramnegative Arten umfassenden Gattung wie auch bei der Speciesbeschreibung als grampositiv (sic!) bezeichnet wurde. Andererseits mußte jeder spätere Untersucher, der bei der Identifizierung von *Bacteroides*-Isolaten auf die grundlegenden Arbeiten von Eggerth u. Gagnon (1933) zurückgriff, aus pathologischem Material isolierte Stämme vornehmlich als *B. convexus* einordnen (vgl. Reinhold, 1964; Werner, 1964). Von Werner (1969c) wurde der Nachweis erbracht, daß *B. convexus* ein späteres und daher ungültiges Synonym von *B. fragilis* ist. Das gleiche gilt für *Eggerthella convexa* nicht ohne weiteres; denn diese Species soll nach Beerens u. Mitarb. (1963) die von Eggerth u. Gagnon (1933) beschriebenen Arten *B. convexus*, *B. vulgatus*, *B. variabilis* u.a. umfassen. Daher ist lediglich bei aus pathologischem Material isolierten Kulturen die Gleichsetzung von *Eggerthella convexa* und *B. fragilis* weitgehend berechtigt.

Ristella[2] *pseudoinsolita* wurde seit der Erstbeschreibung durch Beerens u. Aladame (1949) vor allem von dem Arbeitskreis um Prévot zunehmend als anaerober Sepsis- und Eitererreger nachgewiesen (vgl. z.B. Prévot, 1965 und die Übersicht bei Prévot et al., 1967). Die Art war von Beerens u. Aladame (1949) auf Grund des Fermentationstyps (Bildung von Essig- und Buttersäure aus Glucose) von der angeblich Ameisen- und Propionsäure bildenden Species *Ristella insolita* (= *B. insolitus*, Eggerth u. Gagnon, 1933) abgegrenzt worden. Später wurde *R. pseudoinsolita* jedoch ebenfalls als Propionsäurebildner beschrieben (Prévot et al., 1967). Werner (1969d) untersuchte 20 *Ristella pseudoinsolita*-Stämme aus der Anaerobiersammlung des Pasteur-Institutes in Paris, darunter den Stamm R 376 von Beerens u. Aladame (1949), und wies Identität mit *B. fragilis*-Stämmen nach. Die von dem Arbeitskreis um Prévot herausgestellten Besonderheiten von *R. pseudoinsolita* wie Häminbedürftigkeit und Hämolysinbildung finden sich auch bei *B. fragilis*-Stämmen.

b) Natürlicher Standort und Infektionen des Menschen

B. fragilis gehört zur Gruppe der saccharolytischen intestinalen *Bacteroides*-Arten (s. S. 200 und Tabelle 2).

Die Erstbeschreiber Veillon u. Zuber (1898) fanden *B. fragilis* besonders häufig in appendicitischem Eiter. Zu ähnlichen Befunden kamen Grigoroff (1905) sowie Werner u. Pulverer (1971). Die meisten Berichte betreffen jedoch Septikämien (Debré et al., 1923; Vaucher u. Woringer, 1925; Boez et al., 1927; Richon et al., 1934; Raikoff, 1935; Lemierre et al., 1938; Delbove et al., 1941; Maupéou, 1973). Außerdem ist *B. fragilis* bei Fällen von Lungengangrän (Guillemot, 1899), Lungenabsceß (Cohen, 1932), Hirnabsceß (Werner et al., 1970a), eitriger Pleuritis (Guillemot et al., 1904; Vallée et al., 1932), Cholecystitis mit Cholelithiasis (Gilbert u. Lippman, 1902) und eitrigen Puerperalinfektionen (Jeannin, 1902; Werner u. Pulverer, 1971) isoliert worden.

Als *Eggerthella convexa* identifizierte Erreger wurden bei Sepsis und bei eitrigen Prozessen unterschiedlicher Lokalisation isoliert (Übersicht bei Beerens u. Tahon-Castel, 1965; Werner, 1966, 1968). Auch *Ristella pseudoinsolita* wurde vornehmlich bei Sepsis, Appendicitis und Peritonitis sowie bei Abscessen im Bereich des weiblichen Genitale gefunden (Quinto, 1964, 1966; Prévot, 1965; Prévot et al., 1967).

c) Experimentelle Pathogenität

Nur wenige Autoren haben die Pathogenität ihrer *B. fragilis*-Isolate im Tierversuch geprüft.

In den älteren Arbeiten wurden Kaninchen als Versuchstiere verwendet. Während Guillemot et al. (1904) *B. fragilis* zusammen mit anderen Anaerobiern („flore de Veillon") Kaninchen injizierten und dadurch eitrige Pleuritis und Lungengangrän erzeugten, sahen Thompson u. Beaver (1932) ähnliche Erfolge (putride Lungenabscesse) nach intravenöser Verabfolgung von *B. fragilis*-Reinkulturen. Nach intravenöser Gabe abgetöteter *B. fragilis*-Kulturen gingen die Kaninchen unter den Zeichen einer sich langsam entwickelnden Intoxikation zugrunde (Guillemot et al., 1904).

Der von Richon et al. (1934) bei tödlicher *B. fragilis*-Sepsis isolierte Stamm war für Mäuse nicht pathogen, rief jedoch beim Meerschweinchen nach subcutaner Injektion lokale Abscesse mit Befall der regionären Lymphknoten hervor. In den

---

2 Die Gattungsbezeichnung *Ristella* (Prévot, 1938) ist gleichbedeutend mit *Bacteroides*.

Lymphknoten waren nekrotisch-eitrige Bezirke von Resten normalen Lymphgewebes umgeben. LEMIERRE et al. (1938) erzeugten mit ihrem ebenfalls bei einem Fall von Septikämie isolierten Stamm beim Meerschweinchen lediglich einen kleinen lokalen Absceß.

Die als *Ristella pseudoinsolita* angesprochenen Stämme von QUINTO et al. (1963) waren für Meerschweinchen nicht pathogen. Nach PRÉVOT et al. (1967) bleibt nur bei wenigen Stämmen nach Aufbewahrung in der Kultur Pathogenität für Mäuse und Meerschweinchen nachweisbar. Solche Stämme rufen nach subcutaner Injektion Absceßbildung hervor, die den Tod der Tiere zur Folge hat.

Nach SCHAFFNER (1963) sind Kaninchen und Meerschweinchen für die experimentelle Infektion mit *B. fragilis* (*Eggerthella convexa*) unempfänglich.

Die intravenöse Injektion von 25 ml einer Kultur in Hefeextrakt-Cystein-Glucose-Bouillon zeigte beim Kaninchen keine Folgen. Intraperitoneal ging die Infektion ebenfalls nicht an.

Bei der subcutanen Infektion ging SCHAFFNER (1963) folgendermaßen vor: Dem gleichen Kaninchen wurden 5 verschiedene Stämme unter die rasierte Rückenhaut zwischen Wirbelsäule und Flanken eingespritzt. Die Injektionsstellen lagen auf einer Linie parallel zur Wirbelsäule und waren jeweils 3 cm voneinander entfernt. Auf der linken Seite wurden jeweils 0,5 ml einer 48 Std lang bebrüteten Bouillonkultur, auf der rechten Seite 0,5 ml der gleichen Kultur gemischt mit 0,5 ml einer 30%igen Suspension pulverisierter Kohle in halbflüssigem Hefeextrakt-Cystein-Medium injiziert. Trotz dieses Zusatzes eines Phagocytosehemmers waren nach 30 Tagen Beobachtungszeit keine Abscesse oder dergleichen aufgetreten. Am Injektionsort ließen sich keine *B. fragilis*-Zellen mehr nachweisen.

Ähnliche Versuche beim Meerschweinchen blieben ebenfalls ohne Erfolg.

Die weiße Maus dagegen erwies sich in den Versuchen von SCHAFFNER (1963) als geeignetes Laboratoriumstier für den Pathogenitäts- und Virulenznachweis von *Eggerthella convexa*-(*B. fragilis*-)Stämmen. Der intraperitoneale Infektionsweg ergab die besten Resultate. Nach Injektion von 0,5 ml einer 48 Std bebrüteten Hefeextrakt-Cystein-Bouillonkultur bzw. von 0,5 ml der gleichen Kultur gemischt mit 0,3 ml einer 10%igen Suspension pulverisierter Kohle in halbflüssigem Hefeextrakt-Cystein-Medium überlebten nur wenige Tiere (Tabelle 11). 24 bzw. 27 von

Tabelle 11. Wirkung von 10 *B. fragilis*-(*Eggerthella convexa*-)Stämmen bei jeweils 6 weißen Mäusen nach intraperitonealer Verabfolgung von 0,5 ml einer 48 Std bebrüteten Bouillonkultur (Methode A) bzw. von 0,5 ml der gleichen Kultur gemischt mit 0,3 ml einer 10%igen Suspension pulverisierter Kohle in halbflüssigem Hefeextrakt-Cystein-Medium (Methode B). (Nach SCHAFFNER, 1963, gekürzt)

Lfd. Nr. der *B. fragilis*-(*E. convexa*-) Stämme	Methode A		Methode B		Anzahl der Tiere, bei denen *B. fragilis* (*E. convexa*) nachgewiesen wurde	
	Anzahl der verendeten Tiere	Anzahl der überlebenden Tiere	Anzahl der verendeten Tiere	Anzahl der überlebenden Tiere	im Herzblut	in makroskopisch veränderten Organen
1	3	0	2	1	4	4
2	2	1	3	0	3	4
3	3	0	1	2	3	3
4	2	1	3	0	5	5
5	3	0	3	0	5	5
6	3	0	3	0	4	1
7	3	0	3	0	4	4
8	1	2	3	0	4	3
9	1	2	3	0	2	0
10	3	0	3	0	6	6
	24	6	27	3	40	35

jeweils 30 infizierten Mäusen (vgl. Tabelle 11) verendeten nach 1 bis maximal 35, im Mittel nach 12 Tagen. Bei der Autopsie der Tiere waren Milzabscesse, eitrige Peritonitis und Befall der inguinalen Lymphknoten die häufigsten pathologisch-anatomisch faßbaren Veränderungen. Aus dem Herzblut sowie aus den in üblicher Weise im Mörser mit sterilem Sand zerkleinerten Organen waren nach Anreicherung in Rosenowbouillon (s. S. 189) *Eggerthella convexa-(B. fragilis-)*Keime vielfach noch nachweisbar (Tabelle 11).

SCHAFFNER (1963) zeigte weiter, daß bei tierpathogenen *B. fragilis-(E. convexa-)*Stämmen auch Virulenzunterschiede bestehen:

Zwei gleich lange bebrütete Kulturen von zwei Stämmen wurden in halbflüssigem Hefeextrakt-Cystein-Medium von 10^{-1} bis 10^{-5} verdünnt und mit 1 ml von jeder Verdünnung zwei Mäusen intraperitoneal injiziert. Von einem Stamm wirkte noch die Verdünnung 10^{-3} tödlich, während der andere Stamm nur bis zur Verdünnung 10^{-1} wirksam war.

Die Toxicität abgetöteter Kulturen ließ sich erst von einer beachtlichen Keimdichte an nachweisen (SCHAFFNER, 1963):

Während 1 ml einer durch 10 min Erhitzen auf 60° C abgetöteten *B. fragilis-(E. convexa-)* Kultur nach intraperitonealer Applikation keinerlei Störungen hervorrief, starben 5 Mäuse, denen in 1 ml Suspension die Bakterien aus 10 ml Kulturflüssigkeit, d.h. ungefähr 100 Milliarden Zellen, injiziert worden waren, bereits nach 6 Std. Wurde diese Suspension wieder 1:10 verdünnt, blieben die Tiere erscheinungsfrei.

An Kulturfiltraten konnte keine toxische Wirkung nachgewiesen werden (SCHAFFNER, 1963).

WOLFF (1972) führte Untersuchungen zur Frage der Invasivität, Endotoxicität und Adjuvanswirkung von drei aus Eiter isolierten *B. fragilis*-Stämmen an weiblichen weißen Mäusen des Inzuchtstammes NMRI/Han. durch. Eine Dosis letalis konnte bei intraperitoneal infizierten Tieren auch nach Zusatz virulenzsteigernder bzw. resistenzmindernder Stoffe zum Inoculum nicht ermittelt werden. In Abhängigkeit von der Infektionsdosis ließen sich jedoch vermehrungsfähige *B. fragilis*-Keime bis zu 30 Tage post infectionem in parenchymatösen Organen nachweisen:

WOLFF (1972) überimpfte die *B. fragilis*-Stämme etwa eine Woche vor Beginn der Tierversuche mehrmals in 48stündigem Abstand auf Rosenow-Medium (S. 189). 48 Std vor den Tierversuchen wurden die *B. fragilis*-Kulturen in ein Hefeextrakt-Cystein-Glucose-Medium (Pepton tryptisch 10 g, NaCl 5 g, Fleischextrakt 2 g, Hefeextrakt 5 g, Cysteinchlorhydrat 0,3 g, Glucose 1 g, Bacto-Agar 0,5 g, Aqua dest. ad 1000 ml, pH 7,4) geimpft. Nach 48 Std Bebrütung bei 37° C erfolgte die Keimzahlbestimmung durch mikroskopische Auszählung in der Helber-Zählkammer. Eine 48 Std alte Hefeextrakt-Cystein-Glucose-Kultur wies demnach eine Keimdichte von $8 \cdot 10^9 \pm 10\%$ auf. Geringere Keimdichten wurden durch Zusatz von sterilem Hefeextrakt-Cystein-Glucose-Medium hergestellt. Zur Erzielung höherer Keimdichten wurden die Kulturen 30 min bei 4000 U/min zentrifugiert und entsprechende Mengen des Überstandes verworfen.

In einer ersten Versuchsreihe zur Bestimmung der Dosis letalis überlebten 12 NMRI/Han.-Mäuse die intraperitoneale Verimpfung von $4 \cdot 10^6$ bis $4 \cdot 10^9$ *B. fragilis*-Zellen 60 Tage lang. Nach 60 Tagen wurden alle Tiere durch Äthernarkose getötet und zum Nachweis der injizierten Bakterien folgendermaßen aufbereitet: Nach Eröffnung des Thorax wurde mit der Pasteurpipette Herzblut entnommen, danach wurden Herz und Lungen herauspräpariert. Erst anschließend wurde das Abdomen eröffnet und ein Peritonealabstrich angefertigt. Danach wurden Leber, Milz und beide Nieren herausgenommen. Zur Vermeidung von Kontamination durch Peritonealexsudat wurden die Abdominalorgane nach der Entnahme kurz in siedendes Wasser getaucht. Anschließend wurden die Organe steril zerkleinert und in Rosenow-Bouillon gebracht. Rechte und linke Nieren wurden jeweils gemeinsam untersucht. Nach 48stündiger Bebrütung wurde von jeder Rosenow-

Kultur eine anaerobe und eine aerobe Aussaat auf Schafblutagar angelegt sowie ein Grampräparat angefertigt. Auf diese Weise wurden 89 Organe der 12 mit *B. fragilis* infizierten Mäuse untersucht. *B. fragilis* war in keinem Organ nachweisbar (dagegen fanden sich häufig andere Bakterien, insbesondere Lactobacillen; WOLFF, 1972).

Da durch die intraperitoneale Verimpfung selbst höchster Keimzahlen bei NMRI/Han.-Mäusen keine tödliche Infektion zu setzen war, verwendete WOLFF (1972) in einer zweiten Versuchsreihe virulenzsteigernde bzw. resistenzmindernde Zusätze, nämlich Eisenammoniumcitrat (BULLEN et al., 1968) und pulverisierte medizinische Kohle (SCHAFFNER, 1963). Als Inoculum wurden *B. fragilis*-Kulturen in Hefeextrakt-Cystein-Glucose-Medium und Rosenow-Bouillon verwendet. Zehn Mäusen wurden 0,5 ml der Hefeextrakt-Cystein-Glucose-Kultur mit einem Zusatz von 0,625 mg Eisenammoniumcitrat in 0,1 ml 0,85%iger Kochsalzlösung injiziert (BULLEN et al., 1968). Bei einem Eisengehalt von 20% und einem durchschnittlichen Mausgewicht von 25 g entsprach dies der Gabe von 5 mg Eisen pro kg Körpergewicht. Eine Kontrollgruppe von ebenfalls 10 Mäusen erhielt die gleiche Menge Hefeextrakt-Cystein-Glucose-Medium und Eisenammoniumcitrat ohne *B. fragilis*-Keime. Einer weiteren Gruppe von 20 Tieren wurden 0,5 ml einer 48 Std bei 37° C bebrüteten Rosenow-Bouillonkultur intraperitoneal injiziert. Zehn Mäuse dieser Gruppe erhielten zu der Keimsuspension 0,3 ml Hefeextrakt-Cystein-Glucose-Medium mit 10% medizinischer Kohle. Lediglich eine Maus starb am 6. Versuchstag, die übrigen Tiere überlebten die experimentelle Infektion mit dem verwendeten *B. fragilis*-Stamm 75 Tage lang. In den Organen des einen verendeten Tieres ließ sich in anaerober Kultur *B. fragilis* nachweisen.

Weitere Versuche von WOLFF (1972) dienten dem Studium der Ausbreitung intraperitoneal verimpfter *B. fragilis*-Keime und ihrer Haftung in den tierischen Organen:

Von insgesamt 36 mit $4 \cdot 10^9$, $8 \cdot 10^9$ und $1{,}6 \cdot 10^{10}$ *B. fragilis*-Zellen intraperitoneal infizierten Mäusen wurden jeweils 3 nach 6 Std sowie 1, 2, 3, 5, 10, 15, 20, 25, 30, 35 und 85 Tagen getötet. Bakteriologisch in der oben (S. 208) beschriebenen Weise untersucht wurden 252 Organe. Nach 5tägiger anaerober Bebrütung bei 37° C auf Schafblutagarplatten gewachsene grauweiß-glänzende, etwas transparente, flach gewölbte Kolonien mit 0,5—2 mm Durchmesser wurden in Rosenow-Bouillon geimpft und kulturell-biochemisch geprüft (s. S. 195). Auf diese Weise gelangen Retrokultur und Identifizierung von *B. fragilis* aus 88 Organen (Tabelle 12). Die Häufigkeit der *B. fragilis*-Funde nahm mit zunehmender Versuchsdauer ab: Während die mit $4 \cdot 10^9$ Keimen infizierten Mäuse nur bis zum 3. Tag positive Organkulturen aufwiesen, blieb *B. fragilis* bei Tieren, die mit $8 \cdot 10^9$ bzw. $1{,}6 \cdot 10^{10}$ Zellen infiziert worden waren, teilweise bis zum 15. bzw. 30. Versuchstag nachweisbar (Tabelle 12). Bei der Sektion am 85. Tag waren alle untersuchten Organe frei von *B. fragilis*. Von den 88 *B. fragilis*-Funden entfielen 17 auf das Peritoneum und jeweils 10—13 auf Lungen, Blut, Herz, Milz, Leber und Nieren (Tabelle 12). Der größte Teil der untersuchten Organe enthielt allerdings neben *B. fragilis* noch andere Keime (*Escherichia coli*, Lactobacillen, Corynebakterien, Mikrokokken, nichthämolysierende Streptokokken u.a.).

Die Endotoxinwirkung abgetöteter *B. fragilis*-Zellen prüfte WOLFF (1972) an 20 Mäusen mit einem Durchschnittsgewicht von 22 g und an 36 Mäusen mit einem Gewicht von etwa 35 g (Tabelle 13). Die *B. fragilis*-Kulturen wurden vor der intraperitonealen Injektion 30 min auf 56° C erwärmt. Die injizierten Keimmengen betrugen bei der leichteren Versuchstiergruppe $4 \cdot 10^9$ bis $8 \cdot 10^{10}$, bei der schwereren $4 \cdot 10^9$ bis $2 \cdot 10^{11}$. Die Mäuse von etwa 22 g Gewicht überlebten die intraperitoneale Injektion von $4 \cdot 10^9$ und $2 \cdot 10^{10}$ hitzeinaktivierten Zellen, die

Tabelle 12. Nachweis von *B. fragilis* in den Organen intraperitoneal infizierter NMRI/Han.-Mäuse. (Nach WOLFF, 1972)

Untersuchungs-material	Versuchs-tiergruppe[a]	Tage nach der intraperitonealen Infektion												Positive Befunde pro Versuchstier-Gruppe	Gesamtzahl der positiven Befunde
		$^1/_4$	1	2	3	5	10	15	20	25	30	35	85		
Peritoneal-abstrich	A	+	+	+	+	−	−	−	−	−	−	−	−	4	
	B	+	+	+	+	+	−	+	−	−	−	−	−	6	17
	C	−	+	+	+	+	+	+	−	−	+	−	−	7	
Blut	A	+	+	+	+	−	−	−	−	−	−	−	−	4	
	B	+	+	−	+	−	−	−	−	−	−	−	−	3	11
	C	+	+	+	+	−	−	−	−	−	−	−	−	4	
Herz	A	+	+	+	+	−	−	−	−	−	−	−	−	4	
	B	+	+	+	+	−	−	−	−	−	−	−	−	4	12
	C	+	+	−	+	−	−	+	−	−	−	−	−	4	
Lunge	A	−	−	+	−	−	−	−	−	−	−	−	−	1	
	B	+	+	+	−	+	−	−	−	−	−	−	−	4	10
	C	+	+	+	+	+	−	−	−	−	−	−	−	5	
Leber	A	+	+	+	+	−	−	−	−	−	−	−	−	4	
	B	−	+	+	+	−	−	+	−	−	−	−	−	4	13
	C	+	+	−	+	−	−	+	−	−	+	−	−	5	
Milz	A	+	+	+	+	−	−	−	−	−	−	−	−	4	
	B	−	−	+	−	+	−	+	−	−	−	−	−	3	12
	C	+	+	+	+	+	−	−	−	−	−	−	−	5	
Nieren	A	+	+	+	+	−	−	−	−	−	−	−	−	4	
	B	+	−	+	+	−	−	+	−	−	−	−	−	4	13
	C	+	+	+	−	+	−	−	−	−	+	−	−	5	

[a] A = Infektionsdosis $4 \cdot 10^9$ Keime; B = Infektionsdosis $8 \cdot 10^9$ Keime; C = Infektionsdosis $1,6 \cdot 10^{10}$ Keime.

Tabelle 13. Endotoxinwirkung abgetöteter Zellen eines *B. fragilis*-Stammes.
(Nach WOLFF, 1972)

Intraperitoneal injizierte Keimmenge	Anzahl der Mäuse von 22 g Gewicht	Davon innerhalb Tagesfrist verendet	Anzahl der Mäuse von 35 g Gewicht	Davon innerhalb Tagesfrist verendet
$4 \cdot 10^9$	4	0	4	0
$2 \cdot 10^{10}$	4	0	4	0
$4 \cdot 10^{10}$	4	1	4	0
$6 \cdot 10^{10}$	4	4	4	0
$8 \cdot 10^{10}$	4	4	4	1
$1 \cdot 10^{11}$	nicht durchgeführt	nicht durchgeführt	4	3
$1,2 \cdot 10^{11}$	desgl.	desgl.	4	3
$1,6 \cdot 10^{11}$	desgl.	desgl.	4	3
$2 \cdot 10^{11}$	desgl.	desgl.	4	4

schwereren Mäuse vertrugen $4 \cdot 10^9$ bis $6 \cdot 10^{10}$ Keime (Tabelle 13). Nach der Injektion von $4 \cdot 10^{10}$ Zellen starb eines der leichteren, nach Gabe von $8 \cdot 10^{10}$ Zellen eines der schwereren Tiere. Die Gabe von $6 \cdot 10^{10}$ und $8 \cdot 10^{10}$ *B. fragilis*-Zellen wirkte bei den Mäusen von 22 g ausnahmslos tödlich. Von den jeweils 4 behandelten Tieren der höheren Gewichtsklasse starben jeweils nur 3 nach Injektion von $1 \cdot 10^{11}$, $1,2 \cdot 10^{11}$ und $1,6 \cdot 10^{11}$ Zellen. Der Gabe von $2 \cdot 10^{11}$ Zellen erlagen alle 4 Tiere (Tabelle 13).

Eine Erhöhung der anaphylaktischen Schockbereitschaft war bei intraperitoneal mit Rinderserumalbumin und *B. fragilis* immunisierten NMRI/Han.-Mäusen nicht nachweisbar; Adjuvanswirkung kommt daher dem *B. fragilis* wohl nicht zu (WOLFF, 1972). Nach intraperitonealer Immunisierung mit *B. fragilis*-Zellen allein stellte WOLFF (1972) eine mäßige Erhöhung des Milzgewichtes als Ausdruck einer vorübergehend vermehrten Tätigkeit des RES fest.

α) Endotoxin

Aus dem Stamm NCTC 9343 von *B. fragilis* (s. S. 205) extrahierten HOFSTAD u. KRISTOFFERSEN (1970) mit Hilfe der Phenol-Wasser-Methode von WESTPHAL et al. (1952) Lipopolysaccharide, die im Kaninchentest endotoxische Aktivität entfalteten:

Gleiche Volumina von wäßrigen *B. fragilis*-Suspensionen und 90%igem Phenol wurden 15 min bei Laboratoriumstemperatur homogenisiert. Nach Zentrifugation (30 min $3000 \times g$) wurde der wäßrige Überstand abpipettiert und die Extraktion mit der gleichen Menge destilliertem Wasser wiederholt. Die gesammelten wäßrigen Extrakte wurden 3 Tage gegen dest. Wasser dialysiert und anschließend mit 2,5 Vol. kaltem Aceton gefällt. Der Niederschlag wurde in destilliertem Wasser aufgenommen. Die entstandene homogene, leicht opalescente Suspension wurde 1 Std bei $100000 \times g$ in der präparativen Ultrazentrifuge zentrifugiert. Der Bodensatz wurde in kristalline Ribonuclease und Desoxyribonuclease enthaltendem 0,1 mol Phosphat-Puffer pH 7,0 so aufgenommen, daß ein Enzym-Substrat-Verhältnis von ungefähr 1:50 entstand, und 1 Std bei $37° C$ bebrütet. Nach erneuter Ultrazentrifugation wurde der das gereinigte Lipopolysaccharid enthaltende Bodensatz in dest. Wasser aufgenommen und lyophilisiert.

Durch Variation der Extraktionszeiten (15 bzw. 30 min, s. oben) gewannen HOFSTAD u. KRISTOFFERSEN (1970) insgesamt 3 Lipopolysaccharid-Präparationen, deren chemische Zusammensetzung und Endotoxicität geprüft wurden.

Es zeigte sich, daß Heptose und 2-Keto-3-desoxy-octonat, die charakteristischen Bausteine des Endotoxins aerober gramnegativer Bakterien, in den phenol-wasser-extrahierten Lipopolysacchariden von *B. fragilis* NCTC 9343 fehlten. Als Kohlenhydratbausteine wurden Glucosamin, Galaktosamin, Glucose, Galaktose, Fructose, Rhamnose und — in Spuren — Mannose nachgewiesen (HOFSTAD u. KRISTOFFERSEN, 1970).

Von den nach 15 bzw. 30 min Extraktion gewonnenen Lipopolysaccharid-Präparationen wurden in steriler physiologischer Kochsalzlösung Verdünnungsreihen hergestellt und jeweils 6 Albino-Kaninchen von 2,6—3,7 kg Gewicht intracutan in Mengen von 0,2 ml in die rasierte Bauchhaut injiziert. Die intravenösen Erfolgsinjektionen von 400 µg Lipopolysaccharid pro Tier wurden 24 Std später verabfolgt. Am folgenden Tag wurde das Auftreten hämorrhagischer Läsionen (Shwartzman-Reaktion) kontrolliert. Auf diese Weise wurde eine dosisabhängige, mäßige Endotoxicität festgestellt (Tabelle 14).

Tabelle 14. Lokale Shwartzman-Reaktion bei jeweils 6 mit 2 Lipopolysaccharid-Präparationen aus *B. fragilis* NCTC 9343 behandelten Albino-Kaninchen. (Nach Hofstad u. Kristoffersen, 1972)

Lipopolysaccharid-Präparationen	Dosis der intracutanen Erstinjektion					
	400 µg	200 µg	100 µg	50 µg	25 µg	12,5 µg
A (15 min Extraktion)	6/6[a]	6/6	3/6	1/6	0/6	0/6
B (30 min Extraktion)	4/6	3/6	3/6	3/6	1/6	0/6

[a] Positive Shwartzman-Reaktion/Anzahl der geprüften Tiere.

Gereinigte Endotoxin-(Lipopolysaccharid-)Partikeln von *B. fragilis* NCTC 9343 erwiesen sich elektronenoptisch als stäbchenförmig (Hofstad et al., 1972).

β) Neuraminidase und Fibrinolysin

Weil sich die Methoden leicht auch für tierexperimentelle Fragestellungen anwenden lassen, sollen hier anhangsweise Untersuchungen über die Einwirkung von *B. fragilis* auf menschliche Plasmaproteine erwähnt werden.

Werner u. Müller (1971) züchteten anaerobe gramnegative sporenlose Stäbchen, u.a. auch 24 *B. fragilis*-Stämme, auf einem 50% Humanplasma (von Blutkonserven der Blutgruppe AB) enthaltenden Medium und analysierten den unter den Bakterienkolonien gelegenen Plasma-Agar immunelektrophoretisch unter Verwendung spezifischer Plasmaprotein-Antisera. Die 24 *B. fragilis*-Stämme bewirkten bei Glykoproteinen, und zwar insbesondere bei Hämopexin, α_2-HS-Glykoprotein, γA-Globulin, Transferrin und saurem α_1-Glykoprotein, Veränderungen der immunelektrophoretischen Wanderungsgeschwindigkeit, die auf bakterielle Neuraminidasen zurückzuführen waren (Müller u. Werner, 1970a). Fibrinolytische Aktivität (Abb. 10) wiesen 13 *B. fragilis*-Stämme auf.

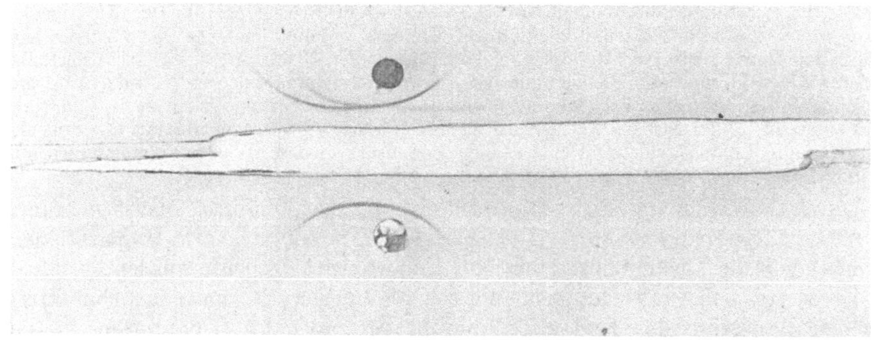

Abb. 10. Immunelektrophoretischer Nachweis der fibrinolytischen Aktivität eines *B. fragilis*-Stammes. Oben: aufgespaltenes Fibrinogen aus dem unter einer *B. fragilis*-Kolonie gelegenen Plasmaagar nach 19 Tagen Bebrütung bei 37° C. Unten: unverändertes Fibrinogen aus unbewachsenem Plasmaagar als Kontrolle. (Nach Werner u. Müller, 1971)

Neuraminidaseeinwirkung war immunelektrophoretisch auch an 6 von 10 Glykoproteinen im Eiter eines durch *B. fragilis* bedingten Abscesses nachweisbar (MÜLLER u. WERNER, 1970b). Ein Zusammenhang zwischen Neuraminidasebildung und Virulenz wurde daher von den genannten Autoren für möglich gehalten.

2. Bacteroides thetaiotaomicron

B. thetaiotaomicron wurde von DISTASO (1912) als *Bacillus thetaiotaomicron* erstmals beschrieben. EGGERTH u. GAGNON (1933) legten die noch gegenwärtig zur Identifizierung benutzten Merkmale, insbesondere die Spaltung zahlreicher Kohlenhydrate (s. S. 200), fest. Im Gegensatz zu DISTASO (1912), der *B. thetaiotaomicron* als beweglich beschrieben hatte, machten EGGERTH u. GAGNON (1933) deutlich, daß die Species unbeweglich ist. PRÉVOT (1938) übernahm die ursprüngliche Angabe von DISTASO (1912) und ordnete die Species als *Sphaerocillus thetaiotaomicron* bei den beweglichen sphaerophorusähnlichen Stäbchen ein. *B. thetaiotaomicron* wurde erst von REINHOLD (1964) und WERNER (1966, 1967) in größerer Zahl in pathologischem Material und gehäuft in Stuhlproben nachgewiesen.

In der National Collection of Type Cultures in London ist unter der Nummer NCTC 10582 von WERNER ein Stamm (E_{50}) deponiert worden, den das Subkomitee für gramnegative anaerobe Stäbchen des Internationalen Komitees für bakteriologische Nomenklatur als Neotyp der Species *B. thetaiotaomicron* vorschlagen will.

B. thetaiotaomicron ist die einzige Species aus der Gruppe der saccharolytischen intestinalen Bacteroides-Arten, deren medizinische Bedeutung (als Erreger eitriger Prozesse unterschiedlicher Lokalisation) mit der von *B. fragilis* vergleichbar ist (WERNER u. PULVERER, 1971).

Zu *B. thetaiotaomicron* gehört der als *Sph. necrophorus* bezeichnete Stamm 12290 der American Type Culture Collection (ATCC), den SUTER et al. (1955) als *B. funduliformis* beschrieben hatten. Nach SUTER et al. (1955) war der Stamm „pathogen für Mäuse und rief meist Leberabscesse hervor".

WOLFF (1972) gelang es nicht, durch intraperitoneale Injektion eines *B. thetaiotaomicron*-Stammes in Keimzahlen bis zu $4 \cdot 10^9$ bei weiblichen weißen NMRI/Han.-Mäusen eine tödliche Infektion zu setzen.

Der Bericht von HOFSTAD u. KRISTOFFERSEN (1971) über „Präparation und chemische Eigenschaften des endotoxischen Lipopolysaccharids von 3 *Sph. necrophorus*-Stämmen" bezieht sich u.a. auf den oben erwähnten Stamm ATCC 12290, d.h. also auf *B. thetaiotaomicron*. Die gereinigten Lopopolysaccharid-Präparationen dieses Stammes (Herstellung s. S. 211) waren wie bei *B. fragilis* NCTC 9343 frei von Heptose und 2-Keto-3-desoxyoctonat und riefen als Ausdruck schwacher Endotoxicität nur wenige positive Shwartzman-Reaktionen im Kaninchentest (Methode s. S. 212) hervor.

Nach WERNER u. MÜLLER (1971) weisen *B. thetaiotaomicron*-Kulturen nur teilweise Neuraminidase-Aktivität auf. Die für mehr als 50% der *B. fragilis*-Stämme charakteristische fibrinolytische Wirksamkeit ist bei *B. thetaiotaomicron* nicht nachweisbar (WERNER u. MÜLLER, 1971).

3. Bacteroides melaninogenicus

a) Definition, systematische Stellung und Synonyme

Die Keimart wurde von OLIVER u. WHERRY (1921) erstmals beschrieben und wegen der vermeintlich durch Melanin bedingten Schwarzbraunfärbung der Kolonie *Bacterium melaninogenicum* genannt. Nach SCHWABACHER et al. (1947) soll das schwarze Pigment jedoch nicht Melanin, sondern ein bakterielles Parahämatin sein, das nach dem Abbau des Globinanteils des im Blutagar vorhandenen Hämoglobins durch Anlagerung der Hämatinkomponente an ein bakterielles Protein entsteht. Die genannten Autoren schlugen daher vor, das Epitheton speciei *melaninogenicus* durch *nigrescens* zu ersetzen und die Art gemäß der Einteilung von WILSON u. MILES (1946) in die Gattung *Fusiformis* zu überführen. Demgegenüber wurde in der 7. Auflage von BERGEYs Manual (BREED et al., 1957) geltend gemacht, daß das Epitheton speciei *melaninogenicus* die Priorität besitze und nach den internationalen Nomenklaturregeln beizubehalten sei. Nach TRACY (1969) ist die charakteristische schwarze oder schwarzbraune Farbe der *B. melaninogenicus*-Kolonien auf die Bildung von Eisensulfid zurückzuführen.

In neuerer Zeit ist der Verdacht aufgekommen, daß unter der Bezeichnung *B. melaninogenicus* heterogene, letztlich nicht zu derselben Species gehörige Vertreter von schwarz wachsenden, strikt anaeroben Bakterien subsumiert worden sind. WERNER et al. (1971c) haben daher versucht, *B. melaninogenicus* ohne Berücksichtigung der Pigmentbildung lediglich auf Grund biochemischer Eigenschaften zu definieren. Danach ist *B. melaninogenicus* durch die Bildung von Essig-, Propion-, Isobutter-, Butter- und Isovaleriansäure (s. S. 197) sowie durch Fehlen der Threoninspaltung und der Glutaminatdecarboxylase-Aktivität gekennzeichnet, bildet Indol und verflüssigt Gelatine. Da in 1% Glucose oder andere Kohlenhydrate enthaltenden Medien pH-Werte von 6,2—6,6 beobachtet werden, kann die Species als asaccharolytisch gelten (WERNER et al., 1971c). Die Zugehörigkeit saccharolytischer pigmentbildender Kulturen, die HOLDEMAN u. MOORE (1972) als Subspecies von *B. melaninogenicus* aufführen, bleibt noch zu klären.

b) Natürlicher Standort und Infektionen des Menschen

Die Erstbeschreiber OLIVER u. WHERRY (1921) züchteten *B. melaninogenicus* von der Mundschleimhaut, den Tonsillen, infizierten chirurgischen Wunden sowie aus Stuhl- und Urinproben. Seitdem wurde der Keim von zahlreichen Autoren gefunden (Übersicht bei WERNER, 1966, 1968).

B. melaninogenicus gehört zur normalen Bakterienflora der menschlichen Mundhöhle. Im Coloninhalt sowie in Stuhlproben scheint die Species dagegen nicht häufig zu sein. In der normalen Appendix reichert sie sich offenbar an (WERNER u. SEELIGER, 1963). So gut wie regelmäßig gelingt der Nachweis des *B. melaninogenicus* im Lochialsekret (WERNER, 1966).

Aus pathologischem Material ist *B. melaninogenicus* nur sehr selten in Reinkultur züchtbar (HEINRICH u. PULVERER, 1960, fanden den Keim nur in 4 von 621 Fällen in Reinkultur). Pathogen wirkt *B. melaninogenicus* demnach so gut wie ausschließlich in Vergesellschaftung mit anderen Bakterien (s. auch weiter unten).

Die meisten bekannt gewordenen Beobachtungen betreffen Mischinfektionen im cervicofacialen Bereich (BURDON, 1928; SCHWABACHER et al., 1947; TEUSCH, 1949; HEINRICH u. PULVERER, 1960); aber auch in Lungenabscessen (VARNEY, 1929; COHEN, 1932), bei Peritonitis (ALTEMEIER, 1938a, b; WEISS, 1943), in einem Schläfenlappenabsceß nach Mastoiditis (BEERENS u. TAHON-CASTEL, 1965) und in multiplen, im Verlaufe einer Septikämie aufgetretenen Hirnabscessen (OEHRING et al., 1967) wurde *B. melaninogenicus*, meist zusammen mit anderen Keimen, nachgewiesen. Die offenbar nicht seltene Beteiligung des *B. melaninogenicus* bei Puerperalinfektionen (SCHWARZ u. DIECKMANN, 1927) ist eine Folge der häufigen Besiedlung des Lochialsekrets (WERNER, 1966).

c) Bereitung eines infektionstüchtigen Inoculums

B. melaninogenicus stellt weitreichende Ansprüche an Medien und Kulturverfahren, seine Nährstoffbedürfnisse sind außerordentlich komplex. Daher sind viele Stämme in Reinkultur nur schwer, in Mischkultur mit anderen Bakterien dagegen recht gut haltbar (Übersicht WERNER, 1966, 1968).

Nach SCHWABACHER et al. (1947) sowie PETER (1963) wirkt Kohlendioxyd wachstumsfördernd. Der Faktor X (= Hämin) soll das Wachstum stärker stimulieren als der Faktor V (dem Medium z.B. in Form von Hefeextrakt zugesetzt); optimales Wachstum tritt jedoch nur in Anwesenheit beider Faktoren auf (SCHWABACHER et al., 1947). Die wachstumsfördernde Wirkung des Serums dürfte u.a. auf die im Serum vorhandenen Häminmengen zurückgehen (WERNER, 1966). LEV (1958) wies bei einem aus dem Pansen isolierten *Fusiformis nigrescens*-Stamm Bedürftigkeit für Vitamin K nach. Nach GIBBONS u. MACDONALD (1960) benötigen viele *B. melaninogenicus*-Stämme außer Hämin einen von bestimmten Bakterien, vor allem *Staphylococcus aureus*, gebildeten, in den Nährboden diffundierenden Wachstumsfaktor. Dieser Faktor kann durch Substanzen der Vitamin K-Gruppe und Naphthalin-Abkömmlinge mit einer Sauerstoff-, Hydroxyl- oder Carboxyl-Gruppe in α-Stellung ersetzt werden. Der menschliche Speichel entfaltet ebenfalls wachstumsfördernde Eigenschaften, wofür die durch Mikroben gebildeten Vitamine verantwortlich gemacht werden (GIBBONS u. MACDONALD, 1960).

Zur Züchtung des *B. melaninogenicus* ist der hämolysierte Blutagar nach SCHÄFER (1948; s. S. 188) besonders zu empfehlen. Auf diesem Medium wächst *B. melaninogenicus* in 2—4 Tagen in zunächst hellbraunen, bald dunkelbraunen bis schwarzen Kolonien. Auf nichthämolysiertem Blutagar sowie auf Hefeextrakt-Cystein-Blutagar (s. S. 188) tritt die Schwärzung der Kolonien langsamer und vielfach erst nach Ausbildung einer Hämolysezone ein. Die Schwarzfärbung der Kolonien ist bei verschiedenen Stämmen unterschiedlich stark ausgeprägt. In Mischkulturen wächst *B. melaninogenicus* besonders gut. Für die Erhaltung der Stämme u.ä. empfiehlt sich gelegentlich geradezu die gemeinsame Verimpfung mit *Staphylococcus aureus*.

In anaerober Oberflächenkultur stirbt *B. melaninogenicus* schnell ab. 10 Tage bei 37° C bebrütete Kulturen sind meist schon nicht mehr überimpfbar. Dagegen sind nach WERNER (1966) Rosenow-Bouillonkulturen (s. S. 189) mit Zusatz von 1 ml hämolysiertem Blut pro Röhrchen unter Paraffinsiegel länger als 2 Monate bei Laboratoriumstemperatur haltbar. Zur Erhöhung der Anwachsrate von Subkulturen empfiehlt sich die Verimpfung des gesamten Inhalts der Kulturröhrchen mit Pasteurpipetten auf frische Rosenow-Bouillon. Für Infektionsversuche bestimmte Kulturen sollten möglichst nicht länger als 2—4 Tage bebrütet werden.

d) Experimentelle Pathogenität

Mit Reinkulturen von *B. melaninogenicus* wurde in Tierversuchen meist keine Wirkung erzielt (BURDON, 1932; SHEVKY et al., 1934; LIEBETRUTH, 1935; SCHWABACHER et al., 1947). Dagegen wurden durch experimentelle Mischinfektionen, z.B. durch Injektion der gesamten aus pathologischen Prozessen gezüchteten Mischflora (ALTEMEIER, 1942) oder durch gleichzeitige Verimpfung von *Streptococcus-*, *Staphylococcus-* und *Sph. necrophorus*-Stämmen (HITE et al., 1949) synergistische Wirkungen mit Bildung lokaler oder expansiver Gangrän beobachtet.

WEISS (1937) sah nach experimenteller Infektion des Bronchialbaumes von *Macacus irus* mit einem aus Lungenabsceß isolierten Stamm keine Wirkung. Wurde *B. melaninogenicus* gemeinsam mit *Staphylococcus aureus* verabfolgt, treten nur die Eiterkokken in die Blutbahn über. Durch gleichzeitige Gabe von Staphylokokkentoxin in den Bronchialbaum wurde jedoch der Übertritt des *B. melaninogenicus* in die Blutbahn ermöglicht. Diese experimentelle *B. melaninogenicus*-Bakteriämie dauerte 44—48 Std und führte zur Bildung miliarer Lungenabscesse. Nach diesen Versuchen schien der Übertritt von *B. melaninogenicus* in die Blutbahn nur auf Grund von toxischen Lungenveränderungen möglich zu sein (s. auch S. 218).

Später stellte Weiss (1943) fest, daß der Erfolg der experimentellen Infektion von der Applikationsart abhängig ist. Nach intracutaner Injektion von Reinkulturen trat beim Meerschweinchen eine zunächst lokale, später fortschreitende putride Gangrän mit Exulcerationen auf, die durch vorherige Verabfolgung von Mucin oder Staphylokokkentoxin intensiviert werden konnte. Dagegen hatten subcutane und intraperitoneale Injektionen von *B. melaninogenicus* nur geringfügige Erscheinungen zur Folge.

Pulverer u. Heinrich (1960) prüften 29 *B. melaninogenicus*-Stämme an insgesamt 40 Meerschweinchen, 60 weißen Mäusen und 3 Kaninchen. Die Tiere erhielten 1 Woche alte Reinkulturen, auf hämolysiertem Blutagar nach Schäfer (1948) gezüchtet, in Keimdichten von 10^8 bis 19^9 Zellen pro ml physiologischer Kochsalzlösung subcutan appliziert, und zwar Kaninchen 2,0 ml, Meerschweinchen 1,0 ml und Mäuse 0,5 ml. Bei 2 Kaninchen und 5 Meerschweinchen gelang es, mit *B. melaninogenicus* einen fortschreitenden Entzündungsprozeß und folgende Septicopyämien hervorzurufen (Einzelheiten in Tabelle 15). Die übrigen Tiere, insbesondere die 60 Mäuse, erwiesen sich als unempfänglich.

Tabelle 15. *Subcutane Infektion von Kaninchen und Meerschweinchen mit Reinkulturen von* B. melaninogenicus. *(Nach* Pulverer u. Heinrich, *1960)*

Versuchstier	Verlauf der experimentellen Infektion und pathologisch-anatomische Befunde	Retrokultur des *B. melaninogenicus* aus
Kaninchen	Tod nach 8 Tagen. Nekrotisierende Gangrän der Bauchwand von der Injektionsstelle in der rechten Leistenbeuge bis zur Axilla mit reichlich fötidem Eiter	Herzblut, Gangräneiter
Kaninchen	Tod nach 10 Tagen. Nekrotisierende Gangrän der gesamten Bauchwand	Herzblut, Milz, Gangräneiter
Meerschweinchen	Tod nach 3 Tagen. Schwere nekrotisierende Gangrän der gesamten Bauchwand mit reichlich fötidem Eiter	Herzblut, Milz, Gangräneiter
Meerschweinchen	Tod nach 5 Tagen. Schwere nekrotisierende Gangrän der gesamten Bauchwand mit reichlich fötidem Eiter	Milz, Gangräneiter
Meerschweinchen	Tod nach 7 Tagen. Ausgedehnte Gangrän der gesamten Bauchwand mit fötidem Eiter; keine Exulcerationen der Haut. Abscesse in Milz, Leber und Nebennieren	Herzblut, Milz, Leber, Nebennieren, Gangräneiter
Meerschweinchen	Tod nach 9 Tagen. Nekrotisierende Gangrän der gesamten Bauchwand mit reichlich fötidem Eiter. Innere Organe makroskopisch o. B.	Herzblut, Gangräneiter
Meerschweinchen	Nach 23 Tagen getötet. An der Injektionsstelle in der rechten Leistenbeuge pflaumengroßer, abgekapselter Absceß mit zähem fötiden Eiter. Entzündlicher Milztumor	Milz, Absceßeiter

Tabelle 16. Synergistische Wirkung des *B. melaninogenicus* auf die Infektiosität von oralen Bakterien. (Nach SOCRANSKY u. GIBBONS, 1965)

Inoculum, bestehend aus einer Mischung von	Anzahl der Meerschweinchen, bei denen das verabfolgte Inoculum Infektiosität aufwies	
	ohne *B. mela-ninogenicus*	mit *B. mela-ninogenicus*
56 Kulturen, die zu ca. 9 Species gehören	0 (von 24)	24 (von 24)
5 grampositive[a] und 5 gramnegative[b] Kulturen	1 (von 12)	12 (von 12)
5 grampositive[a] Kulturen	0 (von 8)	7 (von 8)
5 gramnegative[b] Kulturen		0 (von 12)
Grampositive[a] Kulturen (4) ohne den „Coccobacillus"		0 (von 6)
„Coccobacillus"	0 (von 10)	9 (von 10)

[a] Jeweils 1 Kultur von *Streptococcus mitis*, *Peptostreptococcus* species, mikroaerophilen und anaeroben Corynebakterien und einem grampositiven „Coccobacillus".
[b] 3 Kulturen von *Vibrio sputorum* und jeweils 1 Kultur von *B. oralis* und *Veillonella alcalescens*.

SOCRANSKY u. GIBBONS (1965) bestimmten die Infektiosität von Rein- und Mischkulturen durch Inoculation von 1 ml einer dichten Suspension subcutan in die Leistenbeuge von 200—250 g schweren Meerschweinchen. Die Tiere wurden täglich auf Absceß- und Nekrosebildung kontrolliert. Von Abscessen wurde Exsudat aspiriert und zum Nachweis der Übertragbarkeit in Mengen von 0,2 ml in frische Meerschweinchen injiziert. Das Exsudat wurde außerdem kulturell auf seinen Bakteriengehalt geprüft. Als Beweis für Infektiosität wurde der Tod der Tiere, fortschreitende nekrotisierende Veränderungen oder Entwicklung eines übertragbaren lokalen Abscesses angenommen. Harte, knotenförmige, nichtübertragbare, käsige Abscesse oder geringfügige Entzündungen wurden nicht als positiv gewertet. Mit einer Mischung von 56 aus Zahnbelag gewonnenen Kulturen die zu etwa 9 Species, u. a. zu *Streptococcus mitis*, *Peptostreptococcus* spec., *Veillonella alcalescens* und *B. oralis*, gehörten, wurde bei 24 Meerschweinchen keine Wirkung erzielt. Mit *B. melaninogenicus* zusammen war diese Mischung jedoch bei allen geprüften Tieren infektiös (s. Tabelle 16).

Danach war festzustellen, welche Keime in der Mischkultur eine wesentliche Rolle spielten. Zunächst wurden 10 die in der Originalmischung vorhandenen Species repräsentierende Kulturen geprüft (s. Tabelle 16). Ohne *B. melaninogenicus* zeigte das Gemisch nur bei 1 von 12, mit *B. melaninogenicus* bei allen geprüften Meerschweinchen Infektiosität in dem oben definierten Sinn. Anschließend wurde diese Gruppe in 5 grampositive und 5 gramnegative Kulturen aufgeteilt. Die 5 gramnegativen Kulturen (der Species *Vibrio sputorum*, *B. oralis* und *Veillonella alcalescens*) waren auch mit *B. melaninogenicus* zusammen nicht infektiös. Dagegen zeigte sich bei der grampositiven Gruppe der zuvor schon beobachtete Synergismus. In dieser Gruppe war, wie die weiteren Versuche zeigten (Tabelle 16), ein von SOCRANSKY u. GIBBONS (1965) Coccobacillus genannter Keim gemeinsam mit *B. melaninogenicus* für die Infektiosität verantwortlich (*B. melaninogenicus* allein war ebenfalls unwirksam!). Die Autoren hielten diesen „Coccobacillus" für einen teils den Enterokokken, teils der Viridans-Gruppe nahestehenden *Streptococcus*. Diese Versuche veranlaßten SOCRANSKY u. GIBBONS (1965) zu der Schlußfolgerung, daß *B. melaninogenicus* von allen normalen Epiphyten des Menschen in mischinfizierten Prozessen die vergleichsweise größte Pathogenität entfaltet.

Zu den Enzymen, die mit der Pathogenität des *B. melaninogenicus* in Verbindung gebracht werden, gehören Hämotoxine, Proteasen, Fibrinolysine, eine Plasmakoagulase (Weiss, 1943; Pulverer u. Heinrich, 1960) und eine Kollagenase (Gibbons u. Macdonald, 1961). Durch immunelektrophoretische Untersuchungen zeigten Werner u. Müller (1971), daß *B. melaninogenicus* menschliches Albumin, α_1-Antitrypsin, α_1-Lipoprotein, α_2-HS-Glykoprotein, Coeruloplasmin, Haptoglobin, Transferin, Fibrinogen sowie IgG, IgM und IgA (nach längerer Einwirkungszeit vollständig) abbaut.

Endotoxin

In Kulturfiltraten von *B. melaninogenicus* wies Cohen (1933) eine toxische Substanz nach, die beim Kaninchen das Shwartzman-Phänomen hervorrief. Die sensibilisierende Injektion wurde subcutan, die Erfolgsinjektion 24 Std danach intravenös verabfolgt: Am Orte der Erstinjektion entstand dann eine hämorrhagische Nekrose. Das präparierende Toxin konnte auch heterolog sein, z. B. das Endotoxin von *Neisseria meningitidis* oder *Salmonella typhi*; dabei wurden jedoch nur in 80% positive Resultate erzielt. Mit anderen aus Lungengangrän züchtbaren Anaerobiern ließ sich das Shwartzman-Phänomen nicht erzeugen. Cohen (1933) meinte daraus schließen zu dürfen, daß bei der Entstehung der Lungengangrän ein dem Shwartzman-Phänomen analoger Mechanismus beteiligt ist und daß dem *B. melaninogenicus* somit eine wesentliche pathogene Bedeutung zukommt.

Mergenhagen et al. (1961) wiesen in Phenol-Wasser-Extrakten von *B. melaninogenicus* Endotoxinwirkung nach.

Zur Gewinnung des Endotoxins wurden 5 g acetongetrocknete Zellen in 45 ml destilliertem Wasser suspendiert und in einen Homogenisator gegeben, der 110 g Phenol und 65 ml destilliertes Wasser enthielt (Phenol : Wasser = 1 : 1). Das Gemisch wurde 10—15 min homogenisiert, dann auf 3° C abgekühlt und in Plastikröhrchen 5 min bei 9000 rpm zentrifugiert. Danach wurden die obere wäßrige Phase und die untere Phenolphase getrennt gewonnen. Die wäßrige Phase wurde ausgiebig gegen destilliertes Wasser bei 3° C dialysiert. Der endotoxische Lipoprotein-Polysaccharid-Nucleinsäuren-Komplex wurde durch Hinzufügen von etwas NaCl und 2 Vol. kaltem Aceton gefällt. Das Präcipitat wurde zentrifugiert, dreimal in kaltem Aceton gewaschen, wiederum zentrifugiert und im Vakuum über Calciumsulfatanhydrid getrocknet (= Lipopolysaccharid-Fraktion). In diesen Präparaten wurden im UV-Absorptionsspektrum stets noch Nucleinsäuren nachgewiesen. Die Aufbereitung der Phenolphase erwies sich angesichts ihrer geringen Wirksamkeit im Tierversuch als überflüssig.

Die Lipopolysaccharid-Fraktion zeigte im Versuch am Kaninchen primäre Dermotoxicität und Pyrogenität und sensibilisierte die Kaninchenhaut für das lokale Shwartzman-Phänomen. Die minimale Vorbereitungsdosis für das lokale Shwartzman-Phänomen lag bei *B. melaninogenicus* höher als bei anderen oralen Bakterien, z. B. *F. nucleatum* und *Selenomonas sputigena* (s. Tabelle 17). Während demnach *B. melaninogenicus*-Endotoxin in der Shwartzman-Reaktion nur schwach wirksam war, wies die Lipopolysaccharid-Fraktion von *B. melanino-*

Tabelle 17. Endotoxinwirksamkeit von Phenol-Wasser-Extrakten aus *B. melaninogenicus* und anderen oralen Bakterien. (Nach Mergenhagen et al., 1961)

Keimart	Prozentgehalt der Lipopolysaccharid-Fraktion des Endotoxins an		Minimale Vorbereitungsdosis für das lokale Shwartzman-Phänomen in µg
	N	P	
B. melaninogenicus	6,0	5,7	100
F. nucleatum	8,0	3,5	25
Selenomonas sputigena	2,6	2,2	4
Orale Treponemenart	4,0	3,5	100

genicus — in Mengen von 1 μg 1,5 kg schweren weißen Neuseeländern intravenös injiziert — eine größere Pyrogenität als die *Selenomonas-* und *Treponema*-Extrakte auf.

Nach HOFSTAD (1968) sind Heptose und 2-Keto-3-desoxyoctonat, die charakteristischen Bausteine des Endotoxins aerober gramnegativer Bakterien, in dem endotoxischen Lipopolysaccharid von *B. melaninogenicus* nicht vorhanden.

4. Sphaerophorus necrophorus (Sph. funduliformis)

a) Definition und Synonyme

Sph. necrophorus, die Typspecies der von PRÉVOT (1938) geschaffenen Gattung *Sphaerophorus*, ist die am längsten bekannte Bakteroidazeen-Art (= *Bacillus necrophorus*, FLÜGGE, 1886). Spätere und daher ungültige Synonyme sind *Streptothrix cuniculi* (SCHMORL, 1891) und *Bacillus funduliformis* (HALLÉ, 1898). Die Einordnung bei anderen Gattungen (*Actinomyces necrophorus*, LEHMANN u. NEUMANN, 1899; *Necrobacterium necrophorum*, JONSEN u. THJØTTA, 1948; *Fusiformis necrophorus*, WILSON u. MILES, 1964) hat sich nicht durchgesetzt.

Während die französische Schule (BEERENS, 1954; PRÉVOT, 1957, 1961) *Sph. necrophorus* (meist tierischer Herkunft) und *Sph. funduliformis* (in der Regel humane Stämme) als getrennte Species auffaßt und nach dem Besitz eines Hämagglutinins differenziert, wurde die von DACK et al. (1938) begründete und in der 7. Auflage von Bergey's Manual of Determinative Bacteriology (BREED et al., 1957) vertretene Lehre, daß als *Sph. funduliformis* bezeichnete Kulturen mit *Sph. necrophorus* identisch sind, in neuerer Zeit von den meisten Bakteriologen übernommen. Nach WERNER (1972d) weisen humane *Sph. necrophorus*-Kulturen und Stämme tierischer Herkunft untereinander den gleichen Grad von Antigenverwandtschaft auf.

Sph. necrophorus ist kulturell-biochemisch durch Bildung von Indol, H_2S und reichlich Buttersäure sowie Threoninspaltung (unter Bildung von Propionat und Butyrat) und außerdem durch Penicillin-, Cephalosporin- und Colistin-Empfindlichkeit gekennzeichnet (s. S. 203).

b) Natürlicher Standort und Infektionen des Menschen

Sph. necrophorus kommt auf der Schleimhaut des Oropharynx (WERNER et al., 1971a) und in geringer Zahl auch im Dickdarm des Menschen vor.

Sph. necrophorus ist in zahlreichen Fällen als Erreger von Septikämien, Meningitis, Pleuritis und Lungenabsceß sowie Infektionen im Bereich des weiblichen Genitale nachgewiesen worden (Literaturübersicht bei WERNER, 1968). Pathogene Bedeutung wurde den Keimen auch im Zusammenhang mit der Colitis ulcerosa zugeschrieben.

c) Experimentelle Pathogenität

Von allen anaeroben gramnegativen sporenlosen Stäbchen weisen *Sph. necrophorus*-Keime die größte Tierpathogenität auf. Die Virulenz der einzelnen Stämme ist jedoch unterschiedlich. Virulenzunterschiede sollen vor allem zwischen den vom Menschen und den von Tieren isolierten Kulturen bestehen: Stämme von menschlichen Infektionen sollen nach subcutaner Verimpfung bei Kaninchen nur lokale Abscesse, nicht jedoch fortschreitende Nekrosen hervorrufen (DACK et al., 1938). Bei Aufbewahrung in der Kultur geht die Pathogenität in der Regel schnell verloren (PRÉVOT et al., 1967).

Kaninchen, Meerschweinchen, Mäuse, Hunde und Affen gehen nach intravenöser Injektion von *Sph. necrophorus*-Stämmen unter Bildung von Lungen- und Leberabscessen an Sepsis zugrunde (Grumbach et al., 1939; Grumbach, 1958; Prévot et al., 1967). Das Ausmaß der Veränderungen ist abhängig von der wechselnden Virulenz der Stämme und der unterschiedlichen Resistenz der Versuchstiere. Die Resistenz von Meerschweinchen kann durch Vitamin C-arme Diät herabgesetzt werden (McCullough, 1938).

Durch intravenöse Injektionen von 0,5 ml Kulturbouillon eines aus Leberabscessen des Menschen isolierten Stammes erzeugte Rivalier (1930) bei Affen eine tödliche Infektion. Autoptisch fanden sich in der Leber zahlreiche Abscesse, im Blut waren massenhaft Erreger nachweisbar. Ein Stamm, der bei einem Fall von Septikämie mit metastatischer Arthritis isoliert worden war, rief beim Affen tödliche Sepsis mit Symphysenabsceß und beim Kaninchen tödliche Sepsis mit Gelenkabscessen hervor (Rivalier, 1930). Da die Manifestationen der tierexperimentellen Infektionen und der Sphärophorose des Menschen weitgehend übereinstimmten, besaßen diese Stämme offenbar einen beachtlichen Gewebstropismus (Rivalier, 1930).

Nach Pham Huu Chi (1935) ist auch der Hund sehr empfänglich. Die intravenöse Injektion von 1—2 ml Kulturbouillon führte in 30—36 Std den Tod der Tiere herbei. Autoptisch zeigte sich eine nekrotisierende Pneumonie.

Beveridge (1934) erzeugte durch subcutane Injektionen mehrerer *Sph. necrophorus*-Stämme bei Schafen lokale Abscesse, die keine Tendenz zur Ausbreitung zeigten. Von zwei Schafen, die 1 ml Kulturbouillon intravenös erhalten hatten, blieb eins unbeeinflußt; das andere starb 12 Std post infectionem. Autoptisch waren ausgedehnte Hämorrhagien in verschiedenen Organen nachweisbar. Beim Wallaby, einer Känguruhart, traten nach subcutaner Infektion ausgebreitete Nekrosen auf, die den Tod des Tieres zur Folge hatten.

Prévot (1940) untersuchte die Therapie experimenteller *Sph. necrophorus-* (*Sph. funduliformis-*)Septikämien des Kaninchens durch Sulfonamide:

Als Teststamm diente eine Isolierung aus Mastoiditis-Eiter, die, in Mengen von 0,5 ml Kulturbouillon intravenös verabfolgt, bei Kaninchen regelmäßig in 15—18 Tagen tödlich wirkte. In einer ersten Versuchsreihe erhielten 4 Kaninchen von 2,5 kg Gewicht intravenös 2 ml einer 24 Std bebrüteten Kultur. Von den beiden unbehandelten Tieren starb das erste in 24 Std, das zweite innerhalb von 5 Tagen. Die beiden anderen Kaninchen erhielten die erste subcutane Sulfonamidgabe (0,25 g in öliger Suspension) 1 Std nach intravenöser Injektion der *Sph. necrophorus*-Kultur, d.h. als die septikämische Symptomatik (Schüttelfrost, gesträubtes Fell, Bewegungsarmut, Dyspnoe, Fieber, Inappetenz) bereits voll ausgebildet war. Die Sulfonamid-Injektion wurde 1× täglich 12 Tage lang wiederholt. Vom 3. Tag an boten die behandelten Kaninchen keinerlei Krankheitszeichen mehr, fraßen normal und nahmen an Gewicht zu. 15 Tage nach der letzten Sulfonamid-Injektion wurde ein Tier getötet; autoptisch wurden keine Läsionen festgestellt, das Herzblut war steril.

In einer zweiten Versuchsreihe wurden 12 weitere Kaninchen von 2,5 kg Gewicht in der beschriebenen Weise experimentell mit *Sph. necrophorus* infiziert. Die 6 unbehandelten Kaninchen starben in 8 und 12 Std (2 trächtige Tiere) bzw. 3, 4, 5 und 6 Tagen. Die 6 übrigen Kaninchen erhielten die erste Sulfonamid-Injektion 2 Std nach der intravenösen Gabe von 2 ml *Sph. necrophorus*-Kulturbouillon. Zu diesem Zeitpunkt erschien der Zustand der beiden trächtigen Tiere bereits hoffnungslos. Die Sulfonamid-Injektion wurde 1× täglich 14 Tage lang wiederholt. Eines der behandelten Kaninchen starb 12, ein weiteres 14 Tage nach Beginn der Versuche. Die 4 übrigen Tiere waren vom 5. Tag an erscheinungsfrei.

Diese in der Anfangsphase der chemotherapeutischen Ära durchgeführten Versuche demonstrierten eindeutig die Wirksamkeit der Sulfonamidgabe, die — in Abhängigkeit vom Zeitpunkt des Therapiebeginns — bis zu 75% Heilungen bei unbehandelt 100%ig letaler experimenteller *Sph. necrophorus*-Septikämie herbeiführte (Prévot, 1940).

α) Endotoxin

Nach Prévot et al. (1967) soll von den beiden besonders empfänglichen Laboratoriumstieren: Meerschweinchen und Kaninchen, ersteres vor allem auf die Endotoxicität von *Sph. necrophorus* ansprechen, letzteres vorzugsweise der Infektiosität der Keime erliegen. Während intravenös infizierte Kaninchen in der Regel erst nach 6—15 Tagen an Septikämie sterben und kurz nach der Injektion keine toxischen Symptome zeigen, verenden Meerschweinchen unmittelbar nach der intravenösen Injektion von *Sph. necrophorus*-Bouillonkulturen. Auch nach intraperitonealer Verabfolgung von 1—2 ml Kulturbouillon gehen Meerschweinchen innerhalb von 6—12 Std zugrunde. Das Kulturfiltrat allein hat die gleiche Wirkung; gewaschene Kulturen sollen dagegen nicht tödlich wirken (Prévot et al., 1967).

Prévot u. Kirchheiner (1939) extrahierten mit Trichloressigsäure entsprechend der von Boivin u. Mesrobeanu (1937) beschriebenen Methode aus *Sph. necrophorus* ein Lipopolysaccharid (Endotoxin), das in destilliertem Wasser leicht löslich und durch absoluten Alkohol und Aceton sowie die homologen und heterologen Antiseren präcipitierbar war. Dieses endotoxische Lipopolysaccharid rief nach subcutaner, intramuskulärer oder intraperitonealer Injektion bei der Maus charakteristische lokale Nekrosen hervor. Nach intravenöser Verabfolgung von 0,1 mg trat bei dem gleichen Tier der Tod ein.

Mit Hilfe der Phenol-Wasser-Extraktion (s. S. 211) isolierten Hofstad u. Kristoffersen (1971) aus 3 Stämmen, von denen wahrscheinlich lediglich N 167 Fiévez zur Species *Sph. necrophorus* gehörte, Lipopolysaccharide, die durch Ribonuclease- und Desoxyribonuclease-Behandlung (s. S. 211) sowie durch Gelfiltration und Ionenaustauschchromatographie auf DEAE-Cellulose weiter gereinigt wurden. Das Lipopolysaccharid des Stammes N 167 Fiévez enthielt kleine Mengen von 2-Keto-3-desoxy-octonat. Die hauptsächlichen Kohlenhydratbausteine waren Heptose, Galaktose, Glucose und Glucosamin. Das endotoxische Lipopolysaccharid von *Sph. necrophorus* ist damit chemisch deutlich verschieden von dem Endotoxin der *Bacteroides*-Arten (s. S. 211, 213 u. 219).

Hofstad u. Kristoffersen (1971) stellten von dem gereinigten Lipopolysaccharid des Stammes N 167 Fiévez in steriler physiologischer Kochsalzlösung Verdünnungsreihen her, die insgesamt 10 Albinokaninchen in Mengen von 0,2 ml intracutan in die rasierte Bauchhaut injiziert wurden. Jedes Tier erhielt 24 Std später die intravenöse Erfolgsinjektion von 125 µg Lipopolysaccharid N 167. Eine positive Shwartzman-Reaktion trat, in Abhängigkeit von der Dosis, nur bei wenigen Tieren auf:

Tabelle 18. Lokale Shwartzman-Reaktion bei 10 mit verschiedenen Dosen des endotoxischen Lipopolysaccharids aus *Sph. necrophorus* N 167 Fiévez behandelten 6 Monate alten Albino-Kaninchen. (Nach Hofstad u. Kristoffersen, 1971)

Dosis der intracutanen Erstinjektion	100 µg	50 µg	25 µg	12,5 µg	6,25 µg	3,12 µg
Positive Shwartzman-Reaktion/Anzahl der geprüften Tiere	5/10	4/10	3/10	1/10	0/10	0/10

Elektronenoptisch erwies sich das gereinigte Lipopolysaccharid des Stammes N 167 Fiévez als stäbchenförmig (Hofstad et al., 1972).

β) Leukocidin

Bei experimenteller *Sph. necrophorus*-Infektion der Haut von Kaninchen, Schafen und Meerschweinchen stellte Roberts (1967) fest, daß die Migration der Leukocyten aus den Blutgefäßen innerhalb der inokulierten Bezirke unterbunden war und Leukocyten andererseits bei Einwanderung von außerhalb an der Peripherie des infizierten Bereiches durch ein von wachsenden *Sph. necrophorus*-Zellen freigesetztes Leukocidin immobilisiert und zerstört wurden. Das Leukocidie bewirkende Exotoxin war ein nichtdialysierbares Makromolekül, das erst bei 100° C langsam inaktiviert wurde. Da die Aktivität des Leukocidins durch Anti-Hämolysin-Serum nicht beeinträchtigt wurde, ist dieses Exotoxin mit dem *Sph. necrophorus*-Hämolysin nicht identisch (Roberts, 1967). Andere Bakterien konnten durch das *Sph. necrophorus*-Leukocidin vor der Phagocytose durch Leukocyten geschützt werden. Bei experimenteller Mischinfektion mit *Sph. necrophorus* und *Corynebacterium pyogenes* war die erhöhte Invasivität des *C. pyogenes* auf die phagocytosehemmende Wirkung des *Sph. necrophorus*-Leukocidins zurückzuführen (Roberts, 1967).

Anhang:

Sphaerophorus pseudonecrophorus

Die Keimart wurde von Harris u. Brown (1927) als *Actinomyces pseudonecrophorus* beschrieben und von Prévot (1938) in die Gattung *Sphaerophorus* überführt. In der 7. Auflage von Bergey's Manual (Breed et al., 1957) ist die Species, die lediglich das Fehlen eines Hämolysins von *Sph. necrophorus* bzw. *Sph. funduliformis* unterscheidet, nicht berücksichtigt. Werner (1972c) ordnete einen *Sph. pseudonecrophorus*-Stamm der Anaerobiersammlung des Institut Pasteur de Paris als Angehörigen der Species *Sph. necrophorus* ein. Die Eigenständigkeit des sog. *Sph. pseudonecrophorus* muß daher als zweifelhaft gelten.

Als Sph. pseudonecrophorus angesprochene Keime wurden im Darmtrakt des Menschen nachgewiesen. Die Erstbeschreiber Harris u. Brown (1927) isolierten 6 Stämme bei Fällen von Puerperalfieber aus dem Uterus. Später wurde die Species in eitrigen Prozessen und bei Sepsis nachgewiesen (Übersicht bei Prévot et al., 1967).

Tierversuche. Beim Kaninchen entsteht nach intravenöser Injektion virulenter Stämme eine tödliche Sepsis mit Leberabscessen, d.h. ein der tierexperimentellen *Sph. necrophorus*- bzw. *Sph. funduliformis*-Infektion entsprechendes Bild (Prévot et al., 1967).

Robin (1948) erzeugte durch intravenöse Injektion eines von einer Halsphlegmone isolierten Stammes beim Kaninchen eine tödliche Sepsis mit nekrotisierenden Lungenveränderungen. Der bakterienfreie Überstand der Kulturflüssigkeit erwies sich als toxisch, nach Injektion gewaschener Bakterienzellen trat das oben beschriebene Krankheitsbild auf.

Tardieux u. Nabonne (1949) isolierten einen Stamm aus dem Blut eines 17jährigen Mädchens, bei dem nach einer Angina Sepsis und eitrige Metastasen in der linken Temporomaxillargegend aufgetreten waren. Der zunächst serophile Stamm wuchs bei Subkultur auch auf serumfreien Medien. Er erwies sich als pathogen für Kaninchen und Meerschweinchen: Die intravenöse Injektion von 2 ml Kulturbouillon tötete Kaninchen in 24 Std. Autoptisch wurden zahlreiche miliare Leber- und Milzabscesse nachgewiesen. Aus den Herden ließen sich die Erreger in Reinkultur gewinnen. Die gestauten Lungen waren frei von Metastasen. An Nieren und Darm fanden sich keine Veränderungen. Beim Meerschweinchen rief die subcutane Injektion von 1 ml der Kultur lokale Absceßbildung hervor.

Die Wand der Abscesse war nekrotisch, der Eiter bröckelig. Am 10. Tag trat der Tod ein. Autoptisch zeigten sich zahlreiche viscerale Abscesse, besonders in den Lungen, der Leber und der Milz.

5. Fusobacterium fusiforme

a) Definition, natürlicher Standort und Infektionen des Menschen

WERNER et al. (1971 b), die 17 aus pathologischem Material isolierte *Fuso-bacterium*-Stämme mit 8 als *F. fusiforme, F. nucleatum* und *F. polymorphum* bezeichneten Sammlungskulturen verglichen, stellten bei den 25 geprüften Kulturen nur geringfügige morphologische und biochemische Unterschiede fest. Die strikt anaeroben butyratbildenden Fusobakterien dürften demnach als Angehörige einer Species zu betrachten sein, deren legitime Bezeichnung *F. fusiforme* ist (WERNER et al., 1971 b). Berichte über Tierexperimente mit als *F. polymorphum, F. nucleatum* usw. angesprochenen Kulturen werden daher in diesem Kapitel besprochen.

Die französische Schule verwendete lange Zeit statt *Fusobacterium* den Gattungsnamen *Fusiformis* (vgl. z.B. PRÉVOT, 1957). Einem Vorschlag von SEBALD (1962) folgend, haben PRÉVOT et al. (1967) die ehemaligen *Fusiformis*-Arten in die Gattung *Sphaerophorus* überführt.

F. fusiforme-Stämme haben schlanke, stäbchen- oder fadenförmige Zellen mit abgerundeten oder sich verjüngenden Zellenden, sind nur schwach saccharolytisch, bauen jedoch Aminosäuren ab und bilden reichlich Butyrat (s. S. 198). Von *Sph. necrophorus*-Keimen unterscheiden sich Angehörige der Species *F. fusiforme* mikroskopisch-morphologisch und durch Fehlen der Gasbildung (WERNER et al., 1971 a, b).

Anaerobe butyratbildende Stäbchen der Species *F. fusiforme* finden sich auf der Schleimhaut der Mundhöhle und im Zahnbelag. Im Darmtrakt kommen sie nur gelegentlich vor.

Zusammen mit Schraubenbakterien (Borrelien) sind Fusobakterien für das Zustandekommen einer einseitigen nekrotisierenden, fötiden, ulceromembranösen Tonsillitis (Plaut-Vincentsche Angina) verantwortlich. Vermehrt nachweisbar sind fusiforme Stäbchen auch bei ulceröser Gingivostomatitis und bei Noma. Außerdem wurden als *F. fusiforme, F. plauti-vincenti* usw. angesprochene Stämme, meist zusammen mit anderen Keimen, aus Lungenabscessen und aus pleuritischem Eiter isoliert (BEERENS u. TAHON-CASTEL, 1965; Übersichten bei PRÉVOT et al., 1967; WERNER, 1968).

b) Tierversuche

Tierversuche wurden vor allem mit dem Fusobakterien und Schraubenbakterien enthaltenden nativen Material von Plaut-Vincentscher Angina durchgeführt. VESZPRÉMI (1905, 1907) erzielte damit Abscesse beim Kaninchen, SHPUNTOFF u. ROSEBURY (1949) setzten mit Fusobakterien und „Spirochäten" enthaltendem Eiter beim Meerschweinchen subcutane Abscesse, die sich über mehrere Passagen übertragen ließen. Bei Hamstern, Mäusen und Hühnerembryonen gingen die Infektionen dagegen nur schlecht an. Versuche, ähnliche Ergebnisse mit Reinkulturen beim Meerschweinchen zu erreichen, hatten wenig Erfolg (ROSEBURY et al., 1950 a—c).

DICKER (1938) erzielte mit einem aus Pleuraempyem in Reinkultur gezüchteten als *F. nucleatum* angesprochenen Stamm sowie nach Injektion des Eiters bei Meerschweinchen und Kaninchen subcutane Abscesse. Im Serum der infizierten Tiere wurden, ebenso wie im Serum des Patienten, komplementbindende Antikörper nachgewiesen.

Durch *intracutane* Verimpfung von *F. nucleatum* und *F. polymorphum* erzeugten Hampp u. Mergenhagen (1963) bei Kaninchen regelmäßig Veränderungen, die nach 24 Std in Abscesse übergingen. Die Keime waren in den Läsionen 4 Tage lang nachweisbar. Histologisch waren die durch die beiden *Fusobacterium*-Stämme verursachten intracutanen Läsionen ähnlich:

Bald nach der Injektion trat eine lokale entzündliche Reaktion auf. Unter Vermehrung des Exsudats bildete sich eine lokale Nekrose. Danach griffen die entzündlichen Veränderungen auf die Muskelschicht der Haut und das umgebende Bindegewebe über. An den Rändern der Abscesse traten bereits innerhalb von 48 Std reichlich Fibroblasten auf.

Nach intracutaner Applikation von Fusobakterien zusammen mit oralen Schraubenbakterien zeigte sich eine synergistische Wirkung (Hampp u. Mergenhagen, 1963). Von Macdonald et al. (1954, 1956) wurde dagegen gezeigt, daß die Kombination von Fusobakterien mit oralen Schraubenbakterien zur Erzeugung einer *subcutanen* nekrotisierenden Veränderung nicht unbedingt erforderlich ist, sondern die gleichen Läsionen auch durch das Zusammenwirken eines der beiden Keimanteile mit anderen anaeroben Bakterien zustande kommen.

Mit der Phenol-Wasser-Extraktion gewannen Mergenhagen et al. (1961) unter anderem auch aus *F. nucleatum* eine wasserlösliche, Reste von Nucleinsäuren enthaltende Fraktion mit Endotoxinwirkung (vgl. S. 218). Die Lipopolysaccharid-Fraktion von *F. nucleatum* hatte, in Mengen von 1 µg 1,5 kg schweren Kaninchen intravenös verabfolgt, von den geprüften oralen Bakterienarten (u.a. *Selenomonas sputigena, B. melaninogenicus*) die stärkste pyrogene Wirkung.

Nach Kristoffersen u. Hofstad (1970) enthält das durch Phenol-Wasser-Extraktion gewonnene Lipopolysaccharid oraler Fusobakterien u.a. Heptose und 2-Keto-3-desoxy-octonat, die charakteristischen Bausteine des Endotoxins aerober gramnegativer Bakterien.

Literatur

Altemeier, W.: The bacterial flora of acute perforated appendicitis. Ann. Surg. **107**, 517 (1938a).

Altemeier, W.: The cause of the putrid odor of perforated appendicitis with peritonitis. Ann. Surg. **107**, 634 (1938b).

Altemeier, W.: The pathogenicity of the bacteria of appendicitis peritonitis. Surgery **11**, 374 (1942).

Araujo, W. C. de, Gibbons, R. J.: Ineffectiveness of streptomycin as a selective agent in the cultivation of oral fusobacteria. J. Bact. **84**, 593—594 (1962).

Baird-Parker, A. C.: Isolation of Leptotrichia buccalis and Fusobacterium species from oral material. Nature (Lond.) **180**, 1056—1057 (1957).

Beerens, H.: Procédé de différenciation entre Spherophorus necrophorus (Schmorl, 1891) et Spherophorus funduliformis (Hallé, 1898). Ann. Inst. Pasteur **86**, 384—386 (1954).

Beerens, H.: Milieux sélectifs pour l'isolement de quelques espèces de bactéries anaérobies à Gram négatif. Ann. Inst. Pasteur Lille **9**, 86—89 (1957).

Beerens, H.: Les bactéries anaérobies. In: Manuel de techniques bactériologiques, von R. Buttiaux, H. Beerens, A. Tacquet. Paris: Flammarion 1962.

Beerens, H., Aladame, N.: Sur une nouvelle bactérie anaérobie: Ristella pseudo-insolita nov. sp. Ann. Inst. Pasteur **76**, 476—478 (1949).

Beerens, H., Guillaume, J., Petit, H.: Étude de la fermentation propionique de la L(-)thréonine par 45 souches de bactéries non sporulées à Gram négatif. Ann. Inst. Pasteur **96**, 211—216 (1959).

Beerens, H., Schaffner, Y., Guillaume, J., Castel, M. M.: Les bacilles anaérobies non sporulés à Gram négatif favorisés par la bile. Leur appartenance au genre Eggerthella (nov. gen.). Ann. Inst. Pasteur Lille **14**, 5—48 (1963).

Beerens, H., Tahon-Castel, M.: Infections humaines à bactéries anaérobies non toxigènes. Brüssel: Presses Académiques Européennes 1965.

Beerens, H., Wattre, P., Shinjo, T., Romond, C.: Premiers résultats d'un essai de classification sérologique de 131 souches de Bacteroides du groupe fragilis (Eggerthella). Ann. Inst. Pasteur **121**, 187—198 (1971).

BERGER, U.: Untersuchungen an Fusobakterien. I. Mitteilung: Systematik, Züchtung und Morphologie. Zbl. Bakt., I. Abt. Orig. **166**, 484—497 (1956).

BERGEY, D. H., HARRISON, F. C., BREED, R. S., HAMMER, B. W., HUNTOON, F. M.: Bergey's manual of determinative bacteriology. A key for the identification of organisms of the class schizomyzetes. Baltimore: Williams & Wilkins 1923.

BEVERIDGE, W. J. B.: A study of 12 strains of Bacillus necrophorus with observations on the oxygen intolerance of the organism. J. Path. Bact. **38**, 467 (1934).

BOEZ, L., KELLER, R., KEHLSTADT, A.: Bactériemies à Bacillus fragilis (trois observations). Bull. Soc. Méd. Hôp. Paris **51**, 1148—1189 (1927).

BØE, J.: Fusobacterium. Studies on its bacteriology, serology and pathogenicity. Skr. norske Vidensk.-Akad. I. Mat. nat. Kl. **9**, 1—191 (1941).

BOIVIN, A., MESROBEANU, L.: Sur l'antigène O, endotoxine des pyocyaniques. C. R. Soc. Biol. (Paris) **125**, 273 (1937).

BREED, R. S., MURRAY, E. G. D., SMITH, N. R.: Bergey's manual of determinative bacteriology, 7th ed. Baltimore: Williams & Wilkins 1957.

BULLEN, J. J., LEIGH, L. C., ROGERS, H. J.: The effect of iron compounds on the virulence of Escherichia coli for guinea-pigs. Immunology **15**, 581—588 (1968).

BURDON, K.: Bacterium melaninogenicum from normal and pathologic tissues. J. infect. Dis. **42**, 161—171 (1928).

BURDON, K.: Isolation and cultivation of Bacterium melaninogenicum. Proc. Soc. exp. Biol. (N.Y.) **29**, 1144—1145 (1932).

CASTELLANI, A., CHALMERS, A.: Manual of tropical medicine, 3rd ed. New York: Wood 1919.

COHEN, J.: The bacteriology of abscess of the lung and methods for its study. Arch. Surg. **24**, 171 (1932).

COHEN, J.: Anaerobic gram-negative bacilli isolated from abscess of the lung. J. infect. Dis. **52**, 185 (1933).

DACK, G. M., DRAGSTEDT, L. R., JOHNSON, R., McCULLOUGH, N. B.: Comparison of Bacterium necrophorum from ulcerative colitis in man with strains isolated from animals. J. infect. Dis. **62**, 169 (1938).

DEBRÉ, R., HAGUENAU, J., BONNET, H.: Infection à allure septicémique par microbe anaérobie. Bull. Soc. Méd. Hôp. Paris **47**, 1578—1580 (1923).

DELBOVE, P., ELICHE, J., NGUYEN-VAN-HUONG: Bactériemie post-partum à Bacillus fragilis. Bull. Soc. Path. exot. **34**, 58—61 (1941).

DICKER, H.: Fusobakterien als echte Krankheitserreger beim Menschen. Zbl. Bakt., I. Abt. Orig. **141**, 37—45 (1938).

DISTASO, A.: Contribution à l'étude sur l'intoxication intestinale. Zbl. Bakt., I. Abt. Orig. **62**, 433—468 (1912).

EGGERTH, A. A., GAGNON, B. H.: The Bacteroides of human feces. J. Bact. **25**, 389—413 (1933).

FINEGOLD, S. M., MILLER, A. B., POSNICK, D. J.: Further studies on selective media for Bacteroides and other anaerobes. Ernährungsforschung **10**, 517—528 (1965).

FLÜGGE, C.: Die Mikroorganismen, 2. Aufl. Leipzig 1886.

GIBBONS, R. J., MACDONALD, J. B.: Hemin and vitamin K compounds as required factors for the cultivation of certain strains of Bacteroides melaninogenicus. J. Bact. **80**, 164—170 (1960).

GIBBONS, R. J., MACDONALD, J. B.: Degradation of collageneous substrates by Bacteroides melaninogenicus. J. Bact. **81**, 614—621 (1961).

GILBERT, A., LIPMAN, A.: Bactériologie des cholecystites. C. R. Soc. Biol. (Paris) **54**, 1189—1191 (1902).

GRIGOROFF, S.: Contribution à la pathogénie de l'appendicite. Thèse, Genève 1905.

GRUMBACH, A.: Die Ristellosen, Ramibakteriosen, Vibriosen, Sphaerophorosen und Corynebakteriosen. In: Die Infektionskrankheiten des Menschen und ihre Erreger, von A. GRUMBACH und W. KIKUTH, Bd. II, S. 1073—1088. Stuttgart: Thieme 1958.

GRUMBACH, A., LIEBMANN, E., SCHINDLER, H.: Über eine durch Bac. funduliformis bedingte, gutartige Angina mit Milztumor. Schweiz. med. Wschr. **20**, 1198—1200 (1939).

GUILLEMOT, L.: Recherches sur les gangrènes pulmonaires. Thèse, Paris 1899.

GUILLEMOT, L., HALLÉ, J., RIST, E.: Recherches bactériologiques et expérimentales sur les pleurésies putrides. Arch. Méd. exp. **16**, 571—576 (1904).

HALLÉ, J.: Recherches sur la bactériologie du canal génital de la femme (état normal et pathologique). Thèse, Paris 1898.

HAMPP, E. G., MERGENHAGEN, S. E.: Experimental intracutaneous fusobacterial and fusospirochetal infections. J. infect. Dis. **112**, 84—99 (1963).

HARRIS, J. W., BROWN, J. H.: Description of a new organism that may be a factor in the causation of puerperal infections. Bull. J. Hopk. Hosp. **40**, 203 (1927).

HEINRICH, S., PULVERER, G.: Über den Nachweis des Bacteroides melaninogenicus in Krankheitsprozessen bei Mensch und Tier. Z. Hyg. Infekt.-Kr. 146, 331—340 (1960).

HITE, K. E., LOCKE, M., HESSELTINE, H. C.: Synergism in experimental infections with non sporulating anaerobic bacteria. J. infect. Dis. 84, 1—9 (1949).

HOFSTADT, T.: Chemical characteristics of Bacteroides melaninogenicus endotoxin. Arch. oral Biol. 13, 1149—1155 (1968).

HOFSTADT, T., KRISTOFFERSEN, T.: Chemical characteristics of endotoxin from Bacteroides fragilis NCTC 9343. J. gen. Microbiol. 61, 15—19 (1970).

HOFSTADT, T., KRISTOFFERSEN, T.: Preparation and chemical characteristics of endotoxic lipopolysaccharide from three strains of Sphaerophorus necrophorus. Acta path. microbiol. scand., Section B 79, 385—390 (1971).

HOFSTADT, T., KRISTOFFERSEN, T., SELVIG, K. A.: Electron microscopy of endotoxic lipopolysaccharide from Bacteroides, Fusobacterium and Sphaerophorus. Acta path. microbiol. scand., Section B 80, 413—419 (1972).

HOLDEMAN, L. V., MOORE, W. E. C. (Editors): Anaerobe Laboratory Manual. Virginia Polytechnic Institute and State University Anaerobe Laboratory, Blacksburg, Virginia 1972.

JEANNIN, C.: Étiologie et pathologie des infections puerpérales putrides. Thèse, Paris 1902.

JONSEN, J., THJØTTA, T.: Studies on Bacteroides. II. B. funduliformis and its relation to Necrobacterium necrophorum (Actinomyces necrophorus). Acta path. microbiol. scand. 25, 688—702 (1948).

KRISTOFFERSEN, T., HOFSTADT, T.: Chemical composition of lipopolysaccharide endotoxins from human oral fusobacteria. Arch. oral Biol. 15, 909—916 (1970).

LEHMANN, K. B., NEUMANN, R. O.: Atlas und Grundriß der Bakteriologie und Lehrbuch der speziellen bakteriologischen Diagnostik, 2. Aufl. München: Lehmann 1899.

LEMIERRE, A., REILLY, J., DAUM, S.: Septicémie à Bacillus fragilis. Bull. Soc. Méd. Hôp. Paris 54, 436—439 (1938).

LEV, M.: Apparent requirement for vitamin K of rumen strains of Fusiformis nigrescens. Nature (Lond.) 181, 203—204 (1958).

LEWIS, K. H., BEDELL, M., RETTGER, L. F.: Non sporulating anaerobic bacteria of the intestinal tract. II. Growth-facilitating factors. J. Bact. 40, 309—320 (1940).

LIEBETRUTH, E.: Untersuchungen über das Bacterium melaninogenicum. Z. Hyg. Infekt.-Kr. 116, 611—616 (1935).

MACDONALD, J. B., SUTTON, R. M., KNOLL, M. L.: The production of fusospirochetal infections in guinea pigs with recombined pure cultures. J. infect. Dis. 95, 275 (1954).

MACDONALD, J. B., SUTTON, R. M., KNOLL, M. L., MADLARER, E. M., GRAINGER, R. M.: The pathogenic components of an experimental fusospirochetal infection. J. infect. Dis. 98, 15 (1956).

MAUPÉOU, E. DE: Les septicémies à Ristella fragilis (à propos de 10 observations). Thèse, Montpellier 1973.

McCARTHY, C., SNYDER, M. L.: Selective medium for fusobacteria and leptotrichia. J. Bact. 86, 158—159 (1963).

McCULLOUGH, N. B.: Vitamin C and resistance of the guinea pig to infection with Bacterium necrophorum. J. infect. Dis. 63, 34 (1938).

MERGENHAGEN, S. E., HAMPP, E. G., SCHERP, H. W.: Preparation and biological activities of endotoxins from oral bacteria. J. infect. Dis. 108, 304—310 (1961).

MITSUOKA, T., SEGA, T., YAMAMOTO, S.: Ein neuer Selektivnährboden für Bacteroides. Zbl. Bakt., I. Abt. Orig. 195, 69—79 (1964).

MÜLLER, H. E., WERNER, H.: In vitro-Untersuchungen über das Vorkommen von Neuraminidase bei Bacteroides-Arten. Path. et Microbiol. (Basel) 36, 135—152 (1970a).

MÜLLER, H. E., WERNER, H.: Die Neuraminidase als pathogenetischer Faktor bei einem durch Bacteroides fragilis bedingten Absceß. Z. med. Mikrobiol. Immunol. 156, 98—106 (1970b).

NACESCU, N., BRANDIS, H., WERNER, H.: Isolierung von zwei Bacteroides fragilis-Phagen aus Abwasser und Nachweis lysogener B. fragilis-Stämme. Zbl. Bakt. Hyg., I. Abt. Orig. A 219, 522—529 (1972).

OEHRING, H., SCHULZ, H., KRAMER, B., EHRHARDT, G.: Bacteroides melaninogenicus als Ursache multipler Hirnabscesse. Med. Klin. 62, 1347—1349 (1967).

OLIVER, W., WHERRY, W.: Notes on some bacterial parasites of the human mucous membranes. J. infect. Dis. 28, 341—344 (1921).

OMATA, R. R., DISRAELY, M. N.: A selective medium for oral fusobacteria. J. Bact. 72, 677—680 (1956).

PETER, A.: Der Einfluß von CO_2 auf das Wachstum von Bacteroides melaninogenicus. Zbl. Bakt., I. Abt. Orig. 189, 189—202 (1963).

PHAM HUU CHI: Les septicémies dues au Bacillus funduliformis. Thèse en Médicine, Paris 1935.

PRÉVOT, A. R.: Études de systématique bactérienne. III. Invalidité du genre Bacteroides Castellani et Chalmers. Démembrement et reclassification. Ann. Inst. Pasteur 60, 285—307 (1938).

PRÉVOT, A. R.: Chimiothérapie des septicémies expérimentales du lapin à Spherophorus funduliformis. C. R. Soc. Biol. (Paris) 134, 90—91 (1940).

PRÉVOT, A. R.: Manuel de classification et de détermination des bactéries anaérobies. Paris: Masson 1957.

PRÉVOT, A. R.: Traité de systématique bactérienne. Paris: Dunod 1961.

PRÉVOT, A. R.: Une nouvelle entité bactério-clinique: l'infection à Ristella pseudoinsolita. Bull. Acad. Nat. Méd. (Paris) 149, 689—696 (1965).

PRÉVOT, A. R., KIRCHHEINER, E.: Existence d'un antigène commun aux deux espèces Spherophorus funduliformis et Spherophorus necrophorus. C. R. Acad. Sci. (Paris) 209, 182—184 (1939).

PRÉVOT, A. R., TURPIN, A., KAISER, P.: Les bactéries anaérobies. Paris: Dunod 1967.

PULVERER, G., HEINRICH, S.: Infektionsversuche an Laboratoriumstieren und in vitro-Untersuchungen zur Fermentausstattung des Bacteroides melaninogenicus. Z. Hyg. Infekt.-Kr. 146, 341—349 (1960).

QUINTO, G.: Identification of non-sporulating anaerobes. Amer. J. med. Technol. 30, 304—312 (1964).

QUINTO, G.: Fermentation studies of non-sporulating anaerobes. Amer. J. med. Technol. 32, 195—199 (1966).

QUINTO, G., SEBALD, M., PRÉVOT, A. R.: Étude sur le pouvoir pathogène de Ristella pseudo-insolita. Role de l'hemine dans sa croissance. Ann. Inst. Pasteur 105, 455—459 (1963).

RAIKOFF, R.: Septicémie à B. fragilis. Thèse, Nancy 1935.

REINHOLD, L.: Stoffwechselleistungen bei Stämmen des Genus Bacteroides. Zbl. Bakt., I. Abt. Orig. 193, 491—501 (1964).

Report of the International Committee on Nomenclature of Bacteria Taxonomic Subcommittee for Gram-negative anaerobic rods. Int. J. System. Bact. 20, 297—300 (1970).

RICHON, L., KISSEL, P., LEPOIRE, F.: Septicémie mortelle à Bacillus fragilis consécutive à une angine phlegmoneuse. Rev. Méd. de l'Est 62, 289—294 (1934).

RIVALIER: Le B. funduliformis et les septicémies primitives dues à ce germe. Ier Congrès Internat. Microbiol. Paris 1930. Tome II, p. 388.

ROBERTS, D. S.: The pathogenic synergy of Fusiformis necrophorus and Corynebacterium pyogenes. I. Influence of the leucocidal exotoxin of F. necrophorus. Brit. J. exp. Path. 48, 665—673 (1967).

ROBIN, L. A.: Étude de deux Spherophoraceae: Sph. pseudonecrophorus et Fusiformis nucleatus. Ann. Inst. Pasteur 74, 258—260 (1948).

ROSEBURY, T., CLARK, A. R., ENGEL, S. G., TERGIS, F.: Studies of fusospirochetal infection. I. Pathogenicity for guinea pigs of individual and combined cultures of spirochetes and other anaerobic bacteria derived from the human mouth. J. infect. Dis. 87, 217—225 (1950a).

ROSEBURY, T., CLARK, A. R., MACDONALD, J. B., O'CONNELL, D. C.: Studies of fusospirochetal infection. III. Further studies of a guinea pig passage strain of fusospirochetal infection, including the infectivity of sterile exudate filtrates, of mixed cultures through ten transfers, and of recombined pure cultures. J. infect. Dis. 87, 234 (1950c).

ROSEBURY, T., CLARK, A. R., TERGIS, F., ENGEL, S. G.: Studies of fusospirochetal infection. II. Analysis and attempted quantitative recombination of the flora of fusospirochetal infection after repeated guinea pig passage. J. infect. Dis. 87, 226—233 (1950b).

SCHÄFER, B.: Über das Bacterium melaninogenicum. Inaug.-Diss., Erlangen 1948.

SCHAFFNER, Y.: Les bacilles anaérobies non sporulés à Gram négatif favorisés par la bile. Thèse en Médicine, Lille 1963.

SCHMORL: Über ein pathogenes Fadenbakterium, Streptothrix cuniculi. Dtsch. Z. Tiermed. 17, 376 (1891); ref. Zbl. Bakt., I. Abt. Orig. 11, 666 (1892).

SCHWABACHER, H., LUCAS, D., RIMINGTON, C.: Bacterium melaninogenicum. — A misnomer. J. gen. Microbiol. 1, 109—120 (1947).

SCHWARZ, O., DIECKMANN, W.: The puerperal infection due to anaerobic streptococci. J. Obstet. Gynaec. (N. Dehli) 13, 467 (1927).

SEBALD, M.: Étude sur les bactéries anaérobies Gram-négatives Asporulées. Thèse de Sciences, Paris 1962.

SHEVKY, M., KOHL, C., MARSHALL, M.: Bacterium melaninogenicum. J. Lab. clin. Med. 19, 689—694 (1934).

SHPUNTOFF, H., ROSEBURY, T.: Infectivity of fuso-spirochetal exudates for guinea pigs, hamsters, mice and chick embryos by several routes of inoculation. J. dent Res. 28, 7—16 (1949).

Smith, W., Crabb, W. E.: The faecal bacterial flora of animals and man: its development in the young. J. Path. Bact. 82, 53—66 (1961).

Socransky, S. S., Gibbons, R. J.: Required role of Bacteroides melaninogenicus in mixed anaerobic infections. J. infect. Dis. 115, 247—253 (1965).

Suter, L. S., Ulrich, E. W., Vaughan, B. F.: Observation on a strain of Bacteroides. J. Bact. 69, 604—605 (1955).

Sutter, V. L., Sugihara, P. T., Finegold, S. M.: Rifampin-blood-agar as a selective medium for the isolation of certain anaerobic bacteria. Appl. Microbiol. 22, 777—780 (1971).

Suzuki, S., Ushijima, T., Ichinose, H.: Differentiation of Bacteroides from Sphaerophorus and Fusobacterium. Jap. J. Microbiol. 10, 193—200 (1966).

Tardieux, P., Nabonne, A.: Nouveau cas de septicémie à Spherophorus pseudonecrophorus. Ann. Inst. Pasteur 76, 181—183 (1949).

Teusch, W.: Bacterium melaninogenicum — Saprophyt oder pathogener Keim? Dtsch. med. Rdsch. 3, 1210—1212 (1949).

Thompson, L., Beaver, D. C.: Bacteriemia due to anaerobic gram-negative organisms of the genus Bacteroides. Med. Clin. N. Amer. 15, 1611 (1932).

Tracy, O.: Pigment production in Bacteroides. J. med. Microbiol. 2, 309—315 (1969).

Vallée, A., Guirard, J., Giroud, M.: Pleurésie purulente à Bacillus fragilis. Bull. Med. Québec 4, 112—115 (1932).

Varney, P.: The bacterial flora of treated and untreated abscesses of the lung. Arch. Surg. 19, 1602 (1929).

Vaucher, E., Woringer, P.: Bactériemies et septicémies dues à des anaérobies. J. Méd. Franç. 4, 141—155 (1925).

Veillon, A., Zuber, A.: Recherches sur quelques microbes strictement anaérobies et leur rôle en pathologie. Arch. Méd. exp. 10, 517—545 (1898).

Veszprémi, D.: Kultur- und Tierversuche mit dem Bacillus fusiformis und dem Spirillum. Zbl. Bakt., I. Abt. Orig. 38, 136—137 (1905).

Veszprémi, D.: Züchtungs- und Tierversuche mit Bacillus fusiformis, Spirochaete gracilis und Cladothrix putridogenes. Beiträge zur Bakteriologie und Histogenese der experimentellen gangränösen Entzündungen. Zbl. Bakt., I. Abt. Orig. 44, 332—339, 408—415, 515—523, 648—665 (1907).

Weinberg, M., Nativelle, R., Prévot, A. R.: Les microbes anaérobies. Paris: Masson 1937.

Weiss, C.: Observations on Bacterium melaninogenicum: Demonstration of fibrinolysin, pathogenicity and serological types. Proc. Soc. exp. Biol. (N.Y.) 37, 473—476 (1937).

Weiss, C.: The pathogenicity of Bacteroides melaninogenicus and its importance in surgical infections. Surgery 13, 683—691 (1943).

Werner, H.: Otogener Hirnabsceß und Meningitis durch Eggerthella convexa. Zbl. Bakt., I. Abt. Orig. 194, 203—211 (1964).

Werner, H.: Zum gegenwärtigen Stand der Diagnostik der gramnegativen anaeroben sporenlosen Stäbchen. Zbl. Bakt., I. Abt. Ref. 197, 137—158 (1965).

Werner, H.: Untersuchungen über die gramnegativen anaeroben sporenlosen Stäbchenbakterien des Menschen. Habilitationsschrift, Bonn 1966.

Werner, H.: Eggerthella-Arten aus pathologischem Material und aus Stuhlproben. Arch. Hyg. (Berl.) 151, 492—508 (1967).

Werner, H.: Die gramnegativen anaeroben sporenlosen Stäbchen des Menschen. Jena: Fischer 1968.

Werner, H.: Das serologische Verhalten von Stämmen der Species Bacteroides convexus, B. thetaiotaomicron, B. vulgatus und B. distasonis. Zbl. Bakt., I. Abt. Orig. 210, 192—201 (1969a).

Werner, H.: Sphaerophorus intermedius Bergan und Hovig 1968 ein späteres und illegitimes Homonym von Bacteroides fragilis (Veillon und Zuber 1898) Castellani und Chalmers 1919. Zbl. Bakt., I. Abt. Orig. 211, 107—110 (1969b).

Werner, H.: Bacteroides convexus Eggerth und Gagnon 1933 identisch mit Bacteroides fragilis (Veillon und Zuber 1898) Castellani und Chalmers 1919. Zbl. Bakt., I. Abt. Orig. 211, 344—353 (1969c).

Werner, H.: Vergleichende Untersuchungen an Stämmen von Ristella pseudoinsolita Beerens und Aladame 1949. Path. et Microbiol. (Basel) 34, 352—359 (1969d).

Werner, H.: Glutaminsäuredecarboxylaseaktivität bei Bacteroides-Arten. Zbl. Bakt., I. Abt. Orig. 215, 320—326 (1970a).

Werner, H.: Das kulturell-biochemische Verhalten und die Antibiotikaempfindlichkeit des Bacteroides putredinis (Weinberg et al., 1937) Kelly 1957. Zbl. Bakt., I. Abt. Orig. 215, 327—332 (1970b).

Werner, H.: Anaerobierdifferenzierung durch gaschromatographische Stoffwechselanalysen. Zbl. Bakt. Hyg., I. Abt. Orig. A 220, 446—451 (1972a).

WERNER, H.: The susceptibility of Bacteroides, Fusobacterium, Leptotrichia, and Sphaerophorus strains to rifampicin. Arzneimittel-Forsch. (Drug Res.) **22**, 1043—1045 (1972b).

WERNER, H.: A comparative study of 55 Sphaerophorus strains. Differentiation of 3 species: Sphaerophorus necrophorus, Sph. varius, and Sph. freundii. Med. Microbiol. Immunol. **157**, 299—314 (1972c).

WERNER, H.: A serological study of strains belonging to Sphaerophorus necrophorus, Sph. varius, and Sph. freundii. Med. Microbiol. Immunol. **157**, 315—324 (1972d).

WERNER, H., BOLL, G.: Die Antibiotikaempfindlichkeit von Bacteroides(Eggerthella)-Stämmen. Zbl. Bakt., I. Abt. Orig. **208**, 437—448 (1968).

WERNER, H., HUSSELS, H., NEUHAUS, F.: Pleuraempyem durch die anaerobe nichtsporenbildende Bakterienart Sphaerophorus necrophorus. Dtsch. med. Wschr. **96**, 202—205 (1971a).

WERNER, H., MÜLLER, H. E.: Immunelektrophoretische Untersuchungen über die Einwirkung von Bacteroides-, Fusobacterium-, Leptotrichia- und Sphaerophorus-Arten auf menschliche Plasmaproteine. Zbl. Bakt., I. Abt. Orig. **216**, 96—113 (1971).

WERNER, H., NEUHAUS, F., HUSSELS, H.: A biochemical study of fusiform anaerobes. Med. Microbiol. Immunol. **157**, 10—16 (1971b).

WERNER, H., NEUHAUS, F., REICHERTZ, C.: Otogener Hirnabsceß durch die darmbewohnende Bacteroides-Art B. fragilis. Dtsch. med. Wschr. **95**, 343—345 (1970a).

WERNER, H., PULVERER, G.: Häufigkeit und medizinische Bedeutung der eitererregenden Bacteroides- und Sphaerophorus-Arten. Dtsch. med. Wschr. **96**, 1325—1329 (1971).

WERNER, H., PULVERER, G., REICHERTZ, C.: The biochemical properties and antibiotic susceptibility of Bacteroides melaninogenicus. Med. Microbiol. Immunol. **157**, 3—9 (1971c).

WERNER, H., REICHERTZ, C.: Buttersäurebildende Bacteroides-Kulturen. Zbl. Bakt., I. Abt. Orig. **217**, 206—216 (1971).

WERNER, H., REICHERTZ, C., SCHRÖTER, G.: Der Bacteroides-Anteil der menschlichen Darmflora. Zbl. Bakt., I. Abt. Orig. **212**, 530—537 (1970b).

WERNER, H., SEBALD, M.: Étude sérologique des anaérobies Gram négatifs asporulés, et particulièrement de Bacteroides convexus et Bacteroides melaninogenicus. Ann. Inst. Pasteur **115**, 350—366 (1968).

WERNER, H., SEELIGER, H. P. R.: Kulturelle Untersuchungen über den Keimgehalt der Appendix unter besonderer Berücksichtigung der Anaerobier. Zbl. Bakt., I. Abt. Orig. **188**, 345—364 (1963).

WESTPHAL, O., LÜDERITZ, O., BISTER, F.: Über die Extraktion von Bakterien mit Phenol/Wasser. Z. Naturforsch. **7B**, 148—155 (1952).

WILSON, G. S., MILES, A. A.: Topley and Wilson's principles of bacteriology and immunity. London: Arnold 3rd ed. 1946, 5th ed. 1964.

WOLFF, R.: Untersuchungen an NMRI/Han-Mäusen zur Frage der tierexperimentellen Pathogenität von Bacteroides fragilis-Stämmen. Inaug.-Diss., Bonn 1972.

Verhütung von Laboratoriumsinfektionen

RICHARD-ERNST BADER[1]

Mit 4 Abbildungen

A. Einleitung

Alle Arbeiten mit Reinkulturen von pathogenen Mikroorganismen, mit infektiösem Material und infizierten Versuchstieren sind für den Untersucher, seine Mitarbeiter und einen erweiterten Personenkreis mit Gefahren verbunden, die eine breite Skala von banalen Infektionskrankheiten bis zu gemeingefährlichen Seuchen umfassen. Um diese Risiken auf ein Minimum zu reduzieren, wurden in den meisten Staaten Gesetze und Verordnungen erlassen, die die Anforderungen an das Laboratoriumspersonal, die Ausstattung der Arbeitsräume und die beim Umgang mit Krankheitserregern notwendigen Sicherheitsmaßnahmen festlegen. Sie zu kennen und strikt zu befolgen ist zur Verhütung von Schäden unerläßlich.

Eine Vielzahl von nationalen gesetzlichen Vorschriften zu zitieren würde den Rahmen dieses Beitrags sprengen und zudem wenig Konkretes zur Erweiterung der Thematik beitragen, da die Probleme der Infektionsverhütung im mikrobiologischen Laboratorium überall ähnlich sind und ihre Lösung mit adäquaten Mitteln angestrebt wird. Der Darstellung werden deshalb im wesentlichen die sehr ausführlichen Regelungen der Bundesrepublik Deutschland zugrunde gelegt. Eine Sammlung der wichtigsten hier geltenden Gesetze und Verordnungen findet sich bei ETMER u. LUNDT (1969ff.), eine ähnliche Zusammenstellung für den Gebrauch in der Deutschen Demokratischen Republik bei HEILMANN et al. (1969). Es empfiehlt sich jedoch, bei Arbeiten in anderen Staaten die dort geltenden Vorschriften zu beachten, um sich vor Schäden sowie zivil- und strafrechtlichen Konsequenzen zu schützen.

Erschwert werden die Sicherheitsbemühungen durch die geringe Größe der Mikroorganismen, die sich — abgesehen von ihrer Anordnung in Kolonien — der direkten Beobachtung entziehen. Kontaminationen der menschlichen Haut und Schleimhäute, der Kleidung und Arbeitsgeräte, der Laboratoriumseinrichtungen und Räume sind deshalb nicht unmittelbar zu erkennen. Hinzu kommt die Vielfalt der Eintrittspforten in den menschlichen Organismus. Die meisten Krankheitserreger dringen über die Verdauungs- und Atemwege, andere durch die Haut und die Schleimhäute ein, ein kleiner Teil ist auf den Transport durch tierische Überträger angewiesen.

Schließlich erfordern die Kleinheit der Mikroorganismen und Besonderheiten ihrer Vermehrung und ihrer Stoffwechselleistungen spezielle, von anderen biologischen Methoden abweichende Techniken, deren exakte Anwendung im Laboratorium unter Beachtung der Sicherheitsvorschriften selbstverständlich sein muß.

---

1 Herrn Ehrensenator ALFRED TEUFEL, dem verdienstvollen Förderer lufthygienischer Untersuchungen, dankbar gewidmet.

B. Häufigkeit von Laboratoriumsinfektionen

Die *Statistiken* der Laboratoriumsinfektionen sind lückenhaft, da von deren Publikation aus begreiflichen, wenn auch nicht immer zu billigenden Gründen meist Abstand genommen wird. Es ist das Verdienst von Kisskalt (1915), am Beispiel des Typhus abdominalis als einer der ersten auf die Häufigkeit derartiger Ereignisse hingewiesen zu haben. Von 50 ihm durch eine Umfrage zur Kenntnis gelangten Erkrankungen waren 6 tödlich verlaufen. In der Folgezeit wurde in mehreren hundert Mitteilungen über etwa 6000 Erkrankungen berichtet (Phillips, 1965, 1969). Zahlreiche Fälle wurden von Müller (1950) gesammelt.

In einer Veröffentlichung von Wundt (1964) finden sich statistische Angaben der Berufsgenossenschaft für Gesundheitsdienst und Wohlfahrtspflege über entschädigungspflichtige Infektionskrankheiten in der Bundesrepublik Deutschland in den Jahren 1949—1960, allerdings unter Einschluß der auch außerhalb von Laboratorien erworbenen Infektionen. Ihre Zahl schwankte jährlich zwischen etwa 800 und 1200, die der Todesfälle zwischen 0,9 und 5,3%. Hepatitis und Tuberkulose standen weit an erster Stelle. Wie aus Tabelle 1 (persönliche Mitteilung der Berufsgenossenschaft, 1967) hervorgeht, sind in den Jahren 1950—1965 die gegenläufigen Zahlen für diese beiden Krankheiten bemerkenswert. Gemessen an den Erhebungen von 1959—1961 und von 1965 ist die Hepatitis in etwa 11—16% auf Infektionen in Laboratorien zurückzuführen.

Für das Jahr 1971 wies die Statistik aus gleicher Quelle insgesamt 1385 Infektionskrankheiten aus, davon 1028 Virushepatitiden und 223 Tuberkulosen. Salmonellosen standen mit 48 an dritter Stelle.

Eine umfangreiche Statistik mit 1342 Erkrankungen und 39 Todesfällen in den USA erstellten Sulkin u. Pike (1951). Als Ursachen wurden 69 verschiedene Krankheitserreger erwähnt. In einer späteren Publikation konnte sie auf 2262 Erkrankungen mit 96 Todesfällen (Sulkin et al., 1961) und kurz darauf auf 2348 Erkrankungen, davon 107 mit tödlichem Ausgang, erweitert werden (Sulkin, 1961).

Einer Veröffentlichung von Pike et al. (1965) kann der Anteil der verschiedenen Gruppen von Mikroorganismen am Zustandekommen von Laboratoriumsinfek-

Tabelle 1. Als Berufskrankheiten gemeldete Laboratoriumsinfektionen

| | Infektionskrankheiten | | |
| | insgesamt | davon | |
		Tuberkulose	Hepatitis
1950	1367	684	141
1951	1146	588	151
1952	964	542	146
1953	790	415	143
1954	764	367	160
1955	693	339	167
1956	646	276	192
1957	609	254	207
1958	579	256	217
1959	682	264	240
1960	755	257	267
1961	689	242	305
1962	618	201	321
1963	641	187	316
1964	743	195	416
1965	685	177	414

Tabelle 2. Laboratoriumsinfektionen 1930—1963. (Nach PIKE et al., 1965)

Erreger	USA 1930—1950				Welt 1950—1963			
	Zahl der Fälle	insge- samt %	ver- öffent- licht %	Zahl der Todes- fälle	Zahl der Fälle	insge- samt %	ver- öffent- licht %	Zahl der Todes- fälle
Bakterien	775	57	30	19	191	30	85	1
Viren	265	20	49	12	250	39	85	11
Rickettsien	200	15	49	6	107	17	67	0
Pilze	63	5	13	2	58	9	100	0
Parasiten	39	3	5	0	35	5	100	1
Insgesamt	1 342	100	35	39	641	100	84	13

Tabelle 3. Häufigkeit bakterieller Erkrankungen. (Nach PIKE et al., 1965)

USA 1930—1950		Welt 1950—1963	
Brucellose	224	Tularämie	64
Tuberkulose	153	Brucellose	50
Tularämie	65	Tuberkulose	21
Typhus abdominalis	58	Leptospirose	16
Streptokokkenerkrankungen	55	Shigellose	11
Shigellose	31	Pest	4
Milzbrand	30	Salmonellose	3
Erysipeloid	27	Milzbrand	3
Unspezifische lokale Erkrankungen	23	Syphilis	3
Rückfallfieber	17	Rattenbißkrankheit	3
Staphylokokkenerkrankungen	16	Staphylokokkenerkrankungen	3
Diphtherie	15	Streptokokkenerkrankungen	3
Rattenbißkrankheit	11	Typhus abdominalis	2
11 andere	50	Erysipeloid	2
		PPLO	1
		Vibriose (Vibrio fetus)	1
		Tetanus	1
Insgesamt	775	Insgesamt	191

tionen in den Jahren 1930—1950 (USA) und 1950—1963 (Welt) entnommen werden (Tabelle 2). Im ersten Zeitraum waren Bakterien die häufigsten Ursachen. In weitem Abstand folgten Viren, Rickettsien, Pilze und Parasiten. Im zweiten Zeitraum rückten Viren an die erste Stelle.

Unter den bakteriellen Erkrankungen lagen von 1930—1950 die Brucellosen und die Tuberkulose, von 1950—1963 die Tularämie vor diesen an der Spitze (Tabelle 3). Die Angaben über die Häufigkeit der Tularämie sind allerdings irreführend, weil sich fast alle Infektionen in nur zwei Laboratorien ereigneten.

Unter den Viruserkrankungen dominierte die Hepatitis bzw. die Encephalitis (Tabelle 4), unter den Rickettsiosen eindeutig das Q-Fieber (Tabelle 5) (s. auch TIGERTT et al., 1961).

Mykosen waren relativ selten und überwiegend auf außereuropäische Pilze zurückzuführen (Tabelle 6).

Die Zahlen der parasitären Erkrankungen finden sich in Tabelle 7.

Tabelle 4. Häufigkeit von Viruserkrankungen. (Nach Pike et al., 1965)

USA 1930—1950		Welt 1950—1963	
Hepatitis	95	Encephalitis	46
Psittacose	44	Hepatitis	31
Lymphocytäre Choriomeningitis	19	Coxsackie-Erkrankung	29
Encephalitis	17	Psittacose	26
Gelbfieber	14	Newcastle-Erkrankung	21
Newcastle-Erkrankung	11	B-Virus-Erkrankung	11
Rifttal-Fieber	11	Kyasanur Forest-Erkrankung	8
Lymphogranuloma inguinale	6	Adenovirus-Erkrankung	8
Coxsackie-Erkrankung	6	Vesiculäre Stomatitis	8
Poliomyelitis	4	Bunyamwera-Erkrankung	6
11 andere	38	Colorado-Zeckenfieber	6
		Poliomyelitis	5
		Trachom	5
		21 andere	40
Insgesamt	265	Insgesamt	250

Tabelle 5. Häufigkeit von Rickettsiosen. (Nach Pike et al., 1965)

USA 1930—1950		Welt 1950—1963	
Q-Fieber	104	Q-Fieber	80
Fleckfieber	64	Fleckfieber	18
Rocky Mountains Fleckfieber	16	Rocky Mountains Fleckfieber	7
Tsutsugamushifieber	12	Akaririckettsiose	2
Akaririckettsiose	4	Tsutsugamushifieber	0
Insgesamt	200	Insgesamt	107

Tabelle 6. Häufigkeit von Mycosen. (Nach Pike et al., 1965)

USA 1930—1950		Welt 1950—1963	
Coccidioidomycose	49	Histoplasmose	46
Trichophytie	4	Coccidioidomycose	8
Blastomycose	2	Trichophytie	4
Sporotrichose	2		
Moniliasis	2		
Nicht diagnostiziert	2		
Insgesamt	61	Insgesamt	58

Tabelle 7. Häufigkeit von Erkrankungen durch Parasiten. (Nach Pike et al., 1965)

USA 1930—1950		Welt 1950—1963	
Amoebiasis	18	Toxoplasmose	21
Malaria	9	Trypanosomiasis	5
Ascaridiasis	2	Malaria	4
Strongyloidiasis	2	Coccidiosis	3
8 andere	8	Leishmaniasis	1
		Giardiasis	1
Insgesamt	39	Insgesamt	35

Tabelle 8. Laboratoriumsepidemien. (Nach PHILLIPS, 1969)

Erkrankung	Jahr	Zahl der infizierten Personen
Psittacose	1930	11
Brucellose	1938	94
Q-Fieber	1940	15
Murines Fleckfieber	1942	6
Q-Fieber	1946	47
Coccidioidomycose	1950	13
Histoplasmose	1955	18
Venezuela-Encephalitis	1959	24
Tularämie	1961	5

Obwohl sich Laboratoriumsinfektionen in der Regel auf einzelne Personen beschränken, scheinen manche Krankheitserreger die Tendenz zu haben, sich auf mehrere Laboratorien, gelegentlich auf ganze Gebäude, auszubreiten und umfangreiche Epidemien zu verursachen. Von PHILLIPS (1969) wurden aus der Literatur 9 derartige Ereignisse zusammengestellt (Tabelle 8). Bemerkenswert sind in diesem Zusammenhang auch die Publikationen von KIKUTH u. BOCK (1949) über gehäufte Q-Fieber-Erkrankungen, von SLEPUSHKIN (1959) über Infektionen mit dem Erreger der Venezuela-Pferdeencephalitis und von SIEGERT et al. (1967) über eine Epidemie mit dem FMS-Virus.

In den Literaturverzeichnissen der genannten Arbeiten finden sich zahlreiche Hinweise auf Laboratoriumsinfektionen verschiedenster Art, weitere kasuistische Mitteilungen über Brucellosen bei MEYER u. EDDIE (1941), über Tuberkulose bei JENSEN (1959), ALBRECHT (1961, 1968), JEANJEAN u. JEANJEAN (1969) und LIEBKNECHT (1971, mit einer Literaturzusammenstellung über Inoculationstuberkulose durch Spritzen), über Typhus abdominalis bei ALBRECHT (1967), über Rotlauf bei AJMAL (1969).

Auf virologischem Gebiet berichteten HUEBNER (1947), ROSEBURY et al. (1947) und SULKIN u. PIKE (1949) über Laboratoriumsinfektionen. Kasuistische Beiträge lieferten JOHNSON u. KADULL (1967) und CALIA et al. (1970) über Rocky Mountain spotted fever und REID et al. (1972) über louping-ill. Eine umfangreiche Zusammenstellung von Erkrankungen durch Arboviren findet sich bei HANSON et al. (1967). In 91 Laboratorien von 38 Ländern erkrankten 428 Personen, davon 16 tödlich, durch 36 Virusarten.

Ausgehend von importierten Grünen Meerkatzen (Cercopithecus aethiops), brach im Herbst 1967 eine Epidemie aus, die in Marburg, Frankfurt und Belgrad 31 Personen erfaßte, von denen 7 verstarben. Das FMS-Virus wurde teils vom Tier bzw. seinen Organen auf den Menschen, teils von Mensch zu Mensch übertragen (SIEGERT et al., 1967; SHU et al., 1968; HAAS et al., 1968).

Über Laboratoriumsinfektionen mit Pilzen berichteten KAFFKA u. RIETH (1958), FURCOLOW (1961) und SMITH et al. (1961), mit Blastomyces dermatitidis DENTON et al. (1967) und BAUM u. LERNER (1970), mit Microsporum cookei bei der Isolierung von Dermatophyten aus Erde SCHICK (1968) und über Pilzinfektionen in Finnland SONCK (1961).

Zur Infektionsgefährdung durch Toxoplasma gondii äußerten sich PIEKARSKI (1967, 1968), ALBRECHT (1968), ANDERS u. LEWANDOWSKI (1968) sowie PIETSCH u. BAUMGARTEN (1969), zur Gefährdung durch Mycobacterium tuberculosis LURIE (1930), LONG (1951), JENSEN (1959, 1968), RILEY (1961) und ALBRECHT (1961, 1968).

Die durchschnittliche *Letalität* aller Laboratoriumsinfektionen schätzte PHILLIPS (1969) auf etwa 4%. Aus den Angaben von PIKE et al. (1965) lassen sich für den Zeitraum von 1930—1950 2,9%, für 1950—1963 2,0% errechnen. Nach SULKIN (1961) betrug die Letalität bei Virusinfektionen 7,3%, bei bakteriellen Erkrankungen 4,0% und bei Rickettsien- bzw. Pilzinfektionen 2,6 bzw. 2,3%.

Die *Infektionsquellen* blieben überwiegend im dunkeln, nach WEDUM (1953) konnten sie nur bei etwa 20% der Zwischenfälle geklärt werden. Als häufigste Ursachen erwähnte PHILLIPS (1969) bei 3700 Infektionen das Pipettieren (4,7%), den Stich mit Injektionsnadeln (4%), Tierbisse (1,4%), das Versprühen von Material mit Spritzen (1,2%) und Zentrifugenunfälle (0,8%). PIKE et al. (1965) fanden bei 1342 Erkrankungen als häufigste wahrscheinliche Infektionsquellen das Hantieren mit dem Erreger (454), Unfälle (373), Aerosole (334) und infizierte Tiere oder Ektoparasiten (222). Bei der Auswertung von 371 durch Unfälle verursachten Erkrankungen aus den Jahren 1930—1963 kamen sie zu etwas anderen Ergebnissen als PHILLIPS (1969). Unfälle durch Nadeln und Spritzen waren mit 26,5 bzw. 22,4% am häufigsten, durch Pipettieren mit 15,3 bzw. 5,8% wesentlich seltener. Nach SULKIN u. PIKE (1961) waren 16% der Infektionen auf Unfälle zurückzuführen. Bei 428 Infektionen mit Arboviren ermittelten HANSON et al. (1967) folgende Ursachenskala: Tierversuche 21,7%, unbekannte Infektionsquellen 19,6%, Aerosole 17,3%, Hantieren mit Erregern 16,4%, Unfälle 10%, Herstellen von Vaccinen und Antigenen 8,2%, Beimpfen von Bruteiern 2,1% und Glasverletzungen 2,1%. WEDUM (1961) maß der Aerosolbildung besondere Bedeutung bei.

Ursachenanalysen sind für die Verhütung von Laboratoriumsinfektionen von unschätzbarem Wert, da sie die Grundlagen für Unfallverhütungsvorschriften bilden.

C. Anforderungen an das Personal

1. Ausbildung

Arbeiten mit Krankheitserregern sollen Personen vorbehalten sein, die eine fachliche Ausbildung nachweisen können. Diese soll theoretische Kenntnisse auf den Gebieten der Morphologie und Physiologie der Mikroorganismen, der Immunologie, der Pathogenese und Epidemiologie der Infektionskrankheiten, insbesondere der Infektkettenbildung einschließlich der Erregerreservoire, Austrittspforten, Übertragungswege und Eintrittspforten, der Sicherheitsvorschriften und Schutzmaßnahmen vermitteln und eine fundierte praktische Unterweisung in den mikrobiologischen und serologischen Techniken umfassen.

In der Bundesrepublik Deutschland ist das „Arbeiten und der Verkehr mit Krankheitserregern" durch die §§ 19—29 des Bundes-Seuchengesetzes von 1961 ausführlich geregelt. „Den Vorschriften liegt der Gedanke zugrunde, daß beim Arbeiten und beim Verkehr mit Krankheitserregern eine Krankheitsverbreitung nur vermeidbar ist, wenn die entsprechenden Tätigkeiten auf fachlich vorgebildete und zuverlässige Personen beschränkt bleiben und wenn geeignete Räume zur Verfügung stehen" (ETMER u. LUNDT, 1969ff.). Besonders streng sind die Bestimmungen hinsichtlich der Erreger von Cholera, Fleckfieber, Gelbfieber, Kinderlähmung, Milzbrand, Ornithosen, Pest, Pocken, Toxoplasmose und Tularämie. Arbeiten mit diesen, ihre Ein- und Ausfuhr, Aufbewahrung und Abgabe sind an eine staatliche Erlaubnis gebunden, die Sachkenntnis, Zuverlässigkeit sowie geeignete Laboratorien und Einrichtungen voraussetzt. Die Sachkenntnis wird durch die Bestallung als Arzt, Zahnarzt, Tierarzt oder Apotheker oder den Abschluß eines naturwissenschaftlichen Hochschulstudiums und eine mindestens dreijährige einschlägige Tätigkeit nachgewiesen. Außerdem werden die Personenkreise und Institutionen definiert, die ohne besondere Erlaubnis unter bestimmten Bedingungen mikrobiologische und serologische Arbeiten durchführen dürfen, sofern sich diese nicht auf die namentlich erwähnten Erreger erstrecken und die Einfuhr, Ausfuhr und Abgabe ausschließen. Die Erleichterungen gelten insbesondere für Ärzte, Zahnärzte und Tierärzte.

Arbeiten und Verkehr mit Krankheitserregern

§ 19 (Erlaubnis)

(1) Wer 1. die lebenden Erreger von Cholera, Fleckfieber, Gelbfieber, Kinderlähmung, Milzbrand, Ornithosen, Pest, Pocken, Toxoplasmose oder Tularämie, 2. die lebenden Erreger anderer auf den Menschen übertragbarer Krankheiten, ausgenommen Maul- und Klauenseuche und Rotz, einführen, ausführen, aufbewahren, abgeben oder mit ihnen arbeiten will, bedarf einer Erlaubnis der zuständigen Behörde.

(2) Als Arbeiten mit Krankheitserregern sind insbesondere anzusehen 1. Versuche mit vermehrungsfähigen Krankheitserregern, 2. mikrobiologische und serologische Untersuchungen zur Feststellung übertragbarer Krankheiten, 3. Fortzüchtung von Krankheitserregern.

(3) Als Arbeiten mit Krankheitserregern gelten ferner die serologischen Untersuchungen zur Feststellung der Syphilis.

§ 20 (Befreiung)

Der Erlaubnis zum Arbeiten mit den in § 19 Abs. 1 Nr. 2 bezeichneten Krankheitserregern sowie zu ihrer Aufbewahrung bedürfen nicht

1. Ärzte, Zahnärzte und Tierärzte, soweit sie sich auf diagnostische Untersuchungen oder therapeutische Maßnahmen für die eigene Praxis beschränken,
2. Ärzte in Gefangenenanstalten, soweit sie sich auf diagnostische Untersuchungen oder therapeutische Maßnahmen bei den Gefangenen beschränken,
3. Krankenhäuser, Polikliniken oder Tierkliniken, soweit sie sich unter ärztlicher Leitung auf diagnostische Untersuchungen oder therapeutische Maßnahmen in ihrem Arbeitsbereich beschränken,
4. ärztlich geleitete staatliche oder kommunale Hygiene-Institute, Medizinaluntersuchungsämter und Veterinäruntersuchungsämter sowie Gesundheitsämter, Veterinärämter, Tiergesundheitsämter und solche öffentliche Forschungsinstitute, deren Aufgaben das Arbeiten mit Krankheitserregern erfordern.

§ 21

Der Erlaubnis nach § 19 Abs. 1 bedarf nicht, wer für denjenigen, der eine Erlaubnis besitzt oder nach § 20 keiner Erlaubnis bedarf, tätig ist.

§ 22 (Versagung der Erlaubnis)

(1) Die Erlaubnis ist zu versagen,
   1. wenn der Antragsteller a) die erforderliche Sachkenntnis nicht besitzt, b) sich als unzuverlässig in bezug auf die Tätigkeiten erwiesen hat, für deren Ausübung die Erlaubnis begehrt wird, oder
   2. wenn geeignete Räume oder Einrichtungen nicht vorhanden sind.

(2) Wenn der Antragsteller nicht selbst die Leitung der Tätigkeiten übernimmt, so darf bei ihm der Versagungsgrund nach Absatz 1 Nr. 1 Buchstabe b und dürfen bei der von ihm mit der Leitung beauftragten Person die Versagungsgründe nach Absatz 1 Nr. 1 nicht vorliegen. Bei juristischen Personen darf der Versagungsgrund nach Absatz 1 Nr. 1 Buchstabe b bei den nach Gesetz oder Satzung zur Vertretung berufenen Personen nicht vorliegen.

(3) Die erforderliche Sachkenntnis wird durch
   1. die Bestallung als Arzt, Zahnarzt, Tierarzt oder Apotheker oder den Abschluß eines naturwissenschaftlichen Hochschulstudiums und
   2. eine mindestens dreijährige Tätigkeit auf dem Gebiete der Mikrobiologie und Serologie nachgewiesen.

(4) Bei Antragstellern, die nicht die Bestallung als Arzt, Zahnarzt oder Tierarzt besitzen, ist die Erlaubnis auf die in § 19 Abs. 2 Nr. 1 und 3 bezeichneten Arbeiten zu beschränken. Im übrigen kann die Erlaubnis auf bestimmte Tätigkeiten und auf bestimmte Krankheitserreger beschränkt und mit Auflagen verbunden werden, soweit dies zur Verhütung übertragbarer Krankheiten erforderlich ist.

§ 23 (Zurücknahme der Erlaubnis)

Die Erlaubnis ist zurückzunehmen, wenn ein Versagungsgrund nach § 22 vorhanden ist und wenn im Falle des § 22, Abs. 1 Nr. 2 dem Mangel nicht innerhalb einer von der zuständigen Behörde zu setzenden angemessenen Frist abgeholfen wird.

§ 24 (Anzeigepflichten des Erlaubnisinhabers)

Der Inhaber einer Erlaubnis hat jeden Wechsel der mit der Leitung der Tätigkeiten beauftragten Person sowie jede wesentliche Änderung der Räume oder Einrichtungen unverzüglich der zuständigen Behörde anzuzeigen. Das gleiche gilt beim Wechsel der Vertretungsberechtigten juristischer Personen.

§ 25 (Aufsicht)

Wer eine Erlaubnis erhalten hat, untersteht der Aufsicht der zuständigen Behörde. Er ist insoweit verpflichtet, den von der zuständigen Behörde beauftragten Personen das Betreten seines Grundstücks zu gestatten, Räume, Anlagen und Einrichtungen zugänglich zu machen, Bücher und sonstige Unterlagen vorzulegen, die Einsicht in diese zu gewähren und die notwendigen Prüfungen zu dulden. Das Grundrecht der Unverletzlichkeit der Wohnung (Artikel 13 Abs. 1 Grundgesetz) wird insoweit eingeschränkt.

§ 26 (Abgabe von Krankheitserregern)

Krankheitserreger der in § 19 Abs. 1 bezeichneten Art sowie Material, das solche Krankheitserreger enthält, dürfen nur an denjenigen abgegeben werden, der eine Erlaubnis besitzt oder einer solchen nach § 20 oder 21 nicht bedarf.

§§ 27—29

(Schädlingsbekämpfung durch Krankheitserreger, gewerbsmäßige Herstellung von Seren und Impfstoffen, Ermächtigung zum Erlaß einer Rechtsverordnung über die Anforderungen an Räume und Einrichtungen sowie über Vorsichtsmaßregeln usw.).

Die einen theoretischen und praktischen Unterricht in Mikrobiologie und Serologie umfassenden Ausbildungsgänge der Ärzte, Zahnärzte, Tierärzte und Apotheker sind in der Bestallungsordnung bzw. Approbationsordnung für Ärzte von 1953 bzw. 1970, im Gesetz über die Ausübung der Zahnheilkunde von 1952, in der Bestallungsordnung für Tierärzte von 1967 und in der Approbationsordnung für Apotheker von 1971 niedergelegt.

Eine Vertiefung der Kenntnisse vermittelt die Weiterbildung zum Laborarzt, für die im Rahmen einer fünfjährigen Ausbildung eine vierjährige mikrobiologische und immunologische Tätigkeit vorgeschrieben ist (Berufsordnungen der Landesärztekammern).

Die für die Deutsche Demokratische Republik geltenden Vorschriften für das Arbeiten mit Krankheitserregern finden sich in der „Dritten Durchführungsbestimmung zum Gesetz zur Verhütung und Bekämpfung übertragbarer Krankheiten beim Menschen — Arbeit mit Erregern von übertragbaren Krankheiten —" von 1966 und in dem genannten Gesetz von 1965.

Für die nichtakademischen Mitarbeiter in mikrobiologischen Laboratorien gelten besondere Regelungen. Das „Gesetz über technische Assistenten in der Medizin" von 1971 macht eine Tätigkeit unter der Berufsbezeichnung „medizinisch-technischer Laboratoriumsassistent" von einer Erlaubnis abhängig, die neben persönlicher Zuverlässigkeit und Eignung einen zweijährigen Lehrgang an einer staatlich anerkannten Lehranstalt mit staatlicher Prüfung voraussetzt. Von besonderer Bedeutung ist die Bestimmung, daß auf dem Gebiet der Human- und Veterinärmedizin mikrobiologische, parasitologische und serologische Arbeiten solchen Personen vorbehalten sind, die die erwähnte Erlaubnis besitzen. Sie findet allerdings keine Anwendung auf einen aus § 10 ersichtlichen Personenkreis.

§ 1 [2]

Der Erlaubnis bedarf, wer eine Tätigkeit unter der Berufsbezeichnung
1. ,,medizinisch-technischer Laboratoriumsassistent'' oder ,,medizinisch-technische Laboratoriumsassistentin'',
3. ,,veterinärmedizinisch-technischer Assistent'' oder ,,veterinärmedizinisch-technische Assistentin''
ausüben will.

§ 2

Eine Erlaubnis nach § 1 wird erteilt, wenn der Antragsteller
1. sich nicht eines Verhaltens schuldig gemacht hat, aus dem sich die Unzuverlässigkeit zur Ausübung des Berufs ergibt,
2. nicht wegen eines körperlichen Gebrechens, wegen Schwäche seiner geistigen oder körperlichen Kräfte oder wegen einer Sucht zur Ausübung des Berufs unfähig oder ungeeignet ist,
3. in der Fachrichtung, für die die Erlaubnis beantragt wird, nach einem zweijährigen Lehrgang die staatliche Prüfung bestanden hat.

§ 7

(1) Die Lehrgänge nach diesem Gesetz werden an Lehranstalten durchgeführt, die als zur Ausbildung geeignet staatlich anerkannt sind. Sie umfassen jeweils eine theoretische und praktische Ausbildung.
(2) Zu den Lehrgängen nach § 2 Nr. 3 wird zugelassen, wer eine abgeschlossene Realschulbildung oder eine andere gleichwertige Ausbildung nachweist.

§ 9 [3]

(1) Auf dem Gebiet der Humanmedizin dürfen
   1. die folgenden Tätigkeiten nur von Personen mit einer Erlaubnis nach § 1 Nr. 1 ausgeübt werden:
      d) Arbeiten auf dem Gebiet der Mikrobiologie (einschließlich Parasitologie) und auf dem Gebiet der Serologie.
(2) Auf dem Gebiet der Veterinärmedizin dürfen die folgenden Tätigkeiten nur von Personen mit einer Erlaubnis nach § 1 Nr. 3 ausgeübt werden:
   1. Arbeiten, die den in Absatz 1 Nr. 1 genannten entsprechen.

§ 10 [4]

(1) § 9, Abs. 1 findet keine Anwendung auf
   1. Personen, die auf Grund einer abgeschlossenen Hochschulbildung über die erforderlichen Fachkenntnisse zur Ausübung der genannten Tätigkeiten verfügen, Zahnärzte, die die Bestallung gemäß den §§ 8 bis 10 des Gesetzes über die Ausübung der Zahnheilkunde erhalten haben, sowie Heilpraktiker,
   5. Personen mit einer staatlich geregelten, staatlich anerkannten oder staatlich überwachten abgeschlossenen Ausbildung, wenn sie eine der vorbehalteneu Tätigkeiten nach § 9 ausüben, sofern diese Tätigkeit Gegenstand ihrer Ausbildung und Prüfung war,
   6. Personen, die unter Aufsicht und Verantwortung einer der in Nr. 1 genannten Personen tätig werden.

Ergänzt wird dieses Gesetz durch die ,,Ausbildungs- und Prüfungsordnung für technische Assistenten in der Medizin'' von 1972, die neben anderen Bestimmungen den Ausbildungsgang und die Prüfungsanforderungen für medizinisch-technische Assistenten verbindlich festlegt.

---

2 Gekürzt.
3 Gekürzt.
4 Gekürzt.

Den Schülern sind mindestens 170 Std theoretischer Unterricht in Mikrobiologie (einschließlich Virologie und Parasitologie), Serologie, Hygiene und allgemeiner Krankheitslehre und mindestens 325 Std Praktikum in Mikrobiologie (einschließlich Virologie und Parasitologie) und Serologie zu erteilen. Die Fächer sind, mit Ausnahme der allgemeinen Krankheitslehre, Gegenstand von mündlichen, schriftlichen oder praktischen Prüfungen.

2. Eignung

Die Erlaubnis zum Arbeiten mit Krankheitserregern ist nach § 22 des Bundes-Seuchengesetzes von 1961 (Kommentar s. Etmer u. Lundt, 1969 ff. und Seyf-fertitz u. Thomaschewski, 1968) zu versagen, wenn der Antragsteller sich als unzuverlässig erwiesen hat (s. S. 237).

Nach dem „Gesetz über technische Assistenten in der Medizin" von 1971 wird eine Erlaubnis zur Tätigkeit unter der Berufsbezeichnung „medizinisch-technischer Laboratoriumsassistent" oder „medizinisch-technische Laboratoriumsassistentin" nur erteilt, wenn der Antragsteller „nicht wegen eines körperlichen Gebrechens, wegen Schwäche seiner geistigen oder körperlichen Kräfte oder wegen einer Sucht zur Ausübung des Berufs unfähig oder ungeeignet ist" (s. S. 239). Abgesehen von diesen Hinderungsgründen ist nach den Forderungen der Berufsgenossen-schaften jeweils vor Antritt einer Tätigkeit im Laboratorium ein ärztliches Zeugnis über den einwandfreien Gesundheitszustand vorzulegen (Merkblatt „Eignungs-untersuchung und Gesundheitsüberwachung des Personals von Krankenanstalten", 1955, das sinngemäß auch für alle medizinisch-mikrobiologisch tätigen Personen gilt). Falls eine Beschäftigung in Laboratorien vorgesehen ist, in denen mit Tuberkelbakterien oder tuberkelbakterienhaltigem Material gearbeitet wird, sind in die ärztliche Untersuchung eine Röntgenaufnahme der Lunge auf Film und ein Tuberkulintest einzubeziehen. Personen mit negativem Tuberkulintest dürfen nicht beschäftigt werden (Unfallverhütungsvorschrift „Behandlung, Pflege und sonstige Betreuung von Kranken und Siechen", 1961).

Während der Tätigkeit mit infektiösem Material sind im Rahmen der Gesund-heitsüberwachung mindestens halbjährlich, bei stärker gefährdetem Personal in mikrobiologischen Laboratorien in kürzeren Abständen Nachuntersuchungen durchzuführen. Die Ergebnisse sind aktenkundig zu machen.

Nach dem „Gesetz zum Schutze der erwerbstätigen Mutter" von 1968 müssen Schwangeren und stillenden Müttern durch besondere Gestaltung des Arbeits-platzes Erleichterungen gewährt werden. Für mikrobiologische Laboratorien ist zusätzlich von Bedeutung, daß werdende Mütter nicht beschäftigt werden dürfen, „soweit nach ärztlichem Zeugnis Leben oder Gesundheit von Mutter oder Kind bei Fortdauer der Beschäftigung gefährdet ist". Das Beschäftigungsverbot gilt schließ-lich auch für „Arbeiten, bei denen Berufserkrankungen im Sinne der Vorschriften über Ausdehnung der Unfallversicherung auf Berufskrankheiten entstehen können, sofern werdende Mütter infolge ihrer Schwangerschaft bei diesen Arbeiten in besonderem Maße der Gefahr einer Berufserkrankung ausgesetzt sind".

Besondere Vorsicht ist bei Arbeiten mit solchen Mikroorganismen aus der Gruppe der Viren, Bakterien und Protozoen geboten, die Embryopathien ver-ursachen können. Eine ausführliche Darstellung der pränatalen Infektionen des Menschen findet sich bei Flamm (1959), Übersichten über Virusembryopathien bei Deibel (1966) und Haas (1971).

3. Impfungen

Nach den Bestimmungen der Berufsgenossenschaften ist vor Beginn mikro-biologischer Arbeiten zu prüfen, ob Schutzimpfungen erforderlich sind (Merkblatt „Eignungsuntersuchung und Gesundheitsüberwachung des Personals von Kran-

Tabelle 9. Impfabstände (Richtlinien des Bundesgesundheitsamtes, 1972)

Nach Schutzimpfung gegen	Mindestabstand zu Schutzimpfungen gegen		
	Pocken (Erstimpfung)	Pocken (Wiederimpfung), Gelbfieber, Polio oral, Masern, Röteln, Mumps, BCG	Cholera, Typhus-Paratyphus, Pertussis, Influenza, Polio parenteral, Diphtherie, Tetanus, Masern (Spaltimpfstoff)
Pockenerstimpfung[a]	—	1 Monat	1 Monat
Pockenwiederimpfung[a]	—	1 Woche	kein
Gelbfieber	1 Monat	2 Wochen	kein
Polio oral Masern Röteln Mumps BCG[a]	1 Monat	1 Monat	kein
Cholera Typhus-Paratyphus Pertussis Influenza Polio parenteral Masern (Spaltimpfstoff) Diphtherie Tetanus	1 Monat	kein	kein

[a] Sofern eine etwaige Reaktion vollständig abgeklungen ist und keine Komplikationen aufgetreten sind.

kenanstalten", 1955). Sie können nicht erzwungen, die Einstellung eines Mitarbeiters jedoch von ihrer Duldung abhängig gemacht werden. Es ist so rechtzeitig zu immunisieren, daß bei Eintritt des Risikos die erhoffte Schutzwirkung vorhanden ist. Wiederholungen sind nach ärztlicher Indikation anzuberaumen. Alle Impfungen sind aus medizinischen und juristischen Gründen aktenkundig zu machen.

Immunisierungen machen die Präzision mikrobiologischer Technik und die üblichen Vorsichtsmaßnahmen keinesfalls überflüssig, da der Schutz immer relativ ist, nur eine begrenzte Zeit dauert und von der aufgenommenen Erregermenge und individuellen Faktoren abhängt. Zusammenfassende Darstellungen des Impfwesens finden sich bei EHRENGUT (1964), HARTUNG (1966), SPIESS (1966) und ROHDE et al. (1968), eine ausführliche Würdigung der BCG-Impfung bei GRIESBACH (1954).

In der Bundesrepublik Deutschland sind Impfstoffe gegen Typhus und Paratyphus (TAB-Impfstoff, Typhoral), Cholera, Tetanus, Diphtherie und Tuberkulose, ferner gegen Influenza, Pocken, Poliomyelitis, Tollwut und Gelbfieber erhältlich. In Pestlaboratorien zu beschäftigende Personen sollten gegen Pest aktiv immunisiert werden (,,Bekanntmachung betreffend Vorschriften über Krankheitserreger" von 1917, s. S. 263).

Um die Gefährdung beim Arbeiten mit Tuberkelbakterien, tuberkelbakterienhaltigem Material und infizierten Versuchstieren zu reduzieren, dürfen nach den Bestimmungen der Berufsgenossenschaften nur solche Personen mit einschlägigen Arbeiten betraut werden, bei denen der Tuberkulintest positiv ist (s. S. 240). Andernfalls kann eine BCG-Impfung durchgeführt werden, deren Wirksamkeit erneut mit Tuberkulin zu überprüfen ist. Literaturangaben zur Diskussion über die Notwendigkeit der Impfung finden sich bei Neumann (1970).

Werden mehrere Schutzimpfungen für notwendig erachtet, so sind zur Vermeidung gesundheitlicher Schäden die vom Bundesgesundheitsamt (1972) aufgestellten Richtlinien zu beachten (s. Tabelle 9).

1. Zwischen Schutzimpfungen mit vermehrungsfähigen abgeschwächten Krankheitserregern (Pocken, Polio oral, Gelbfieber, Masern, Röteln, Mumps, BCG) wird ein Mindestabstand von einem Monat empfohlen unter der Voraussetzung, daß die Impfreaktion abgeklungen ist und Komplikationen nicht aufgetreten sind.
2. Bei Schutzimpfungen mit inaktivierten Krankheitserregern, ihren Spaltprodukten (Cholera, Typhus-Paratyphus, Pertussis, Influenza, Polio parenteral, Masernspaltimpfstoff) oder mit Toxoiden (Diphtherie, Tetanus) sind Zeitabstände untereinander und zu anderen Impfungen nicht erforderlich.
3. Ausnahmen:
   a) Eine gleichzeitige Verabfolgung von Impfstoff aus vermehrungsfähigen und Impfstoff aus inaktivierten Krankheitserregern der gleichen Art soll bei Erstimpfungen vermieden werden.
   b) Eine Pockenschutzerstimpfung soll mindestens einen Monat vor oder nach einer anderen Schutzimpfung durchgeführt werden.
   c) Nach einer Pockenschutzwiederimpfung können Impfungen mit vermehrungsfähigen abgeschwächten Krankheitserregern frühestens nach 1 Woche durchgeführt werden, nachdem die Impfreaktion vollständig abgeklungen ist und wenn Komplikationen nicht aufgetreten sind.
   d) Nach einer Gelbfieberschutzimpfung kann bereits nach zwei Wochen eine andere Schutzimpfung mit vermehrungsfähigen, abgeschwächten Krankheitserregern vorgenommen werden.
   e) Nach einer Tollwutschutzimpfung sollen mit Ausnahme der Tetanusprophylaxe bis sechs Wochen nach der letzten Injektion keine anderen Schutzimpfungen vorgenommen werden.

Weitere Ratschläge über die Durchführung von Impfungen finden sich in den vom Bundesgesundheitsamt herausgegebenen Merkblättern Nr. 1 (Poliomyelitis, 1963), Nr. 3 (Tollwut, 1970), Nr. 11 (Grippe, 1963), Nr. 18 (Pocken, 1971), Nr. 25 (Cholera, 1972) und Nr. 30 (Röteln, 1972).

D. Anforderungen an Laboratorien

1. Räume

An Räume, in denen mit Krankheitserregern gearbeitet wird, sind Anforderungen zu stellen, die sich an den Vorschriften des § 120a (Betriebssicherheit) der Gewerbeordnung (1967), der Gefährlichkeit der Organismen und der Art der Untersuchungen orientieren. Mindestforderungen sind in den Unfallverhütungsvorschriften der Berufsgenossenschaft für Gesundheitsdienst und Wohlfahrtspflege „Medizinische Laboratoriumsarbeiten" (1956) und „Allgemeine Unfallverhütungsvorschriften" (1969) aufgestellt.

§ 2: Der Unternehmer hat, soweit es nach dem Stand der Technik möglich ist, alle Baulichkeiten, Arbeitsstätten, Betriebseinrichtungen, Maschinen und Gerätschaften so einzurichten und zu erhalten, daß die Versicherten gegen Unfälle und Berufskrankheiten geschützt sind. Solange die genannten Betriebsmittel Mängel aufweisen, die eine Gefahr für Leben und Gesundheit der Versicherten bedeuten, sind sie der Benutzung zu entziehen.

Nach § 710 der Reichsversicherungsordnung sind bei vorsätzlichen oder grobfahrlässigen Verstößen gegen die Unfallverhütungsvorschriften Ordnungsstrafen bis zu 10000,— DM festzusetzen.

Außerdem wird durch das Bundes-Seuchengesetz von 1961 bestimmt, daß die Erlaubnis zum Arbeiten mit Krankheitserregern zu versagen ist, „wenn geeignete

Tabelle 10. Gefahrenquellen im mikrobiologischen Laboratorium

A. Aerosole

Auftropfen von Flüssigkeiten
Ausblasen von Pipetten
Ausglühen von Ösen
Beimpfen von Nährböden
Homogenisatoren
Injektionsspritzen
Objektträgeragglutination
Öffnen von Gefäßen
Öffnen von lyophilisierten Kulturen

B. Pipettieren

Aerosolbildung beim Ausblasen
Aufsaugen von Flüssigkeit
Kontamination des Mundstücks

C. Stich- und Schnittverletzungen

Deckgläser
Schadhafte Glasgeräte
Zerbrechende Glasgeräte
Injektionsspritzen
Kanülen
Objektträger
Scheren
Skalpelle

D. Versuchstiere

Aerogene Übertragung
Ausscheidungen (Kot, Urin, Speichel,
  Sekrete)
Biß
Injektionen
Kratzwunden
Sektionen
Wunden

E. Ungeziefer

Ameisen
Fliegen
Flöhe
Läuse
Milben
Schaben
Zecken

Räume oder Einrichtungen nicht vorhanden sind" (s. S. 237). Für Arbeiten mit
Pest-, Tularämie-, Rotz-, Rinderpest- und Maul- und Klauenseuche-Erregern
gelten die besonders strengen Maßstäbe der „Bekanntmachung betreffend Vorschriften über Krankheitserreger" von 1917 (s. S. 262). Schließlich wurden von
der Weltgesundheitsorganisation 1957 Richtlinien über die allgemeinen Anforderungen an Laboratorien erarbeitet.

2. Fußböden, Wände

Für Fußböden und Wände sind auch bei Arbeiten mit wenig gefährlichen
Krankheitserregern Materialien zu wählen, die glatt, möglichst fugenlos, abwasch-
bar und gegen Desinfektionsmittel resistent sind.

3. Arbeitstische

An Arbeitstische sind die gleichen Anforderungen wie an Fußböden zu stellen.
Zusätzlich müssen sie unempfindlich gegen die Wärmeentwicklung von Bunsen-
brennern und elektrischen Geräten sein. Für besonders gefährliche Arbeiten sind
Tische aus V4A-Stahl zu empfehlen, die abgeflammt werden können.

4. Waschbecken

In jedem Laboratorium muß eine Waschgelegenheit vorhanden sein. Zur Vermeidung von Kontaktinfektionen soll sie das Waschen der Hände ohne Berührung
von Wasserhähnen ermöglichen. Für ihre Bedienung sind mit dem Knie oder

Tabelle 11. Liste der vom Bundesgesundheitsamt geprüften und

Wirkstoff	Name	Wäschedesinfektion	
		Gebrauchs-verdünnung %	Ein-wirkungs-zeit Std
Phenol oder Phenolderivate	Amocid	1,0	12
	Bac	0,5	12
	Bacillotox	1,0	12
	Baktol	1,5	12
	Baktolan		
	Delegol	1,5	12
	Gevisol	0,5	12
	Gründesin	3,0	12
	Korsyl·Bacillol	1,5	12
	Kresolseifenlösung DAB 6	1,0	12
	Lysolin	1,5	12
	Neosept	1,5	12
	Phenol	1,0	12
	Sagrotan	1,5	12
	Tb-Bacillol		
	Tb-Lysoform	1,0	12
	Wasapon	1,5	12
	Xynolan	1,5	12
Formaldehyd und/oder sonstige Aldehyde bzw. Derivate	Buraton	3,0	12
	Fomaldehyd-Lösung DAB 7 (Formalin)	1,5	12
	Incidin GG	2,0	12
	Korsoform	2,0	12
	Korsolin	2,0	12
	Lysoform	4,0	12
	Lysoformin	3,0	12
Chlor, organische oder anorganische Substanzen mit aktivem Chlor	Chloramin 80 „Heyden"	2,0	12
	Chloramin-T DAB 7	1,5	12
	Clorina „Heyden"	1,5	12
	Halamid	1,5	12
	Para-Caporit[b]		
Amphotensid	Estella 100	2,0	12
	Tego 103 G	2,0	12
	Tego 103 S	2,0	12
Lauge	Kalkmilch[a]		

[a] unbrauchbar bei Tuberkulose.   [b] Grobdesinfektion.

Fuß zu betätigende Armaturen vorzusehen. Lichtstrahlgesteuerte Anlagen sind zu empfehlen, wenn ihre Elektronik nicht störanfällig und ihre mechanischen Teile robust sind. Die Wassertemperatur ist mit einem Thermostaten zu regeln.

Für die Entnahme von Händedesinfektionsmitteln sind ohne Handberührung zu bedienende Spender anzubringen. Besondere Becken dienen als Ausgüsse.

anerkannten Desinfektionsmittel (Stand vom 1. Oktober 1971, 5. Ausgabe)

Scheuerdesinfektion		Desinfektion von Ausscheidungen 1 Teil Auswurf oder Stuhl + 2 Teile Gebrauchsverdünnung bzw. 1 Teil Harn + 1 Teil Gebrauchsverdünnung					
		Auswurf		Stuhl		Harn	
Gebrauchs-verdünnung	Ein-wirkungs-zeit	Gebrauchs-verdünnung	Ein-wirkungs-zeit	Gebrauchs-verdünnung	Ein-wirkungs-zeit	Gebrauchs-verdünnung	Ein-wirkungs-zeit
%	Std	%	Std	%	Std	%	Std
6	6	5	4	5	6	5	2
5	4	5	4	5	6	5	2
6	4	5	4	5	6	5	2
5	4	5	4	5	6	5	2
5	4	5	4	5	6	5	2
5	4						
3	2						
		5	4	5	6	5	2
5	6	5	4	5	6	5	2
5	6						
3	4						
3	4						
4	4						
3	4						
5	6						
5	6						
3	2	6	4				
2,5	2	5	4				
2,5	2	5	4				
2,5	2	5	4				
1	2						
		20	6				

Für das Abtrocknen der Hände sind nur Einmalhandtücher zulässig. Sofern
sie aus Zellstoff hergestellt sind, werden sie in Plastikbeuteln gesammelt und verbrannt. Einmalhandtücher aus Textilien werden in koch- oder autoklavenfesten
Säcken nach einem anerkannten Verfahren desinfiziert und gewaschen (Liste des
Bundesgesundheitsamtes, 1971, und Liste der Deutschen Gesellschaft für Hygiene
und Mikrobiologie, 1966—1972).

Tabelle 12. Liste der Deutschen Gesellschaft für Hygiene und Mikrobiologie

Name	Händedesinfektion		Wäschedesinfektion auch bei Tuberkulose	Flächendesinfektion[b]		Sputumdesinfektion bei Tuberkulose	Stuhldesinfektion außer Tuberkulose	Flächendesinfektion bei Hautpilzerkrankungen	Flächendesinfektion bei Tuberkulose
	hygienische[a]	chirurgische		bei übertragbaren Krankheiten außer Tuberkulose	bei Staphylokokken (Hospitalismus)				
A. Zubereitungen des Deutschen Arzneibuches und chemisch einheitliche Desinfektionsmittel									
Chlorkalkmilch				10%					
Formalin			3%—4 h 1,5%—12 h	2%	3%			3%	3%
Kalkmilch 20%							20%—6 h (2 Teile Kalkmilch, 1 Teil Stuhl)		
Kresolseifenlösung			2%—4 h 1%—12 h	5%					5%
Phenol (Karbolsäure)			2%—4 h 1%—12 h						3%
Sublimat	0,1%—2 min								
Quecksilberoxycyanat	0,5%—2 min								
Äthylalkohol	70%—1 min	80%—5 min							
Isopropylalkohol	60%—1 min	70%—5 min							
n-Propylalkohol	50%—1 min	60%—5 min							

[a] Präparate auf der Basis chlorierter Phenole, die in 2%iger Konzentration zur Händedesinfektion angeführt sind, können zu Hautreizungen führen.
[b] Die angegebenen Konzentrationen gelten für eine Einwirkungszeit von 4 bis 6 Stunden und sichern den in den „Richtlinien für die Prüfung chemischer Desinfektionsmittel" festgelegten Desinfektionserfolg bei einmaliger Anwendung.
Bei der Phenolresistenz der Staphylokokken an der Fläche sind für die Bekämpfung des Staphylokokkenhospitalismus höhere Konzentrationen von mindestens 5% erforderlich, die erfahrungsgemäß zu Schäden führen können. Bei einzelnen besonders hochwertigen Präparaten auf phenolischer Basis wird eine 2- bis 3%ige Lösung als ausreichend angesehen.

Tabelle 12 (Fortsetzung)

| Name | Wirkstofftyp | Händedesinfektion | | Flächendesinfektion | | |
| | | hygienische, Wirksamkeit geprüft nach | chir-urgische | bei über-tragbaren Krank-heiten (außer Tbc) | bei Staph.-Hospita-lismus | bei Tbc |
		1 min 2 min				
B. Handelspräparate[a]						
Amocid	halogenierte Phenole	1%		0,5%	2%	6%
Bac	halogenierte Alkyl- und Arylphenole			0,5%	2%	5%
Bacillol-Spray[b]	Alkohole und Formal-dehyddepotstoffe			konzentriert wirksam bei voller Be-netzung der Fläche		
Bacillotox	halogenierte Alkyl- und Arylphenole	2%		1,5%	3—4%	6%
Baktol	Chlorkresol und Arylphenole	2%		1,5%	4—5%	
Baktonium	quartäre Ammonium-verbindung	2%				
Baktosept	Propanol, quartäre Ammoniumverbin-dung und Alkyl-aminsalze	3 ml	2 × 5 ml 5 min			
Battikon	halogenierte Phenole			1,5%	4—5%	
Blankazid	Preventol			2%	5%	
Buraton	Formaldehyd			1%	1,5%	3%
Chirosept	Alkohol	5 ml	2 × 5 ml 5 min			
Chloramin 80	aktives Chlor 20%	0,5%		0,5%	1%	
Clorina	aktives Chlor 25%	0,5%		0,5%	1%	
Creolin	Kresolhomologe			2%	5%	
Delegol	o-Benzylphenol			1,5%	4—5%	
Dyocid	Propylalkohol, quar-täre Ammonium-verbindung	3 ml	2 × 5 ml 5 min			
Eossan	Natriumorthophenyl-phenolat			2,5%	10%	
Galosept	Chlorkresol, Chlor-xylenol-Seifen-lösung			3%	7,5%	
Gevisol	arylierte und haloge-nierte Phenole			0,5%	2%	5%
Gründesin	arylierte und chlorierte Phenole	2%		1,5%	5%	
H5-Hände-desinfizienz	Alkohol	3 ml	2 × 5 ml 5 min			
Havisol	arylierte und halo-genierte Phenole	2%				

[a] gekürzt.
[b] Bacillol als Kresolseife wird seitens der Herstellerfirma nicht mehr angeboten.

Tabelle 12 (Fortsetzung)

Name	Wirkstofftyp	Händedesinfektion			Flächendesinfektion		
		hygienische, Wirksamkeit geprüft nach		chirurgische	bei übertragbaren Krankheiten (außer Tbc)	bei Staph.-Hospitalismus	bei Tbc
		1 min	2 min				
Helotil HL 10	organischer Chlorträger				50 Vol.-%	50 Vol.-%	50 Vol.-%
Hycolin	arylierte Phenole				2%	5%	
Incidin	Organozinnverbindungen, Formaldehyd und Formaldehydderivate				0,5%	1,5%	2%
Incidin-Spray	Organozinnverbindungen, Formaldehyd und Formaldehydderivate				konzentriert wirksam bei voller Benetzung der Fläche		
Izal	Phenolderivate				2%	4—5%	
Jonirol	Ampholytseife	2%	2 × 5 ml 5 min				
Killavon	quartäres Ammoniumsalz	2%					
Korsoform	Formaldehyd				0,5—1%	2%	4%
Korsyl-Bacillol	Alkylarylphenole teilweise halogeniert				1,5%	4—5%	
Laud-amonium	quartäres Ammoniumsalz	2%					
Liquidosept-Spray	Alkohol, Glykolderivate				konzentriert wirksam bei voller Benetzung der Fläche		
Luzol-Spray	i-Propanol, arylierte und halogenierte Phenole				konzentriert wirksam bei voller Benetzung der Fläche		
Lysoform	Formaldehyd				2%	3%	5%
Lysoformin	Formaldehyd				1,5%	2—3%	5%
Lysol	Kresol				2%	4—5%	
Lysolin	arylierte und aralkylierte Phenole				1,5%	4—5%	
Ma 614	halogenierte und arylierte Phenole				1%	3%	
Manusept-Emulsion	halogenierte Alkyl- und Arylphenole		3 ml				
Manusept-Gel	Propanol, Phenole	3 cm Salbenstrang	2 × 3 cm Salbenstrang 5 min				
MC-905	Chlorbasis				2%	3%	

Tabelle 12 (Fortsetzung)

Name	Wirkstofftyp	Händedesinfektion			Flächendesinfektion		
		hygienische, Wirksamkeit geprüft nach		chirurgische	bei übertragbaren Krankheiten (außer Tbc)	bei Staph.-Hospitalismus	bei Tbc
		1 min	2 min				
MC Pursept HD	Alkoholbasis mit hautfreundlichen Zusätzen zur Rückfettung	3 ml = 3 Spritzer		2 × 5 ml 5 min			
Morbicid	Formaldehyd				1%	2%	4%
Myxal-S-Konzentrat	quartäre Phosphoniumverbindung				3%	5%	
Neosept	halogenierte Phenole		2%		1,5%	4—5%	
Para-Caporit	35—38% aktives Chlor				0,5%	1%	
Parmetol	halogeniertes Kresol und Alkali				2%	3%	
Primasept	Phenolderivate	2 ml					
Qdf-Seife	quartäre Ammoniumsalze			konz.			
Quartamon	quartäre Ammoniumverbindung		2%				
Rapidosept	Dichlorbenzylalkohol und Glykolderivat	3 ml		2 × 5 ml 5 min			
Rutisept	Isopropanol		3 ml	2 × 5 ml 5 min			
Sagrotan	alkylierte, arylierte, aralkylierte und halogenierte Phenole		2%		2%	4—5%	
Satinazid	Propylalkohol		3 ml	2 × 5 ml 5 min			
Septanin	Chlorkresol, Chlorxylenol und Formaldehyd				1,5%	3%	
Septikal	n-Propanol und kationenaktive Stickstoffverbindung	3 ml		2 × 5 ml 5 min			
Skinsept	Alkohole, Adamatanderivat	3—5 ml		2 × 5 ml 5 min			
Spitacid	Alkohole, Glykolderivat	3 ml		2 × 5 ml 5 min			
Sterillium	Isopropanol und n-Propanol	3 ml		2 × 5 ml 5 min			
Tego 103 G	Ampho-Tensid				2%	5%	
Tego 103 S	Ampho-Tensid		2%	2 × 5 ml 5 min	2%	5%	

Tabelle 12 (Fortsetzung)

Name	Wirkstofftyp	Händedesinfektion			Flächendesinfektion		
		hygienische, Wirksamkeit geprüft nach		chir-urgische	bei übertragbaren Krankheiten (außer Tbc)	bei Staph.-Hospitalismus	bei Tbc
		1 min	2 min				
Tegolan	Ampho-Tensid		3 ml				
Therapogen „Neu"	Mischung verschiedener chlorierter Phenole mit speziellen Netzmitteln				1,5%	5%	
Tolix-Anti	o-Benzylphenol				1,5%	4—5%	
W-1-Z	chlorierte Phenole		2%				
Wasapon	halogenierte Phenole		2%		1,5%	4%	
Xynolan	chlorierte Phenole		2%		2%	5%	
Zephirol	quartäre Ammoniumverbindung		2%				
Stand: Juni 1967							
Ahabin	Formaldehyd, Organozinnverbindung				0,5%	1,5%	
Mucocit	halogenierte Alkyl- und Arylphenole				1%	3%	
Peresam	Propanol und halogeniertes Karbonsäureamid	5 cm Paste					
Stand: Dezember 1967							
Halamid	Tosylchloramidumnatricum (nach DAB VI pharm. rein)	0,5%			0,3%	1%	
Includal-Spray	quaternäre Phosphonium- und Ammonium-Verbindungen				konzentriert wirksam bei voller Benetzung der Fläche		
Stand: November 1968							
Incidin GG	Aldehyde, Alkylzinnverbindungen, Alkohole				0,25%	1,5%	1,5%
Lysoform-Spray	Formalin				konzentriert wirksam bei voller Benetzung der Fläche		
Peresam-HD	Propylalkohol und halogenisiertes Karbonsäureamid	3 ml	2 × 5 ml 5 min				
Tb-Lysoform	arylierte Phenole				1,5%	3%	5%

Tabelle 12 (Fortsetzung)

Name	Wirkstofftyp	Händedesinfektion		Flächendesinfektion		
		hygienische, Wirksamkeit geprüft nach	chirurgische	bei bakteriellen Darmkrankheiten (außer Tbc)	bei Staph.-Hospitalismus	bei Tbc
		1 min 2 min				
Stand: 1. Juli 1970						
Apesin A 3	kationaktive Ammoniumbasen und Phenolderivate			2,5%	2,5%	
Apesin A4	quartäre Ammoniumverbindungen, chlorierte Amide und Aldehyd			50%	50%	
Desderman	Äthanol und Tetrabrom-o-methylphenol	3 ml	2 × 5 ml 5 min			
Dibromol-Tinktur	Isopropylalkohol und halogenierte Phenole	3 ml	2 × 5 ml 5 min			
Korsolin	Formaldehyd und Formaldehydderivate			0,25%	1%	3%
Minutil	Formaldehyd und Formaldehydderivate			0,25%	1%	2%
Stand: 1. April 1971						
Amphisept	alkoholische Amphitensidlösung	3 ml	2 × 5 ml 5 min			
Buraton 25	Gemisch von Aldehyden			0,25%	0,5%	
Buraton-Spray	Isopropanol und Aldehydgemisch			konzentriert wirksam bei voller Benetzung der Fläche		
Estella 100	amphotere oberflächenaktive Aminosäurederivate			3%	6%	
Fugaten-Spray	Alkohol			konzentriert wirksam bei voller Benetzung der Fläche		
Lysoformin-Spray Konzentrat	aktive Aldehydgruppen			2%ig wirksam bei voller Benetzung der Fläche		4—5%ig[a] bzw. 3%ig[b] wirksam bei voller Benetzung der Fläche
MedWasch 65	Alkohol, quartäre Ammoniumbasen	3 ml	2 × 5 ml 5 min			
Orbiphen 25	Gemisch von chlorierten Alkylphenolen und einem Arylphenol			0,25%	2%	5%

[a] Verdünnung mit Wasser.
[b] Verdünnung mit 50% Isopropylalkohol.

Tabelle 12 (Fortsetzung)

Name	Wirkstofftyp	Händedesinfektion			Flächendesinfektion		
		hygienische, Wirksamkeit geprüft nach		chirurgische	bei bakteriellen Darmkrankheiten (außer Tbc)	bei Staph.-Hospitalismus	bei Tbc
		1 min	2 min				
Stand: 1. Dezember 1971							
Apesin AP1	Phenolderivate und Formaldehyd abgebende Mittel				5%	50%	
Blankazid	Preventol				2%	5%	
Formosapol	aktive Aldehydgruppen				0,25%	0,5%	
Gevisol	substituierte Phenole				0,25%	2%	2%
H5-Händedesinfiziens	Alkohol	3 ml					
Hospisept	Alkohol	3 ml					
Korsolin	Formaldehyd und Formaldehydderivate					0,5%	
Lomades N	Isopropanol, quartäre Ammoniumbasen		5 ml	2 × 5 ml 5 min			
Lysoformin	aktive Aldehydgruppen				0,25%	1%	
Neosept	halogenierte Phenole	2%					
Spitacid	Alkohole, Glykolderivat	3 ml					
Tego 103 F	Amphotensid und Formaldehyd				0,25%	1%	3%

5. Abwasser

Bei einwandfreier mikrobiologischer Technik dürfen keine Krankheitserreger in das Abwasser von Laboratorien gelangen. Wenn dies durch Besonderheiten der Arbeiten nicht gewährleistet ist und mit gefährlichen Organismen experimentiert wird, kann die Möglichkeit einer Abwasserdesinfektion vorgesehen werden. Am sichersten ist die thermische Behandlung nach Homogenisierung grober Bestandteile. Sie ist deshalb der chemischen Desinfektion vorzuziehen, allerdings aufwendig und erfordert sorgfältige Wartung (DIN 19520 „Abwasser aus Krankenanstalten", 1964, Liste des Bundesgesundheitsamtes, 1971).

6. Fenster

Die Fenster sollen von mittlerer Größe sein (DIN 5034 „Innenraumbeleuchtung mit Tageslicht", 1963, 1966, 1969). Überdimensionierte Glasflächen sind aus thermischen Gründen unzweckmäßig. Ihre Erwärmung im Sommer und Abkühlung im Winter wirken sich störend auf das Raumklima aus, fördern konvektive Luftströmungen und damit den Transport von Staub und Mikroorganismen. Es empfiehlt sich deshalb der Einbau von wärmedämmenden Doppelfenstern oder Thermopanescheiben. Da Arbeitstische in der Regel unmittelbar vor den Fenstern angeordnet sind, sollen diese aus Sicherheitsgründen durch eine Kippvorrichtung zu öffnen sein.

Als Schutz vor zu starker Besonnung und unfallfördernder Blendung dienen Außenjalousien. Durch Fliegengitter werden Insekten ferngehalten, die sich mit Krankheitserregern beladen und diese über weite Entfernungen verschleppen können (MARTINI, 1952).

7. Lärm

Lärm am Arbeitsplatz ist der Konzentration abträglich und erhöht die Unfall- und Infektionsgefahr. Schallpegel zwischen 30 und 65 dB können schon als Belästigung empfunden werden. Zwischen 65 und 90 dB verursachen sie meßbare Veränderungen am Kreislauf und bewirken psychische Reaktionen (KNAPP, 1969).

8. Beleuchtung

Zur Verminderung der Infektionsgefahr sind an die Beleuchtung hohe bis außergewöhnlich hohe Ansprüche zu stellen (LIESE, 1957, 1964). In allen Teilen der Laboratorien soll die Beleuchtungsstärke 250—1000 Lux betragen. Für die Arbeitsplatzbeleuchtung sind mindestens 1000 Lux anzustreben (DIN 5034 ,,Innenraumbeleuchtung mit Tageslicht", 1963, 1966, 1969; DIN 5035 ,,Innenraumbeleuchtung mit künstlichem Licht", 1972). Zu starke Kontraste zwischen der Allgemein- und Arbeitsplatzbeleuchtung sind wegen der damit verbundenen Adaptationsschwierigkeiten zu vermeiden. Sie fördern, wie auch die Blendung, Unfallgefahren. Andererseits ist eine gewisse Schattenwirkung für das plastische Sehen unerläßlich (RODENWALDT u. BADER, 1951).

Bei Verwendung von Kunststoffleuchten ist auf die Möglichkeit elektrostatischer Aufladungen und der Ansammlung von infektiösem Staub zu achten, der sich bei Luftbewegungen oder Erschütterungen ablöst und das Personal gefährdet.

9. Lüftungs- und Klimaanlagen

In allen Laboratorien entstehen Wärme, Dämpfe, Aerosole, Staub und andere unerwünschte Luftbeimengungen, die durch einen 5—15maligen Luftwechsel pro Stunde entfernt werden müssen (LIESE, 1964). Außerdem ist es notwendig, den Keimgehalt der Luft möglichst niedrig zu halten (s. S. 255).

Eine Raumtemperatur von ca. 22° C, bei hohen Außentemperaturen etwas höher, und eine relative Luftfeuchtigkeit zwischen 35 und 65% sind als günstig anzusehen. Diese Bedingungen fördern die Behaglichkeit und mindern deshalb das Unfallrisiko. Von SPRENGER (1955) werden höhere Feuchtigkeitswerte als zulässig angegeben.

Ist die freie Lüftung durch Fenster und Schächte nicht ausreichend, müssen *Lüftungsanlagen* eingebaut werden, in denen die Zu- oder Abluft durch Ventilatoren bewegt wird. Umluftbetrieb ist in mikrobiologischen Laboratorien nicht statthaft. Es ist dafür zu sorgen, daß Krankheitserreger weder in andere Räume noch in die Außenwelt gelangen können (s. S. 254).

Die klimatischen Gegebenheiten und die Art der mikrobiologischen Arbeiten können eine *Klimatisierung* erforderlich machen, die neben der Erneuerung der Raumluft und der Konstanthaltung ihrer Temperatur und Feuchtigkeit die Reduzierung von Staub und Mikroorganismen bezweckt. Die Anforderungen an Lüftungs- und Klimaanlagen sind deshalb besonders hoch.

In der Bundesrepublik Deutschland gelten die Empfehlungen der DIN 1946, Blatt 1 „Lüftungstechnische Anlagen, Grundregeln" (1960) in Verbindung mit Blatt 4 „Lüftung in Krankenanstalten" (1963). Weitere Erkenntnisse fanden in den VDI-Richtlinien 2051 „Lüftung von Laboratorien" (1958) ihren Niederschlag. Technische Einzelheiten sind ihnen zu entnehmen. Ausführliche Darstellungen der Grundlagen und Anwendungen der Heiz- und Lüftungstechnik finden sich bei KOLLMAR u. LIESE (1954) und RAISS (1960), der Klimatechnik bei LOEWER (1968).

Für hochinfektiöse Räume, z. B. Pockenlaboratorien, sind Sonderregelungen zu treffen.

Klimaanlagen müssen so gestaltet sein, daß von außen keine Mikroorganismen in die Laboratorien gelangen können. Die Ansaugöffnungen dürfen deshalb weder in der Nähe des Erdbodens noch auf dem Dach angeordnet sein (BOTZENHART u. SATTEL, 1972; THOMSEN u. KREBS, 1972; WINKLE et al., 1972). Wie bei Lüftungsanlagen muß ein Keimtransport in andere Räume und die Außenwelt vermieden werden.

Die zur Luftbefeuchtung häufig verwendeten Wäscherkästen sind ideale Brutstätten für Mikroorganismen. Sie können auch zur Quelle allergischer Erkrankungen werden. Sie müssen mikrobiologisch überwacht, gereinigt und desinfiziert werden. Dampfbefeuchter sind deshalb vorzuziehen. Grundsätzlich sind Wasseransammlungen in Klimaanlagen zu vermeiden.

Die Abluft ist bei Arbeiten mit gefährlichen Erregern zu filtern oder durch UV-Bestrahlung bzw. thermisch zu desinfizieren. In diesem Fall ist die Möglichkeit von Explosionen bei Verwendung von organischen Lösungsmitteln zu bedenken.

Die besonderen Aufgaben eines Laboratoriums können die Erzeugung eines Unter- oder Überdrucks notwendig machen. Bei Arbeiten mit hochinfektiösen Mikroorganismen ist ein geringer Unterdruck zu empfehlen, um sie am Übertritt in die Außenwelt zu hindern, zur Vermeidung einer Kontamination des Laboratoriums mit Keimen der Außenluft ein geringer Überdruck (WEDUM, 1961). In jedem Fall sind Filter in den Luftkanälen, am besten an den Auslaßöffnungen, unerläßlich. Sie müssen trocken gehalten werden, um ein Durchwachsen von Bakterien und Pilzen zu verhindern (SCHICHT, 1971).

Grobstaubfilter haben ein Rückhaltevermögen für Partikel bis etwa 10 μ, Feinstaubfilter bis etwa 1 μ und Feinststaubfilter unter 1 μ Durchmesser. Bei besonders hohen Anforderungen sind Hochleistungs-Schwebstoff-Filter (HOSCH-Filter, Sonderstufe S) zu verwenden. Über die Eigenschaften von Filtern und ihre Prüfung wurden vom Staubforschungsinstitut des Hauptverbandes der gewerblichen Berufsgenossenschaften Richtlinien (1961) aufgestellt, die als DIN 24185 herausgegeben werden sollen. Über die Technologie moderner Filter s. WALTER (1965).

Die Filter sind sorgfältig zu warten und regelmäßig auszuwechseln, die Luftkanäle zu reinigen und auf das Vorhandensein von Krankheitserregern zu untersuchen. Gegebenenfalls sind die Anlagen zu desinfizieren, um sie als Infektionsquellen auszuschalten (SCHICHT, 1971). Über die dabei auftretenden Probleme s. bei GRÜN (1972).

Um einen orientierenden Überblick über die in der Laboratoriumsluft vorhandenen Mikroorganismen zu erhalten, werden geöffnete Petrischalen mit Bakterien- und Pilznährböden an verschiedenen Stellen des Raumes während einer bestimmten Zeit aufgestellt. Nach Bebrütung werden die Kolonien gezählt (SCHMIDT-MENDE et al., 1968). Für exakte Keimzahlbestimmungen wird eine gemessene Menge Luft durch Gelatinefilter gesaugt (SATTEL u. NELSON, 1972) oder auf Nährböden geblasen und aus der Zahl der sich bildenden Kolonien auf den Keimgehalt geschlossen. Die Probleme der Luftdesinfektion mit physikalischen und chemischen Verfahren sowie der Keimzahlbestimmung wurden von GRÜN (1955) dargestellt.

10. Ultraviolett-Strahler

Um den Keimpegel eines Laboratoriums zu senken, können Ultraviolett-Strahler eingebaut werden. Die besten Erfolge werden mit Wellenlängen um 254 nm (240—280 nm, Absorptionsbereich der Thymonucleinsäure, HETTCHE, 1954) erzielt.

Bei der wirkungsvollsten, *direkten Bestrahlung* werden alle Raumteile aus verschiedenen Richtungen ausgeleuchtet. Für eine optimale Wirkung sind eine nicht zu hohe Luftfeuchtigkeit, peinliche Sauberkeit und Staubfreiheit wesentliche Voraussetzungen (BÖNICKE u. BAYHA, 1952; HETTCHE, 1954), da Mikroorganismen im Schatten auch kleinster Partikeln von Ultraviolett nicht erreicht werden. Da die direkte Exposition die Augen schädigen kann, ist die Bestrahlung des gesamten Raumes nur während der arbeitsfreien Zeit, z.B. während der Nacht, möglich. Bei Betreten während der Bestrahlung müssen Schutzbrillen getragen und ungeschützte Hautpartien bedeckt werden.

Zur Keimreduktion während der Arbeitszeit wird die Methode der *indirekten Bestrahlung* gewählt, bei der Personen kaum einer Belastung ausgesetzt sind. Durch Montage der Geräte über Augenhöhe und entsprechende Stellung der Reflektoren bleiben die Augen außerhalb des Strahlungsbereichs. Die die Augen gefährdende, von der Decke und den Wänden reflektierte Strahlung kann durch Kunstharzbinder oder Ölfarbenanstriche (Reflexion 3—10%, HETTCHE, 1954) unterdrückt werden. Die Wirkung der indirekten Bestrahlung ist geringer. Sie beschränkt sich auf die Abtötung der durch Konvektion am Strahler vorbeigeführten Organismen.

Die Bestrahlungsstärke sollte beim Menschen in 24 Std 0,1 μW/cm^2 nicht überschreiten. FRIEDERISZICK (1954) sah bei Kleinkindern bis zu Werten von 0,75 μW/cm^2 auch bei Dauereinwirkung keine Schädigungen.

UV-Geräte lassen sich zur Keimreduktion auch über Arbeitsplätzen, in Impfkästen oder als UV-Schranken an Durchgängen zur Verhinderung von Keimtransporten in benachbarte Laboratorien oder Verkehrsräume einsetzen. Schließlich werden sie zur Entkeimung der Zu- oder Abluft in die Kanäle von Belüftungs- und Klimaanlagen eingebaut (PARTMANN u. MONFORT, 1951/52; MATZ u. SCHASSAN, 1968).

Die für eine 90%ige Reduzierung von Bakterien und Sproßpilzen notwendige *Bestrahlungsdosis* liegt zwischen etwa 2000 und 8000 μW sec/cm^2, bei manchen Arten höher. Für die gleiche Wirkung bei Schimmelpilzen werden zum Teil über 100000 μW sec/cm^2 benötigt (HART u. NICKS, 1961).

11. Impfkästen, Reine Werkbänke

Für gefährliche Arbeiten kann es zweckmäßig sein, Impfkästen zu verwenden, die in der Regel durch UV-Strahler entkeimt werden. Ein mit Unterdruck arbeitendes Gerät für gefahrloses Arbeiten mit größeren Versuchstieren wurde von TAURASO et al. (1969) konstruiert.

Eine Weiterentwicklung sind die „Reinen Werkbänke" (CORIELL u. McGARRITY, 1968; FAVERO u. BERQUIST, 1968; LÖER u. FUNNEKÖTTER, 1972). Diese aufwendigen Geräte gestatten mikrobiologische Manipulationen in einem vertikal oder horizontal von ultrafiltrierter Luft durchströmten Raum, deren Geschwindigkeit etwa 0,45 m/sec beträgt. Verwendet werden Hochleistungs-Schwebstoff-(HOSCH-)Filter (s. S. 254). Wichtig ist die ständige Erhaltung des laminaren Luftstroms. Turbulenzen entstehen besonders thermisch, z.B. durch Leuchtstoffröhren oder Bunsenbrenner, und durch alle in den Luftstrom eingebrachten festen Körper, auch die Hände des Untersuchers. Sorgfältige Wartung, Prüfung der Luftgeschwindigkeit, des Filterzustandes, der Partikelzahl und der bakteriologischen Reinheit sind in regelmäßigen Abständen unerläßlich. Bei Verdoppelung des Anfangsdruckverlustes ist ein Filterwechsel angebracht (Schicht, 1972). Die Filter sind unter Umständen hochinfektiös und müssen entsprechend vernichtet werden.

12. Reine Räume

Für extrem hohe Reinheitsansprüche werden „Reine Räume" eingerichtet, in denen die Luft klimatisiert und ihr Gehalt an Staub und Mikroorganismen durch Hochleistungs-Schwebstoff-Filter auf ein Minimum reduziert wird. Angaben über die technischen Grundlagen finden sich bei Schicht (1972). Sie werden nach dem Prinzip der turbulenten Mischströmung oder der wirksameren turbulenzarmen Kolbenströmung (laminar air-flow) mit Fallstrom- oder Querstrom-Luftführung gebaut. Im ersten Fall werden keine Anforderungen an die Gleichförmigkeit von Strömungsbild und Geschwindigkeit gestellt, im zweiten wird der Raum von einem Luftstrom mit gleichförmiger Geschwindigkeit und parallelen Stromlinien mit einem Minimum an Turbulenzen durchflossen. Die Geschwindigkeit beträgt $0{,}45 \pm 0{,}1$ m/sec. Die Luft wird durch Hochleistungs-Schwebstoff-Filter mit einem Abscheidungsgrad von mindestens 99,97% gereinigt. Mit modernen Filtern wird bereits eine Wirkung von 99,999% erzielt, gemessen mit dem DOP-Test (Dioctyl-phtalatnebel mit einer Teilchengröße von 0,3 Mikron).

Das Arbeiten in derartigen Räumen stellt an ihre Ausstattung und den Betriebsablauf, z.B. das Ein- und Ausschleusen von Personen und deren Verhalten, höchste Anforderungen. Eine besondere Kleidung ist unerläßlich (Kratel, 1971).

E. Arbeitsablauf, Sicherheitsvorkehrungen

1. Versand von Krankheitserregern

Für den Versand von Krankheitserregern gelten die Bestimmungen der „Bekanntmachung betreffend Vorschriften über Krankheitserreger" von 1917. Sie wurden von der Deutschen Bundespost übernommen und sind in Anhang 3 der Postordnung von 1963 abgedruckt. Besondere Vorsichtsmaßnahmen sind beim Versand von lebenden Kulturen der Erreger der Cholera, Pest und Tularämie, des Rotzes, der Rinder- und Schweinepest sowie der Maul- und Klauenseuche zu treffen.

B. Vorschriften über die Versendung von Krankheitserregern

§ 9

(1) Die Versendung von lebenden Kulturen der Erreger der Cholera, der Pest, der Tularämie oder des Rotzes, oder von Material, das die Erreger der Rinderpest, der Maul- und Klauenseuche oder der Schweinepest enthält oder zu enthalten verdächtig ist — dieses nur insofern, als es nach seiner Beschaffenheit für eine solche Versendungsart in Betracht kommen kann (z.B. Bläscheninhalt, Serum) —, hat in zugeschmolzenen Glasröhren zu erfolgen, die, umgeben von einer weichen Hülle (Filtrierpapier und Watte oder Holzwolle), in einem durch übergreifenden Deckel gut verschlossenen Blechgefäß stehen; das letztere ist seinerseits noch in einer Kiste mit Holzwolle oder Watte zu verpacken; es empfiehlt sich, nur frisch angelegte, noch nicht im Brutschrank behaltene Aussaaten auf festem Nährboden zu versenden.

(2) Die Sendungen müssen mit starkem Bindfaden umschnürt, versiegelt und mit der deutlich geschriebenen Adresse sowie mit dem Vermerk „Vorsicht" versehen werden. Zur Beförderung durch die Post sind die Sendungen als „dringendes Paket" aufzugeben; sie sind den Empfängern telegraphisch anzukündigen. Bei Sendungen an Anstalten ist nicht deren Leiter, sondern die Anstalt als Empfänger zu bezeichnen. Dasselbe gilt hinsichtlich der telegraphischen Ankündigung.

(3) Der Empfänger hat dem Absender den Eingang der Sendung sofort mitzuteilen.

Die Bestimmungen der §§ 10—17 regeln im einzelnen den Versand von Erregern anderer als der in § 9 aufgeführten Krankheiten sowie von Untersuchungsmaterial, das Erreger enthält oder dessen verdächtig ist.

§ 10

(1) Die Versendung von lebenden Kulturen anderer als der in § 9 bezeichneten Erreger von Krankheiten, welche auf den Menschen übertragbar sind, oder von Tierkrankheiten, deren Anzeigepflicht, sei es auch nur für einen Teil des Reichsgebietes, eingeführt ist, hat in wasserdicht verschlossenen Glasröhren zu erfolgen. Diese Röhren sind entweder in angepaßten Hülsen oder, mit einer weichen Hülle (Holzwolle, Watte oder dergleichen) umgeben, derart in festen Kästen zu verpacken, daß sie unbeweglich liegen und nicht aneinanderstoßen. Die Sendungen müssen fest verschlossen und mit deutlicher Adresse sowie mit dem Vermerk „Vorsicht" versehen werden. Bei Sendungen an Anstalten ist nicht deren Leiter, sondern die Anstalt als Empfänger zu bezeichnen.

(2) Der Empfänger hat dem Absender den Eingang der Sendung sofort mitzuteilen.

§ 11

Sonstiges Material, welches lebende Erreger von Krankheiten, die auf den Menschen übertragbar sind, oder lebende Erreger von Tierkrankheiten, deren Anzeigepflicht, sei es auch nur für einen Teil des Reichsgebietes, eingeführt ist, enthält oder zu enthalten verdächtig erscheint, ist vor der Versendung unter Beobachtung der nachstehenden Vorschriften so zu verpacken, daß eine Verschleppung von Krankheitskeimen ausgeschlossen ist.

§ 12

(1) Größere Körperteile und kleinere Tierkadaver sind zunächst in ein mit einem geeigneten Desinfektionsmittel, am besten mit Sublimatlösung durchtränktes und dann gründlich ausgewrungenes Tuch einzuhüllen. Sie sind alsdann mit einem undurchlässigen Stoff (Pergamentpapier oder dergleichen) zu umwickeln und fest zu verschnüren; saftreiche Gegenstände sind außerdem in Tücher einzuschlagen oder in Säcke zu verpacken. Die Gegenstände sind sodann in starke, undurchlässige, sicher verschlossene Behälter (Fässer, Kübel, Kisten) zu bringen und in Sägemehl, Kleie, Torfmull, Lohe, Häcksel, Heu, Holzkohle oder ähnlichen Feuchtigkeit aufsaugenden Stoffen fest und so einzubetten, daß sie sich nicht verschieben können und ein Durchsickern von Flüssigkeit verhindert wird.

(2) Für Köpfe tollwutverdächtiger Tiere ist als Desinfektionsmittel, mit dem die Tücher getränkt werden, ausschließlich Sublimatlösung zu verwenden. Die Versendung solcher Köpfe hat mit der Post als „dringendes Paket" zu geschehen.

(3) Material, das Rotzerreger enthält oder zu enthalten verdächtig ist, muß zunächst unter Beachtung der in Absatz 1 gegebenen Vorschriften in einen dichten, sicher verschlossenen Behälter verpackt werden; dieser ist in eine starke, dichte Kiste zu bringen. Der Raum zwischen dem Behälter und der Kiste ist mit aufsaugenden Stoffen (Absatz 1) fest auszufüllen.

(4) Werden menschliche oder tierische Körperteile mit der Eisenbahn verwandt, so muß der Absender im Frachtbrief bescheinigen, daß Zweck und Verpackung der Sendung denjenigen Vorschriften, welche in der Anlage C der Eisenbahn-Verkehrsordnung für ekelerregende oder ansteckungsgefährliche Stoffe der in Rede stehenden Art ergangen ist, entsprechen. Die Beförderung solcher Gegenstände als Eilgut oder als beschleunigtes Eilgut ist nach den Eisenbahntarifen ausgeschlossen.

§ 13

(1) Zur Aufnahme kleinerer Gegenstände, welche lebende Erreger der Cholera, der Pest, der Tularämie, des Rotzes, der Rinderpest, der Maul- und Klauenseuche oder der Schweinepest enthalten oder zu enthalten verdächtig sind, eignen sich am besten starkwandige Pulvergläser mit eingeschliffenem Glasstöpsel und weitem Hals oder, falls sich diese nicht beschaffen lassen, Gläser mit glattem zylindrischem Hals, die mit gut passenden, frisch ausgekochten Korken zu verschließen sind. Die Gläser müssen vor dem Gebrauch in reinem Wasser frisch ausgekocht und dann durch kräftiges Ausschwenken möglichst vom Wasser befreit sein; sie dürfen aber nicht mit einer Desinfektionsflüssigkeit ausgespült werden. Auch darf zu dem Untersuchungsmaterial Flüssigkeit irgendwelcher Art nicht hinzugesetzt werden. Die Gläser sind durch Überbinden der Öffnung oder des Stöpsels mit Schweinsblase oder Pergamentpapier zu verschließen. An jedem Glase ist ein Zettel fest aufzukleben oder sicher anzubinden, der genaue Angaben über den Inhalt enthält. Deckgläschen werden in signierte Stückchen Fließpapier eingeschlagen und mit Watte fest in einem besonderen Schächtelchen verpackt.

(2) Bei Cholera, Pest und Tularämie darf in eine Sendung in der Regel nur Untersuchungsmaterial von *einem* Kranken oder *einer* Leiche gepackt werden. Handelt es sich jedoch um gleichzeitige Übersendung zahlreicher Proben, insbesondere zu Massenuntersuchungen der Umgebung von Cholerakranken, so werden zweckmäßig nur 1—2 cm der Ausleerungen entnommen, in die üblichen kleinen Glasgefäße gebracht und, wie unten angegeben, verpackt. Dabei ist durch eine entsprechende Kennzeichnung jedes einzelnen Gegenstandes dafür Sorge zu tragen, daß seine Herkunft leicht erkennbar ist (vgl. § 15).

(3) Die Gefäße und Schächtelchen sind in einem widerstandsfähigen Behälter, am besten einer festen Kiste, unter Verwendung von Watte, Sägemehl, Holzwolle oder dergleichen (vgl. § 12 Abs. 1) so zu verpacken, daß sie unbeweglich liegen und nicht aneinanderstoßen. Zigarrenkisten, Pappschachteln und dergleichen dürfen nicht verwendet werden. Die Sendungen müssen mit starkem Bindfaden umschnürt und versiegelt sein.

(4) Enthalten kleinere Gegenstände andere lebende Seuchenerreger oder scheinen sie verdächtig, solche zu enthalten, so können sie in dicht schließenden Gefäßen aus Metall, Steingut oder Glas untergebracht werden. Metallgefäße sind durch einen übergreifenden Deckel, der am Rande mit einem Streifen Heftpflaster verklebt wird, Steingut- und Glasgefäße in der in Absatz 1 angegebenen Weise zu verschließen und zu verpacken.

(5) Falls kleinere Gegenstände mit der Eisenbahn versandt werden, so finden die Bestimmungen des § 12 Abs. 4 Anwendung.

§ 14

(1) Cholera-, Pest-, Tularämie-, Rotz-, Rinderpest- oder Maul- und Klauenseuche- oder Schweinepestmaterial darf nicht mit der Briefpost versandt werden. Dagegen darf in dieser Weise Material, welches lebende Erreger von anderen Krankheiten, die auf den Menschen übertragbar sind, oder von anderen Tierkrankheiten, deren Anzeigepflicht, sei es auch nur für einen Teil des Reichsgebietes, eingeführt ist, enthält oder verdächtig ist, solche Erreger zu enthalten, verschickt werden; dabei ist folgendermaßen zu verfahren:

(2) Trockene Gegenstände, insbesondere mit Untersuchungsmaterial beschickte Deckgläschen, Objektträger, Fließpapier, Gipsstäbchen, Seidenfäden, Räudeborken usw. sind in mehrere Lagen Fließpapier einzuschlagen, alsdann in Pergamentpapier oder einen anderen undurchlässigen Stoff einzuwickeln und, umhüllt mit Watte, in feste Kästchen aus Holz, Blech oder dergleichen mit gut schließendem Deckel zu legen.

(3) Feuchtes oder flüssiges Material (Auswurf, Erbrochenes, Stuhl, Harn, Eiter oder sonstiges Wundsekret, Punktionsflüssigkeit, Blut, Serum, Abstriche von der Rachenschleimhaut, abgeschnittene oder abgeschabte Gewebsteile usw.) ist in ein Gefäß aus hinreichend starkem Glase mit Korkstöpselverschluß zu bringen. Dieses Gefäß ist in einen Blechbehälter zu verpacken. Um aber das Glasgefäß vor Zertrümmerung zu schützen und etwa aus dem Glasgefäß austretende Flüssigkeit aufzusaugen, ist sowohl auf den Boden als auch in den Deckel des Blechbehälters eine Scheibe Asbestpappe oder eine hinreichend starke Schicht von Fließpapier, Watte oder dergleichen zu legen. Der Blechbehälter wird sodann in einen ausgehöhlten, durch einen Deckel verschließbaren Holzblock gebracht. Bei Versendung von Schutzpockenlymphe genügt es, wenn das Glasgefäß unmittelbar in den Holzblock oder in Kästchen von Holz, Blech oder dergleichen gelegt wird; jedoch ist dann die Aushöhlung des Blockes oder das Kästchen besonders sorgfältig mit einem weichen, aufsaugenden Stoff auszupolstern. Die Kästchen oder Holzblöcke sind mit einem roten Zettel zu bekleben, der die Aufschrift „Vorsicht! Infektiöses Material!" enthält.

(4) Die Holzblöcke oder Kästchen sind in den Briefumschlägen derartig unterzubringen, daß sie bei deren Abstempelung nicht beschädigt werden. Am besten geeignet sind an der Innenseite mit Stoffbezug versehene Briefumschläge aus festem Papier, die nur an der einen Schmalseite offen und etwa doppelt so lang wie die Behälter sind; sie werden nicht durch Zukleben, sondern zweckmäßig durch eine kleine Metallklammer geschlossen. Die zum Abstempeln bestimmte Stelle wird am besten durch einen vorgezeichneten Kreis oder den Vermerk „Hier stempeln" gekennzeichnet.

(5) Die Briefsendungen sollen nicht in den Briefkasten geworfen, sondern an den Postschaltern oder auf dem Lande dem Briefträger übergeben werden.

§ 15

(1) Jeder Sendung ist ein Begleitschein so beizulegen, daß er gegen Durchfeuchtung und Beschmutzung geschützt ist und bei der Öffnung des Behälters leicht in die Augen fällt. Dieser Schein hat genaue Angaben über den Inhalt unter Bezeichnung der Person (Name, Geschlecht, Alter, Wohnort) oder der Tiere, von denen er stammt, zu enthalten. Außerdem sind bei Material von kranken Menschen oder Tieren anzugeben: die mutmaßliche Art der Erkrankung, der Tag des Beginns der Erkrankung, der Tag des Todes, der Zeitpunkt der Entnahme des

Materials, der Name und der Wohnort des Arztes oder Tierarztes, der die Einsendung veranlaßt hat, der Zweck der Einsendung.

(2) Bei Untersuchungsmaterial ist auf dem Scheine auch die Stelle anzugeben, welcher das Ergebnis der Untersuchung mitgeteilt werden soll.

(3) Enthält die Sendung Material von verschiedenen Menschen oder Tieren, so ist durch eine entsprechende Kennzeichnung jedes einzelnen Gegenstandes Sorge zu tragen, daß seine Herkunft leicht erkennbar ist.

§ 16

(1) Auf den Sendungen ist außer der deutlichen Adresse der Name und die Wohnung des Absenders anzugeben und der Vermerk „Vorsicht!" „Menschliche (Tierische) Untersuchungsstoffe!" anzubringen.

(2) Bei Sendungen an Anstalten ist nicht deren Leiter, sondern die Anstalt als Empfänger zu bezeichnen. Dasselbe gilt hinsichtlich der telegraphischen Ankündigung (§ 17).

§ 17

Postsendungen mit Material von Cholera, Pest, Tularämie, Rotz oder Rinderpest oder mit Material, das lebende Erreger einer dieser Krankheiten zu enthalten verdächtig ist, sind als „dringendes Paket" aufzugeben und den Empfängern rechtzeitig telegraphisch anzukündigen. Diese telegraphische Anzeige hat auch dann zu erfolgen, wenn der Versand von Rotzmaterial mit der Eisenbahn erfolgt.

Die meisten Krankheitserreger können von Stammsammlungen bezogen werden. Eine der bedeutendsten ist The American Type Culture Collection (ATCC), Rockville, Maryland (USA), die bestimmte Stämme, z.B. aus den Gattungen Bacillus, Brucella, Clostridium, Francisella, Mycobacterium, Neisseria, Pseudomonas, Salmonella, Vibrio und Yersinia, wegen ihrer besonderen Gefährlichkeit nur an qualifizierte Untersucher abgibt. Für ihre Bestellung ist deshalb eine vorgeschriebene Form einzuhalten: "Requests for these pathogenic agents should be made on the institution's official stationery (purchase order) and signed by the director of the institution, the chairman of the department concerned, or the scientist in charge of the project."

Die Verantwortung für die Kulturen trägt ausschließlich der Empfänger: "The ATCC requires that the persons or organizations receiving cultures from this repository assume all risks and responsibility in connection with their receipt, handling, storage and use."

Dem technischen Fortschritt entsprechend werden häufig lyophilisierte Kulturen versandt. Da in den zugeschmolzenen Ampullen ein geringer Unterdruck herrscht, besteht beim Öffnen die Gefahr der Aerosolbildung aus dem gefriergetrockneten Material (s. S. 263). Besondere Vorsicht ist daher bei der Entnahme von Krankheitserregern geboten, die über den Respirationstrakt aufgenommen werden. Sie müssen für die Rehydration sorgfältig nach den der Sendung beigefügten Anweisungen behandelt werden.

Richtlinien für Bakterien

"To open the freeze-dried culture:

a) Double-Vial preparation (soft-glass) — Heat the pointed end of the outer container vigorously in a Bunsen flame and while still hot add a drop or two of water to crack the glass; remove the tip of the container with an sharp blow from an pencil or similar object and remove the inner vial.

b) Single-Vial preparation (borosilicate glass) — These preparations may be enclosed in a thin skin of cellulose; this skin must be removed (either with a sharp blade or by soaking in water for a few minutes); score the ampule once briskly with a sharp file about one inch from the tip; disinfect the ampule with alcohol-dampened gauze; wrap gauze around the ampule, and break at the scored area."

Richtlinien für Bakteriophagen

"With a small, three-edged file cut a groove in the ampule approximately one inch from the sealed tip. Wipe ampule with alcohol-soaked gauze. Using two pieces of dry sterile gauze grasp each end of the ampule, one in each hand, and with the groove outward, snap open. Rehydrate material in the ampule at once."

Die einschlägigen Bestimmungen der Deutschen Demokratischen Republik finden sich in der „Dritten Durchführungsbestimmung zum Gesetz zur Verhütung und Bekämpfung übertragbarer Krankheiten beim Menschen. — Arbeit mit Erregern von übertragbaren Krankheiten —" von 1966. Sie weisen gegenüber den Vorschriften in der Bundesrepublik Deutschland einige Besonderheiten auf. So ist der Versand von Kulturen der Erreger von Pest, Pocken, Cholera, Afrikanischer Schweinepest, Rotz, exotischer Maul- und Klauenseuche sowie Rinderpest unzulässig.

Die für Österreich gültigen Bestimmungen finden sich in der „Verordnung des Bundesministeriums für soziale Verwaltung vom 2. April 1948, betreffend die Befugnis zur Vornahme medizinisch-diagnostischer Untersuchungen und die hiebei bei Arbeiten mit Krankheitserregern zu beobachtenden Vorsichtsmaßnahmen".

Die in den amerikanischen Bundesstaaten geltenden Bestimmungen über die Verpackung und den Versand von Krankheitserregern wurden von Alexander u. Brandon (1970) zusammengestellt.

Von der Weltgesundheitsorganisation werden für den internationalen Versand von Krankheitserregern violette Klebezettel empfohlen, die aus Genf bezogen werden können.

2. Arbeiten mit Krankheitserregern

Die *mikrobiologische Technik* ist so hoch entwickelt, daß Laboratoriumsinfektionen bei Beachtung der Vorschriften relativ selten sind (s. S. 232), jedoch kann mangelnde Übung im Umgang mit Krankheitserregern für den in der Ausbildung Befindlichen ebenso zur Gefahrenquelle werden wie abgestumpfte Vorsicht, Unachtsamkeit, Gleichgültigkeit, ungenügende Konzentration oder exogene Störfaktoren für den Erfahrenen. Hinzu kommt, daß Laboratoriumsarbeiten trotz weitgehender physiologischer Automatisierung relativ hohe Anforderungen an die geistige Leistung stellen (Klosterkötter, 1969). Schließlich dürfte auch der Grad der tageszeitlich bedingten Leistungsbereitschaft nicht ohne Bedeutung für das Unfallgeschehen sein.

Die wenigsten Infektionen lassen sich nachträglich auf ein bestimmtes Ereignis zurückführen, z.B. auf das Zerbrechen oder Auslaufen eines Kulturgefäßes, das Verspritzen oder Verschlucken von Krankheitserregern, Schnitt- oder Stichverletzungen bzw. Verwundungen durch Versuchstiere. Meist sind es kleine Nachlässigkeiten, unbemerkte technische Fehler und Mängel, nicht zuletzt die Aerosolbildung bei verschiedensten Tätigkeiten, die Laboratoriumsinfektionen bedingen (s. S. 243). Diese auch versicherungstechnisch wichtige Erfahrung (s. S. 273) macht deutlich, daß Konzentration auf die Arbeit, einwandfreie Technik und genaue Beachtung der Vorschriften den besten Schutz bieten.

Grundsätzlich ist in mikrobiologischen Laboratorien der *Leiter* für den ordnungsgemäßen Zustand der Räume und ihrer Einrichtung, den Arbeitsablauf und die Aufbewahrung oder Vernichtung der Kulturen und des infektiösen Materials verantwortlich.

Entsprechende Vorschriften finden sich in den §§ 6 und 8 der „Bekanntmachung betreffend Vorschriften über Krankheitserreger" von 1917 (s. S. 261) und in § 2 der „Allgemeinen Unfallverhütungsvorschriften der Berufsgenossenschaft für Gesundheitsdienst und Wohlfahrtspflege" (1969): „Der Unternehmer hat die für eine gefahrlose Regelung des Betriebes und die für das Verhalten des Versicherten erforderlichen Anweisungen zu geben und die Durchführung der Unfallverhütungsvorschriften zu überwachen."

Über die Bestellung von Sicherheitsbeauftragten, die den Leiter jedoch nicht von seiner Verantwortung entbindet, s. S. 269. Unbefugten ist der Zutritt zu infektiösen Laboratorien verboten.

Als *obligatorische Schutzkleidung* genügt in der Regel ein hochgeschlossener Mantel aus kochfestem Material. Er gilt als infiziert und ist entsprechend zu behandeln. Für männliches Personal empfehlen sich zusätzlich kochfeste Beinkleider. Das Tragen von besonderen Schuhen verhindert den Transport von Mikroorganismen aus den Laboratorien in die Außenwelt.

Bei erhöhter Gefährdung müssen nach Anweisung des verantwortlichen Leiters weitere Schutzmaßnahmen getroffen werden. Gummi- oder Plastikhandschuhe, Mund-Nasenschutz, dessen Wirksamkeit nicht überschätzt werden darf (WEDUM, 1961), Atemmasken, allseitig geschlossene Schutzbrillen und Kopfbedeckungen sind vorrätig zu halten. Zur Desinfektion von Arbeitsschutzgeräten äußerte sich WEICHARDT (1968).

Besonders gefährliche Arbeiten sind in Impfkästen oder auf Reinen Werkbänken durchzuführen (s. S. 255).

Alle Personen, die mit Krankheitserregern arbeiten, haben dafür Sorge zu tragen, daß diese nicht verschleppt und Kulturen und infiziertes Material nach Versuchsende vernichtet oder desinfiziert werden. Zur Desinfektion von kleinen Geräten (Instrumenten, Pipetten usw.) sind am Arbeitsplatz kippsichere Behälter mit Desinfektionslösung aufzustellen. Dies entbindet nicht von der anschließenden Sterilisation im Autoklaven oder mit einem anderen, ebenso wirksamen Verfahren.

Besonders strenge Vorschriften sind wegen der Gemeingefährlichkeit für Arbeiten mit den Erregern der Pest, der Tularämie, des Rotzes, der Rinderpest und der Maul- und Klauenseuche erlassen. In der Bundesrepublik Deutschland gilt für einschlägige Arbeiten die „Bekanntmachung betreffend Vorschriften über Krankheitserreger" von 1917.

§ 6

(1) Wer (mit Krankheitserregern) arbeitet, hat — auch wenn er von der Einholung der Erlaubnis oder von der Anzeigepflicht entbunden ist — die Erreger so aufzubewahren, daß sie Unberufenen unzugänglich sind; auch hat er sonst alle Vorkehrungen zu treffen, um eine Verschleppung der Krankheitserreger, insbesondere durch Versuchstiere, zu verhüten. Kulturen, infizierte Versuchstiere und deren Organe sowie sonstiges die Krankheitserreger enthaltendes Material müssen, sobald sie entbehrlich geworden sind, derart beseitigt werden, daß jede Verschleppung der Krankheitskeime ausgeschlossen wird. Instrumente, Gefäße usw., die mit infektiösen Gegenständen in Berührung waren, sind sorgfältig zu desinfizieren.

(2) Insbesondere müssen alle Personen, welche die Räume betreten, in denen mit den Erregern der Pest, der Tularämie, des Rotzes, der Rinderpest oder der Maul- und Klauenseuche oder mit Material, das solche Erreger enthält oder zu enthalten verdächtig ist, gearbeitet wird, leicht desinfizierbare und waschbare Schutzüberkleider anlegen, die vor dem Verlassen der Räume wieder abzulegen sind; diese Schutzkleider sind vor der Ausgabe zur Wäsche in den Arbeitsräumen selbst zu desinfizieren. In den Räumen darf nur bei geschlossenen Türen und Fenstern gearbeitet werden; das Rauchen in den Räumen ist verboten. Sämtliche mit infektionstüchtigem Material in Berührung gekommene Gegenstände, ausgenommen das zur Aufbewahrung bestimmte Material, sind möglichst sofort zu desinfizieren oder zu vernichten. Bei den Arbeiten mit Versuchstieren ist namentlich sorgfältig darauf zu achten, daß ein Entweichen von Tieren oder eine Verstreuung von infektionstüchtigem Material nicht stattfindet. Tiere, welche in den Arbeitsräumen untergebracht waren, sind in diesen selbst zu vernichten; die Kadaver werden zweckmäßig entweder verbrannt oder in konzentrierter Schwefelsäure aufgelöst oder mittels Dampfes sterilisiert. Die Arbeitsräume sind außerhalb der Zeit ihrer Benutzung sicher verschlossen zu halten. Vor dem Verlassen der Räume hat sich der Leiter oder sein Vertreter zu vergewissern, daß die Versuchstiere und Kulturen sicher untergebracht sind und das Infektionsmaterial nicht verstreut ist.

(3) Untersuchungsmaterial und Kulturen der Erreger der in Absatz 2 genannten Krankheiten dürfen in den Räumen nur in besonderen festverschließbaren Schränken aufbewahrt werden.

(4) Versuchsstallungen für größere Tiere, an welchen Versuche mit Rotz, Rinderpest oder mit Maul- und Klauenseuche ausgeführt werden, müssen von anderen Stallungen getrennt sein. Für sie muß besonderes Stallpersonal vorhanden sein. Auch müssen dort Vorrichtungen getroffen werden, welche gestatten, den Mist, die Streu und die Kadaver der Tiere sofort an

Ort und Stelle unschädlich zu beseitigen. Wer diese Stallungen betreten will, hat ein waschbares Überkleid sowie Gummischuhe anzulegen, die beim Verlassen des Stalles abzulegen sind. Diese Schutzkleider sind in allen Stallungen selbst zu desinfizieren. Zweckmäßig werden vor die Ausgänge der Räume und Ställe in Sublimat getränkte dicke Matten gelegt, auf denen alle, die diese Räume verlassen, ihre Schuhsohlen zu desinfizieren haben.

§ 7

(1) Die zur Aufbewahrung von lebenden Erregern der Pest und der Tularämie oder zum Arbeiten mit Pest-, Tularämie-, Rotz-, Rinderpest- und Maul- und Klauenseuche-Material oder einer dieser Krankheiten verdächtigem Material bestimmten Räume dürfen nur in der Zeit zu anderen bakteriologischen Untersuchungen benutzt werden, während der dort nicht mit Pest-, Tularämie-, Rotz-, Rinderpest- oder Maul- und Klauenseuche-Material gearbeitet wird. Sie müssen bezüglich ihrer Beschaffenheit, Einrichtung und Ausstattung folgende Anforderungen erfüllen:

1. Die Räume sollen durch eine in Stein ausgeführte Wand (ohne Tür) getrennt von anderen Räumen liegen und für sich einen eigenen, sicher abschließbaren Eingang besitzen. Das Schloß der Eingangstür darf sich nur mittels des dazugehörigen Schlüssels öffnen lassen, nicht durch sogenannte Hauptschlüssel. Grundsätzlich sollen wenigstens zwei Räume vorhanden sein, von denen der eine hauptsächlich für die Züchtung der Erreger und für mikroskopische Untersuchungen und dergleichen, der andere hauptsächlich für Unterbringung, Sektion und Vernichtung der kleinen Versuchstiere zu verwenden ist. Die Räume sollen unmittelbar nebeneinander liegen und durch eine abschließbare Zwischentür verbunden sein. Wenn nur ein einziger Raum zur Verfügung steht und ausnahmsweise für ausreichend erachtet wird, so empfiehlt es sich, diesen so herzurichten, daß eine sichere, gesonderte Unterbringung der Versuchstiere darin gewährleistet wird.
2. Diese Räume sollen gut lüftbar und für Licht überall, namentlich auch in den Winkeln, leicht zugänglich sein, glatte, undurchlässige, leicht zu reinigende und zu desinfizierende Fußböden und Wände haben; sie sollen keine Öffnungen besitzen, durch welche kleinere Tiere oder Ratten schlüpfen können. Lüftungsöffnungen sind mit dichten Drahtnetzen zu überziehen. Die Fenster müssen dicht schließen; werden sie geöffnet, so sind Einsätze mit engmaschigem Drahtgitter einzufügen.
3. Die Räume sollen für sich allein mit allen denjenigen Einrichtungen und Instrumenten ausgestattet sein, welche für die Züchtung von Mikroorganismen und zur Anstellung von Tierversuchen erforderlich sind; namentlich dürfen nicht fehlen:
   a) ein mit sicherem Schlosse versehener Behälter zur Aufbewahrung lebender Kulturen und verdächtigen Materials (vgl. § 6 Abs. 3), b) Einrichtungen für sichere Unterbringung der Versuchstiere (am zweckmäßigsten hohe, in Wasserdampf sterilisierbare Glasgefäße mit Drahtumhüllung und fest anschließendem Drahtdeckel mit Watteabschluß), ferner Einrichtungen für die Öffnung der Tiere, für die Vernichtung der Kadaver und sonstiger infizierter Gegenstände, wie Streumaterialien und Futterreste (z.B. Verbrennungsofen, Dampfsterilisator, Gefäße mit konzentrierter Schwefelsäure), c) ein hinreichend großes Gefäß mit breiter Öffnung für Kresolwasser, in welches Kadaver und Kadaverteile vor der Sektion zur Vernichtung des an ihnen haftenden Ungeziefers gelegt werden können, d) Einrichtungen zur Desinfektion und Reinigung der Hände (Waschvorrichtung) und aller bei den Arbeiten gebrauchten Gegenstände (z.B. Autoklav oder Dampfsterilisator, Heißluftsterilisator).
4. Andere Gegenstände, als die zur Ausführung der Untersuchung erforderlichen, dürfen in den Räumen nicht untergebracht werden.

(2) Die Verwendung von Dienern bei den Arbeiten mit den Erregern der Pest, der Tularämie, des Rotzes, der Rinderpest oder der Maul- und Klauenseuche oder mit Material, das solche Erreger enthält oder zu enthalten verdächtig ist, ist nur dann gestattet, wenn sie über die aus einer Verschleppung dieser Krankheitserreger entstehenden Gefahren wohl unterrichtet und in der sachgemäßen Behandlung bakteriologischer Geräte, Kulturen und infizierter Tiere gut ausgebildet sind.

(3) Alle dem Diener etwa übertragenen Arbeiten (wie Reinigung des Laboratoriums, Fütterung der Tiere, Desinfektion und Reinigung der Käfige, Unschädlichmachung und Vernichtung des Mistes, der Streu und der Kadaver) haben nach genauer Anweisung des Leiters zu geschehen.

(4) Der Diener darf nur zur Ausführung von Anordnungen des Leiters oder seines Vertreters in den Arbeitsräumen sich aufhalten, sobald dort mit Pestmaterial gearbeitet wird.

(5) Die Kulturen der Erreger der Pest, der Tularämie, des Rotzes, der Rinderpest und der Maul- und Klauenseuche sowie das mit solchen behaftete oder verdächtige Material sollen unter sicherem Verschluß aufbewahrt werden und dürfen dem Diener nicht zugänglich sein.

§ 8

(1) Der Leiter der Arbeiten mit Krankheitserregern hat für die dauernde ordnungsgemäße Instandhaltung und für den gesamten Betrieb in den Arbeitsräumen, namentlich für die Durchführung der bei dem Aufbewahren von Kulturen, insbesondere solchen der Pesterreger, sowie bei Tierversuchen zu beobachtenden Maßregeln Sorge zu tragen. Er darf in Behinderungsfällen sowie für einzelne Arbeiten und Verrichtungen nur solche Persönlichkeiten mit seiner Vertretung betrauen oder zu seiner Hilfe heranziehen, welche nach Vorbildung und persönlichen Eigenschaften (Zuverlässigkeit usw.) imstande sind, die volle Verantwortlichkeit zu übernehmen.

Ist aus besonderen Gründen anderen Personen der Zutritt zu den Räumen zu gestatten, so hat der Leiter die zur Sicherung gegen Ansteckungsgefahr erforderlichen Maßregeln zu treffen.

(2) Es ist darauf hinzuwirken, daß die in Pestlaboratorien zu beschäftigenden Personen (Leiter, Vertreter, Diener) sich aktiv gegen Pest immunisieren lassen.

Durch den „Runderlaß des Reichs- und Preußischen Ministers des Innern betreffend Laboratoriumsinfektionen mit Erregern der Weilschen Krankheit" vom 22. August 1936 wird ergänzend geregelt, daß bei Arbeiten mit den genannten Mikroorganismen oder bei Versuchen mit Ratten oder Hunden Schutzbrillen und Gummihandschuhe zu tragen sind. Besondere Vorsicht ist auch bei der Untersuchung von Rattenurin geboten (s. S. 265).

In der Deutschen Demokratischen Republik gilt für das Arbeiten mit Krankheitserregern die „Dritte Durchführungsbestimmung zum Gesetz zur Verhütung und Bekämpfung übertragbarer Krankheiten beim Menschen. — Arbeit mit Erregern von übertragbaren Krankheiten —" von 1966. Sie nimmt Bezug auf das „Gesetz zur Verhütung und Bekämpfung übertragbarer Krankheiten beim Menschen" von 1965. Die Vorschriften unterscheiden sich inhaltlich nicht wesentlich von denen der Bundesrepublik Deutschland, jedoch dürfen z. B. Kulturen bestimmter Erreger nicht versandt werden (s. S. 260).

3. Besondere Gefahrenquellen

Nach den Vorschriften der Berufsgenossenschaft für Gesundheitsdienst und Wohlfahrtspflege ist in Laboratorien das Pipettieren mit dem Mund untersagt (Unfallverhütungsvorschrift „Medizinische Laboratoriumsarbeiten", 1956). Auch die Verwendung von zweikugeligen Sicherheitspipetten, die zusätzlich mit Watte „gestopft" werden können, ist nach dem Wortlaut der Vorschrift nicht zulässig. Gefahren drohen von der zu pipettierenden Flüssigkeit und vom kontaminierten Mundstück der Pipette. Leider haben jedoch mechanische Pipettiergeräte so große Nachteile, daß ihr allgemeiner Gebrauch, vor allem bei Reihenuntersuchungen, heute noch auf erhebliche Schwierigkeiten stößt.

Eine vielfach unterschätzte Infektionsquelle ist die Bildung von *Aerosolen*, deren Gefährlichkeit mit abnehmender Partikelgröße zunimmt (HATCH, 1961; WRIGHT, 1961). Sie können beim Ausblasen von Pipetten, Mischen von Flüssigkeiten durch Einblasen von Luft, Auftropfen von Flüssigkeiten (Abb. 1—3), Dekantieren von Zentrifugengläsern, Öffnen von lyophilisierten Kulturen (ROSEBURY et al., 1947, s. S. 259) oder von Gefäßen entstehen, die mit Gummi-, Plastik- oder Korkstopfen versehen sind (TOMLINSON, 1957; BADER et al., 1971). Auch Homogenisatoren und schnellaufende Zentrifugen neigen zur Aerosolbildung. Modelle mit Windkessel sind deshalb zu bevorzugen. Die Zentrifugengläser sind zu verschließen (WHITWELL et al., 1957, Unfallverhütungsvorschrift der Berufsgenossenschaft für Gesundheitsdienst und Wohlfahrtspflege „Schleudermaschinen — Zentrifugen und Separatoren —", 1971). Beim Ausglühen von Ösen und Nadeln in der Bunsenflamme werden kleine bis kleinste bakterienhaltige Tröpfchen verspritzt. Die Verwendung von Schutzglocken aus Glas oder Metall ist

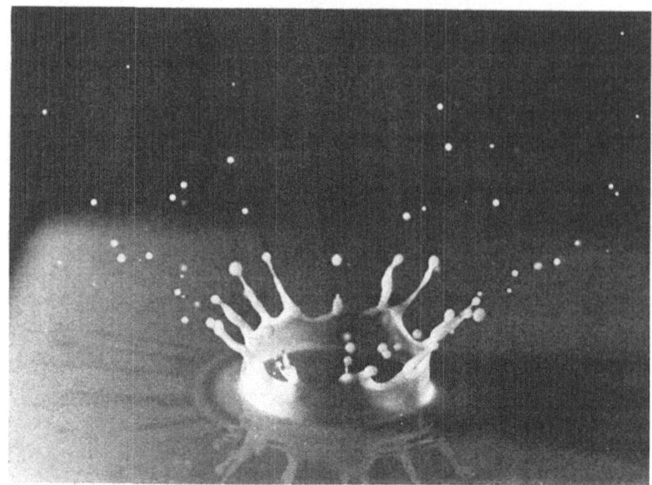

Abb. 1

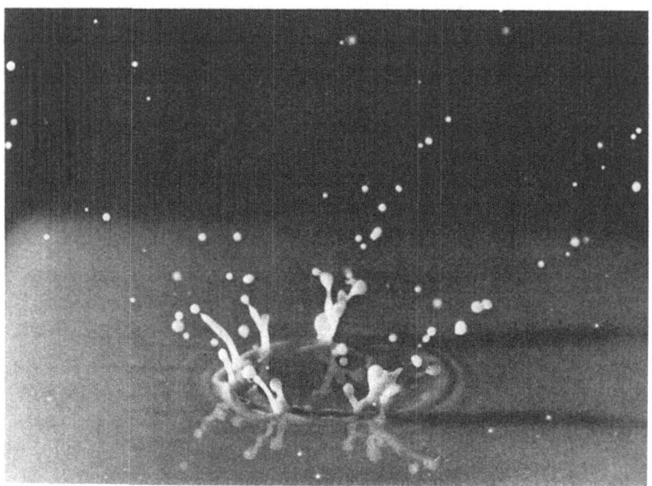

Abb. 2

Abb. 1 u. 2. Bildung eines Aerosols beim Aufprall eines Flüssigkeitstropfens auf eine Fläche. (Phot. Huhn)[5]

deshalb dringend anzuraten. Mit einer Aerosolbildung ist auch bei der Beimpfung von Nährböden (Johansson u. Ferris, 1946) und der Objektträgeragglutination zu rechnen. Nach derartigen Arbeiten ist deshalb eine sorgfältige Desinfektion der Hände, der Geräte und des Arbeitsplatzes unerläßlich. Vor Injektion infektiöser Flüssigkeit ist auf einen festen Sitz der Kanüle auf dem Konus der Spritze zu achten. Durch Sicherheitsspritzen wird diese Gefahrenquelle vermieden. Ein auf die Spitze der Injektionsnadel gesteckter, mit Alkohol getränkter Wattebausch verhindert die Aerosolbildung beim Entfernen von Luftblasen.

Zahlreiche Beiträge zur Theorie und Praxis der Aerosolbildung und deren Bedeutung für Laboratoriumsinfektionen finden sich in den gesammelten Berichten

5 Für die freundliche Überlassung der Abb. 1—3 bin ich Herrn Bernd Huhn, Kiel, zu besonderem Dank verpflichtet.

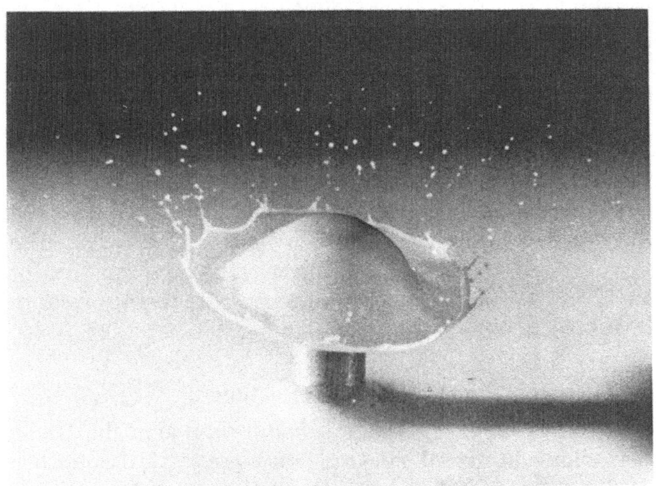

Abb. 3. Bildung eines Aerosols beim Aufprall eines Flüssigkeitstropfens auf einen cylindrischen Körper. (Phot. HUHN)

der Conference on Airborne Infection (McDermott, 1961), eine umfassende Aufzählung von Gefahrenquellen mit besonderer Berücksichtigung der Aerosole und ihrer Verhütung mit einer reichhaltigen Literaturzusammenstellung über diese Themen bei WEDUM (1961).

Gelegentlich siedeln sich in mikrobiologischen Laboratorien *Milben* an, die in Petrischalen kriechen und Mikroorganismen verschleppen. Als Spuren ihrer Wanderungen hinterlassen sie auf der Nährbodenoberfläche Keime, die lange Straßen von Kolonien bilden können. Auch *Schaben* (Phyllodromia germanica, Blatta orientalis, Periplaneta americana) verbreiten bei ihren Wanderungen Mikroorganismen. Sie sind, insbesondere in alten Gebäuden, kaum ausrottbar. Durch Verwendung von Insecticiden läßt sich jedoch ihre Zahl niedrighalten. *Fliegen* und *Ameisen* sind unnachsichtig zu bekämpfen. Über die Rolle von Gliederfüßlern bei der Verbreitung von Mikroorganismen s. MARTINI (1952) und BUSVINE (1966).

Im Gegensatz zur In-vitro-Technik, deren Gefahren sich bei sorgfältiger Beachtung der Regeln reduzieren lassen, sind *Tierversuche* mit erhöhten Risiken belastet. Viele Krankheitserreger werden mit dem Kot oder Urin, über die Atemwege oder Operationswunden ausgeschieden und finden sich, oft in großer Zahl, in den Käfigen der Tiere. Bei ihrer Wartung kann es zur direkten oder indirekten Kontaktübertragung oder, falls die Mikroorganismen sich an flugfähigen Staub anheften, zur aerogenen Übertragung kommen (s. S. 254). Entsprechend der Gefährlichkeit der Mikroorganismen müssen deshalb besondere Schutzmaßnahmen getroffen werden. Außer peinlicher Sauberkeit während der Arbeit und gründlicher Desinfektion nach deren Beendigung kann das Tragen von Handschuhen, Mund- und Nasenschutz, Atemmasken oder Brillen angezeigt sein.

Weiterhin ist zu berücksichtigen, daß Laboratoriumstiere natürliche Reservoire von Mikroorganismen sein können, die auf den genannten Wegen, aber auch durch Biß auf den Menschen übertragen werden. Besonderer Erwähnung bedürfen Ratten, Mäuse, Meerschweinchen und Hamster als Infektionsquellen für Leptospiren (MASON, 1937; VAN THIEL, 1948; WOLFF et al., 1949; MOCHMANN u. SCHMUTZLER, 1956; BROOME u. NORRIS, 1957; POPOVA u. AMOSENKOWA, 1957;

Stoenner u. Maclean, 1958; Kleinschmidt u. Christ, 1959; Goley et al., 1960; Kappeler et al., 1961, s. S. 263) und die Ratte als Reservoir für Spirillum minus als Erreger einer Rattenbißkrankheit. Hunde und Katzen sind Reservoire besonders für Pasteurella multocida (Helm u. Stille, 1972).

Zahlreiche kasuistische Mitteilungen zeigen, daß auch infizierte Bruteier Infektionsquellen sein können (Olitzky u. Morgan, 1939; Helwig, 1940; McKee et al., 1940; Harrop et al., 1941; Koprowski u. Cox, 1947; Goley et al., 1960).

Schließlich kann das Arbeiten mit Parasiten, z.B. Proglottiden von Cestoden (Bader, 1951), für den Menschen gefährlich werden. Zahlreiche Hinweise finden sich bei Piekarski (1954). Einige typische Gefahrenquellen sind ohne Berücksichtigung der Häufigkeit in Tabelle 9 zusammengestellt. Ihre Kenntnis weist den Weg zur Prophylaxe.

4. Händedesinfektion

Bei Arbeiten im mikrobiologischen Laboratorium sind die Hände bevorzugt einer Kontamination mit Krankheitserregern ausgesetzt. Dennoch ist es nur in besonderen Fällen notwendig, sie durch Handschuhe aus Gummi oder Plastik zu schützen (s. S. 263). Um das Eindringen von Krankheitserregern in den menschlichen Organismus zu verhindern, dürfen jedoch Mund, Nase und Augen nicht berührt werden. Es ist selbstverständlich, daß im Laboratorium Rauchen, Essen und Trinken untersagt sind. Um die von den Händen ausgehenden Gefahren zu verringern, ist ihre Desinfektion nach besonderen Verrichtungen und grundsätzlich nach Beendigung der Arbeit unerläßlich.

Unter Desinfektion wird zwar die Abtötung der Krankheitserreger, also auch ihrer Sporen, verstanden, jedoch wirken die üblichen Händedesinfektionsmittel nur auf vegetative Formen. Mit der Abtötung von Sporen kann während der üblichen Einwirkungszeiten nicht gerechnet werden. Dies ist besonders bei Arbeiten mit Bacillus anthracis zu berücksichtigen.

Für die Händedesinfektion dürfen ausschließlich *geprüfte Mittel* verwendet werden, die in Listen des Bundesgesundheitsamtes (1971) und der Deutschen Gesellschaft für Hygiene und Mikrobiologie (1966—1972) veröffentlicht sind. Ein Kommentar zur Liste des Bundesgesundheitsamtes findet sich bei Heicken (1966). Bei Arbeiten mit Mycobakterien (Mycobacterium tuberculosis, M. leprae, M. ulcerans, Kieninger et al., 1972) sind außerdem die Hinweise des Merkblatts des Deutschen Zentralkomitees zur Bekämpfung der Tuberkulose „Desinfektionsmaßnahmen bei Tuberkulose" (1967) zu beachten. Eine Beurteilung sog. desinfizierender Seifen findet sich bei Kanz u. Kanz (1969), üblicher Seifen bei Eschment u. Lutz-Dettinger (1970).

Die Mittel sind in der vom Hersteller vorgeschriebenen Gebrauchsverdünnung täglich frisch anzusetzen und vorrätig zu halten. Da ihre Hautverträglichkeit neben der bactericiden Wirkung eine der wichtigsten Eigenschaften ist, dürfen die vorgeschriebenen Konzentrationen nicht überschritten, um ihre Wirksamkeit nicht zu mindern allerdings auch nicht unterschritten werden. Außerdem sollten sie von Zeit zu Zeit gegen solche mit anderen Wirkstoffgruppen ausgetauscht werden. Hinweise für die Praxis finden sich bei Grün u. Preuner (1964), Grün (1955, 1965), über die theoretischen Grundlagen bei Sykes (1965), Roemer (1969) und Horn et al. (1972).

In Laboratorien wird in der Regel die *hygienische Händedesinfektion* durchgeführt, die die Abtötung der Anflug- und Kontaktkeime, der transienten Flora, bewirken soll. Die Hände werden zunächst je nach Vorschrift 1—2 min mit der Gebrauchsverdünnung des Desinfiziens sorgfältig behandelt und in der Regel anschließend mit Seife gewaschen. Dies soll unterbleiben, wenn eine nachhaltige Wirkung des Mittels erwünscht ist.

Beispiele einer hygienischen Händedesinfektion:

a) 70 vol.-%iges Äthanol (bzw. 60%iges Isopropanol oder 60%iges n-Propanol)   1 min
70 vol.-%iges Äthanol wird durch Mischen von 100 ml Äthanol mit 25 ml Wasser und Einstellen des spezifischen Gewichtes auf 0,8658 bei 25° C hergestellt (BORNEFF, 1971).

b) Gebrauchsverdünnung eines Handelspräparates   1—2 min
In der Regel waschen mit oder ohne Seife

c) Nach Arbeiten mit Mycobakterien:
Abreiben der Hände mit einem alkoholgetränkten Wattebausch   5 min
(80%iges Äthanol, 70%iges Isopropanol bzw. 60%iges n-Propanol), der anschließend verbrannt wird.

d) Für die Desinfektion der mit Pockenviren infizierten Hände:
Einwirkung von 80 vol.-%igem Äthanol oder 60 vol.-%igem n-Propanol (GROSS-GEBAUER, 1967)   5 min

Das Ziel der *chirurgischen Händedesinfektion* ist es, die an der Oberfläche der Haut haftenden Anflug- und Kontaktkeime und die Haftkeime, die residente Flora, abzutöten. Dies ist weitaus schwieriger, da die Cutis ein Biotop für zahlreiche Bakterien ist, die, für chemische Mittel kaum erreichbar, in den Haarbälgen, Talg- und Schweißdrüsen angesiedelt sind. Eine Sterilisation der Hände ist deshalb nicht möglich, wohl aber neben der Abtötung der transienten Flora eine Reduktion der residenten Flora um über 99%.

Die chirurgische Händedesinfektion kann im Laboratorium vor Operationen an Tieren notwendig werden. Sie wird, im Gegensatz zur hygienischen Händedesinfektion, durch gründliches Waschen mit Seife und Bürste eingeleitet und mit der anschließenden Anwendung des Desinfektionsmittels beendet.

Beispiele einer chirurgischen Händedesinfektion:

a) Waschen mit warmem Wasser, Seife und weicher Bürste   3 min
Desinfizieren mit 80 vol.-%igem Äthanol (bzw. 70%igem Isopropanol oder 60%igem n-Propanol)   5 min
Nicht abspülen

b) Waschen mit warmem Wasser, Seife und weicher Bürste   3 min
Desinfizieren mit einer Gebrauchsverdünnung eines Handelspräparates   5 min
Nicht abspülen.

Die während des Arbeitens aus der Tiefe der Haut an die Oberfläche gelangenden Mikroorganismen werden durch das Tragen von sterilen Operationshandschuhen unschädlich gemacht. Diese schützen andererseits den Operateur vor einer Infektion.

Für die Desinfektion der Haut von Versuchstieren eignet sich besonders Jodtinktur oder Sepsotinktur. Ihre Anwendung ist nach Injektion von Krankheitserregern notwendig, um an der Einstichstelle haftende Keime abzutöten. SCHENKER et al. (1972) ziehen Jodtinktur wegen ihrer besseren Wirksamkeit vor. Benzin und Äther sind ungeeignet.

5. Flächendesinfektion

In mikrobiologischen Laboratorien ist eine tägliche Desinfektion der Fußböden und Arbeitstische, nach Bedarf auch anderer Einrichtungsgegenstände und Geräte, notwendig. Die geeigneten Mittel, ihre Konzentration und Einwirkungszeiten sind den vom Bundesgesundheitsamt und der Deutschen Gesellschaft für Hygiene und Mikrobiologie veröffentlichten Listen zu entnehmen (s. S. 244, 246). Bei Arbeiten mit Tuberkelbakterien ist auf die Verwendung besonders gekennzeichneter Mittel zu achten. Sie sind in dem Merkblatt „Desinfektionsmaßnahmen bei Tuberkulose" (1967) zusammengestellt.

Für die Desinfektion der Fußböden ist die Zwei-Eimer-Methode unter Verwendung eines Soogers zu empfehlen. Eine trockene Reinigung ist nicht zulässig.

Die in einem Eimer bereitgehaltene Desinfektionsmittellösung wird mit einem Sooger auf den Fußboden aufgebracht, sorgfältig verteilt, anschließend wieder aufgenommen und in den zweiten Eimer ausgedrückt. Dieser Vorgang wird so oft wiederholt, bis der gesamte Boden aufgewischt ist. Der Sooger verbleibt anschließend zur Desinfektion 4 Std im zweiten Eimer.

Auf Arbeitstische und andere Flächen kann das Desinfiziens mit einem Tuch oder Sprühgerät aufgebracht werden. Anschließend wird die physikalisch und chemisch wirkende Scheuerdesinfektion durchgeführt. Die Reinigungsgeräte sind chemisch, durch Kochen oder Autoklavieren zu entkeimen.

Der Innenraum von Brut- und Kühlschränken ist in regelmäßigen Abständen zu desinfizieren.

Über die Möglichkeiten der Desinfektion großer ärztlicher Geräte berichteten PREUNER et al. (1963).

Bei allen Arbeiten mit Desinfektionsmitteln sind zum Schutz vor Hautschädigungen Plastik- oder Gummihandschuhe zu tragen.

6. Raumdesinfektion

Nach Arbeiten mit besonders gefährlichen Krankheitserregern kann eine Formaldehyd-Raumdesinfektion angezeigt sein. Im sorgfältig abgedichteten Laboratorium werden 5 g Formaldehyd/m³ Luftraum in einem besonderen Gerät (Flügge-, Breslau-Gerät) verdampft. Nach 6stündiger Einwirkung wird der Formaldehyd mit Ammoniak zu Hexamethylentetramin neutralisiert. Die für die jeweiligen Raumgrößen benötigten Mengen von Formaldehyd, Wasser, Ammoniak und Spiritus sind Tabellen zu entnehmen (KIRSTEIN, 1944). Über den Einfluß der relativen Feuchtigkeit auf die Wirksamkeit des Verfahrens berichteten HOFFMAN u. SPINER (1970). Anstelle des genannten Verdampfers kann auch ein Hochleistungssprühgerät eingesetzt werden. Es empfiehlt sich, diese Arbeiten geprüften Desinfektoren zu überlassen. Über weitere Möglichkeiten der Raumdesinfektion s. SCHMIDT-MENDE et al. (1968).

7. Vernichten von infektiösem Material

Alle infektiösen Materialien müssen autoklaviert, Tierkadaver in Verbrennungsöfen verbrannt werden. Größere Versuchstiere werden unter Beachtung aller Vorsichtsmaßnahmen von einer Tierkörperbeseitigungsanstalt möglichst innerhalb 24 Std nach Eintreffen der Anzeige abgeholt (Tierkörperbeseitigungsgesetz von 1939).

Das Autoklavieren ist durch Richtlinien des Deutschen Arzneibuchs (DAB 7, 1968) geregelt. Sie schreiben eine Sterilisiertemperatur von mindestens 120° C und eine Sterilisierzeit von mindestens 20 min vor. Geräte mit einer Betriebstemperatur von 134° C sind jedoch vorzuziehen.

Die „Sterilisierzeit" darf nicht mit der „Betriebszeit" verwechselt werden. Diese setzt sich aus Anheizzeit, Ausgleichszeit, Sterilisierzeit und Abkühlungszeit zusammen. Die Sterilisierzeit beginnt nach Beendigung der Ausgleichszeit, wenn an allen Punkten des Sterilisationsraumes einschließlich der eingebrachten Objekte die vorgeschriebene Betriebstemperatur erreicht ist. Sie beträgt bei 120° C, wie erwähnt, 20 min, bei 134° C etwa 10 min.

Begriffsbestimmungen der Dampf- und Heißluftsterilisation mit allerdings abweichender Nomenklatur finden sich in DIN 58946, „Dampf- und Heißluftsterilisation" (1967), die sicherheitstechnischen Festlegungen in Blatt 2 (Anforderungen, 1972) der gleichen Norm.

Aus Sicherheitsgründen darf ein Autoklav erst nach Absinken der Temperatur auf 80° C geöffnet werden (LÜDDE, 1972).

Die Funktionstüchtigkeit von Autoklaven sollte mindestens jährlich und zusätzlich nach jeder größeren Reparatur überprüft werden. Als Kriterium dient die sichere Abtötung von Mikroorganismen der Resistenzstufe III (native Erdsporen).

Testobjekt ist Sporenerde, die nach DIN 58947 ,,Sporenerde zur Prüfung von Dampf- und Heißluft-Sterilisatoren'' (1969) aufbereitet, geprüft und in Filterpapierbriefchen verpackt wird. Diese werden im Sterilisationsgut, vor allem auf die vermuteten Kälteinseln, verteilt. Nach beendeter Sterilisation werden sie entnommen und 2 Wochen in flüssigen Nährböden bebrütet. Deren Freisein von vermehrungsfähigen Keimen gilt als Kriterium für die einwandfreie Funktion des Sterilisators. Bei diesem Vorgehen wird auf die Einbeziehung der höchstresistenten thermophilen Mikroorganismen in den Test verzichtet (BÖHME u. HARTKE, 1969; BADER, 1973).

Neben dieser direkten Prüfung, deren Vorteil die Sicherheit des Verfahrens und deren Nachteil die lange Beobachtungsdauer der Kulturen ist, können indirekte Methoden angewendet werden. In der Regel dient der Farbumschlag einer chemischen Verbindung bei bestimmten Kombinationen von Temperatur und Zeit als Indicator für eine einwandfreie Funktion des Sterilisators. Sie bieten den Vorteil, den Effekt jedes Sterilisationsgangs unmittelbar nach seiner Beendigung anzuzeigen.

Die genannten Funktionsprüfungen sind Aufgabe des Mikrobiologen und Hygienikers. Die technische Prüfung der Autoklaven gehört dagegen zum Arbeitsbereich der Technischen Überwachungsvereine.

Glas-, Porzellan- und andere hitzebeständige Geräte können in Heißluftsterilisatoren keimfrei gemacht werden. Das Deutsche Arzneibuch (DAB 7, 1968) nennt eine Sterilisierzeit von mindestens 30 min bei 180° C. Wegen der schlechten Leitfähigkeit der Luft sind in der Regel sehr lange Betriebszeiten notwendig.

Zu den Begriffen Sterilisierzeit und Betriebszeit s. S. 268 und DIN 58946 ,,Dampf- und Heißluftsterilisation'' (1967). Heißluftsterilisatoren werden wie Autoklaven geprüft.

Ausführliche Darstellungen der Theorie und Praxis von Desinfektions- und Sterilisationsmaßnahmen finden sich bei RUBBO u. GARDNER (1965), WALLHÄUSER u. SCHMIDT (1967), HORN (1968), STUTZ (1968) und PERKINS (1969).

8. Unfallverhütungsvorschriften, Erste Hilfe

In der Bundesrepublik Deutschland ist die Berufsgenossenschaft für Gesundheitsdienst und Wohlfahrtspflege bemüht, durch die Herausgabe von *Unfallverhütungsvorschriften*, Richtlinien und Merkblättern Unfälle und Infektionskrankheiten in mikrobiologischen Laboratorien zu verhüten. Zu erwähnen sind insbesondere die ,,Allgemeinen Unfallverhütungsvorschriften'' (1969), in denen die drei Merkblätter ,,Allgemeine Vorschriften'', ,,Erste Hilfe und Verhalten bei Unfällen'' und die ,,Übergangs- und Ausführungsbestimmungen'' zusammengefaßt wurden, sowie die Unfallverhütungsvorschrift ,,Medizinische Laboratoriumsarbeiten'' (1956) mit Anweisungen über Geltungsbereich, Meldepflicht, Kenntnisse der Beschäftigten, Vorbeugung gesundheitlicher Schäden, Räume für Laboratoriumsarbeiten, Einrichtung der Laboratorien, Laboratoriumsarbeiten, Arbeiten mit infektiösem Material, Versuchstieren und Tierkadavern, Erste Hilfe bei Verletzungen und Infektionen und schließlich der Ausführungsbestimmungen.

Nach § 7 der genannten ,,Allgemeinen Unfallverhütungsvorschriften'' (1969) ist mindestens *ein Sicherheitsbeauftragter* zu bestellen (Merkblätter ,,Die Bestellung von Sicherheitsbeauftragten'', 1969, und ,,Der Sicherheitsbeauftragte'', 1969).

In der Deutschen Demokratischen Republik sind die ,,Arbeitsschutzbestimmungen'' von 1953 zu beachten, in denen sich eingehende Anweisungen für das Verhalten in mikrobiologischen Laboratorien finden.

In Großbritannien wurden vom Medical Research Council (1960) die ,,Safety Precautions in Laboratories'' erarbeitet.

Als *Warnung* vor biologischen Gefahren wurde von BALDWIN u. RUNKLE (1967) ein in fluorescierender orangeroter Farbe ausgeführtes Symbol vorgeschlagen (Abb. 4). Es hat bereits in zahlreichen Laboratorien der USA Eingang gefunden.

Abb. 4. Biologische Gefahren: Warnsymbol. (BALDWIN u. RUNKLE, 1967)

Allen in mikrobiologischen Laboratorien beschäftigten Personen müssen die bei Unfällen zu treffenden Maßnahmen geläufig sein. Unregelmäßigkeiten sind unverzüglich dem Dienstvorgesetzten zu melden. Verzögerungen oder Verschweigen können schwerwiegende Folgen für die unmittelbar Betroffenen, die Mitarbeiter und weitere Personen haben.

Die Befolgung der von der Berufsgenossenschaft für Gesundheitsdienst und Wohlfahrtspflege auch als Aushängetafel herausgegebenen Merksätze „Erste Hilfe bei Laboratoriumsinfektionen" (1955) ist allen Beschäftigten zur Pflicht zu machen.

Erste Hilfe bei Laboratoriumsinfektionen

Vorbemerkungen

Bei Infektionen ist so bald wie möglich ärztliche Hilfe in Anspruch zu nehmen. Die nachstehenden Anordnungen sind daher nur als erste Schutzmaßnahmen aufzufassen.

Jede Laboratoriumsinfektion, jede Verletzung durch infizierte Instrumente, jede Sektionsverletzung, jede Beschmutzung von Hautwunden und Schrunden mit infiziertem Material sowie jede Biß- und sonstige Verletzung durch infizierte oder gesunde Tiere ist ebenso wie jeder Unfall unverzüglich dem Laboratoriumsleiter zu melden. Ist der Betroffene hierzu nicht imstande, hat die Meldepflicht der Betriebsangehörige, der zuerst von dem Ereignis erfährt.

Die für die Erste-Hilfe-Leistung erforderlichen Mittel sind in jedem Laboratorium in einem geeigneten Schrank an einer allen Beschäftigten bekannten und leicht zugänglichen Stelle, trocken, kühl, staubfrei und jederzeit erreichbar bereitzuhalten. Die Mittel sind regelmäßig daraufhin zu prüfen, ob sie einwandfrei (genügend frisch) und vollzählig vorhanden sind.

In den Arbeitsräumen müssen Einrichtungen zum Waschen mit fließendem Wasser und zum Trocknen der Hände (Einzel- oder Papierhandtücher) bereitgestellt und benutzt werden. Für Hand- und Hautdesinfektionen sind gebrauchsfertige Desinfektionsmittel bereitzuhalten.

Allgemeine Schutzmaßnahmen

Mund

Nicht schlucken!   Ausspucken!   Spülen!

1. Infektiöses Material ist in den Mund gelangt, aber noch nicht geschluckt worden:

Nicht schlucken! Sofort ausspucken! Darauf wiederholt gründlich Mund ausspülen und gurgeln mit frisch angesetzter 0,1%iger Kaliumpermanganatlösung oder 1%iger Wasserstoffsuperoxydlösung. Jedes Schlucken vermeiden! Zweckmäßig ist, nunmehr wiederholt Brot zu kauen und das zerkaute Brot unter Nachspülen und Gurgeln mit Wasser auszuspucken. Speichel ausspucken! Abschließend soll man zwecks Anregung der Salzsäureabsonderung im Magen Fleischextrakt einnehmen. Mundspülungen sind während der ersten Stunden noch mehrfach zu wiederholen.

2. Infektiöses Material ist geschluckt worden:

Kurze kräftige Mundspülung und Gurgeln mit 0,1%iger frisch angesetzter Kaliumpermanganatlösung. Anschließend zwecks Anregung der Salzsäureabsonderung im Magen Fleischextrakt und salzsäure-pepsinhaltiges Mittel einnehmen.

Auge

Nicht reiben!

3. Infektiöses Material ist in das Auge gelangt:

Bindehautsack mit 1⁰/₀₀iger (promilliger) Oxycyanatlösung gründlich ausspülen (mit der Pipette in das durch Abspreizen der Lider offen gehaltene Auge reichlich und wiederholt eintropfen). Darauf 1⁰/₀₀ige (promillige) Oxycyanatvaseline mit Glasstäbchen einstreichen. In den Augenbindehautsack geratene Krankheitserreger können auf dem Wege des Tränenkanals in die Nase und weiterhin in den Rachen, Mund und Magen gelangen. An die Desinfektion des Auges sind deshalb die unter 1. (Mund) aufgeführten Maßnahmen anzuschließen.

Nase

Ausschnauben! Einatmen durch den Mund, ausatmen durch die Nase!

4. Infektiöses Material ist in die Nase gelangt:

Wiederholtes energisches Ausschnauben in Zellstoff, unter Vermeidung von Einziehen durch die Nase (Luft durch den Mund einholen und bei geschlossenem Munde kräftig durch die Nase ausstoßen). Einstreichen von 1⁰/₀₀iger (promilliger) Oxycyanatvaseline in die Nase. Außerdem sind anschließend die unter 1. (Mund) angegebenen Maßnahmen vorzunehmen.

Haut
Wunden ausbluten lassen!

5. Verletzungen der Haut durch infizierte Instrumente, Biß- und Kratzwunden, durch infizierte oder gesunde Tiere, Beschmutzung von Hautwunden mit infektiösem Material:

Oberflächliche Kratzwunden sofort mit Jodersatzlösung überpinseln. Darauf die Umgebung der Wunde abspülen und nach Abtupfen mit Zellstoff die Wunde nochmals mit Jodersatzlösung überpinseln. Anschließend Schutzverband!

Auf Stichverletzungen, die schlecht bluten, setzt man zweckmäßig den Saugschlauch einer Wasserstrahlluftpumpe und saugt aus. Ausbluten lassen! Einstichstelle wiederholt mit Jodersatzlösung betupfen. Anschließend Schutzverband!

Stark blutende Schnittwunden u. dgl. erst ausbluten lassen, dann Wundumgebung (nicht Wunde selbst) mit Jodersatzlösung desinfizieren. Anschließend Schutzverband!

Sondermaßnahmen
Versuchstiere

6. Zu beachten ist, daß scheinbar gesunde Ratten, Mäuse, Hamster und Hunde mit Leptospiren infiziert sein können. Treten bei Laboratoriumspersonen, die mit solchen Tieren gearbeitet haben, fieberhafte Erkrankungen auf, so ist an Leptospirose zu denken und entsprechend zu handeln. Eintrittspforten sind vorzugsweise Biß- und Kratzwunden, daneben auch Hautdefekte und Schleimhäute, wenn sie durch Tierharn oder Blut verunreinigt werden.

Besondere Infektionen

7. Bei Infektionen von Wunden mit Milzbrand, Rotz[6], Starrkrampf, Gasbrand und anderen besonders gefährlichen Erregern ist die sofortige Abtötung der in die Wunde gelangten Keime anzustreben und die Wunde deshalb je nach Lage der Dinge mit Jodersatzlösung auszupinseln oder mit rauchender Salpetersäure vorsichtig zu ätzen. Anschließend ist unverzüglich ein Krankenhaus oder ein Spezialarzt aufzusuchen, da eine Sonderbehandlung, z. B. eine Serumtherapie, häufig erforderlich sein wird.

Bei allen Verletzungen, insbesondere bei Sektionsverletzungen, ist über die angegebenen Schutzmaßnahmen hinaus das verletzte Glied für mindestens 24 Std ruhig zu stellen.

Zur Durchführung der in dem Merkblatt empfohlenen Prophylaxe ist ein *Erste-Hilfe-Schrank* mit folgenden Medikamenten erforderlich:

1 l	0,25%ige (prozentige) Kaliumpermanganatlösung
1 l	1⁰/₀₀ige (promillige) Lösung von Hydrargyrum oxycyanatum
10 g	1⁰/₀₀ige (promillige) Oxycyanatvaseline
10 g	Jodtinktur oder Sepsotinktur
20 g	Lugolsche Lösung
2 ml	rauchende Salpetersäure
50 g	Carbo medicinalis
50	Acidol-Pepsin-Tabletten
50 g	Fleischextrakt

Glasstäbe, Augenpipetten, Verbandmaterial, Zellstoff, Brandbinden.

---

6 Auf Grund neuerer Erkenntnisse wurde vom Verfasser Tollwut aus der Aufzählung gestrichen.

Besteht die Gefahr, daß Laboratorien zur Quelle von Infektionskrankheiten werden, so können die Vorschriften des § 10 des Bundes-Seuchengesetzes von 1961 Anwendung finden.

§ 10

(1) Wenn Tatsachen festgestellt werden, die zum Auftreten einer übertragbaren Krankheit führen können, so hat die zuständige Behörde die notwendigen Maßnahmen zur Abwendung der dem einzelnen oder der Allgemeinheit hierdurch drohenden Gefahren zu treffen. Den Beauftragten der zuständigen Behörde und des Gesundheitsamtes ist der Zutritt zu Grundstücken, Räumen und Einrichtungen, von denen die Gefahr ausgeht, zu gestatten. Das Grundrecht der Unverletzlichkeit der Wohnung (Artikel 13 Abs. 1 Grundgesetz) wird insoweit eingeschränkt.

(2) Erhält das Gesundheitsamt Kenntnis von einer der in Absatz 1 bezeichneten Tatsachen, so hat es die zuständige Behörde hiervon unverzüglich zu unterrichten und die geeigneten Maßnahmen vorzuschlagen. Bei Gefahr im Verzuge hat das Gesundheitsamt die erforderlichen Maßnahmen selbst anzuordnen und die zuständige Behörde hiervon sofort zu unterrichten. Diese kann die Anordnung ändern oder aufheben. Wird die Anordnung nicht innerhalb von zwei Tagen seit ihrem Erlaß aufgehoben, so gilt sie als von der zuständigen Behörde getroffen.

Die Vorschriften über die Bekämpfung übertragbarer Krankheiten finden sich in den §§ 30—43 des Bundes-Seuchengesetzes von 1961.

9. Meldepflicht

Das Bundes-Seuchengesetz von 1961 schreibt für die in § 3 erwähnten Infektionskrankheiten eine Meldepflicht vor, die bei sinngemäßer Auslegung des § 4 auch dem verantwortlichen Leiter des Laboratoriums und „jeder sonstigen mit der Behandlung oder der Pflege des Betroffenen berufsmäßig beschäftigten Person" obliegt. Die Meldung ist nach § 5 unverzüglich, spätestens innerhalb von 24 Std, dem Gesundheitsamt zu erstatten.

Zu beachten ist außerdem die Vorschrift des § 9, nach der „die Leiter von Medizinaluntersuchungsämtern und sonstigen öffentlichen oder privaten Untersuchungsstellen jeden Untersuchungsbefund, der auf einen meldepflichtigen Fall schließen läßt, unverzüglich dem für den Aufenthaltsort des Betroffenen zuständigen Gesundheitsamt zu melden haben".

Die Anzeigepflicht von Laboratoriumsinfektionen ist — unbeschadet der Meldepflicht nach dem Bundes-Seuchengesetz — zusätzlich in der „Siebenten Berufskrankheiten-Verordnung" von 1968 geregelt.

„§ 5 (1) Hat ein Arzt oder Zahnarzt den begründeten Verdacht, daß bei einem Versicherten eine Berufskrankheit besteht, so hat er dies dem Träger der Unfallversicherung oder der für den medizinischen Arbeitsschutz zuständigen Stelle unverzüglich anzuzeigen."

In der Deutschen Demokratischen Republik sind die einschlägigen Vorschriften in der „Verordnung über Melde- und Entschädigungspflicht bei Berufskrankheiten" vom 14. November 1957 enthalten.

F. Versicherungstechnische Aspekte

Unter den in Anlage 1 zur „Siebenten Berufskrankheiten-Verordnung" von 1968 (Erläuterungen bei Lederer, 1968) aufgezählten Krankheiten finden sich unter Nr. 37 „Infektionskrankheiten, wenn der Versicherte im Gesundheitsdienst, in der Wohlfahrtspflege oder in einem Laboratorium tätig oder durch eine andere Tätigkeit der Infektionsgefahr in ähnlichem Maße besonders ausgesetzt war", und unter Nr. 38 „Von Tieren auf Menschen übertragbare Krankheiten".

Eine Infektionskrankheit kann jedoch nur als Berufskrankheit anerkannt werden, wenn der ursächliche Zusammenhang zwischen der versicherten Tätigkeit, dem schädigenden Ereignis und den Folgen der Schädigung wahrscheinlich ist. Dies bedeutet, daß für die Berufsbedingtheit bestimmte Voraussetzungen gegeben sein müssen (VALENTIN et al., 1971):

„a) Die tatsächliche Infektionsquelle mit den entsprechenden Erregern muß mit Sicherheit oder Wahrscheinlichkeit im Bereich der Berufstätigkeit gegeben sein.

b) Es muß wahrscheinlich sein, daß die Berufstätigkeit mit besonderen, über das verkehrsübliche Maß hinausgehenden Infektionsgefahren verbunden war, und zwar speziell im Hinblick auf die Infektionskrankheit, an welcher der Versicherte erkrankt ist. Die Gefahr der berufsbedingten Ansteckung kann durch die ausgeübte Tätigkeit dauernd und gewohnheitsmäßig oder gelegentlich und vorübergehend gegeben sein. Die Verursachung einer Infektionskrankheit durch die berufliche Beschäftigung erfordert nicht in jedem Falle den Nachweis der tatsächlichen Infektionsquelle.

c) Der zeitliche Zusammenhang zwischen der Gefährdung im Beruf und dem Auftreten der ersten Symptome bzw. dem Zeitpunkt der Diagnosestellung muß gewahrt sein. Hierbei ist die Beachtung der jeweiligen Inkubationszeit von besonderer Bedeutung.

d) Der bei Feststellung der Infektionserkrankung erhobene Befund muß für eine Neuansteckung während der Berufstätigkeit sprechen."

Die besonderen, sich für die Tuberkulose als Berufskrankheit ergebenden Aspekte sind in dem Merkblatt „Gesichtspunkte für die Begutachtung der Tuberkulose als Berufskrankheit, Arbeits- und Dienstunfall" (1972) behandelt. Ein weiterer, auf die besonderen Gefahren in Pathologischen Instituten eingehender Beitrag findet sich bei PURRMANN (1964). Über die Anerkennung der Virushepatitis als Berufskrankheit s. bei PIESBERGEN (1967) und RUOF (1968).

Literatur

Autorenregister

AJMAL, M.: A laboratory infection with Erysipelothrix rhusiopathiae. Vet. Rec. 85, 688 (1969).

ALBRECHT, J.: Infektionsgefährdung im Tuberkuloselaboratorium. Tuberk.-Arzt 15, 563—566 (1961).

ALBRECHT, J.: Ungewöhnlicher Verlauf einer Laboratoriumsinfektion durch Salmonella typhi. Zbl. Bakt., I. Abt. Orig. 204, 299—301 (1967).

ALBRECHT, J.: Diskussionsbeitrag zur Arbeit von G. PIEKARSKI 10 (1967): 345 dieser Zeitschrift. Bundesgesundheitsblatt 11, 121—122 (1968a).

ALBRECHT, J.: Gefährdung des Personals in Tuberkuloselaboratorien. Prax. Pneumol. 22, 332 (1968b).

ALEXANDER, M. T., BRANDON, B. A.: The packaging and shipping of living reference cultures. ATCC Publ. Number 1. Rockville, Maryland, U.S.A.: American Type Culture Collection 1970.

ANDERS, W., LEWANDOWSKI, G.: Zur Infektionsgefährdung des Personals in Toxoplasmoselaboratorien. Bundesgesundheitsblatt 11, 140—141 (1968).

BADER, R.-E.: Ist das Arbeiten mit Bandwurmgliedern gefährlich? Röntgen- u. Lab.-Prax. 4, 115—116 (1951).

BADER, R.-E.: Untersuchungen zur Leistungsfähigkeit von handelsüblichen Sterilisatoren gegenüber thermophilen Sporenbildnern. Mitt. öst. Sanit.-Verwalt. (im Druck).

BADER, R.-E., GERTH, H.-J., HOFFMANN, R.: Akzidentelle Revakzination mit ungewöhnlichem Krankheitsverlauf. Münch. med. Wschr. 113, 677—679 (1971).

BALDWIN, CH. L., RUNKLE, R. S.: Biohazards symbol: Development of a biological hazards warning signal. Science 158, 264—265 (1967).

BAUM, G. L., LERNER, PH. I.: Primary pulmonary blastomycosis: A laboratory-acquired infection. Ann. intern. Med. 73, 263—265 (1970).

BÖHME, H., HARTKE, K.: Deutsches Arzneibuch, 7. Ausg. 1968. Kommentar. Stuttgart: Wiss. Verl.-Ges.; Frankfurt: Govi-Verl. 1969.

BÖNICKE, R., BAYHA, H.: Die Raumentkeimung mit UV-Strahlen unter Berücksichtigung des Mycobacterium tuberculosis. Beitr. Klin. Tuberk. 107, 71—77 (1952).

BORNEFF, J.: Hygiene. Stuttgart: Thieme 1971.

BOTZENHART, K., SATTEL, W.: Luftkeime und Infektionsverhütung in Operations- und Behandlungsräumen mit hohen Reinheitsansprüchen. Krankenhaus 64, 55—63 (1972).

BROOME, J. C., NORRIS, T. S.: Failure of prophylactic oral penicillin to inhibit a human laboratory case of leptospirosis. Lancet 1957 I, 721—722.

Bundesgesundheitsamt: Liste der vom Bundesgesundheitsamt geprüften und anerkannten Desinfektionsmittel und -verfahren (5. Ausg.). Bundesgesundheitsblatt 14, 309—312 (1971).

Bundesgesundheitsamt: Zeitabstände zwischen Schutzimpfungen. Bundesgesundheitsblatt 15, 252—253 (1972).

Busvine, J. R.: Insects and hygiene, 2nd. ed. London: Methuen 1966.

Calia, F. M., Bartelloni, P. J., McKinney, R. W.: Rocky Mountain spotted fever. Laboratory infection in a vaccinated individual. J. Amer. med. Ass. 211, 2012—2014 (1970).

Coriell, L. L., McGarrity, G. J.: Biohazard hood to prevent infection during microbiological procedures. Appl. Microbiol. 16, 1895—1900 (1968).

Deibel, R.: Virusembryopathien. Dtsch. med. Wschr. 91, 1792—1799 (1966).

Denton, J. F., DiSilva, A. F., Hirsch, M. L.: Laboratory acquired North American blastomycosis. J. Amer. med. Ass. 199, 935—936 (1967).

Deutsche Gesellschaft für Hygiene und Mikrobiologie: III. Liste der nach den „Richtlinien für die Prüfung chemischer Desinfektionsmittel" geprüften und von der Deutschen Gesellschaft für Hygiene und Mikrobiologie als wirksam befundenen Desinfektionsmittel. Stand: 1. März 1966. Gesundh.-Wes. Desinfekt. 58, 92—99 (1966).
1. Nachtrag, Stand: Juni 1967. Gesundh.-Wes. Desinfekt. 59, 119 (1967).
2. Nachtrag, Stand: Dezember 1967. Gesundh.-Wes. Desinfekt. 60, (1968).
3. Nachtrag, Stand: November 1968. Gesundh.-Wes. Desinfekt. 61, 28 (1969).
4. Nachtrag, Stand: 1. Juli 1970. Gesundh.-Wes. Desinfekt. 62, 140 (1970).
5. Nachtrag, Stand: 1. April 1971. Gesundh.-Wes. Desinfekt. 63, 112 (1971).
6. Nachtrag, Stand: 1. Dezember 1971. Gesundh.-Wes. Desinfekt. 64, 44—45 (1972).

Deutsches Arzneibuch: 7. Ausgabe 1968. Stuttgart: Deutscher Apotheker-Verl.; Frankfurt: Govi-Verl. 1968.

Ehrengut, W.: Impffibel. Stuttgart: Schattauer 1964.

Eschment, R., Lutz-Dettinger, U.: Die Überlebensdauer von Bakterien auf Gebrauchsseifen. Öff. Gesundh.-Wes. 32, 527—529 (1970).

Etmer, F., Lundt, P. V. (Bearb.): Deutsche Seuchengesetze. München-Percha: Schulz 1969ff.

Favero, M. S., Berquist, K. R.: Use of laminar air-flow equipment in microbiology. Appl. Microbiol. 16, 182—183 (1968).

Flamm, H.: Die pränatalen Infektionen des Menschen. Stuttgart: Thieme 1959.

Friederiszick, F. K.: Neue Erfahrungen mit der UV-Luftentkeimung in der Kinderklinik. Strahlentherapie 95, 491—495 (1954).

Furcolow, M. L.: Airborne histoplasmosis. Bact. Rev. 25, 301—309 (1961).

Goley, A. F., Alexander, A. D., Thiel, J. F., Chappell, V. E.: A case of human infection with Leptospira mini Georgia. Publ. Hlth Rep. (Wash.) 75, 922—924 (1960).

Griesbach, R. (Hrsg.): Die BCG-Schutzimpfung. Stuttgart: Thieme 1954.

Grossgebauer, K.: Zur Desinfektion der mit Pockenviren kontaminierten Hand. Gesundh.-Wes. Desinfekt. 59, 1—4 (1967).

Grün, L.: Zum Problem der Luftdesinfektion unter besonderer Berücksichtigung neuerer physikalischer und chemischer Verfahren. Ergebn. Hyg. Bakt. 29, 623—689 (1955).

Grün, L.: Desinfektion und Sterilisation in der Praxis. Dtsch. med. Wschr. 90, 566—570 (1965).

Grün, L.: Desinfektion medizinischer Spezialgeräte. Zbl. Bakt., I. Abt. Orig. B 156, 129—137 (1972).

Grün, L., Preuner, R.: Desinfektion. Fortschr. Med. 82, 374—376 (1964).

Haas, R.: Der Virusinfekt in der Schwangerschaft. Arch. Gynäk. 211, 100—108 (1971).

Haas, R., Maass, G., Müller, J., Oehlert, W.: Experimentelle Infektionen von Cercopithecus aethiops mit dem Erreger des Frankfurt-Marburg-Syndroms (FMS). Z. med. Mikrobiol. Immunol. 154, 210—220 (1968).

Hanson, R. P., Sulkin, S. E., Buescher, E. L., Hammon, W. McD., McKinney, R. W., Work, T. H.: Arbovirus infections of laboratory workers. Science 158, 1283—1286 (1967).

Harrop, G. A., Rake, G., Shaffer, M. F.: Group of laboratory infections ascribed to lymphogranuloma venereum. Trans. Amer. clin. climat. Ass. 56, 154—159 (1941).

Hart, D., Nicks, J.: Ultra-violette Bestrahlung im Operationssaal. Angewandte Intensitäten und bakterizide Wirkungen. Arch. Surg. 82, 449—465 (1961).

Hartung, K. (Hrsg.): Praktikum der Schutzimpfungen, 2. Aufl. Berlin: Hoffmann 1966.

Hatch, T. F.: Distribution and deposition of inhaled particles in respiratory tract. Bact. Rev. 25, 237—240 (1961).

Heicken, K.: Die Desinfektionsmittelliste des Bundesgesundheitsamtes. Kommentar. Bundesgesundheitsblatt 9, 65—72 (1966).

Heilmann, S., Kühn, H., Laue, F., Meyer, W., Rische, H., Rohne, K., Ziesché, K. (Hrsg.): Seuchenschutz, 2. Aufl. Leipzig: Thieme 1969.

Helm, E. B., Stille, W.: Über die Erreger bei infizierten Tierbissen. Münch. med. Wschr. 114, 922—924 (1972).

HELWIG, F. C.: Western equine encephalomyelitis following accidental inoculation with chick embryo virus: report of fatal human case with necropsy. J. Amer. med. Ass. 115, 291—292 (1940).

HETTCHE, H. O.: Die Entseuchung der Luft durch UV-Strahlen in der ärztlichen Praxis. Strahlentherapie 95, 484—490 (1954).

HOFFMAN, R. K., SPINER, D. R.: Effect of relative humidity on the penetrability and sporicidal activity of formaldehyde. Appl. Microbiol. 20, 616—619 (1970).

HORN, H.: Biologische Prüfung und Leistungskriterien der Sterilisation. Berlin: Verlag Volk u. Gesundheit 1968.

HORN, H., PŘÍVORA, M., WEUFFEN, W. (Hrsg.): Handbuch der Desinfektion und Sterilisation, Bd. 1. Berlin: Verlag Volk u. Gesundheit 1972.

HUEBNER, R. J.: Report of an outbreak of Q fever at the National Institutes of Health. II. Epidemiological features. Amer. J. publ. Hlth 37, 431—440 (1947).

HUHN, B.: Lichtfalle ohne Verzögerung. Kosmos 68, 474—476 (1972).

JEANJEAN, R., JEANJEAN, O.: Problèmes posés par les risques de contamination chez les employés de laboratoire chargés de la recherche du bacille de Koch et de l'étude de leur résistance. Arch. Mal. prof. 30, 632—634 (1969).

JENSEN, E.: Medizinisch-klinische Erfahrungen über die Tuberkulose als Berufskrankheit durch Laborinfektion. Tuberk.-Arzt 13, 473—478 (1959).

JENSEN, E.: Gefährdung des Personals in Tuberkuloselaboratorien. Prax. Pneumol. 22, 129—130 (1968).

JOHANSSON, K. R., FERRIS, D. H.: Photograph of airborne particles during bacteriological plating operations. J. infect. Dis. 78, 238—252 (1946).

JOHNSON, J. E., KADULL, P. J.: Rocky Mountain spotted fever acquired in a laboratory. New Engl. J. Med. 277, 842—847 (1967).

KAFFKA, A., RIETH, H.: Laboratoriumstiere als Ursache einer Berufsdermatomykose und Maßnahmen zur Verhütung weiterer Pilzinfektionen. Zbl. Bakt., I. Abt. Orig. 171, 319—321 (1957/58).

KANZ, E., KANZ, C.: Zur Prüfung und Beurteilung „desinfizierender Seifen". Gesundh.-Wes. Desinfekt. 61, 145—158, 161—173 (1969).

KAPPELER, R., BARANDUN, S., LÜTHI, H., WIESMANN, E.: Über eine Laboratoriumsinfektion mit Leptospira ballum, Orchitis als Komplikation. Schweiz. med. Wschr. 91, 810—812 (1961).

KIENINGER, G., SCHUBERT, G. E., ULLMANN, U.: Das Buruli-Ulkus. Z. Tropenmed. Parasit. 23, 342—353 (1972).

KIKUTH, W., BOCK, M.: 23 Fälle von Laborinfektionen mit Q-Fieber. Med. Klin. 44, 1056—1060 (1949).

KIRSTEIN, F.: Leitfaden der Desinfektion für Desinfektoren und Krankenpflegepersonen in Frage und Antwort, 2. Aufl. Berlin: Springer 1944.

KISSKALT, K.: Laboratoriumsinfektionen mit Typhusbazillen. Z. Hyg. Infekt.-Kr. 80, 145—162 (1915).

KLEINSCHMIDT, A., CHRIST, P.: Leptospira ballum als Ursache einer Laboratoriumsinfektion. Z. Immun.-Forsch. 117, 107—113 (1959).

KLOSTERKÖTTER, W.: Der Mensch im Arbeitsleben. In: Lehrbuch der Hygiene, 2. Aufl., hrsg. von GÄRTNER, H., u. REPLOH, H. Stuttgart: Fischer 1969.

KNAPP, W.: Lärm. In: Lehrbuch der Hygiene, 2. Aufl., hrsg. von GÄRTNER, H., u. REPLOH, H. Stuttgart: Fischer 1969.

KOLLMAR, A., LIESE, W. (Bearb.): Die Heiz- und Lüftungsanlagen in den verschiedenen Gebäudearten von KÄMPER, H., HOTTINGER, M., GONZENBACH, W. v., 3. Aufl. Berlin-Göttingen-Heidelberg: Springer 1954.

KOPROWSKI, H., COX, H.: Human laboratory infection with Venezuelan equine encephalomyelitis virus: report of four cases. New Engl. J. Med. 236, 647—654 (1947).

KRATEL, R. D. (Hrsg.): Arbeit und Fertigung in Reinen Räumen. 1. Europäisches Symposium 15. bis 18. Juni 1970, Stuttgart und Frankfurt/Main, B.R. Deutschland. Stuttgart: Eurocontamination 1971.

LEDERER, E.: Die neue (Siebente) Berufskrankheiten-Verordnung. Münch. med. Wschr. 110, 2466—2469 (1968).

LIEBKNECHT, W. L.: Verlauf einer Laboratoriumsinfektion mit Tuberkelbakterien nach BCG-Impfung. Prax. Pneumol. 25, 389—394 (1971).

LIESE, W.: Lüftung von Laboratorien. Gesundheitsing. 78, 300—303 (1957).

LIESE, W.: Gesundheitstechnisches Taschenbuch. München-Wien: Oldenbourg 1964.

LÖER, U., FUNNEKÖTTER, H.: Untersuchungen über die Einsatzmöglichkeiten eines Sterilarbeitsplatzes. Zbl. Bakt., I. Abt. Orig. B 155, 408—419 (1972).

LOEWER, H.: Klimatechnik. Berlin-Heidelberg-New York: Springer 1968.

Long, E. R.: The hazard of acquiring tuberculosis in the laboratory. Amer. J. publ. Hlth 41, 782—787 (1951).

Lüdde, K.-H.: Zwischenfälle mit Autoklaven beim Sterilisieren mit Flüssigkeiten (Infusions-Flaschen usw.). Dtsch. Gesundh.-Wes. 27, 714 (1972).

Lurie, M. B.: Air-borne contagion of tuberculosis in an animal room. J. exp. Med. 51, 743—751 (1930).

Martini, E.: Lehrbuch der medizinischen Entomologie, 4. überarb. Aufl. Jena: Fischer 1952.

Mason, N.: Leptospiral jaundice occurring naturally in a guinea-pig. Lancet 1937 I, 564—565.

Matz, K., Schassan, H.-H.: Der Einfluß von UV-Bestrahlung im Luftkanal von Klima-anlagen auf die Luftkeimzahl im Operationssaal. Krankenhaus 60, 349—352 (1968).

McDermott, W.: Conference on airborne infection, held in Miami Beach, Florida, December 7—10, 1960. Bact. Rev. 25, 173—382 (1961).

McKee, C. M., Rake, G., Shaffer, M. F.: Complement fixation test in lymphogranuloma venereum. Proc. Soc. exp. Biol. (N.Y.) 44, 410—413 (1940).

Meyer, K. F., Eddie, B.: Laboratory infections due to Brucella. J. infect. Dis. 63, 23—32 (1941).

Mochmann, H., Schmutzler, R.: Erfolgreiche Prophylaxe durch Antibiotika bei einer Laboratoriumsinfektion mit virulenten Weil-Leptospiren. Zbl. Bakt., I. Abt. Orig. 165, 148—155 (1956).

Müller, R.: Medizinische Mikrobiologie, 4. neubearb. Aufl. München-Berlin: Urban & Schwarzenberg 1950.

Neumann, G.: BCG-Impfung des Pflegepersonals. Dtsch. med. Wschr. 95, 1995 (1970).

Olitsky, P. K., Morgan, I. M.: Protective antibodies against equine encephalomyelitis virus in serum of laboratory workers. Proc. Soc. exp. Biol. (N.Y.) 41, 212—215 (1939).

Partmann, W., Montfort, L.: Ein neuer Impfkasten. Zbl. Bakt., I. Abt. Orig. 157, 611—619 (1951/52).

Perkins, J. J.: Principles and methods of sterilization in health sciences, 2nd ed. Springfield, Illinois, USA: Thomas 1969.

Phillips, G. B.: Microbiological hazards in the laboratory. J. chem. Ed. 42, A-43, A-117 (1965).

Phillips, G. B.: Control of microbiological hazards in the laboratory. Amer. industr. Hyg. Ass. J. 30, 170—176 (1969).

Piekarski, G.: Zur Infektionsgefährdung des Personals in Toxoplasmose-Laboratorien. Bundesgesundheitsblatt 10, 345—347 (1967). Schlußwort. Bundesgesundheitsblatt 11, 122—123 (1968).

Piekarski, G.: Medizinische Parasitologie, 2. Aufl. Berlin-Heidelberg-New York: Springer 1973.

Piesbergen, H.: Virushepatitis als Berufskrankheit. Münch. med. Wschr. 109, 505—508 (1967).

Pietzsch, O., Baumgarten, H.-J.: Diskussionsbeitrag zum Thema: Zur Infektionsgefährdung des Personals in Toxoplasmose-Laboratorien. Bundesgesundheitsblatt 12, 320 (1969).

Pike, R. M., Sulkin, S. E., Schulze, M. L.: Continuing importance of laboratory-acquired infections. Amer. J. publ. Hlth 55, 190—199 (1965).

Popova, E. M., Amosenkova, N. I.: Reservoirs of leptospiral infection in the northwest regions of the U.S.S.R.: results of an investigation on leptospiral infections of murine rodents. J. Microbiol. Epidem. Immunobiol. 28, 44—49 (1957).

Preuner, R., Roester, U., Richter, A.: Über die Desinfektion großer ärztlicher Geräte. Chirurg 34, 49—52 (1963).

Przyborowski, R., Würfel, G.: Leitfaden für die Sterilisationspraxis. Leipzig: Barth 1966.

Purrmann, W.: Die Tuberkulose als Berufserkrankung bei Beschäftigten Pathologischer Institute. Dtsch. Gesundh.-Wes. 19, 2389—2390 (1964).

Raiss, W.: H. Rietschels Lehrbuch der Heiz- und Lüftungstechnik, 14. verb. Aufl. Berlin-Göttingen-Heidelberg: Springer 1960.

Reid, H. W., Gibbs, C. A., Burrells, C., Doherty, P. C.: Laboratory infections with louping-ill virus. Lancet 1972 I, 592—593.

Riley, R. L.: Airborne pulmonary tuberculosis. Bact. Rev. 25, 243—248 (1961).

Rodenwaldt, E., Bader, R.-E.: Lehrbuch der Hygiene. Berlin-Göttingen-Heidelberg: Springer 1951.

Roemer, G. B.: Desinfektion und Sterilisation. In: Die Infektionskrankheiten des Menschen und ihre Erreger, 2. Aufl., hrsg. von Grumbach, A., u. Bonin, O., Bd. 1. Stuttgart: Thieme 1969.

Rohde, W., Schneeweiss, U., Otto, F. M. G.: Grundriß der Impfpraxis, 2. Aufl. Leipzig: Barth 1968.

ROSEBURY, T., ELLINGSON, H. V., MEIKLEJOHN, G.: Laboratory infection with psittacosis virus treated with penicillin and sulfadiazine, and experimental data bearing on mode of infection. J. infect. Dis. 80, 64—77 (1947).

RUBBO, S. D., GARDNER, J. F.: A review of sterilization and disinfection. London: Lloyd-Luke 1965.

RUOF, H.: Besteht beim Heil- und Pflegepersonal ein erhöhtes Erkrankungsrisiko gegenüber der Bevölkerung? Arch. Hyg. (Berl.) 152, 170—180 (1968).

SATTEL, W., NELSON, J. PH.: Bakteriologische Untersuchungen in einem Querstrom-Operationsraum. Langenbecks Arch. klin. Chir. Suppl. Chir. Forum 1972, S. 3—5.

SCHENKER, U., BÖTTCHER, R. F. H., MLYNEK, H.-J.: Die Hautdesinfektion des Operationsfeldes. Dtsch. Gesundh.-Wes. 27, 1169—1171 (1972).

SCHICHT, H. H.: Die Klimaanlage als Streuquelle von Mikroorganismen. Kälte-Klima-Rdsch. 9, 29—34 (1971).

SCHICHT, H. H.: Grundlagen und Anwendungen der Reinraumtechnik. Gesundh.-Ing. 93, 232—241 (1972).

SCHICK, G.: Durch Mikrosporum cookei verursachte spontane Laboratoriumsdermatomykose. Berufsdermatosen 16, 34—42 (1968).

SCHMIDT-MENDE, M., KANZ, E., THURMAYR, R.: Untersuchungen über den Staphylokokkengehalt der Luft im Operationssaal und seine Beeinflussung durch Luftdesinfektion. Bruns' Beitr. klin. Chir. 216, 115—121 (1968).

SEYFFERTITZ, W., THOMASCHEWSKI, P.: Bundes-Seuchengesetz. Kommentar. München: Schulz 1968.

SHU, H. L., SIEGERT, R., SLENCZKA, W.: Zur Pathogenese und Epidemiologie der Marburg-Virus-Infektion. Dtsch. med. Wschr. 93, 2163—2165 (1968).

SIEGERT, R., SHU, H.-L., SLENCZKA, W., PETERS, D., MÜLLER, G.: Zur Ätiologie einer unbekannten, von Affen ausgegangenen menschlichen Infektionskrankheit. Dtsch. med. Wschr. 92, 2341—2343 (1967).

SLEPUSHKIN, A. N.: An epidemiological study of laboratory infection with Venezuelan equine encephalomyelitis. Probl. Virol. (N.Y.) 4, 54—57 (1959).

SMITH, CH. E., PAPPAGIANIS, D., LEVINE, H. B., SAITO, M.: Human coccidioidomycosis. Bact. Rev. 25, 310—320 (1961).

SONCK, C. E.: Laboratory infections by skin-pathogenic fungi in Finland. Z. Haut- u. Geschl.-Kr. 31, 117—122 (1961).

SPIESS, H. (Hrsg.): Schutzimpfungen, 2. Aufl. Stuttgart: Thieme 1966.

SPRENGER, E. (Hrsg.): Taschenbuch für Heizung und Lüftung, 48. Jg. München: Oldenbourg 1955.

Staubforschungsinstitut des Hauptverbandes der gewerblichen Berufsgenossenschaften: Richtlinien zur Prüfung von Filtern für die Lüftungs- und Klimatechnik. Staub 21, 206—211 (1961).

STOENNER, H. G., MACLEAN, D.: Leptospirosis ballum contracted from Swiss albino mice. Arch. intern. Med. 191, 606—610 (1958).

STUTZ, L.: Leitfaden der praktischen Desinfektion und Sterilisation. Stuttgart: Enke 1968.

SULKIN, S. E.: Laboratory-acquired infections. Bact. Rev. 25, 203—209 (1961).

SULKIN, S. E., PIKE, R. M.: Viral infections contracted in the laboratory. New Engl. J. Med. 241, 205—213 (1949).

SULKIN, S. E., PIKE, R. M.: Survey of laboratory-acquired infections. Amer. J. publ. Hlth 41, 769—781 (1951).

SULKIN, S. E., PIKE, R. M., LONG, E. R., SMITH, C. E., SIGEL, M. M., WEDUM, A. G.: Laboratory infections and accidents. In: Diagnostic procedures and reagents, 4th ed. New York: Amer. Public Health Assoc. 1961.

SYKES, G.: Disinfection and sterilization, 2nd ed. London: Spon 1965.

TAURASO, N. M., NORRIS, G. F., SORG, T. J., COOK, R. O., MYERS, M. L., TRIMMER, R.: Negative-pressure isolator for work with hazardous infectious agents in monkeys. Appl. Microbiol. 18, 294—297 (1969).

THIEL, P. H. VAN: The leptospiroses. Univ. Pers. Leiden. Leiden 1948.

THOMSEN, K., KREBS, D.: Fehlerhafte Klimaanlage infizierte Operationstrakt. Dtsch. Ärztebl. 69, 544—548 (1972).

TIGERTT, W. D., BENENSON, A. S., GOCHENOUR, W. S.: Airborne Q fever. Bact. Rev. 25, 285—293 (1961).

TOMLINSON, A. J. H.: Infected airborne particles liberated on opening screw-cupped bottles. Brit. med. J. 1957 II, 15.

VALENTIN, H., KLOSTERKÖTTER, W., LEHNERT, G., PETRY, H., RUTENFRANZ, J., WITTGENS, H.: Arbeitsmedizin. Stuttgart: Thieme 1971.

WALLHÄUSSER, K. H., SCHMIDT, H.: Sterilisation, Desinfektion, Konservierung, Chemotherapie. Stuttgart: Thieme 1967.

WALTER, E.: Probleme der Luftreinhaltung bei Verwendung moderner Filter. Staub **25**, 441—447 (1965).

WEDUM, A. G.: Bacteriological safety. Amer. J. publ. Hlth **43**, 1428—1437 (1953).

WEDUM, A. G.: Control of laboratory airborne infection. Bact. Rev. **25**, 210—216 (1961).

WEICHARDT, H.: Desinfektion von Arbeitsschutzgeräten und Kleidung. Zbl. Arbeitsmed. **18**, 114—118 (1968).

WHITWELL, F., TAYLOR, P. J., OLIVER, A. J.: Hazards to laboratory staff in centrifuging screw-capped containers. J. clin. Path. **10**, 88—91 (1957).

WINKLE, S., ROEMER, G. B., MATZ, K.: Konstruktion und Wartung der Klimaanlagen verbessern. Dtsch. Ärztebl. **69**, 548—550 (1972).

WOLFF, J. W., BOHLANDER, H., RUYS, A. C.: Researches on leptospirosis ballum: the detection of urinary carriers in laboratory mice. Antonie van Leeuwenhoek **15**, 1—13 (1949).

World Health Organization: Public health laboratory service. First report of the Expert Committee on Health Laboratory Methods. Wld Hlth Org. techn. Rep. Ser. 1957, **128**.

WRIGHT, G. W.: Structure and function of respiratory tract in relation to infection. Bact. Rev. **25**, 219—227 (1961).

WUNDT, W.: Infektion als Berufsrisiko. Dtsch. med. Wschr. **89**, 1577—1582 (1964).

Gesetze, Verordnungen, Normen

Approbationsordnung für Ärzte vom 28. Oktober 1970. BGBl. I S. 1458.

Approbationsordnung für Apotheker vom 23. August 1971. BGBl. I S. 1377.

Arbeitsschutzbestimmungen (ASB) der DDR. GBl. 1953, S. 550. Zit. in: HABS, H.: Bakteriologisches Taschenbuch, 38. neubearb. Aufl. von SEELIGER, H. P. R. München: Barth 1967.

Ausbildungs- und Prüfungsordnung für medizinisch-technische Laboratoriumsassistenten, für medizinisch-technische Radiologieassistenten und für veterinärmedizinisch-technische Assistenten (Ausbildungs- und Prüfungsordnung für technische Assistenten in der Medizin — MTA-APrO) vom 23. Juni 1972. BGBl. I S. 929.

Bekanntmachung betreffend Vorschriften über Krankheitserreger vom 21. November 1917. RGBl. 1917, S. 1069.

Berufsordnung der Landesärztekammer Baden-Württemberg, II. Teil: Weiterbildungsordnung, genehmigt vom Innenministerium Baden-Württemberg am 21. 1. 1970. Ärztebl. Bad.-Württ. **25**, H. 3, 1970.

Bestallungsordnung für Ärzte vom 15. September 1953 mit einer Einführung von KOCH. Köln: Ärzte-Verlag 1953.

Bestallungsordnung für Tierärzte vom 23. März 1967. BGBl. I S. 360.

Dritte Durchführungsbestimmung zum Gesetz zur Verhütung und Bekämpfung übertragbarer Krankheiten beim Menschen — Arbeit mit Erregern von übertragbaren Krankheiten — vom 25. Januar 1966. GBl. II 1966, S. 83 (DDR).

Gesetz über die Ausübung der Zahnheilkunde vom 31. März 1952. BGBl. I S. 221.

Gesetz zum Schutze der erwerbstätigen Mutter in der Fassung vom 18. April 1968. BGBl. I S. 315.

Gesetz über technische Assistenten in der Medizin (MTA-G) vom 8. September 1971. BGBl. I S. 1515.

Gesetz zur Verhütung und Bekämpfung übertragbarer Krankheiten beim Menschen (Bundes-Seuchengesetz) vom 18. Juli 1961. BGBl. I vom 22. 7. 1961, S. 1012.

Gesetz zur Verhütung und Bekämpfung übertragbarer Krankheiten beim Menschen vom 20. Dezember 1965. GBl. I S. 29 (DDR).

Gewerbeordnung in der Fassung vom 26. Juli 1900 (RGBl. S. 871), zuletzt geändert durch die Änderungsverordnung vom 24. August 1967 (BGBl. I S. 933).

Laboratoriums-Infektionen mit Erregern der Weilschen Krankheit. Runderlaß des RuPrMdI vom 22. August 1936. In: Die Reagenzien der Behringwerke. Düsseldorf: Bagel 1949.

Siebente Berufskrankheiten-Verordnung vom 20. Juni 1968. BGBl. I S. 721. In: VALENTIN, H., KLOSTERKÖTTER, W., LEHNERT, G., PETRY, H., RUTENFRANZ, J., WITTGENS, H.: Arbeitsmedizin. Stuttgart: Thieme 1971.

Tierkörperbeseitigungsgesetz vom 1. Februar 1939. Reichsgesetzbl. I S. 187, BGBl. III 7831-7. In: Deutsche Seuchengesetze, bearb. von ETMER, F., u. LUNDT, P. V. München-Percha: Schulz 1969 ff.

Verordnung des Bundesministeriums für soziale Verwaltung vom 2. April 1948, *betreffend die Befugnis zur Vornahme medizinisch-diagnostischer Untersuchungen und die hierbei bei Arbeiten mit Krankheitserregern zu beobachtenden Vorsichtsmaßnahmen.* BGBl. f. d. Republik Österreich S. 321.

Verordnung über Melde- und Entschädigungspflicht bei Berufskrankheiten vom 14. 11. 1957. GBl. S. 1, mit Änderungen vom 18. 9. 1968. GBl. II S. 821 (DDR).

Merkblätter, Vorschriften

Berufsgenossenschaft für Gesundheitsdienst und Wohlfahrtspflege: Unfallverhütungsvorschriften (UVV), Richtlinien und Merkblätter. VBG 1, 109: Allgemeine Unfallverhütungsvorschriften (1969). VOG .7z: Schleudermaschinen (1971). VBG 103a: Behandlung, Pflege und sonstige Betreuung von Kranken und Siechen (1961). VBG 114: Medizinische Laboratoriumsarbeiten (1956). Eignungsuntersuchung und Gesundheitsüberwachung des Personals von Krankenanstalten (1955). 020/1/M: Die Bestellung von Sicherheitsbeauftragten (1969). 020/2/M.: Der Sicherheitsbeauftragte (1969). A6: Erste Hilfe bei Laboratoriumsinfektionen (Aushang) (1955). Hamburg 6, Schäferkampsallee 24.

Bundesgesundheitsamt: Merkblätter. Nr. 1: Verhütung und Bekämpfung der übertragbaren Kinderlähmung (Poliomyelitis anterior acuta) (1963). Nr. 3: Tollwut. Verhütung und Bekämpfung (1970). Nr. 11: Verhütung und Bekämpfung der Grippe (Influenza) (1963). Nr. 18: Pocken. Verhütung und Bekämpfung (1971). Nr. 25: Cholera. Verhütung und Bekämpfung (1972). Nr. 30: Rötelnschutzimpfung (1972). Köln: Deutscher Ärzte-Verlag.

Deutscher Normenausschuß: DIN 1946 Bl. 1: Lüftungstechnische Anlagen (VDI-Lüftungsregeln); Grundregeln (1960). Bl. 4: Lüftung in Krankenanstalten (1963). DIN 5034: Innenraumbeleuchtung mit Tageslicht; Leitsätze (1969). Bbl. 1: Berechnung und Messung (1963). Bbl. 2: Vereinfachte Bestimmung lichttechnisch ausreichender Fensterabmessungen (1966). DIN 5035: Innenraumbeleuchtung mit künstlichem Licht. Bl. 1: Allgemeine Richtlinien (1972). Bl. 2: Spezielle Empfehlungen für verschiedene Beleuchtungsaufgaben (1972). DIN 19520: Abwasser aus Krankenanstalten; Richtlinien für die Behandlung (1964). DIN 58946: Dampf- und Heißluftsterilisation; Begriffe (1967). Bl. 2: Sterilisation; Dampf-Sterilisatoren, Anforderungen (1972). Bl. 2 Bbl. 2 Entwurf: Dampf- und Heißluftsterilisation; Dampf-Sterilisation, Anforderungen, Technisches Datenblatt (1971). DIN 58947: Sporenerde zur Prüfung von Dampf- und Heißluft-Sterilisatoren; Prüfung (1969). Berlin-Köln: Beuth-Vertrieb.

Deutsches Zentralkomitee zur Bekämpfung der Tuberkulose: Desinfektionsmaßnahmen bei Tuberkulose, Stand 1967, ergänzt durch die Liste der vom Bundesgesundheitsamt geprüften und anerkannten Desinfektionsmittel und -verfahren vom 1. 10. 1971. Gesichtspunkte für die Begutachtung der Tuberkulose als Berufskrankheit, Arbeits- und Dienstunfall. Merkblatt 1972. Hamburg 33, Poppenhusenstr. 14c.

Medical Research Council: Safety precautions in laboratories. London 1960.

Verein Deutscher Ingenieure: VDI 2051: Lüftung von Laboratorien (1958). Berlin-Köln: Beuth-Vertrieb.

Namensverzeichnis

Die kursiven Seitenzahlen beziehen sich auf die Literatur.

Handbuch der experimentellen Pharmakologie /
Handbook of Experimental Pharmacology

Heffter – Heubner. New Series

Reprint from
Handbuch der experimentellen Pharmakologie
Handbook of Experimental Pharmacology
New Series

Edited by: **O. Eichler, A. Farah, H. Herken, A. D. Welch**

Volume XVI/11 B
Editor: Oskar Eichler

Springer-Verlag Berlin · Heidelberg · New York 1973

Experimental Infections by Spirochaetas

B. Babudieri

With 8 Figures

Reprint from
Handbuch der experimentellen Pharmakologie
Handbook of Experimental Pharmacology
New Series

Edited by: **O. Eichler, A. Farah, H. Herken, A. D. Welch**

Volume XVI/11 B
Editor: Oskar Eichler

Springer-Verlag Berlin · Heidelberg · New York 1973

Experimental Infections by Spirilla

B. Babudieri

With 1 Figure

Reprint from
Handbuch der experimentellen Pharmakologie
Handbook of Experimental Pharmacology
New Series

Edited by: **O. Eichler, A. Farah, H. Herken, A. D. Welch**

Volume XVI/11 B
Editor: **Oskar Eichler**

Springer-Verlag Berlin · Heidelberg · New York 1973

A Study of the Chemotherapeutics Active on Syphilis

B. Babudieri

Sonderdruck aus
Handbuch der experimentellen Pharmakologie
Handbook of Experimental Pharmacology
Neue Serie

Herausgegeben von: **O. Eichler, A. Farah, H. Herken, A. D. Welch**

Band XVI/11 B
Herausgeber: Oskar Eichler

Springer-Verlag Berlin · Heidelberg · New York 1973

Experimentelle Infektionen durch Vibrionen

H. Winkler und U. Ullmann

Mit 6 Abbildungen

Sonderdruck aus
Handbuch der experimentellen Pharmakologie
Handbook of Experimental Pharmacology
Neue Serie

Herausgegeben von: **O. Eichler, A. Farah, H. Herken, A. D. Welch**

Band XVI/11 B
Herausgeber: Oskar Eichler

Springer-Verlag Berlin · Heidelberg · New York 1973

Experimentelle Infektionen durcd Bakteroidazeen

Herbert Werner

Mit 10 Abbildungen

Sonderdruck aus
Handbuch der experimentellen Pharmakologie
Handbook of Experimental Pharmacology
Neue Serie

Herausgegeben von: **O. Eichler, A. Farah, H. Herken, A. D. Welch**

Band XVI/11 B
Herausgeber: Oskar Eichler

Springer-Verlag Berlin · Heidelberg · New York 1973

Verhütung von Laboratoriumsinfektionen

Richard-Ernst Bader

Mit 4 Abbildungen

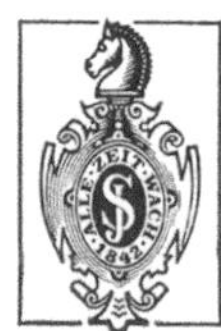

Springer-Verlag
Berlin · Heidelberg · New York
München Johannesburg London New Delhi Paris
Rio de Janeiro Sydney Tokyo Wien

**Archiv für Toxikologie
Archives of Toxicology**
Herausgegeben von der
Deutschen Pharmakologi-
schen Gesellschaft unter
Mitwirkung der Deutschen
Gesellschaft für Rechts-
medizin/Edited for the
Deutsche Pharmakologi-
sche Gesellschaft and the
Deutsche Gesellschaft für
Rechtsmedizin
Subscription Information:
1974, Vol. 33 (4 issues):
DM 108,—
approx. US $44.30
plus postage and handling

**Archives
of Environmental
Contamination and
Toxicology**
Subscription Information:
1974, Vol. 2 (4 issues):
DM 105,—
approx. US $43.10
plus postage and handling

**Berichte Biochemie
und Biologie**
Referierendes Organ der
Deutschen Botanischen
Gesellschaft und der
Zoologischen Gesellschaft
1974, etwa 18 Bände
(je 6 Hefte).
Je Band: DM 218,—
approx. US $89.40
zuzüglich Porto und
Verpackung

**Berichte Physiologie,
physiologische Chemie
und Pharmakologie**
1974, etwa 7 Bände
(je 6 Hefte).
Je Band: DM 218,—
approx. US $89.40
zuzüglich Porto und
Verpackung

**Bulletin of Environmental
Contamination
and Toxicology**
Subscription Information:
1974, Vols. 11-12
(6 issues each):
DM 160,—
approx. US $65.60
plus postage and handling

**European Journal
of Biochemistry**
Published on behalf of
the Federation of European
Biochemical Societies
Subscription Information:
1974, Vols. 41-50
(3 issues each):
DM 1050,—
approx. US $430.50
plus postage and handling

**European Journal of
Clinical Pharmacology**
Subscription Information:
1974, Vol. 7 (6 issues):
DM 150,—
approx. US $61.50
plus postage and handling

**Naunyn-Schmiedeberg's
Archives of Pharmacology**
Organ of the
Deutsche Gesellschaft
für Pharmakologie
Subscription Information:
1974, Vols. 281-285
(4 issues each): DM 540,—
approx. US $221.40
plus postage and handling

Psychopharmacologia
Subscription Information:
1974, Vols. 34-39
(4 issues each): DM 576,—
approx. US $236.20
plus postage and handling

**Research in Experimental
Medicine/Zeitschrift für
die gesamte experimen-
telle Medizin einschließlich
experimenteller Chirurgie**
Subscription Information:
1974, Vols. 162-164
(4 issues each): DM 468,—
approx. US $191.90
plus postage and handling

Preisänderungen
vorbehalten
Prices are subject
to change without notice